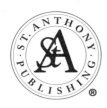

December 2000

Dear HCPCS Level II Code Book Subscriber:

Thank you for purchasing your 2001 *Premier HCPCS Level II Code Book*. Because you are a valued subscriber, we want to keep you up to date on the most current HCPCS Level II codes, modifiers, and Medicare coverage information.

Your code book features 936 new HCPCS Level II codes. It also includes 128 code deletions and 189 code revisions, administrative changes and numerous Medicare coverage clarifications and changes. This year's changes take effect on Jan. 1 (although the deleted codes will be accepted by Medicare carriers and fiscal intermediaries [FIs] through March 31, 2001).

The most significant changes for 2001 include:

- Color coding with St. Anthony's traditional highlighting bars

- 2 new modifiers

- Current revisions and additions to the Medicare Coverage Issues Manual and the Medicare Carriers Manual references

- A new section containing the "C" codes for use with Outpatient PPS

- A new section containing the "H" codes — government codes other than Medicare and Medicaid for reporting substance abuse or therapies

To help ensure that your claims are processed quickly and accurately, we have provided a color key located on the bottom of each page spread to indicate when HCPCS Level II codes are covered, noncovered, may require a certificate of medical necessity, or coverage is at your Medicare FI's or carrier's discretion.

Thank you for choosing this easy-to-use code book. If you have any questions about your 2001 *Premier HCPCS Level II Code Book* — or about any St. Anthony publication—please don't hesitate to call our customer service department. The call is free: (800) 632-0123.

Sincerely,

Elizabeth Boudrie

Elizabeth Boudrie
Publisher

HBK — 031101

11410 Isaac Newton Square • Reston, VA 20190 • (800) 632-0123

Premier

HCPCS
LEVEL II CODE BOOK

2001
EDITION

11410 Isaac Newton Square • Reston, VA 20190 • (800) 632-0123

Disclaimer

The 2001 *Premier HCPCS Level II Code Book* has been prepared for use with codes published by the federal government. It is designed to provide accurate and authoritative information in regard to the subject covered, and every reasonable effort has been made to ensure the accuracy of the information contained within these pages. Nevertheless, the ultimate responsibility for correct coding lies with the provider of services.

St. Anthony Publishing, its employees, agents and staff make no representation, warranty or guarantee that this compilation of codes and narratives is error-free or that the use of this code book will prevent differences of opinion or disputes with Medicare or other third-party payers as to the amounts that will be paid to providers of services, and will bear no responsibility or liability for the results or consequences of this code book.

This presentation includes only CPT codes selected by St. Anthony Publishing, for inclusion in this publication. The AMA assumes no responsibility for consequences attributable to or related to any use or interpretation of any information or views contained or not contained in this publication.

HCPCS Disclaimer

HCPCS is designed to promote uniform medical services reporting and statistical data collection. Inclusion of a service, product or supply does not constitute endorsement by either CPT or alphanumeric panels that it is noninvestigational or is commonly or customarily recognized as appropriate for medical care and treatment. Inclusion or exclusion of a procedure, product or supply does not imply any health insurance coverage or reimbursement policy.

The following staff contributed to this book:

Sheri Poe Bernard, CPC, *Director of Essential Regulatory Products*
Lynn Speirs, *Senior Director of Publishing*
Cathy Hopkins, CPC, *Technical Consultant*
Sharon Bench, LPN, RHIT, CPC, *Technical Consultant*
Christine B. Fraizer, MA, CPC, *Project Editor*
Kerrie Hornsby, *Desktop Publishing Manager*

ISBN 1-56329-726-4

Table of Contents

Preface

Prior to 1983, there was no uniform system for coding a procedure, service or supply for reimbursement. Blue Cross/Blue Shield created and required use of its own coding system; many other insurance companies created their own method of coding physician services and procedures.

But in 1983, Medicare created HCPCS, the Health Care Financing Administration's Common Procedure Coding System (pronounced hick picks). Today, HCPCS codes are required when reporting services and procedures provided to Medicare and Medicaid beneficiaries. More importantly, the creation of HCPCS led to the beginning of a national coding system.

HCPCS is a three-level coding system:

Level I — CPT

CPT, published and updated annually by the American Medical Association, is a five-digit system that describes the procedures and services physicians provide to patients. CPT does not provide codes for nonphysician procedures, services and specific supplies.

Modifiers in CPT are two-digit numeric codes that are added to the main procedure code to report that a procedure has been altered by a specific circumstance. Each modifier has an alternative code beginning with 099 that may be used instead. If the five-digit code is used, the modifier always begins with 099.

CPT simplifies the reporting of procedures or services rendered by physicians or health care providers under their supervision. An example of a CPT code is:

    30115   Excision, nasal polyp(s), extensive

If this procedure is performed bilaterally, the correct method to report this service would be 30115-50 or 30115 and 09950.

Level II —National Codes

Level II codes commonly are referred to as national codes, or sometimes by the acronym, HCPCS. These codes are published and updated annually by the Health Care Financing Administration. Because the CPT coding system does not include codes for nonphysician procedures, such as ambulance services, durable medical equipment and specific supplies, HCFA created a series of codes to supplement CPT. In addition, more specific codes were created for the administration of injectable drugs.

In contrast to the five-digit codes found in Level I, national codes consist of one alphabetic character (a letter between A and V), followed by four digits. (All D codes have a copyright by the American Dental Association.)

For example:

    A4245   Alcohol wipes, per box

    J1240   Injection, dimenhydrinate, up to 50 mg

Level II of HCPCS also contains modifiers, which are either alphanumeric or two letters in the range from -AA to -VP. National modifiers can be used with all levels of HCPCS codes.

For example:

-CC   Procedure code change (used when the procedure code submitted was changed either for administrative reasons or because an incorrect code was filed)

-LT   Left side (used to identify procedures performed on the left side of the body). This modifier has no direct effect on payment.

-F1   Left hand, second digit.

A new section, C Codes, was added to HCPCS Level II coding this year. C codes report drugs, biologicals, and devices eligible for transitional pass through payments, and for items classified in "new technology" ambulatory payment classifications (APCs) under the Outpatient Prospective Payment System. These supplies can be billed in addition to the APC for ambulatory surgical center services (ASCs) when billing APCs to Medicare.

Many C codes were effective earlier in 2000, but because HCPCS Level II code books are published annually, these codes are identified as new in the 2001 book with "new" icons (show dot icon here).

The listing of HCPCS codes contained in this instruction does not assure coverage of the specific item or service in a given case. To be eligible for pass-through and new technology payments from Medicare, the items contained in this document must be considered reasonable and necessary.

Level III — Local Codes

Local codes are used to denote new procedures or specific supplies for which there is no national code. These five-digit alphanumeric codes use the letters W through Z.

Local codes, including all HCPCS Level III codes, are scheduled to be eliminated from medical reimbursement reporting by October 16, 2002. The Health Insurance Portability and Accountability Act of 1996 Final Rule (HIPAA), published in the Aug. 17, 2000 *Federal Register,* requires providers, payers and clearinghouses to use a set of uniform standards for submitting claims data electronically. Local codes are eliminated as a part of this rule. Private payers have in the past two years created nearly 200 S codes to replace local codes for reporting services that aren't codified by the government or the AMA. The government will also be creating national codes to replace local HCPCS Level III codes.

Today , each local Medicare carrier may create local codes as the need dictates. However, carriers are required to obtain approval from the HCFA central office before implementing local codes. Your Medicare carrier is responsible for providing you with the local codes.

The following is a local code used by a Medicare carrier in Georgia:

X1025   Amphotericin B Fungizone 50 mg (20 ml)

At some point in your coding, you may find that the same procedure is coded in two or even three coding levels. Which code do you use? There are certain rules to follow if this should occur. First, if there is an overlap between a local code and either a CPT or Level II code, use the local code — it has the highest priority.

When both a CPT and a HCPCS Level II code have virtually identical narratives for a procedure or service, the CPT code should be used. If, however, the narratives are not identical (for example, the CPT code narrative is generic, whereas the HCPCS Level II code is specific), the Level II code should be used.

Be sure to check for a national or local code when a CPT code description instructs you to include additional information, such as describing specific medication. For example, when billing Medicare or Medicaid for supplies, avoid using CPT code 99070, supplies and materials (except spectacles), provided by the physician over and above those usually included with the office visit or other services rendered (list drugs, trays, supplies or materials provided). There are many HCPCS Level II codes that specify supplies in more detail.

Introduction

All too often, HCPCS Level II codes are billed improperly or ignored. As a result, claims are questioned or denied. St. Anthony's HCPCS Level II Code Book will assist you in assigning HCPCS Level II codes for procedures, services and supplies not covered by CPT.

The information in this book is a reproduction of the 2001 Health Care Financing Administration Common Procedure Coding System (HCPCS). According to HCFA, additional information on coverage issues may have been provided to carriers after publication. All carriers periodically update their systems and records throughout the year.

This reproduction has in no way attempted to change the codes or their descriptions found in the original government version. There are some distinct differences in St. Anthony's *Premier HCPCS Level II Code Book,* however. In some instances, St. Anthony's staff has taken HCFA data and translated this information into a more usable format. For example, color bars and reference notes in this book are our way of identifying administrative data fields such as action codes, coverage issues or *Medicare Carriers Manual* instructions. Another important enhancement St. Anthony's expert coding staff has added to the original format includes the creation or revision of headings/subheadings where none were provided. Headings and subheadings have been added to provide consistency throughout the book.

Appendices

Several appendices have been added to the book for your reference. The following is a list of the helpful information added to enhance the St. Anthony's *Premier HCPCS Level II Code Book* and to assist you further.

Appendix 1: Modifiers
Under certain situations, procedures have been altered by a specific circumstance. Modifiers are required to adequately report the procedure. Appendix 1 contains an introduction and a complete listing of modifiers used with HCPCS Level II codes.

Appendix 2: Summary of Additions, Deletions and Revisions

A complete list of all the code changes for the current year is provided in a summary format.

Appendix 3: Table of Drugs

To enhance the official table of drugs, St. Anthony Publishing has added brand names for drugs listed in the table. The brand names are listed in alphabetical order and will refer you to the appropriate specific generic drug for correct code assignment by route of administration and dosage.

Appendix 4: Medicare *Coverage Issues Manual* (CIM) and *Medicare Carriers Manual* (MCM) References

To assist you in understanding coverage issues associated with certain codes, our experts have researched the coverage guidelines using the Medicare *Coverage Issues Manual* (CIM) and the *Medicare Carriers Manual* (MCM), which are published by HCFA. These issues are referenced to the right of the associated codes and are identified by letter symbols and numbers. The letter symbols refer to the most common guidelines and are conveniently located at the bottom of each page as well as in Appendix 4. The number symbol references more specific coverage guidelines listed in the appendix.

Appendix 5: Deleted Codes

St. Anthony's HCPCS Level II Code Book allows you to track codes deleted from the HCPCS Level II coding system. The first year a code is deleted, the book simply places a line through the code number and narrative in the tabular section of the book, additional information concerning a cross-reference code is provided. The second year of deleted status, the code is removed from the tabular list and listed in Appendix 5. A cross-reference code is provided when available for deleted codes.

Appendix 6: Medicare National Average Payment

A table representing commercial and/or Medicare nation average payment for services and/or supplies reported using HCPCS Level II codes.

With an updated version of Level II codes and the important guidelines on how to use them, the appropriate reimbursement you're entitled to from the third-party payer is possible.

Keep in mind, however, that the insurance companies and government do not base payment solely on what was done for the patient. They need to know why the services were performed. That's why, in addition to using the HCPCS coding system for procedures and supplies, you must also use the ICD-9-CM coding system to denote the patient's diagnosis. This book will not discuss ICD-9-CM codes — you should refer to a St. Anthony's ICD-9-CM code book for diagnosis codes.

At the end of the book is an alphabetic index to the codes. Use it to initially locate a code by looking for the type of service or procedure performed. Additional entries include anatomical sites, conditions, eponyms, abbreviations and the name of the drug or supply. Never code directly from the index. Always check the specific code in the appropriate section. To locate additional information concerning specific drugs, refer to the alphabetized table of drugs provided in Appendix 4.

Symbols

The two symbols used in this book are a bullet (●) and a triangle (▲). A bullet indicates a new code. For example:

●A0425 Ground mileage, per statute mile

A triangle means the terminology for a code has been altered significantly from a previous version. For example:

▲A4364 Adhesive, liquid, for use with facial prosthesis only, per ounce

In addition to these two symbols, current deletions are indicated by a line drawn through the code and narrative. A cross-reference to a CPT code or another national code may be given. For example:

A5149 ~~Incontinence/ostomy supply; miscellaneous~~ This code has been deleted in 2001. See A4335, A4421.

Specific modifiers must be used when reporting outpatient services for accuracy in reimbursement, coding consistency, editing and to capture payment data. Modifiers indicated by a ◆ symbol are required by HCFA for reporting outpatient services provided to beneficiaries.

◆-LT Left side (used to identify procedures performed on the left side of the body)

Explanation of References

Throughout the book, *Coverage Issues Manual* and *Mediare Carriers Manual* reference numbers that correspond to references in Appendix 4 are found in the column to the right of a code's description.

Color bars ientify coverage instructions for each code and a key is provided on the bottom of each page spread for your convenience.

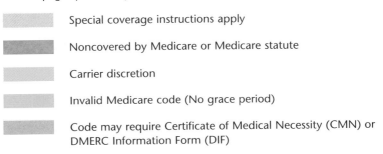

Special coverage instructions apply

Noncovered by Medicare or Medicare statute

Carrier discretion

Invalid Medicare code (No grace period)

Code may require Certificate of Medical Necessity (CMN) or DMERC Information Form (DIF)

ASC

Contained within the proposed rule for Ambulatory Surgical Center (ASC) services is a list of services/supplies for which separate payment could be made. Medicare does not include payment for the item/service in the ASC facility fee. The HCPCS Level II codes identified with the "ASC" symbol can be reported separately when furnished by an ASC.

Notes

A few of the subsections, headings or codes have special instructions that apply only to them. The term "NOTE" sometimes, but not always, is used to identify these instructions. Some notes are found following the subsection, heading or code to which they apply. Others appear as part of a heading's or code's description, separated by a comma or dash or placed within parentheses.

Unlisted Procedures

HCFA does not use consistent terminology when a code for a specific procedure is not listed. The code's description may include any of the following terms: unlisted, not otherwise classified (NOC), unspecified, unclassified, other and miscellaneous. When coding this type of procedure, check with your Medicare carrier in case a specific HCPCS Level III code is available. If one is not available, use the appropriate unlisted procedure code, and submit a special report with the claim.

Special Report

Submit a special report with the claim when a new, unusual or variable procedure is provided or a modifier is used. Include the following information:

- A copy of the appropriate report (e.g., operative, x-ray), explaining the nature, extent and need for the procedure

- Documentation of the medical necessity of the procedure

- Documentation of the time and effort necessary to perform the procedure.

Modifiers

Under certain circumstances, the code chosen may require a modifier. For example, there are modifiers for the side of the body where the procedure was performed, whether the services were performed by a physician assistant or whether the DME provided to the patient was new. Check Appendix 1 for the complete listing.

General Instructions for Use

To locate a HCPCS Level II code, follow these steps:

1. First identify what services or procedures the patient received.
   Ex: Patient receives an implantable neurostimulart pulse generator for intractable pain treatment.

2. Look up the appropriate term in the index.
   Ex: Neurostimulator
         pulse generator, E0756

   Coding Tip: If you can't find the procedure or service in the index, look in the table of contents for the type of procedure or device to narrow your code choices. Also, remember to check the unlisted procedure guidelines for additional choices.

3. Assign a tentative code(s).
   Ex: Code E0756 is tentatively assigned.

   Coding Tip: To the right of the terminology, you may find a single code or multiple codes, a cross-reference or an indication that the code has been deleted. Tentatively assign all codes listed.

4. Locate the code(s) in the appropriate section.

Code	Narrative	Reference Appendix 5
● **E0756**	Implantable neurostimulator pulse generator	*CIM 65-8*

5. Check for color bars, symbols, notes and references.
   Ex:
●	New code for 2001
E0756	Color bar means special coverage instructions apply
CIM 65-8	Coverage Instructions

6. Review Appendix 5 for the reference definitions and other guidelines for coverage issues that apply.
   Ex: CIM 65-8, Two classifications of nerve stimulators are used to treat chronic intractable pain: implanted peripheral nerve stimulators and central nervous system stimulators. Payment is made for implanted peripheral nerve stimulators under the prosthetic device benefit. Use of this stimulator involves implantation of electrodes around a selected peripheral nerve. Implantation requires surgery and usually necessitates an operating room.

7. Determine if any modifiers should be used.

8. Assign the code.
   Ex: The code assigned is E0756

Coding Scenarios

The following coding scenarios illustrate proper selection and billing using HCPCS Level II codes.

Scenario One

A disabled, 46-year-old, established Medicare patient with menopausal syndrome is seen by the clinic's nurse for a 5 mg intramuscular injection of depo-estradiol cypionate. Code the ICD-9 and HCPCS Level I and II codes for this service.

21. DIAGNOSIS OR NATURE OF ILLNESS OR INJURY (RELATE ITEMS 1, 2, 3 OR 4 TO ITEM 24E BY LINE)		
1 627.2	3	
2	4	

24.	A						B	C	D		E
	DATE(S) OF SERVICE						Place of Service	Type of Service	PROCEDURES, SERVICES, OR SUPPLIES (Explain Unusual Circumstances)		DIAGNOSIS CODE
	From			To					CPT / HCPCS	MODIFIER	
MM	DD	YY	MM	DD	YY						
12	5	01	12	5	01		11		99211		1
12	5	01	12	5	01		11		J1000		1
12	5	01	12	5	01		11		90782		

Summary

Medicare bundles the administration of the medication into the E/M service provided, but allows separate payment for the drug administered. Each Medicare carrier has individual requirements for the use of HCPCS Level II codes to describe the drug administered. Some carriers require the use of the CPT code and the HCPCS Level II J code; others use only the J code and require a CPT code to designate the method of administration.

Scenario Two

An elderly established patient presented to his physician with a sore throat. A strep infetion was diagnosed using a quick strep test in the office. The physician administered an injection of 1,200,000 units of penicillin G benzathine to treat the infection. Report the appropriate CPT and HCPCS Level II codes for the office visit, test, and injection.

21. DIAGNOSIS OR NATURE OF ILLNESS OR INJURY (RELATE ITEMS 1, 2, 3 OR 4 TO ITEM 24E BY LINE)						
1 034.0				3		
2				4		

24. A DATE(S) OF SERVICE						B Place of Service	C Type of Service	D PROCEDURES, SERVICES, OR SUPPLIES (Explain Unusual Circumstances) CPT / HCPCS MODIFIER	E DIAGNOSIS CODE
From MM	DD	YY	To MM	DD	YY				
4	1	01	4	1	01	11		99212	1
4	1	01	4	1	01	11		J0570	1
4	1	01	4	1	01	11		86403	1

Scenario Three

A week following a suture repair of a perforated ulcer, a patient is discharged from the hospital. Three days later, she presented at her physician's office as an emergency walk-in patient, having experienced severe vomiting and diarrhea during the past 24 hours. The patient informs the physician during his detailed history and examination that her entire family recently had a bout of severe vomiting and diarrhea, but recovered within a 24-hour period.The physician ordered a "stat" automated CBC with a manual differential WBC count and complete (non-automated) urinalysis. When the results returned from the clinic laboratory, the physician concluded the patient suffered from viral gastroenteritis, dehydration, status post suture repair of perforated gastric ulcer. He placed her in an observation room in the minor surgery suite of the clinic, and started an IV with 1000 ccs of Ringer's lactate, to which he injected 25 mg of IV promethazine hydrochloride for the nausea. The patient remained in observation. The physician and clinic nurses check on her frequently. After six hours, the physician discontinues the IV and examines the patient, who states she feels much better. He gives instructions for her care, makes final notes, writes a prescription, and discharges the patient home. How should these services be coded?

21. DIAGNOSIS OR NATURE OF ILLNESS OR INJURY (RELATE ITEMS 1, 2, 3 OR 4 TO ITEM 24E BY LINE)

1. | 008.8
2. | 276.5
3. | V45.89
4. |

24. A DATE(S) OF SERVICE						B	C	D		E
From MM	DD	YY	To MM	DD	YY	Place of Service	Type of Service	PROCEDURES, SERVICES, OR SUPPLIES (Explain Unusual Circumstances) CPT / HCPCS	MODIFIER	DIAGNOSIS CODE
3	4	01	3	4	01	11		99218	−24	1,2,3
3	4	01	3	4	01	11		90780	−79	1,2,3
3	4	01	3	4	01	11		90781	−79	1,2,3
3	4	01	3	4	01	11		90784	−79	1,2,3
3	4	01	3	4	01	11		85022		1,2,3
3	4	01	3	4	01	11		81000		1,2,3

21. DIAGNOSIS OR NATURE OF ILLNESS OR INJURY (RELATE ITEMS 1, 2, 3 OR 4 TO ITEM 24E BY LINE)		
1	008.8	3	V45.89
2	276.5	4	

24.	A					B	C	D		E
	DATE(S) OF SERVICE					Place of	Type of	PROCEDURES, SERVICES, OR SUPPLIES (Explain Unusual Circumstances)		DIAGNOSIS CODE
	From			To		Service	Service	CPT / HCPCS	MODIFIER	
MM	DD	YY	MM	DD	YY					
3	4	01	3	4	01	11		A4305		1,2,3
3	4	01	3	4	01	11		A4215		1,2,3
3	4	01	3	4	01	11		J7120		1,2,3
3	4	01	3	4	01	11		J2550		1,2,3

Summary

CPT states that 90780 and 90781 may not be used in addition to prolonged services codes. However, CPT does not specify that observation cannot be coded. Coding guidelines listed under initial observation care specify: when observation status is initiated in the course of an encounter in another site of service (e.g., emergency department, physician's office, nursing facility) all E/M services provided by the supervising physician in conjunction with initiating observation status are considered part of the initial observation care when performed on the same date. The observation care level of service reported by the supervising physician should include the services related to initiating observation status provided in the other sites of service as well as in the observation setting. E/M services provided on the same date in sites that are related to initiating observation status should not be reported separately. CPT further states that these codes apply to all evaluation and management services that are provided on the same date of initiating observation status.

Note: Modifiers -24 and -79 have been added to the E/M and medicine codes that indicate the procedure or service by the same physician was unrelated during the postoperative period.

Scenario Four

A 65-year-old patient who was previously seen in an orthopedist's office for another problem was seen on an emergency basis for a minimally displaced closed fracture of the radius and ulna of right forearm. The fracture was diagnosed after anteroposterior and lateral x-rays of the forearm were obtained by the physician's staff. The patient also had a puncture wound of the right, upper arm that occurred when a branch stabbed her as she fell six feet out of a tree she was pruning at home. From the patient's verbal history it had been over 20 years since her last tetanus injection.

The patient's arm was prepped, the fracture site was injected with lidocaine, and the fracture easily reduced. Post-reduction x-rays (taken by the physician's staff) demonstrated good alignment of the bones.

A long arm fiberglass splint was then applied. The patient was given a tetanus toxoid immunization, and instructions to return in one week. Code the ICD-9, CPT, and HCPCS Level II codes.

Orthopedic

21. DIAGNOSIS OR NATURE OF ILLNESS OR INJURY (RELATE ITEMS 1, 2, 3 OR 4 TO ITEM 24E BY LINE)

1. 813.23	3. E884.9	5. E920.8
2. 880.03	4. E849.0	

24.	A					B	C	D		E
	DATE(S) OF SERVICE					Place of Service	Type of Service	PROCEDURES, SERVICES, OR SUPPLIES (Explain Unusual Circumstances)		DIAGNOSIS CODE
	From			To						
MM	DD	YY	MM	DD	YY			CPT / HCPCS	MODIFIER	
9	14	01	9	14	01	11		25565		1,2,3,4,5
9	14	01	9	14	01	11		99058		1,2,3,4,5
9	14	01	9	14	01	11		73090	−76	1,2,3,4,5
9	14	01	9	14	01	11		90703		1,2,3,4,5
9	14	01	9	14	01	11		A4590		1,2,3,4,5

Summary

Five ICD-9 diagnosis codes apply. This forces the coder to make some choices, since only four spaces are available on a HCFA-1500. The codes and sequence should reflect the primary diagnosis and the most resource-intensive codes; in this case, the fracture and its repair. Secondary codes should reflect other conditions for which treatment is provided, in the order of their importance to the clinical picture. In this case, E codes should first report the fall, because it consumed the most resources. Reported second is the place of occurrence, the patient's home. This lets the payer (in this case, Medicare) know that it is the primary insurer. Generally, homeowner's insurance does not cover accidents or injuries to the homeowner.

CPT code 99058 reports office services provided on an emergency basis, but does not include the actual medical or surgical service performed. The musculoskeletal codes for fracture management include medical examination, open or closed treatment of the fracture, application of the first cast or traction device, and normal uncomplicated follow-up care.

There are many variables in managing fractures, e.g., closed or open, non-manipulated or manipulated. Closed management (or reduction) means no surgical incision was necessary and that treatment was in the form of a manipulation, cast, splint, or traction application. Open management (or reduction) requires a surgical reduction with or without internal skeletal fixation. When the initial medical evaluation and/or management of the fracture is provided on the same day, the medical service is included in the surgical package.

When cast application is performed as an initial service, it is not coded. Removal of the first cast and/or traction device is included in the surgical package. X-ray services and expensive casting materials (i.e.,. fiberglass) are not included in the surgical procedure and may be reported when provided by the orthopedist.

Note: Modifier -76 has been added to CPT code 73090 to indicate that a procedure or service was repeated subsequent to the original procedure or service.

Scenario Five

The patient noted a small lump in her right breast, and scheduled an appointment with her local rural physician. After examining the patient, the physician opted to do an open incisional biopsy of the lesion during the same appointment. Code the diagnosis and services.

21. DIAGNOSIS OR NATURE OF ILLNESS OR INJURY (RELATE ITEMS 1, 2, 3 OR 4 TO ITEM 24E BY LINE)		
1 | 611.72	3 |
2 |	4 |

24. A DATE(S) OF SERVICE						B Place of Service	C Type of Service	D PROCEDURES, SERVICES, OR SUPPLIES (Explain Unusual Circumstances) CPT / HCPCS | MODIFIER |		E DIAGNOSIS CODE
From MM	DD	YY	To MM	DD	YY			CPT/HCPCS	MODIFIER	
4	1	01	4	1	01	11		19101	QB RT	1
4	1	01	4	1	01	11		A4550		1
4	1	01	4	1	01	11		99000		1

Summary

The physician correctly reported the biopsy with 19101 and added HCPCS Level II modifier -QB, identifying a physician providing service in a rural health professional shortage area. Modifier -RT indicates the procedure was performed on the right side of the body. Generally, the modifier that will affect reimbursement is listed first when two or more modifiers are used. The physician also reported A4550 for the surgical tray used in this minor surgical procedure. CPT code 19101 is on the Medicare facility-based list of codes that qualify nationally for surgical tray reimbursement. This list is available through your carrier. If the physician had instead made the common mistake of using 99070 Supplies and materials (except spectacles), this charge would likely have been denied. Because the HPSA bonus payment applies only to medical services, the physician did not apply modifier -QB to A4550. Because the tissue sample was to be transported to a laboratory for analysis, the physician also reported 99000 for handling and conveyance of the specimen.

Transportation Services Including Ambulance A0000-A0999

Ambulance Origin and Destination modifiers used with Transportation Service codes are single-digit modifiers used in combination in boxes 12 and 13 of HCFA form 1491. The first digit indicates the transport's place of origin, and the destination is indicated by the second digit. The modifiers most commonly used are:

D	Diagnostic or therapeutic site other than 'P' or 'H' when these codes are used as origin codes
E	Residential, domiciliary, custodial facility (other than an 1819 facility)
G	Hospital-based dialysis facility (hospital or hospital-related)
H	Hospital
I	Site of transfer (e.g., airport or helicopter pad) between types of ambulance
J	Non hospital-based dialysis facility
N	Skilled nursing facility (SNF) (1819 facility)
P	Physician's office (includes HMO non-hospital facility, clinic, etc.)
R	Residence
S	Scene of accident or acute event
X	(Destination code only) intermediate stop at physician's office on the way to the hospital (includes HMO non-hospital facility, clinic, etc.)

Claims for transportation services fall under the jurisdiction of the local carrier.

A0021 Ambulance service, outside state per mile, transport (Medicaid only)

Cross-reference A0430

A0030 ~~Ambulance service, conventional air service, transport, one way~~ This code has been deleted in 2001. See A0430.

A0040 ~~Ambulance service, air, helicopter service, transport~~ This code has been deleted in 2001. See A0431.

A0050 ~~Ambulance service, emergency, water, special transportation services~~ This code has been deleted in 2001. See A0429.

A0080 Nonemergency transportation: per mile — volunteer, with no vested or personal interest

A0090 Nonemergency transportation: per mile — volunteer, interested individual, neighbor

A0100 Nonemergency transportation: taxi — intracity

A0110 Nonemergency transportation and bus, intra- or interstate carrier

A0120 Nonemergency transportation mini-bus, mountain area transports, other non-profit transportation systems

A0130 Nonemergency transportation: wheelchair van

A0140 Nonemergency transportation and air travel (private or commercial), intra- or interstate

A0160 Nonemergency transportation: per mile — caseworker or social worker

---

= Special Coverage Instructions Apply   = Carrier Discretion

= Noncovered by Medicare or Medicare Statute

A0170	Nonemergency transportation: ancillary: parking fees, tolls, other
A0180	Nonemergency transportation: ancillary: lodging — recipient
A0190	Nonemergency transportation: ancillary: meals — recipient
A0200	Nonemergency transportation: ancillary: lodging — escort
A0210	Nonemergency transportation: ancillary: meals — escort
A0225	Ambulance service, neonatal transport, base rate, emergency transport, one way
A0300	~~Ambulance service, basic life support (BLS), non-emergency transport, all inclusive (mileage and supplies)~~ This code has been deleted in 2001. See A0428.
A0302	~~Ambulance service, BLS, emergency transport, all inclusive (mileage and supplies)~~ This code has been deleted in 2001. See A0429.
A0304	~~Ambulance service, advanced life support (ALS), nonemergency transport, no specialized ALS services rendered, all inclusive (mileage and supplies)~~ This code has been deleted in 2001. See A0428.
A0306	~~Ambulance service, ALS, nonemergency transport, specialized ALS services rendered, all inclusive (mileage and supplies)~~ This code has been deleted in 2001. See A0426.
A0308	~~Ambulance service, ALS, emergency transport, no specialized ALS services rendered, all inclusive (mileage and supplies)~~ This code has been deleted in 2001. See A0429.
A0310	~~Ambulance service, ALS, emergency transport, specialized ALS services rendered, all inclusive (mileage and supplies)~~ This code has been deleted in 2001. See A0427.
A0320	~~Ambulance service, BLS, non-emergency transport, supplies included, mileage separately billed~~ This code has been deleted in 2001. See A0428.
A0322	~~Ambulance service, BLS, emergency transport, supplies included, mileage separately billed~~ This code has been deleted in 2001. See A0429.
A0324	~~Ambulance service, ALS, non-emergency transport, no specialized ALS services rendered, supplies included, mileage separately billed~~ This code has been deleted in 2001. See A0428.
A0326	~~Ambulance service, ALS, non-emergency transport, specialized ALS services rendered, supplies included, mileage separately billed~~ This code has been deleted in 2001. See A0426.
A0328	~~Ambulance service, ALS, emergency transport, no specialized ALS services rendered, supplies included, mileage separately billed~~ This code has been deleted in 2001. See A0429.
A0330	~~Ambulance service, ALS, emergency transport, specialized ALS services rendered, supplies included, mileage separately billed~~ This code has been deleted in 2001. See A0427.

= Invalid Medicare Code (no grace period)

= Code may require certificate of medical necessity (CMN) or DMERC information form (DIF)

A0340 ~~Ambulance service, BLS, nonemergency transport, mileage included, disposable supplies separately billed~~ This code has been deleted in 2001. See A0428.

A0342 ~~Ambulance service, BLS, emergency transport, mileage included, disposable supplies separately billed~~ This code has been deleted in 2001. See A0429.

A0344 ~~Ambulance service, ALS, nonemergency transport, no specialized ALS services rendered, mileage included, disposable supplies separately billed~~ This code has been deleted in 2001. See A0428.

A0346 ~~Ambulance service, ALS, nonemergency transport, specialized ALS services rendered, mileage included, disposable supplies separately billed~~ This code has been deleted in 2001. See A0426.

A0348 ~~Ambulance service, ALS, emergency transport, no specialized ALS services rendered, mileage included, disposable supplies separately billed~~ This code has been deleted in 2001. See A0429.

A0350 ~~Ambulance service, ALS, emergency transport, specialized ALS services rendered, mileage included, disposable supplies separately billed~~ This code has been deleted in 2001. See A0427.

A0360 ~~Ambulance service, BLS, nonemergency transport, mileage and disposable supplies separately billed~~ This code has been deleted in 2001. See A0428.

A0362 ~~Ambulance service, BLS, emergency transport, mileage and disposable supplies separately billed~~ This code has been deleted in 2001. See A0429.

A0364 ~~Ambulance service, ALS, nonemergency transport, no specialized ALS services rendered, mileage and disposable supplies separately billed~~ This code has been deleted in 2001. See A0428.

A0366 ~~Ambulance service, ALS, nonemergency transport, specialized ALS services rendered, mileage and disposable supplies separately billed~~ This code has been deleted in 2001. See A0426.

A0368 Ambulance service, ALS, emergency transport, no specialized ALS services rendered, mileage and disposable supplies separately billed

A0370 ~~Ambulance service, ALS, emergency transport, specialized ALS services rendered, mileage and disposable supplies separately billed~~ This code has been deleted in 2001. See A0427.

A0380 ~~BLS mileage (per mile)~~ This code has been deleted in 2001. See A0425.

A0382 BLS routine disposable supplies

A0384 BLS specialized service disposable supplies; defibrillation (used by ALS ambulances and BLS ambulances in jurisdictions where defibrillation is permitted in BLS ambulances)

A0390 ~~ALS mileage (per mile)~~ This code has been deleted in 2001. See A0425.

A0392	ALS specialized service disposable supplies; defibrillation (to be used only in jurisdictions where defibrillation cannot be performed by BLS ambulances)
A0394	ALS specialized service disposable supplies; IV drug therapy
A0396	ALS specialized service disposable supplies; esophageal intubation
A0398	ALS routine disposable supplies

Waiting Time Table

Units		Time	
1	½	to	1 hr.
2	1	to	1½ hrs.
3	1½	to	2 hrs.
4	2	to	2½ hrs.
5	2½	to	3 hrs.
6	3	to	3½ hrs.
7	3½	to	4 hrs.
8	4	to	4½ hrs.
9	4½	to	5 hrs.
10	5	to	5½ hrs.

A0420	Ambulance waiting time (ALS or BLS), one-half (½) hour increments
A0422	Ambulance (ALS or BLS) oxygen and oxygen supplies, life sustaining situation
A0424	Extra ambulance attendant, ALS or BLS (requires medical review)
● A0425	Ground mileage, per statute mile
● A0426	Ambulance service, advanced life support, non-emergency transport, level 1 (ALS 1)
● A0427	Ambulance service, advanced life support, emergency transport, level 1 (ALS 1-emergency)
● A0428	Ambulance service, basic life support, non-emergency transport (BLS)
● A0429	Ambulance service, basic life support, emergency transport (BLS-emergency)
● A0430	Ambulance service, conventional air services, transport, one way (fixed wing)
● A0431	Ambulance service, conventional air services, transport, one way (rotary wing)
● A0432	Paramedic intercept (PI), rural area, transport furnished by a volunteer ambulance company which is prohibited by state law from billing third party payers
● A0433	Advanced life support, level 2 (ALS 2)
● A0434	Specialty care transport (SCT)
● A0435	Fixed wing air mileage, per statute mile
● A0436	Rotary wing air mileage, per statute mile

= Invalid Medicare Code (no grace period)

= Code may require certificate of medical necessity (CMN) or DMERC information form (DIF)

A0888	Non-covered ambulance mileage, per mile (e.g., for miles traveled beyond closest appropriate facility)	*MCM 2125*
A0999	Unlisted ambulance service	*MCM 2120.1, MCM 2125.1*

Medical and Surgical Supplies A4000-A8999

This section covers a wide variety of medical and surgical supplies, and some durable medical equipment (DME), supplies and accessories. DME and the supplies, accessories, maintenance, and repair required to ensure the proper functioning of this equipment is generally covered by Medicare under the prosthetic devices provision.

Miscellaneous Supplies

A4206	Syringe with needle, sterile 1 cc, each	
▲ **A4207**	Syringe with needle, sterile 2 cc, each	
A4208	Syringe with needle, sterile 3 cc, each	
A4209	Syringe with needle, sterile 5 cc or greater, each	
A4210	Needle-free injection device, each	*CIM 60-9*
A4211	Supplies for self-administered injections	*MCM 2049*
A4212	Non coring needle or stylet with or without catheter	
A4213	Syringe, sterile, 20 cc or greater, each	
A4214	Sterile saline or water, 30 cc vial	
A4215	Needles only, sterile, any size, each	
A4220	Refill kit for implantable infusion pump	*CIM 60-14*
A4221	Supplies for maintenance of drug infusion catheter, per week (list drug separately)	
A4222	Supplies for external drug infusion pump, per cassette or bag (list drug separately)	
A4230	Infusion set for external insulin pump, nonneedle cannula type	*CIM 60-14*
A4231	Infusion set for external insulin pump, needle type	*CIM 60-14*
A4232	Syringe with needle for external insulin pump, sterile, 3cc	*CIM 60-14*
A4244	Alcohol or peroxide, per pint	
A4245	Alcohol wipes, per box	
A4246	Betadine or pHisoHex solution, per pint	
A4247	Betadine or iodine swabs/wipes, per box	
A4250	Urine test or reagent strips or tablets (100 tablets or strips)	*MCM 2100*
A4253	Blood glucose test or reagent strips for home blood glucose monitor, per 50 strips	*CIM 60-11*

	= Special Coverage Instructions Apply		= Carrier Discretion
	= Noncovered by Medicare or Medicare Statute		

A4254	Replacement battery, any type, for use with medically necessary home blood glucose monitor owned by patient, each *CIM 60-11*
A4255	Platforms for home blood glucose monitor, 50 per box
A4256	Normal, low, and high calibrator solution/chips
A4258	Spring-powered device for lancet, each
A4259	Lancets, per box of 100 *CIM 60-11*
A4260	Levonorgestrel (contraceptive) implants system, including implants and supplies
A4261	Cervical cap for contraceptive use
A4262	Temporary, absorbable lacrimal duct implant, each
A4263	Permanent, long-term, nondissolvable lacrimal duct implant, each *MCM 15030*
A4265	Paraffin, per pound
A4270	Disposable endoscope sheath, each
A4280	Adhesive skin support attachment for use with external breast prosthesis, each
● **A4290**	Sacral nerve stimulation test lead, each

Vascular Catheters

A4300	Implantable access catheter (venous, arterial, epidural, or peritoneal), external access *MCM 2130*
A4301	Implantable access total system; catheter, port/reservoir (venous, arterial or epidural), percutaneous access
A4305	Disposable drug delivery system, flow rate of 50 ml or greater per hour
A4306	Disposable drug delivery system, flow rate of 5 ml or less per hour

Incontinence Appliances and Care Supplies
Covered by Medicare when the medical record indicates incontinence is permanent, or of long and indefinite duration.

A4310	Insertion tray without drainage bag and without catheter (accessories only) *MCM 2130*
A4311	Insertion tray without drainage bag with indwelling catheter, Foley type, two-way latex with coating (Teflon, silicone, silicone elastomer or hydrophilic, etc.) *MCM 2130*
A4312	Insertion tray without drainage bag with indwelling catheter, Foley type, two-way, all silicone *MCM 2130*
A4313	Insertion tray without drainage bag with indwelling catheter, Foley type, three-way, for continuous irrigation *MCM 2130*
A4314	Insertion tray with drainage bag with indwelling catheter, Foley type, two-way latex with coating (Teflon, silicone, silicone elastomer or hydrophilic, etc.) *MCM 2130*

© 2000 Ingenix Publishing Group

A4315	Insertion tray with drainage bag with indwelling catheter, Foley type, two-way, all silicone	*MCM 2130*
A4316	Insertion tray with drainage bag with indwelling catheter, Foley type, three-way, for continuous irrigation	*MCM 2130*
● **A4319**	Sterile water irrigation solution, 1000 ml	
A4320	Irrigation tray with bulb or piston syringe, any purpose	*MCM 2130*
A4321	Therapeutic agent for urinary catheter irrigation	
A4322	Irrigation syringe, bulb or piston, each	*MCM 2130*
A4323	Sterile saline irrigation solution, 1000 ml	*MCM 2130*
● **A4324**	Male external catheter, with adhesive coating, each	
● **A4325**	Male external catheter, with adhesive strip, each	
A4326	Male external catheter specialty type (e.g., inflatable, faceplate, etc.) each	*MCM 2130*
A4327	Female external urinary collection device; metal cup, each	*MCM 2130*
A4328	Female external urinary collection device; pouch, each	*MCM 2130*
A4329	External catheter starter set, male/female, includes catheters/urinary collection device, bag/pouch and accessories (tubing, clamps, etc.), seven-day supply	*MCM 2130*
A4330	Perianal fecal collection pouch with adhesive, each	*MCM 2130*
● **A4331**	Extension drainage tubing, any type, any length, with connector/adaptor, for use with urinary leg bag or urostomy pouch, each	*MCM 2130*
● **A4332**	Lubricant, individual sterile packet, for insertion of urinary catheter, each	
● **A4333**	Urinary catheter anchoring device, adhesive skin attachment, each	
● **A4334**	Urinary catheter anchoring device, leg strap, each	
A4335	Incontinence supply; miscellaneous	*MCM 2130*
A4338	Indwelling catheter; Foley type, two-way latex with coating (Teflon, silicone, silicone elastomer, or hydrophilic, etc.), each	*MCM 2130*
A4340	Indwelling catheter; specialty type, (e.g., coudé, mushroom, wing, etc.), each	*MCM 2130*
A4344	Indwelling catheter, Foley type, two-way, all silicone, each	*MCM 2130A*
A4346	Indwelling catheter; Foley type, three-way for continuous irrigation, each	*MCM 2130*
A4347	Male external catheter with or without adhesive, with or without anti-reflux device; per dozen	*MCM 2130*
● **A4348**	Male external catheter with integral collection compartment, extended wear, each (e.g., 2 per month)	
A4351	Intermittent urinary catheter; straight tip, each	*MCM 2130*
A4352	Intermittent urinary catheter; coudé (curved) tip, each	*MCM 2130*

= Special Coverage Instructions Apply   = Carrier Discretion

= Noncovered by Medicare or Medicare Statute

A4353	Intermittent urinary catheter, with insertion supplies	
A4354	Insertion tray with drainage bag but without catheter	*MCM 2130*
A4355	Irrigation tubing set for continuous bladder irrigation through a three-way indwelling Foley catheter, each	*MCM 2130*

External Urinary Supplies

A4356	External urethral clamp or compression device (not to be used for catheter clamp), each	*MCM 2130*
A4357	Bedside drainage bag, day or night, with or without anti-reflux device, with or without tube, each	*MCM 2130*
A4358	Urinary leg bag; vinyl, with or without tube, each	*MCM 2130*
A4359	Urinary suspensory without leg bag, each	*MCM 2130*

Ostomy Supplies

	A4361	Ostomy faceplate, each	*MCM 2130A*
	A4362	Skin barrier; solid, four by four or equivalent; each	*MCM 2130*
▲	**A4364**	Adhesive, liquid, for use with facial prosthesis only, per ounce	*MCM 2130*
▲	**A4365**	Adhesive remover wipes, any type, per 50	
	A4367	Ostomy belt, each	*MCM 2130A*
	A4368	Ostomy filter, any type, each	
	A4369	Ostomy skin barrier, liquid (spray, brush, etc), per oz	
	A4370	Ostomy skin barrier, paste, per oz	
	A4371	Ostomy skin barrier, powder, per oz	
	A4372	Ostomy skin barrier, solid 4x4 or equivalent, standard wear, with built-in convexity, each	
	A4373	Ostomy skin barrier, with flange (solid, flexible or accordion), standard wear, with built-in convexity, any size, each	
	A4374	Ostomy skin barrier, with flange (solid, flexible or accordion), extended wear, with built-in convexity, any size, each	
	A4375	Ostomy pouch, drainable, with faceplate attached, plastic, each	
	A4376	Ostomy pouch, drainable, with faceplate attached, rubber, each	
	A4377	Ostomy pouch, drainable, for use on faceplate, plastic, each	
	A4378	Ostomy pouch, drainable, for use on faceplate, rubber, each	
	A4379	Ostomy pouch, urinary, with faceplate attached, plastic, each	
	A4380	Ostomy pouch, urinary, with faceplate attached, rubber, each	
	A4381	Ostomy pouch, urinary, for use on faceplate, plastic, each	
	A4382	Ostomy pouch, urinary, for use on faceplate, heavy plastic, each	
	A4383	Ostomy pouch, urinary, for use on faceplate, rubber, each	
	A4384	Ostomy faceplate equivalent, silicone ring, each	

▬ = Invalid Medicare Code (no grace period)

▬ = Code may require certificate of medical necessity (CMN) or DMERC information form (DIF)

A4385	Ostomy skin barrier, solid 4x4 or equivalent, extended wear, without built-in convexity, each
A4386	Ostomy skin barrier, with flange (solid, flexible or accordion), extended wear, without built-in convexity, any size, each
A4387	Ostomy pouch closed, with standard wear barrier attached, with built-in convexity (1 piece), each
A4388	Ostomy pouch, drainable, with extended wear barrier attached, without built-in convexity (1 piece)
A4389	Ostomy pouch, drainable, with standard wear barrier attached, with built-in convexity (1 piece), each
A4390	Ostomy pouch, drainable, with extended wear barrier attached, with built-in convexity (1 piece), each
A4391	Ostomy pouch, urinary, with extended wear barrier attached, without built-in convexity (1 piece), each
A4392	Ostomy pouch, urinary, with standard wear barrier attached, with built-in convexity (1 piece), each
A4393	Ostomy pouch, urinary, with extended wear barrier attached, with built-in convexity (1 piece), each
A4394	Ostomy deodorant for use in ostomy pouch, liquid, per fluid ounce
A4395	Ostomy deodorant for use in ostomy pouch, solid, per tablet
● **A4396**	Ostomy belt with peristomal hernia support
A4397	Irrigation supply; sleeve, each *MCM 2130*
A4398	Ostomy irrigation supply; bag, each *MCM 2130A*
A4399	Ostomy irrigation supply; cone/catheter, including brush *MCM 2130A*
A4400	Ostomy irrigation set *MCM 2130*
A4402	Lubricant, per ounce *MCM 2130*
A4404	Ostomy ring, each *MCM 2130*
A4421	Ostomy supply; miscellaneous *MCM 2130*

Additional Miscellaneous Supplies

A4454	Tape, all types, all sizes *MCM 2130*
A4455	Adhesive remover or solvent (for tape, cement or other adhesive), per ounce *MCM 2130*
A4460	Elastic bandage, per roll (e.g., compression bandage) *MCM 2079*
A4462	Abdominal dressing holder/binder, each
● **A4464**	Joint supportive device/garment, elastic or equal, each *MCM 2303*
A4465	Nonelastic binder for extremity
A4470	Gravlee jet washer *CIM 50-4, MCM 2320*
A4480	VABRA aspirator *CIM 50-10, MCM 2320*
A4481	Tracheostoma filter, any type, any size, each

= Special Coverage Instructions Apply   = Carrier Discretion

= Noncovered by Medicare or Medicare Statute

A4483	Moisture exchanger, disposable, for use with invasive mechanical ventilation
A4490	Surgical stocking above knee length, each
	CIM 60-9, MCM 2133, MCM 2079
A4495	Surgical stocking thigh length, each *CIM 60-9, MCM 2133, MCM 2079*
A4500	Surgical stocking below knee length, each
	CIM 60-9, MCM 2133, MCM 2079
A4510	Surgical stocking full-length, each *CIM 60-9, MCM 2133, MCM 2079*
A4550	Surgical trays *MCM 15030*
A4554	Disposable underpads, all sizes (e.g., Chux's) *CIM 60-9, MCM 2130*
A4556	Electrodes (e.g., Apnea monitor), per pair
A4557	Lead wires (e.g., Apnea monitor), per pair
A4558	Conductive paste or gel
A4560	~~Pessary~~ This code has been deleted in 2001. See A4561, A4562.
● A4561	Pessary, rubber, any type
● A4562	Pessary, non rubber, any type
A4565	Slings
A4570	Splint *MCM 2079*
A4572	Rib belt
A4575	Topical hyperbaric oxygen chamber, disposable *CIM 35-10*
A4580	Cast supplies (e.g., plaster) *MCM 2079*
A4590	Special casting material (e.g., fiberglass)
A4595	TENS supplies, 2 lead, per month
● A4608	Transtracheal oxygen catheter, each

Supplies for Oxygen and Related Respiratory Equipment

A4611	Battery, heavy duty; replacement for patient-owned ventilator
A4612	Battery cables; replacement for patient-owned ventilator
A4613	Battery charger; replacement for patient-owned ventilator
A4614	Peak expiratory flow rate meter, hand held
A4615	Cannula, nasal *CIM 60-4, MCM 3312*
A4616	Tubing (oxygen), per foot *CIM 60-4, MCM 3312*
A4617	Mouthpiece *CIM 60-4, MCM 3312*
A4618	Breathing circuits *CIM 60-4, MCM 3312*
A4619	Face tent *CIM 60-4, MCM 3312*
A4620	Variable concentration mask *CIM 60-4, MCM 3312*
A4621	Tracheostomy mask or collar
A4622	Tracheostomy or laryngectomy tube *CIM 65-16*

= Invalid Medicare Code (no grace period)

= Code may require certificate of medical necessity (CMN) or DMERC information form (DIF)

A Codes

A4623	Tracheostomy, inner cannula (replacement only)	*CIM 65-16*
A4624	Tracheal suction catheter, any type, each	
A4625	Tracheostomy care kit for new tracheostomy	
A4626	Tracheostomy cleaning brush, each	
A4627	Spacer, bag or reservoir, with or without mask, for use with metered dose inhaler	*MCM 2100*
A4628	Oropharyngeal suction catheter, each	
A4629	Tracheostomy care kit for established tracheostomy	

Supplies for Other Durable Medical Equipment

A4630	Replacement batteries for medically necessary transcutaneous electrical nerve stimulator (TENS) owned by patient	*CIM 65-8, ASC*
A4631	Replacement batteries for medically necessary electronic wheelchair owned by patient	*CIM 60-9, ASC*
A4635	Underarm pad, crutch, replacement, each	*CIM 60-9, ASC*
A4636	Replacement, handgrip, cane, crutch, or walker, each	*CIM 60-9, ASC*
A4637	Replacement, tip, cane, crutch, walker, each	*CIM 60-9, ASC*
A4640	Replacement pad for use with medically necessary alternating pressure pad owned by patient	*CIM 60-9, MCM 4107.6, ASC*

Supplies for Radiologic Procedures

A4641	Supply of radiopharmaceutical diagnostic imaging agent, not otherwise classified	*MCM 15030*
A4642	Supply of satumomab pendetide, radiopharmaceutical diagnostic imaging agent, per dose	*MCM 15030*
A4643	Supply of additional high dose contrast material(s) during magnetic resonance imaging, e.g., gadoteridol injection	*MCM 15030*
A4644	Supply of low osmolar contrast material (100–199 mg of iodine	*MCM 15022, 15030*
A4645	Supply of low osmolar contrast material (200–299 mg of iodine)	*MCM 15022, 15030*
A4646	Supply of low osmolar contrast material (300–399 mg of iodine)	*MCM 15022, 15030*
A4647	Supply of paramagnetic contrast material (e.g., gadolinium)	*MCM 15022, 15030*
A4649	Surgical supply; miscellaneous	

Supplies for ESRD

For DME items for ESRD, see procedure codes E1550–E1669.

A4650	Centrifuge (includes calibrated microcapillary tubes and sealease)	
A4655	Needles and syringes for dialysis	*ASC*

= Special Coverage Instructions Apply	= Carrier Discretion
= Noncovered by Medicare or Medicare Statute	

A4660	Sphygmomanometer/blood pressure apparatus with cuff and stethoscope	*ASC*
A4663	Blood pressure cuff only	*ASC*
A4670	Automatic blood pressure monitor	*CIM 50-42*
A4680	Activated carbon filters for dialysis	*CIM 55-1, ASC*
A4690	Dialyzer (artificial kidneys) all brands, all sizes, per unit	*ASC*
A4700	Standard dialysate solution, each	*ASC*
A4705	Bicarbonate dialysate solution, each	*ASC*
A4712	Water, sterile	*ASC*
A4714	Treated water (deionized, distilled, reverse osmosis) for use in dialysis system	*CIM 55-1, ASC*
A4730	Fistula cannulation set for dialysis only	*ASC*
A4735	Local/topical anesthetic for dialysis only	*ASC*
A4740	Shunt accessory for dialysis only	*ASC*
A4750	Blood tubing, arterial or venous, each	
A4755	Blood tubing, arterial and venous, combined	
A4760	Dialysate standard testing solution, supplies	*ASC*
A4765	Dialysate concentrate additive, each	*ASC*
A4770	Blood testing supplies (e.g., vacutainers and tubes)	
A4771	Serum clotting time tube, per box	
A4772	Dextrostick or glucose test strips, per box	
A4773	Hemostix, per bottle	
A4774	Ammonia test paper, per box	
A4780	Sterilizing agent for dialysis equipment, per gallon	*ASC*
A4790	Cleansing agent for equipment for dialysis only	*ASC*
A4800	Heparin for dialysis and antidote, any strength, porcine or beef, up to 1,000 units, 10–30 ml (for parenteral use, see code B4216)	*ASC*
A4820	Hemodialysis kit supply	*ASC*
A4850	Hemostats with rubber tips for dialysis	*ASC*
A4860	Disposable catheter caps	
A4870	Plumbing and/or electrical work for home dialysis equipment	*Medicaid suspend for medical review, ASC*
A4880	Storage tank utilized in connection with water purification system, replacement tank for dialysis	*CIM 55-1, ASC*
A4890	Contracts, repair and maintenance, for home dialysis equipment (noncovered)	*MCM 2100.4, ASC*
A4900	Continuous ambulatory peritoneal dialysis (CAPD) supply kit	*ASC*
A4901	Continuous cycling peritoneal dialysis (CCPD) supply kit	*ASC*

= Invalid Medicare Code (no grace period)

= Code may require certificate of medical necessity (CMN) or DMERC information form (DIF)

A4905	Intermittent peritoneal dialysis (IPD) supply kit	*ASC*
A4910	Nonmedical supplies for dialysis, (i.e., scale, scissors, stop-watch, etc.) *ASC*	
A4912	Gomco drain bottle	
A4913	Miscellaneous dialysis supplies, not identified elsewhere, by report	*ASC*
A4914	Preparation kit	
A4918	Venous pressure clamp, each	
A4919	Dialyzer holder, each	*ASC*
A4920	Harvard pressure clamp, each	
A4921	Measuring cylinder, any size, each	
A4927	Gloves, sterile or nonsterile, per pair	

Additional Ostomy Supplies

A5051	Pouch, closed; with barrier attached (one piece)	*MCM 2130, ASC*
A5052	Pouch, closed; without barrier attached (one piece)	*MCM 2130, ASC*
A5053	Pouch, closed; for use on faceplate	*MCM 2130, ASC*
A5054	Pouch, closed; for use on barrier with flange (two piece)	*MCM 2130, ASC*
A5055	Stoma cap	*MCM 2130, ASC*
A5061	Pouch, drainable; with barrier attached (one piece)	*MCM 2130, ASC*
A5062	Pouch, drainable; without barrier attached (one piece)	*MCM 2130, ASC*
A5063	Pouch, drainable; for use on barrier with flange (two piece system)	*MCM 2130, ASC*
A5064	Pouch, drainable; with faceplate attached; plastic or rubber	*MCM 2130*
A5065	~~Pouch, drainable; for use on faceplate; plastic or rubber~~ This code has been deleted in 2001.	
A5071	Pouch, urinary; with barrier attached (one piece)	*MCM 2130, ASC*
A5072	Pouch, urinary; without barrier attached (one piece)	*MCM 2130, ASC*
A5073	Pouch, urinary; for use on barrier with flange (two piece)	*MCM 2130, ASC*
A5074	Pouch, urinary; with faceplate attached; plastic or rubber	*MCM 2130*
A5075	Pouch, urinary; for use on faceplate; plastic or rubber	*MCM 2130*
A5081	Continent device; plug for continent stoma	*MCM 2130, ASC*
A5082	Continent device; catheter for continent stoma	*MCM 2130, ASC*
A5093	Ostomy accessory; convex insert	*MCM 2130, ASC*

Medicare claims fall under the jurisdiction of the DME regional carrier, unless otherwise noted.

Additional Incontinence Appliances/Supplies

| A5102 | Bedside drainage bottle, with or without tubing, rigid or expandable, each | *MCM 2130, ASC* |

= Special Coverage Instructions Apply   = Carrier Discretion

= Noncovered by Medicare or Medicare Statute

A5105	Urinary suspensory; with leg bag, with or without tube	*MCM 2130, ASC*
A5112	Urinary leg bag; latex	*MCM 2130, ASC*
A5113	Leg strap; latex, replacement only, per set	*MCM 2130, ASC*
A5114	Leg strap; foam or fabric, replacement only, per set	*MCM 2130, ASC*

Supplies for Either Incontinence or Ostomy Appliances

A5119	Skin barrier; wipes, box per 50	*MCM 2130*
A5121	Skin barrier; solid, 6 x 6 or equivalent, each	*MCM 2130*
A5122	Skin barrier; solid, 8 x 8 or equivalent, each	*MCM 2130*
A5123	Skin barrier; with flange (solid, flexible or accordion), any size, each	*MCM 2130*
A5126	Adhesive or non-adhesive; disk or foam pad	*MCM 2130*
A5131	Appliance cleaner, incontinence and ostomy appliances, per 16 oz.	*MCM 2130*
A5149	~~Incontinence/ostomy supply; miscellaneous~~ This code has been deleted in 2001. See A4335, A4421.	
A5200	Percutaneous catheter/tube anchoring device, adhesive skin attachment	

Medicare jurisdiction: DME regional carrier.

Diabetic Shoes, Fitting, and Modifications

According to Medicare, documentation from the prescribing physician must certify the diabetic patient has one of the following conditions: peripheral neuropathy with evidence of callus formation; history of preulcerative calluses; history of ulceration; foot deformity; previous amputation; or poor circulation. The footwear must be fitted and furnished by a podiatrist, pedorthist, orthotist, or prosthetist.

A5500	For diabetics only, fitting (including follow-up) custom preparation and supply of off-the-shelf depth-inlay shoe manufactured to accommodate multi-density insert(s), per shoe	*MCM 2134, ASC*
A5501	For diabetics only, fitting (including follow-up) custom preparation and supply of shoe molded from cast(s) of patient's foot (custom molded shoe), per shoe	*MCM 2134, ASC*
A5502	For diabetics only, multiple density insert(s), per shoe	*MCM 2134, ASC*
A5503	For diabetics only, modification (including fitting) of off-the-shelf depth-inlay shoe or custom molded shoe with roller or rigid rocker bottom, per shoe	*MCM 2134, ASC*
A5504	For diabetics only, modification (including fitting) of off-the-shelf depth-inlay shoe or custom molded shoe with wedge(s), per shoe	*MCM 2134, ASC*
A5505	For diabetics only, modification (including fitting) of off-the-shelf depth-inlay shoe or custom molded shoe with metatarsal bar, per shoe	*MCM 2134, ASC*

| | = Invalid Medicare Code (no grace period) |
| | = Code may require certificate of medical necessity (CMN) or DMERC information form (DIF) |

A5506	For diabetics only, modification (including fitting) of off-the-shelf depth-inlay shoe or custom molded shoe with off-set heel(s), per shoe *MCM 2134, ASC*
A5507	For diabetics only, not otherwise specified modification (including fitting) of off-the-shelf depth-inlay shoe or custom molded shoe, per shoe *MCM 2134, ASC*
A5508	For diabetics only, deluxe feature of off-the-shelf depth-inlay shoe or custom-molded shoe, per shoe

Dressings

A6020	~~Collagen based wound dressing, each dressing~~ This code has been deleted in 2001.
● A6021	Collagen dressing, pad size 16 sq. in. or less, each
● A6022	Collagen dressing, pad size more than 16 sq. in. but less than or equal to 48 sq in, each
● A6023	Collagen dressing, pad size more than 48 sq. in., each
● A6024	Collagen dressing wound filler, per 6 in
A6025	Silicone gel sheet, each
A6154	Wound pouch, each
A6196	Alginate dressing, wound cover, pad size 16 sq. in. or less, each dressing
A6197	Alginate dressing, wound cover, pad size more than 16 sq. in. but less than or equal to 48 sq. in., each dressing
A6198	Alginate dressing, wound cover, pad size more then 48 sq. in., each dressing
A6199	Alginate dressing, wound filler, per 6 inches
A6200	Composite dressing, pad size 16 sq. in. or less, without adhesive border, each dressing
A6201	Composite dressing, pad size more than 16 sq. in. but less than or equal to 48 sq. in., without adhesive border, each dressing
A6202	Composite dressing, pad size more than 48 sq. in., without adhesive border, each dressing
A6203	Composite dressing, pad size 16 sq. in. or less, with any size adhesive border, each dressing
A6204	Composite dressing, pad size more than 16 sq. in. but less than or equal to 48 sq. in., with any size adhesive border, each dressing
A6205	Composite dressing, pad size more than 48 sq. in., with any size adhesive border, each dressing
A6206	Contact layer, 16 sq. in. or less, each dressing
A6207	Contact layer, more than 16 sq. in. but less than or equal to 48 sq. in., each dressing
A6208	Contact layer, more than 48 sq. in., each dressing

= Special Coverage Instructions Apply   = Carrier Discretion
= Noncovered by Medicare or Medicare Statute

A6209	Foam dressing, wound cover, pad size 16 sq. in. or less, without adhesive border, each dressing
A6210	Foam dressing, wound cover, pad size more than 16 sq. in. but less than or equal to 48 sq. in., without adhesive border, each dressing
A6211	Foam dressing, wound cover, pad size more then 48 sq. in., without adhesive border, each dressing
A6212	Foam dressing, wound cover, pad size 16 sq. in. or less, with any size adhesive border, each dressing
A6213	Foam dressing, wound cover, pad size more than 16 sq. in. but less than or equal to 48 sq. in., with any size adhesive border, each dressing
A6214	Foam dressing, wound cover, pad size more than 48 sq. in., with any size adhesive border, each dressing
A6215	Foam dressing, wound filler, per gram
A6216	Gauze, non-impregnated, non-sterile, pad size 16 sq. in. or less, without adhesive border, each dressing
A6217	Gauze, non-impregnated, non-sterile, pad size more than 16 sq. in. but less than or equal to 48 sq. in., without adhesive border, each dressing
A6218	Gauze, non-impregnated, non-sterile, pad size more than 48 sq. in., without adhesive border, each dressing
A6219	Gauze, non-impregnated, pad size 16 sq. in. or less, with any size adhesive border, each dressing
A6220	Gauze, non-impregnated, pad size more than 16 sq. in. but less than or equal to 48 sq. in., with any size adhesive border, each dressing
A6221	Gauze, non-impregnated, pad size more than 48 sq. in., with any size adhesive border, each dressing
▲ **A6222**	Gauze, impregnated with other than water, normal saline, or hydrogel, pad size 16 sq. in. or less, without adhesive border, each dressing
▲ **A6223**	Gauze, impregnated with other than water, normal saline, or hydrogel, pad size more than 16 sq. in. but less than or equal to 48 sq. in., without adhesive border, each dressing
▲ **A6224**	Gauze, impregnated with other than water, normal saline, or hydrogel, pad size more than 48 sq. in., without adhesive border, each dressing
A6228	Gauze, impregnated, water or normal saline, pad size 16 sq. in. or less, without adhesive border, each dressing
A6229	Gauze, impregnated, water or normal saline, pad size more than 16 sq. in. but less than or equal to 48 sq. in., without adhesive border, each dressing
A6230	Gauze, impregnated, water or normal saline, pad size more than 48 sq. in., without adhesive border, each dressing
● **A6231**	Gauze, impregnated, hydrogel, for direct wound contact, pad size 16 sq. in. or less, each dressing

= Invalid Medicare Code (no grace period)

= Code may require certificate of medical necessity (CMN) or DMERC information form (DIF)

● **A6232** Gauze, impregnated, hydrogel, for direct wound contact, pad size greater than 16 sq. in., but less than or equal to 48 sq. in., each dressing

● **A6233** Gauze, impregnated, hydrogel for direct wound contact, pad size more than 48 sq. in., each dressing

A6234 Hydrocolloid dressing, wound cover, pad size 16 sq. in. or less, without adhesive border, each dressing

A6235 Hydrocolloid dressing, wound cover, pad size more than 16 sq. in. but less than or equal to 48 sq. in., without adhesive border, each dressing

A6236 Hydrocolloid dressing, wound cover, pad size more than 48 sq. in., without adhesive border, each dressing

A6237 Hydrocolloid dressing, wound cover, pad size 16 sq. in. or less, with any size adhesive border, each dressing

A6238 Hydrocolloid dressing, wound cover, pad size more than 16 sq. in. but less than or equal to 48 sq. in., with any size adhesive border, each dressing

A6239 Hydrocolloid dressing, wound cover, pad size more than 48 sq. in., with any size adhesive border, each dressing

A6240 Hydrocolloid dressing, wound filler, paste, per fluid ounce

A6241 Hydrocolloid dressing, wound filler, dry form, per gram

A6242 Hydrogel dressing, wound cover, pad size 16 sq. in. or less, without adhesive border, each dressing

A6243 Hydrogel dressing, wound cover, pad size more than 16 sq. in. but less than or equal to 48 sq. in., without adhesive border, each dressing

A6244 Hydrogel dressing, wound cover, pad size more than 48 sq. in., without adhesive border, each dressing

A6245 Hydrogel dressing, wound cover, pad size 16 sq. in. or less, with any size adhesive border, each dressing

A6246 Hydrogel dressing, wound cover, pad size more than 16 sq. in. but less than or equal to 48 sq. in., with any size adhesive border, each dressing

A6247 Hydrogel dressing, wound cover, pad size more than 48 sq. in., with any size adhesive border, each dressing

A6248 Hydrogel dressing, wound filler, gel, per fluid ounce

A6250 Skin sealants, protectants, moisturizers, ointments, any type, any size

A6251 Specialty absorptive dressing, wound cover, pad size 16 sq. in. or less, without adhesive border, each dressing

A6252 Specialty absorptive dressing, wound cover, pad size more than 16 sq. in. but less than or equal to 48 sq. in., without adhesive border, each dressing

A6253 Specialty absorptive dressing, wound cover, pad size more than 48 sq. in., without adhesive border, each dressing

= Special Coverage Instructions Apply   = Carrier Discretion

= Noncovered by Medicare or Medicare Statute

A6254	Specialty absorptive dressing, wound cover, pad size 16 sq. in. or less, with any size adhesive border, each dressing
A6255	Specialty absorptive dressing, wound cover, pad size more than 16 sq. in. but less than or equal to 48 sq. in., with any size adhesive border, each dressing
A6256	Specialty absorptive dressing, wound cover, pad size more than 48 sq. in., with any size adhesive border, each dressing
A6257	Transparent film, 16 sq. in. or less, each dressing
A6258	Transparent film, more than 16 sq. in. but less than or equal to 48 sq. in., each dressing
A6259	Transparent film, more than 48 sq. in., each dressing
A6260	Wound cleansers, any type, any size
A6261	Wound filler, gel/paste, per fluid ounce, not elsewhere classified
A6262	Wound filler, dry form, per gram, not elsewhere classified
A6263	Gauze, elastic, non-sterile, all types, per linear yard
A6264	Gauze, non-elastic, non-sterile, per linear yard
A6265	Tape, all types, per 18 sq. in.
A6266	Gauze, impregnated, other than water or normal saline, any width, per linear yard
A6402	Gauze, non-impregnated, sterile, pad size 16 sq. in. or less, without adhesive border, each dressing
A6403	Gauze, non-impregnated, sterile, pad size more than 16 sq. in. but less than or equal to 48 sq. in., without adhesive border, each dressing
A6404	Gauze, non-impregnated, sterile, pad size more than 48 sq. in., without adhesive border, each dressing
A6405	Gauze, elastic, sterile, all types, per linear yard
A6406	Gauze, non-elastic, sterile, all types, per linear yard
A7000	Canister, disposable, used with suction pump, each
A7001	Canister, non-disposable, used with suction pump, each
A7002	Tubing, used with suction pump, each
A7003	Administration set, with small volume nonfiltered pneumatic nebulizer, disposable
A7004	Small volume nonfiltered pneumatic nebulizer, disposable
A7005	Administration set, with small volume nonfiltered pneumatic nebulizer, non-disposable
A7006	Administration set, with small volume filtered pneumatic nebulizer
A7007	Large volume nebulizer, disposable, unfilled, used with aerosol compressor
A7008	Large volume nebulizer, disposable, prefilled, used with aerosol compressor

= Invalid Medicare Code (no grace period)

= Code may require certificate of medical necessity (CMN) or DMERC information form (DIF)

A7009	Reservoir bottle, non-disposable, used with large volume ultrasonic nebulizer
A7010	Corrugated tubing, disposable, used with large volume nebulizer, 100 feet
A7011	Corrugated tubing, non-disposable, used with large volume nebulizer, 10 feet
A7012	Water collection device, used with large volume nebulizer
A7013	Filter, disposable, used with aerosol compressor
A7014	Filter, non-disposable, used with aerosol compressor or ultrasonic generator
A7015	Aerosol mask, used with DME nebulizer
A7016	Dome and mouthpiece, used with small volume ultrasonic nebulizer
A7017	Nebulizer, durable, glass or autoclavable plastic, bottle type, not used with oxygen *CIM 60-9*
● **A7018**	Water, distilled, used with large volume nebulizer, 1000 ml
● **A7019**	Saline solution, per 10 ml, metered dose dispenser, for use with inhalation drugs
● **A7020**	Sterile water or sterile saline, 1000 ml, used with large volume nebulizer
● **A7501**	Tracheostoma valve, including diaphragm, each *MCM 2130*
● **A7502**	Replacement diaphragm/faceplate for tracheostoma valve, each *MCM 2130*
● **A7503**	Filter holder or filter cap, reusable, for use in a tracheostoma heat and moisture exchange system, each *MCM 2130*
● **A7504**	Filter for use in a tracheostoma heat and moisture exchange system, each *MCM 2130*
● **A7505**	Housing, reusable without adhesive, for use in a heat and moisture exchange system and/or with a tracheostoma valve, each *MCM 2130*
● **A7506**	Adhesive disc for use in a heat and moisture exchange system and/or with tracheostoma valve, any type each *MCM 2130*
● **A7507**	Filter holder and integrated filter without adhesive, for use in a tracheostoma heat and moisture exchange system, each *MCM 2130*
● **A7508**	Housing and integrated adhesive, for use in a tracheostoma heat and moisture exchange system and/or with a tracheostoma valve, each *MCM 2130*
● **A7509**	Filter holder and integrated filter housing, and adhesive, for use as a tracheostoma heat and moisture exchange system, each *MCM 2130*

A Codes

Administrative, Miscellaneous and Investigational A9000–A9999

A9150	Nonprescription drug	MCM 2050.5
A9160	Noncovered service by podiatrist	Medicare Statute 1861.R3
A9170	Noncovered service by chiropractor	Medicare Statute 1861.R5
A9190	Personal comfort item	Medicare Statute 1862.A6
A9270	Noncovered item or service	MCM 2303
A9300	Exercise equipment	CIM 60-9, MCM 2100.1
A9500	Supply of radiopharmaceutical diagnostic imaging agent, technetium Tc 99m sestamibi, per dose	MCM 15022
A9502	Supply of radiopharmaceutical diagnostic imaging agent, technetium Tc 99m tetrofosmin, per unit dose	MCM 15022, ASC
A9503	Supply of radiopharmaceutical diagnostic imaging agent, technetium Tc 99m, medronate, up to 30 mCi	MCM 15022
A9504	Supply of radiopharmaceutical diagnostic imaging agent, technetium Tc 99m apcitide	MCM 15022
A9505	Supply of radiopharmaceutical diagnostic imaging agent, thallous chloride TL-201, per mCi	MCM 15022
A9507	Supply of radiopharmaceutical diagnostic imaging agent, indium IN 111 capromab pendetide, per dose	MCM 15022
● A9508	Supply of radiopharmaceutical diagnostic imaging agent, iobenguane sulfate I-131, per 0.5 mCi	MCM 15030
● A9510	Supply of radiopharmaceutical diagnostic imaging agent, technetium Tc 99m disofenin, per vial	MCM 15030
A9600	Supply of therapeutic radiopharmaceutical, strontium-89 chloride, per mCi	ASC
A9605	Supply of therapeutic radiopharmaceutical, samarium sm 153 lexidronamm, 50 mCi	
● A9700	Supply of injectable contrast material for use in echocardiography, per study	MCM 15022, 15030
▲ A9900	Miscellaneous DME supply, accessory, and/or service component of another HCPCS code	
▲ A9901	DME delivery, set up, and/or dispensing service component of another HCPCS code	

= Invalid Medicare Code (no grace period)

= Code may require certificate of medical necessity (CMN) or DMERC information form (DIF)

Enteral and Parenteral Therapy
B4000–B9999

Certification of medical necessity is required for coverage. Submit a revision to the certification of medical necessity if the patient's daily volume changes by more than one liter; if there is a change in infusion method; or if there is a change from premix to home mix or parenteral to enteral therapy.

B Codes

Enteral Formulae and Enteral Medical Supplies

B4034 Enteral feeding supply kit; syringe, per day
CIM 65-10, MCM 2130, MCM 4450, ASC

B4035 Enteral feeding supply kit; pump fed, per day
CIM 65-10, MCM 2130, MCM 4450, ASC

B4036 Enteral feeding supply kit; gravity fed, per day
CIM 65-10, MCM 2130, MCM 4450, ASC

B4081 Nasogastric tubing with stylet *CIM 65-10, MCM 2130, MCM 4450, ASC*

B4082 Nasogastric tubing without stylet *CIM 65-10, MCM 2130, MCM 4450, ASC*

B4083 Stomach tube — Levine type *CIM 65-10, MCM 2130, MCM 4450, ASC*

B4084 Gastrostomy/jejunostomy tubing *CIM 65-10, MCM 2130, MCM 4450, ASC*

B4085 Gastronomy tube, silicone with sliding ring, each *ASC*

▲ **B4150** Enteral formulae; category I; semi-synthetic intact protein/protein isolates, administered through an enteral feeding tube, 100 calories = 1 unit *CIM 65-10, MCM 2130, MCM 4450, ASC*

▲ **B4151** Enteral formulae; category I: natural intact protein/protein isolates, administered through an enteral feeding tube, 100 calories = 1 unit *CIM 65-10, MCM 2130, MCM 4450, ASC*

▲ **B4152** Enteral formulae; category II: intact protein/protein isolates (calorically dense), administered through an enteral feeding tube, 100 calories = 1 unit *CIM 65-10, MCM 2130, MCM 4450, ASC*

▲ **B4153** Enteral formulae; category III: hydrolized protein/amino acids, administered through an enteral feeding tube, 100 calories = 1 unit *CIM 65-10, MCM 2130, MCM 4450, ASC*

▲ **B4154** Enteral formulae; category IV: defined formula for special metabolic need, administered through an enteral feeding tube, 100 calories = 1 unit *CIM 65-10, MCM 2130, MCM 4450, ASC*

▲ **B4155** Enteral formulae; category V: modular components, administered through an enteral feeding tube, 100 calories = 1 unit *CIM 65-10, MCM 2130, MCM 4450, ASC*

▲ **B4156** Enteral formulae; category VI: standardized nutrients, administered through an enteral feeding tube, 100 calories = 1 unit *CIM 65-10, MCM 2130, MCM 4450, ASC*

= Special Coverage Instructions Apply = Carrier Discretion

= Noncovered by Medicare or Medicare Statute

Parenteral Nutrition Solutions and Supplies

B4164 Parenteral nutrition solution; carbohydrates (dextrose), 50% or less (500 ml = 1 unit) — home mix   *CIM 65-10, MCM 2130, MCM 4450, ASC*

B4168 Parenteral nutrition solution; amino acid, 3.5%, (500 ml = 1 unit) — home mix   *CIM 65-10, MCM 2130, MCM 4450, ASC*

B4172 Parenteral nutrition solution; amino acid, 5.5% through 7%, (500 ml = 1 unit) — home mix   *CIM 65-10, MCM 2130, MCM 4450, ASC*

B4176 Parenteral nutrition solution; amino acid, 7% through 8.5%, (500 ml = 1 unit) — home mix   *CIM 65-10, MCM 2130, MCM 4450, ASC*

B4178 Parenteral nutrition solution; amino acid, greater than 8.5% (500 ml = 1 unit) — home mix   *CIM 65-10, MCM 2130, MCM 4450, ASC*

B4180 Parenteral nutrition solution; carbohydrates (dextrose), greater than 50% (500 ml = 1 unit) — home mix   *CIM 65-10, MCM 2130, MCM 4450, ASC*

B4184 Parenteral nutrition solution; lipids, 10% with administration set (500 ml = 1 unit)   *CIM 65-10, MCM 2130, MCM 4450, ASC*

B4186 Parenteral nutrition solution; lipids, 20% with administration set (500 ml = 1 unit)   *CIM 65-10, MCM 2130, MCM 4450, ASC*

B4189 Parenteral nutrition solution; compounded amino acid and carbohydrates with electrolytes, trace elements, and vitamins, including preparation, any strength, 10 to 51 grams of protein — premix   *CIM 65-10, MCM 2130, MCM 4450, ASC*

B4193 Parenteral nutrition solution; compounded amino acid and carbohydrates with electrolytes, trace elements, and vitamins, including preparation, any strength, 52 to 73 grams of protein — premix   *CIM 65-10, MCM 2130, MCM 4450, ASC*

B4197 Parenteral nutrition solution; compounded amino acid and carbohydrates with electrolytes, trace elements and vitamins, including preparation, any strength, 74 to 100 grams of protein — premix   *CIM 65-10, MCM 2130, MCM 4450, ASC*

B4199 Parenteral nutrition solution; compounded amino acid and carbohydrates with electrolytes, trace elements and vitamins, including preparation, any strength, over 100 grams of protein — premix   *CIM 65-10, MCM 2130, MCM 4450, ASC*

B4216 Parenteral nutrition; additives (vitamins, trace elements, heparin, electrolytes) — home mix, per day   *CIM 65-10, MCM 2130, MCM 4450, ASC*

B4220 Parenteral nutrition supply kit; premix, per day   *CIM 65-10, MCM 2130, MCM 4450, ASC*

B4222 Parenteral nutrition supply kit; home mix, per day   *CIM 65-10, MCM 2130, MCM 4450, ASC*

B4224 Parenteral nutrition administration kit, per day   *CIM 65-10, MCM 2130, MCM 4450, ASC*

= Invalid Medicare Code (no grace period)

= Code may require certificate of medical necessity (CMN) or DMERC information form (DIF)

B5000 Parenteral nutrition solution; compounded amino acid and carbohydrates with electrolytes, trace elements, and vitamins, including preparation, any strength, renal — amirosyn RF, nephramine, renamine — premix   *CIM 65-10, MCM 2130, MCM 4450, ASC*

B5100 Parenteral nutrition solution; compounded amino acid and carbohydrates with electrolytes, trace elements, and vitamins, including preparation, any strength, hepatic — freamine HBC, hepatamine — premix   *CIM 65-10, MCM 2130, MCM 4450, ASC*

B5200 Parenteral nutrition solution; compounded amino acid and carbohydrates with electrolytes, trace elements, and vitamins, including preparation, any strength, stress — branch chain amino acids — premix   *CIM 65-10, MCM 2130, MCM 4450, ASC*

Submit documentation of the need for the infusion pump. Medicare will reimburse for the simplest model that meets the patient's needs.

Enteral and Parenteral Pumps

B9000 Enteral nutrition infusion pump — without alarm
CIM 65-10, MCM 2130, MCM 4450, ASC

B9002 Enteral nutrition infusion pump — with alarm
CIM 65-10, MCM 2130, MCM 4450, ASC

B9004 Parenteral nutrition infusion pump, portable
CIM 65-10, MCM 2130, MCM 4450, ASC

B9006 Parenteral nutrition infusion pump, stationary
CIM 65-10, MCM 2130, MCM 4450, ASC

B9998 NOC for enteral supplies   *CIM 65-10, MCM 2130, MCM 4450, ASC*

B9999 NOC for parenteral supplies   *CIM 65-10, MCM 2130, MCM 4450, ASC*

B Codes

= Special Coverage Instructions Apply   = Carrier Discretion

= Noncovered by Medicare or Medicare Statute

C Codes — Temporary Codes for Use with Outpatient PPS

C Codes are used exclusively for services paid under the Outpatient PPS and may not be used to bill services paid under other Medicare payment systems.

● **C1000** Closure, arterial vascular device, Perclose Closer Arterial Vascular Closure Device, Prostart Arterial Vascular Closure Device
Medicare Statute 1833(T)

● **C1001** Catheter, diagnostic ultrasound, Acunav Diagnostic Ultrasound Catheter *Medicare Statute 1833(T)*

● **C1003** Catheter, ablation, Livewire Tc Ablation Catheter 402132, 402133, 402134, 402135, 402136, 402137, 402145, 402146, 402147, 402148, 402149, 402150, 402151, 402152, 402153, 402154, 402155, 402156 *Medicare Statute 1833(T)*

● **C1004** Fast-Cath, SWARTZ, SAFL, CSTA, SEPT, RAMP Guiding Introducer *Medicare Statute 1833(T)*

C1005 ~~Intraocular lens, Sensar Soft Acrylic Ultraviolet Light Absorbing Posterior Chamber Intraocular Lens~~ This code was added and deleted in 2000.

● **C1006** Intraocular lens, Array Multifocal Silicone Posterior Chamber Intraocular Lens *Medicare Statute 1833(T)*

● **C1007** Prosthesis, penile, AMS 700 Penile Prosthesis, AMS Ambicor penile prosthesis *Medicare Statute 1833(T)*

● **C1008** Stent, urethral, permanent, Urolume *Medicare Statute 1833(T)*

● **C1009** Plasma, cryoprecipitate reduced, each unit *Medicare Statute 1833(T)*

● **C1010** Blood, leukoreduced CMV-negative, each unit *Medicare Statute 1833(T)*

● **C1011** Platelet, HLA-matched leukoreduced, apheresis/pheresis, each unit *Medicare Statute 1833(T)*

● **C1012** Platelet concentrate, leukoreduced, irradiated, each unit *Medicare Statute 1833(T)*

● **C1013** Platelet concentrate, leukoreduced, each unit *Medicare Statute 1833(T)*

● **C1014** Platelet, leukoreduced, apheresis/pheresis, each unit *Medicare Statute 1833(T)*

● **C1016** Blood, leukoreduced, frozen/deglycerol/washed, each unit *Medicare Statute 1833(T)*

● **C1017** Platelet, leukoreduced, CMV-negative, apheresis/pheresis, each unit *Medicare Statute 1833(T)*

● **C1018** Blood, leukoreduced, irradiated, each unit *Medicare Statute 1833(T)*

● **C1019** Platelet, leukoreduced, irradiated, apheresis/pheresis, each unit *Medicare Statute 1833(T)*

● **C1024** Quinopristin/dalfopristin, 10 ml, Synercid IV *Medicare Statute 1833(T)*

● **C1025** Catheter, Marinr CS Catheter *Medicare Statute 1833(T)*

C Codes

[shaded box] = Special Coverage Instructions Apply   [shaded box] = Carrier Discretion

[shaded box] = Noncovered by Medicare or Medicare Statute

● **C1026** Catheter ablation, RF Performr, 5F RF Marinr *Medicare Statute 1833(T)*

● **C1027** Stent, coronary, Magic Wallstent Extra Short Or Short Coronary Self-Expanding Stent with Delivery System, Radius 14 mm Self Expanding Stent with Over-the Wire-Delivery System *Medicare Statute 1833(T)*

● **C1028** Sling fixation system for treatment of stress urinary incontinence, Precision Twist Transvaginal Anchor System, Precision Tack Transvaginal Anchor System, Vesica Press-In Anchor System, Capio CL (TVB/S) Transvaginal Suturing Device *Medicare Statute 1833(T)*

● **C1029** Catheter, balloon dilatation, controlled radial expansion (CRE) balloon dilatation catheter wire guided and fixed wire *Medicare Statute 1833(T)*

● **C1030** Catheter, balloon dilatation, Marshal, Blue Max 20, Ultra-Thin Diamond *Medicare Statute 1833(T)*

● **C1031** Electrode, needle, ablation, MR Compatible Leveen, modified Leveen needle electrode *Medicare Statute 1833(T)*

● **C1033** Catheter, imaging, Sonicath Ultra Model 37-410 Ultrasound Imaging Catheter *Medicare Statute 1833(T)*

● **C1034** Catheter, coronary angioplasty, Surpass Superfusion Catheter, long 30 Surpass Superfusion Catheter *Medicare Statute 1833(T)*

● **C1035** Catheter, intracardiac echocardiography, Ultra Ice 6F, 12.5 MHz Catheter (with disposable sheath), Ultra Ice 9F, 9 MHz Catheter (with disposable sheath) *Medicare Statute 1833(T)*

● **C1036** Port/reservoir, venous access device, Vaxcel Implantable Vascular Access System, R Port Premier Vascular Access System *Medicare Statute 1833(T)*

● **C1037** Catheter, dialysis, Vaxcel Chronic Dialysis Catheter *Medicare Statute 1833(T)*

● **C1038** Catheter, imaging, Ultracross 2.9F 30MHz Coronary Imaging Catheter, Ultracross 3.2F MHz Coronary Imaging Catheter *Medicare Statute 1833(T)*

● **C1039** Stent, tracheobronchial, Wallstent Tracheobronchial Endoprosthesis (covered), Wallstent Tracheobronchial Endoprosthesis with Permalume Covering and Unistep Plus Delivery System, Wallstent RP Tracheobronchial Endoprosthesis with Unistep Plus Delivery System *Medicare Statute 1833(T)*

● **C1040** Stent, self-expandable for creation of intrahepatic shunts, Wallstent transjugular intrahepatic portosystemic shunt (TIPS) with Unistep Plus Delivery System (40/42/60/68 mm in length), Wallstent RP Endoprosthesis with Unistep Plus Delivery System (42/68 mm in length) *Medicare Statute 1833(T)*

● **C1042** Stent, biliary, Wallstent Biliary Endoprosthesis with Unistep Plus Delivery System, Wallstent Biliary Endoprosthesis with Unistep Delivery System (Biliary Stent and Catheter), Wallstent RP Biliary Endoprosthesis with Unistep Plus Delivery System, Ultraflex Diamond Biliary Stent System, New Microvasive Biliary Stent and Delivery System *Medicare Statute 1833(T)*

= Invalid Medicare Code (no grace period)

= Code may require certificate of medical necessity (CMN) or DMERC information form (DIF)

● C1043 Atherectomy system, coronary, Rotablator Rotalink Atherectomy Catheter and Burr, Rotablator Rotalink Rotational Atherectomy System Advancer and Guide Wire *Medicare Statute 1833(T)*

● C1045 Supply of radiopharmaceutical diagnostic imaging agent, I-131 MIBG [iobenguane sulfate I-131], per 0.5 mCi *Medicare Statute 1833(T)*

● C1047 Catheter, diagnostic, Navi-Star Diagnostic Deflectable TIP Catheter, Noga-Star Diagnostic Deflectable TIP Catheter *Medicare Statute 1833(T)*

● C1048 Generator, bipolar pulse, Cyberonics Neurocybernetic Prosthesis Generator *Medicare Statute 1833(T)*

● C1050 Protein A immunoadsorption, Prosorba Column *Medicare Statute 1833(T)*

● C1051 Catheter, thrombectomy, Oasis Thrombectomy Catheter *Medicare Statute 1833(T)*

● C1053 Catheter, diagnostic, Ensite 3000 Catheter *Medicare Statute 1833(T)*

● C1054 Catheter, thrombectomy, Hydrolyser 6F Mechanical Thrombectomy Catheter, Hydrolyser 7F Mechanical Thrombectomy Catheter *Medicare Statute 1833(T)*

● C1055 Catheter, Transesophageal 210 Atrial Pacing Catheter, Transesophageal 210-S Atrial Pacing Catheter *Medicare Statute 1833(T)*

● C1056 Catheter, ablation, Gynecare Thermachoice II Catheter *Medicare Statute 1833(T)*

● C1057 Tissue marker, 11-Gauge Micromark II Tissue Marker *Medicare Statute 1833(T)*

● C1059 Autologous cultured chondrocytes, implantation, Carticel *Medicare Statute 1833(T)*

● C1060 Stent, coronary, ACS Multi-Link Tristar Coronary Stent System and Delivery System, ACS Multi-Link Ultra Coronary Stent System *Medicare Statute 1833(T)*

● C1061 Catheter, coronary guide, ACS Viking Guiding Catheter *Medicare Statute 1833(T)*

● C1063 Lead, defibrillator, Endotak Endurance EZ, Endotak Endurance RX, Endotak Endurance 0134, 0135, 0136 *Medicare Statute 1833(T)*

● C1067 Stent, biliary, Megalink Biliary Stent *Medicare Statute 1833(T)*

● C1068 Pacemaker, dual chamber, Pulsar DDD *Medicare Statute 1833(T)*

● C1069 Pacemaker, dual chamber, Discover DR *Medicare Statute 1833(T)*

● C1071 Pacemaker, single chamber, Pulsar Max SR, Pulsar SR *Medicare Statute 1833(T)*

● C1072 Catheter, balloon dilatation, coronary, RX Esprit, RX Gemini, RX Solaris, OTW Photon, OTW Solaris *Medicare Statute 1833(T)*

● C1073 Morcellator, laparoscopic, Gynecare X-Tract Laparoscopic Morcellator *Medicare Statute 1833(T)*

C Codes

= Special Coverage Instructions Apply ■ = Carrier Discretion

= Noncovered by Medicare or Medicare Statute

● **C1074** Catheter, peripheral dilatation, RX Viatrac 14 Peripheral Dilatation Catheter, OTW Viatrac 18 Peripheral Dilatation Catheter
Medicare Statute 1833(T)

● **C1075** Lead, pacemaker, Selute Picotip, Selute, Sweet PicoTIP RX, Sweet TIP RX, Fineline, Fineline EZ, Thinline, Thinline EZ *Medicare Statute 1833(T)*

● **C1076** Defibrillator, single chamber, automatic, implantable, Ventak Mini IV, Ventak Mini IV+ (Models 1793, 1796), Ventak Mini III HE, Ventak Mini III HE+ (Models 1788, 1789), Ventak Mini III, Ventak Mini III + (Models 1783, 1786) *Medicare Statute 1833(T)*

● **C1077** Defibrillator, single chamber, automatic, implantable, Ventak Prizm VR, Ventak VR *Medicare Statute 1833(T)*

● **C1078** Defibrillator, dual chamber, automatic, implantable, Ventak Prizm, Ventak AV III DR *Medicare Statute 1833(T)*

● **C1079** Supply of radiopharmaceutical diagnostic imaging agent, cyanocobalamin co 58/57, kit, 0.5 mCi, nycomed cyanoco Co57/cyanoco Co58 *Medicare Statute 1833(T)*

● **C1084** Denileukin diftitox, 300 mcg, Ontak IV *Medicare Statute 1833(T)*

● **C1086** Temozolomide, 5 mg, Temodar *Medicare Statute 1833(T)*

● **C1087** Supply of radiopharmaceutical imaging agent, sodium iodide 1-123 (capsule), per uCi *Medicare Statute 1833(T)*

● **C1088** Laser optic treatment system, Indigo Laseroptic Treatment System *Medicare Statute 1833(T)*

● **C1089** Supply of radiopharmaceutical diagnostic imaging agent, cyanocobalamin Co 57, 0.5 mCi, capsule *Medicare Statute 1833(T)*

● **C1090** Supply of radiopharmaceutical diagnostic imaging agent, indium in 111 chloride, per mCi *Medicare Statute 1833(T)*

● **C1091** Supply of radiopharmaceutical diagnostic imaging agent, indium in 111 oxyquinoline, per 5 mCi *Medicare Statute 1833(T)*

● **C1092** Supply of radiopharmaceutical diagnostic imaging agent, indium in 111 pentetate disodium, per 1.5 mCi *Medicare Statute 1833(T)*

● **C1094** Supply of radiopharmaceutical diagnostic imaging agent, technetium Tc 99m albumin aggregated, per vial *Medicare Statute 1833(T)*

● **C1095** Supply of radiopharmaceutical diagnostic imaging agent, technetium Tc 99m depreotide, per vial *Medicare Statute 1833(T)*

● **C1096** Supply of radiopharmaceutical diagnostic imaging agent, technetium Tc 99m exametazime, per dose *Medicare Statute 1833(T)*

● **C1097** Supply of radiopharmaceutical diagnostic imaging agent, technetium Tc 99m mebrofenin, per vial *Medicare Statute 1833(T)*

● **C1098** Supply of radiopharmaceutical diagnostic imaging agent, technetium Tc 99m pentetate, per vial *Medicare Statute 1833(T)*

● **C1099** Supply of radiopharmaceutical diagnostic imaging agent, technetium Tc 99m pyrophosphate, per vial *Medicare Statute 1833(T)*

= Invalid Medicare Code (no grace period)

= Code may require certificate of medical necessity (CMN) or DMERC information form (DIF)

● **C1100** Guide wire, percutaneous transluminal coronary angioplasty, Medtronic AVE gGTL Guide Wire, Medtronic AVE GT2 Fusion Guide Wire
Medicare Statute 1833(T)

● **C1101** Catheter, percutaneous transluminal coronary angioplasty guide, Medtronic AVE 5F, 6F, 7F, 8F, 9F Zuma Guide Catheter, Medtronic AVE Z2 5F, 6F, 7F, 8F, 9F Zuma Guide Catheter *Medicare Statute 1833(T)*

● **C1102** Generator, pulse, neurostimulator, Medtronic Synergy Neurostimulator Generator and Extension *Medicare Statute 1833(T)*

● **C1103** Defibrillator, implantable, Micro Jewel, Micro Jewel II
Medicare Statute 1833(T)

● **C1104** Catheter, ablation, RF Conductr MC 4 mm, RF Conductr MC 5 mm (Models 6042, 7544) *Medicare Statute 1833(T)*

● **C1105** Pacemaker, dual chamber, Sigma 300 VDD *Medicare Statute 1833(T)*

● **C1106** Neurostimulator, patient programmer, Synergy EZ Patient Programmer
Medicare Statute 1833(T)

● **C1107** Catheter, diagnostic, electrophysiology, Torqr, Soloist
Medicare Statute 1833(T)

● **C1109** Anchor, Implantable, Mitek GII Anchor, Mitek Knotless, Mitek Tacit, Mitek Rotator Cuff, Mitek GLS, Mitek Mini, Mitek Fastin, Mitek Super, Mitek Panalok, Mitek Micro, Mitek Panalok RC, Mitek Fastin RC, Innovasive ROC EZ, Innovasive MiniROC, Innovasive BioROC, Innovasive ROC XS, Innovasive Contack *Medicare Statute 1833(T)*

● **C1110** Catheter, diagnostic, electrophysiology, Stable Mapper
Medicare Statute 1833(T)

● **C1111** Stent graft system, Aneurx Aorto-Uni-Iliac-Stent Graft System
Medicare Statute 1833(T)

● **C1112** Stent graft system, Aneurx Stent Graft System *Medicare Statute 1833(T)*

● **C1113** Stent graft system, Talent Endoluminal Spring Stent Graft System
Medicare Statute 1833(T)

● **C1114** Stent graft system, Talent Spring Stent Graft System
Medicare Statute 1833(T)

● **C1115** Lead, pacemaker, 5038S, 5038, 5038l *Medicare Statute 1833(T)*

● **C1116** Lead, pacemaker, CapSure SP Novus, CapSure SP, CapSure, Excellence +, S+, PS+, CapSure Z Novus, CapSure Z, Impulse
Medicare Statute 1833(T)

● **C1117** Endograft system, Ancure Endograft Delivery System
Medicare Statute 1833(T)

● **C1118** Pacemaker, dual chamber, Sigma 300 DR, Legacy II DR
Medicare Statute 1833(T)

● **C1119** Lead, defibrillator, Sprint 6932, Sprint 6943 *Medicare Statute 1833(T)*

● **C1120** Lead, defibrillator, Sprint 6942, Sprint 6945 *Medicare Statute 1833(T)*

● **C1121** Defibrillator, implantable, Gem *Medicare Statute 1833(T)*

C Codes

= Special Coverage Instructions Apply   = Carrier Discretion

= Noncovered by Medicare or Medicare Statute

● **C1122** Supply of radiopharmaceutical diagnostic imaging agent, technetium Tc 99m arcitumomab, per vial *Medicare Statute 1833(T)*

● **C1123** Defibrillator, implantable, Gem II VR *Medicare Statute 1833(T)*

● **C1124** Lead, neurostimulator, kit, Interstim Test Stimulation Lead Kit *Medicare Statute 1833(T)*

● **C1125** Pacemaker, single chamber, Kappa 400 SR, Topaz II SR *Medicare Statute 1833(T)*

● **C1126** Pacemaker, dual chamber, Kappa 700 DR (all models) *Medicare Statute 1833(T)*

● **C1127** Pacemaker, single chamber, Kappa 700 SR *Medicare Statute 1833(T)*

● **C1128** Pacemaker, dual chamber, Kappa 700 D, Ruby II D *Medicare Statute 1833(T)*

● **C1129** Pacemaker, Kappa 700 VDD *Medicare Statute 1833(T)*

● **C1130** Pacemaker, dual chamber, Sigma 200 D, Legacy II D *Medicare Statute 1833(T)*

● **C1131** Pacemaker, dual chamber, Sigma 200 DR *Medicare Statute 1833(T)*

● **C1132** Pacemaker, single chamber, Sigma 200 SR, Legacy II SR *Medicare Statute 1833(T)*

● **C1133** Pacemaker, single chamber, Sigma 300 SR, Vita SR *Medicare Statute 1833(T)*

● **C1134** Pacemaker, dual chamber, Sigma 300 D *Medicare Statute 1833(T)*

● **C1135** Pacemaker, dual chamber, rate-responsive, Entity DR 5326l, Entity DR 5326R, Entity DR 5326 *Medicare Statute 1833(T)*

● **C1136** Pacemaker, dual chamber, rate-responsive, Affinity DR 5330l, Affinity DR 5330R, Affinity DR 5330 *Medicare Statute 1833(T)*

● **C1137** Septal defect implant system, Cardioseal Septal Occlusion System, Cardioseal Occluder Delivery Catheter *Medicare Statute 1833(T)*

● **C1143** Pacemaker, dual chamber, Addvent 2060BL *Medicare Statute 1833(T)*

● **C1144** Pacemaker, single chamber, rate-responsive, Affinity SR 5130, Affinity SR 5130l, Affinity SR 5130r, Integrity SR 5142 *Medicare Statute 1833(T)*

● **C1145** Vascular closure device, Angio-Seal 6 French Vascular Closure Device 610091, Angio-Seal 8 French Vascular Closure Device 610089, 610097 *Medicare Statute 1833(T)*

● **C1146** Endotracheal tube, Vett Tracheobronchial Tube *Medicare Statute 1833(T)*

● **C1147** Lead, pacemaker, AV PLUS DX 1368/52, AV PLUS DX 1368/58, AV PLUS DX 1368/65 *Medicare Statute 1833(T)*

● **C1148** Defibrillator, single chamber, implantable, Contour MD V-175, Contour MD V-175A, Contour MD V-175AC, Contour MD V-175B, Contour MD V-175C, Contour MD V-175D *Medicare Statute 1833(T)*

● **C1149** Pacemaker, dual chamber, non-rate responsive, Entity DC 5226R, Entity DC 5226 *Medicare Statute 1833(T)*

= Invalid Medicare Code (no grace period)

= Code may require certificate of medical necessity (CMN) or DMERC information form (DIF)

● **C1151** Lead, pacemaker, Passive Plus DX 1343K/46, Passive Plus DX 1343k/52, Passive Plus DX 1345K/52, Passive Plus DX 1345K/58, Passive Plus DX 1336T/52, Passive Plus DX 1336T/58, Passive Plus DX 1342T/46, Passive Plus DX 1342T/52, Passive Plus DX 1346T/52, Passive Plus DX 1346T/58 *Medicare Statute 1833(T)*

● **C1152** Access system, dialysis, Lifesite Access System *Medicare Statute 1833(T)*

● **C1153** Pacemaker, single chamber, Regency SC+ 2402l *Medicare Statute 1833(T)*

● **C1154** Lead, defibrillator, SPL SP01, SP02, SPL04 *Medicare Statute 1833(T)*

● **C1155** Repliform Tissue Regeneration Matrix, per 8 sq cm
Medicare Statute 1833(T)

● **C1156** Pacemaker, single chamber, Affinity SR 5131m/s, Tempo VR 1102, Trilogy SR+ 2260l, Trilogy SR+ 2264l *Medicare Statute 1833(T)*

● **C1157** Pacemaker, dual chamber, Trilogy DC+2318l *Medicare Statute 1833(T)*

● **C1158** Lead, defibrillator, TVL SV01, TVL SV02, TVL SV04 *Medicare Statute 1833(T)*

● **C1159** Lead, defibrillator, TVL RV02, TVL RV06, TVL RV07
Medicare Statute 1833(T)

● **C1160** Lead, defibrillator, TVL-ADX 1559/65 *Medicare Statute 1833(T)*

● **C1161** Lead, pacemaker, Tendril DX 1388K/46, Tendril DX 1388K/52, Tendril DX 1388K/58, Tendril DX 1388T/46, Tendril DX 1388T/52, Tendril DX 1388T/58, Tendril DX 1388T/85, Tendril DX 1388T/100, Tendril DX 1388Tc/46, Tendril DX 1388Tc/52, Tendril DX 1388T/58
Medicare Statute 1833(T)

● **C1162** Pacemaker, dual-chamber, Affinity DR 5331 m/s, Tempo DR 2102, Trilogy DR+ 2360l, Trilogy DR+ 2364l *Medicare Statute 1833(T)*

● **C1163** Lead, pacemaker, Tendril SDX 1488T/46, Tendril SDX 1488T/52, Tendril SDX 1488T/58, Tendril SDX 1488Tc/46, Tendril SDX 1488Tc/52, Tendril SDX 1488Tc/58 *Medicare Statute 1833(T)*

● **C1164** Brachytherapy seed, I-125 seed *Medicare Statute 1833(T)*

● **C1166** Injection, cytarabine liposome, 10 mg, depocyt/liposomal cytarabine
Medicare Statute 1833(T)

● **C1167** Injection, epirubicin hydrochloride, 2 mg *Medicare Statute 1833(T)*

● **C1170** Biopsy device, breast, abbi device *Medicare Statute 1833(T)*

● **C1171** Site marker device, disposable, Auto Suture Site Marker Device
Medicare Statute 1833(T)

● **C1172** Balloon, tissue dissector, Spacemaker Tissue Dissection Balloon, Spacemaker 1000cc Hernia Balloon Dissector *Medicare Statute 1833(T)*

● **C1173** Stent, coronary, S540 Over-the-Wire Coronary Stent System, S670 with Discrete Technology Over-the-Wire Coronary Stent System, S670 with Discrete Technology Rapid Exchange Coronary Stent System
Medicare Statute 1833(T)

● **C1174** Needle, brachytherapy, Bard Brachystar Brachytherapy Needle
Medicare Statute 1833(T)

C Codes

= Special Coverage Instructions Apply   = Carrier Discretion

= Noncovered by Medicare or Medicare Statute

● **C1175** Biopsy device, MIBB device   *Medicare Statute 1833(T)*

● **C1176** Biopsy device, Mammotome HH Hand-Held Probe with Smartvac Vacuum System   *Medicare Statute 1833(T)*

● **C1177** Biopsy Device, 11-Gauge Mammotome Probe with Vacuum Cannister   *Medicare Statute 1833(T)*

● **C1178** Injection, busulfan (busulfex IV) per 6 mg   *Medicare Statute 1833(T)*

● **C1179** Biopsy device, 14-Gauge Mammotome Probe With Vacuum Cannister   *Medicare Statute 1833(T)*

● **C1180** Pacemaker, single chamber, Vigor SR   *Medicare Statute 1833(T)*

● **C1181** Pacemaker, single chamber, Meridian SSI   *Medicare Statute 1833(T)*

● **C1182** Pacemaker, single chamber, Pulsar SSI   *Medicare Statute 1833(T)*

● **C1183** Pacemaker, single chamber, Jade II S, Sigma 300 S   *Medicare Statute 1833(T)*

● **C1184** Pacemaker, single chamber, Sigma 200 S   *Medicare Statute 1833(T)*

● **C1188** Sodium iodide I-131, per uCi   *Medicare Statute 1833(T)*

● **C1200** Supply of radiopharmaceutical diagnostic imaging agent, technetium Tc 99m sodium glucoheptonate, per vial   *Medicare Statute 1833(T)*

● **C1201** Supply of radiopharmaceutical diagnostic imaging agent, technetium Tc 99m succimer, per vial   *Medicare Statute 1833(T)*

● **C1202** Supply of radiopharmaceutical diagnostic imaging agent, technetium Tc 99m sulfur colloid, per dose   *Medicare Statute 1833(T)*

● **C1203** Injection, Visudyne (verteporfin)   *Medicare Statute 1833(T)*

● **C1205** Supply of radiopharmaceutical diagnostic imaging agent, technetium Tc 99m disofenin, per vial   *Medicare Statute 1833(T)*

● **C1207** Octreotide acetate, 1 mg   *Medicare Statute 1833(T)*

● **C1300** Hyperbaric oxygen under pressure, full body chamber, per 30 minute interval   *Medicare Statute 1833(T)*

● **C1302** Lead, defibrillator, TVL SQ01   *Medicare Statute 1833(T)*

● **C1303** Lead, defibrillator, CapSure Fix 6940, CapSure Fix 4068-110   *Medicare Statute 1833(T)*

● **C1304** Catheter, imaging, Sonicath Ultra Model 37-416 Ultrasound Imaging Catheter, Sonicath Ultra Model 37-418 Ultrasound Imaging Catheter   *Medicare Statute 1833(T)*

● **C1305** Apligraf, per 44 sq cm   *Medicare Statute 1833(T)*

● **C1306** Lead, neurostimulator, Cyberonics Neurocybernetic Prosthesis Lead   *Medicare Statute 1833(T)*

● **C1311** Pacemaker, dual chamber, Trilogy DR+/DAO   *Medicare Statute 1833(T)*

● **C1312** Stent, coronary, Magic Wallstent Mini Coronary Self Expanding Stent with Delivery System   *Medicare Statute 1833(T)*

─────────────────────────────

= Invalid Medicare Code (no grace period)

= Code may require certificate of medical necessity (CMN) or DMERC information form (DIF)

● **C1313** Stent, coronary, Magic Wallstent Medium Coronary Self Expanding Stent with Delivery System, Radius 31 mm Self Expanding Stent with Over-the-Wire Delivery System *Medicare Statute 1833(T)*

● **C1314** Stent, coronary, Magic Wallstent Long Coronary Self Expanding Stent with Delivery System *Medicare Statute 1833(T)*

● **C1315** Pacemaker, dual chamber, Vigor DR, Meridian DR *Medicare Statute 1833(T)*

● **C1316** Pacemaker, dual chamber, Meridian DDD *Medicare Statute 1833(T)*

● **C1317** Pacemaker, single chamber, Discovery SR *Medicare Statute 1833(T)*

● **C1318** Pacemaker, single chamber, Meridian SR *Medicare Statute 1833(T)*

● **C1319** Stent, Enteral, Wallstent Enteral Endoprosthesis and Unistep Delivery System (60 mm in length), Enteral Wallstent Endoprosthesis and Unistep Plus Delivery System/Single-Use Colonic And Duodenal Endoprosthesis with Unistep Plus Delivery System (60 mm in length) *Medicare Statute 1833(T)*

● **C1320** Stent, Iliac, Wallstent Iliac Endoprosthesis with Unistep Plus Delivery System, Wallstent RP Iliac Endoprosthesis with Unistep Plus Delivery System *Medicare Statute 1833(T)*

● **C1321** Electrode, disposable, Palate Somnoplasty Coagulating Electrode, Base Of Tongue Somnoplasty Coagulating Electrode *Medicare Statute 1833(T)*

● **C1322** Electrode, disposable, Turbinate Somnoplasty Coagulating Electrode *Medicare Statute 1833(T)*

● **C1323** Electrode, disposable, VAPR Electrode, VAPR T Thermal Electrode *Medicare Statute 1833(T)*

● **C1324** Electrode, disposable, Ligasure Disposable Electrode *Medicare Statute 1833(T)*

● **C1325** Brachytherapy seed, palladium-103 seed *Medicare Statute 1833(T)*

● **C1326** Catheter, thrombectomy, Angiojet Rheolytic Thrombectomy Catheter *Medicare Statute 1833(T)*

● **C1328** External transmitter, neurostimulation system, ANS Renew Spinal Cord Stimulator System *Medicare Statute 1833(T)*

● **C1329** Electrode, disposable, Gynecare Versapoint Resectoscopic System Bipolar Electrode *Medicare Statute 1833(T)*

● **C1333** Stent, biliary, Palmaz Corinthian Transhepatic Biliary Stent and Delivery System *Medicare Statute 1833(T)*

● **C1334** Stent, coronary, Palmaz-Schatz Crown Stent, Mini-Crown Stent, Crossflex LC Stent *Medicare Statute 1833(T)*

● **C1335** Mesh, hernia, Prolene Polypropylene Hernia System *Medicare Statute 1833(T)*

● **C1336** Infusion pump, implantable, non-programmable, Constant Flow Implantable Pump with Bolus Safety Valve Model 3000, Model 3000-16 (16ml), Model 3000-50 (50ml) *Medicare Statute 1833(T)*

C Codes

= Special Coverage Instructions Apply   = Carrier Discretion

= Noncovered by Medicare or Medicare Statute

● **C1337** Infusion pump, implantable, non-programmable, Isomed Infusion Pump Model 8472-20, 8472-35, 8472-60 *Medicare Statute 1833(T)*

● **C1348** Sodium iodide I-131, per mCi *Medicare Statute 1833(T)*

● **C1350** Brachytherapy, per source, Prostaseed I-125 *Medicare Statute 1833(T)*

● **C1351** Lead, pacemaker, CapSureFix, SureFix, Pirouet +, S+ *Medicare Statute 1833(T)*

● **C1352** Defibrillator, dual chamber, implantable, Gem II DR *Medicare Statute 1833(T)*

● **C1353** Neurostimulator, implantable, Itrel II/Soletra Implantable Neurostimulator and Extension, Itrel III Implantable Neurostimulator and Extension, Interstim Neurostimulator (implantable) and Extension *Medicare Statute 1833(T)*

● **C1354** Pacemaker, dual chamber, Kappa 400 DR, Diamond II 820 DR *Medicare Statute 1833(T)*

● **C1355** Pacemaker, dual chamber, Kappa 600 DR, Vita DR *Medicare Statute 1833(T)*

● **C1356** Defibrillator, single chamber, implantable, Profile MD V-186HV3 *Medicare Statute 1833(T)*

● **C1357** Defibrillator, single chamber, implantable, Angstrom MD V-190HV3 *Medicare Statute 1833(T)*

● **C1358** Pacemaker, dual chamber, non-rate responsive, Affinity DC 5230R, Affinity DC 5230 *Medicare Statute 1833(T)*

● **C1359** Pacemaker, dual chamber, Pulsar DR, Pulsar MAX DR *Medicare Statute 1833(T)*

● **C1360** Ocular photodynamic therapy *Medicare Statute 1833(T)*

● **C1361** Recorder, cardiac event, implantable, Reveal, Reveal Plus *Medicare Statute 1833(T)*

● **C1362** Stent, biliary, RX Herculink 14 Biliary Stent, OTW Megalink SDS Biliary Stent *Medicare Statute 1833(T)*

● **C1363** Defibrillator, implantable, dual chamber, Gem DR *Medicare Statute 1833(T)*

● **C1364** Defibrillator, dual chamber, Photon DR V-230HV3 *Medicare Statute 1833(T)*

● **C1365** Guide wire, Peripheral, Hi-Torque Spartacore 14 Guide Wire, Hi-Torque Memcore Firm 14 Guide Wire, Hi-Torque Steelcore 18 Guide Wire, Hi-Torque Steelcore 18 LT Guide Wire, Hi-Torque Supra Core 35 Guide Wire *Medicare Statute 1833(T)*

● **C1366** Guide Wire, Percutaneous Transluminal Coronary Angioplasty, Hi-Torque Iron Man, Hi-Torque Balance Middleweight, Hi-Torque All Star, Hi-Torque Balance Heavyweight, Hi-Torque Balance Trek *Medicare Statute 1833(T)*

● **C1367** Guide Wire, Percutaneous Transluminal Coronary Angioplasty, Hi-Torque Cross-It, Hi-Torque Cross-It 100xt, Hi-Torque Cross-It 200XT, Hi-Torque Cross-It 300XT, Hi-Torque Wiggle *Medicare Statute 1833(T)*

= Invalid Medicare Code (no grace period)

= Code may require certificate of medical necessity (CMN) or DMERC information form (DIF)

● **C1368** Infusion System, On-Q Pain Management System, On-Q Soaker Pain Management System, and Painbuster Pain Management System
Medicare Statute 1833(T)

● **C1369** Internal receiver, neurostimulation system, ANS Renew Spinal Cord Stimulator System
Medicare Statute 1833(T)

● **C1370** Single use device for treatment of female stress urinary incontinence, Tension-Gree Vaginal Tape Single Use Device
Medicare Statute 1833(T)

● **C1371** Stent, Biliary, Symphony Nitinol Stent Transhepatic Biliary System, Symphony Nitinol Biliary Stent with Radiopaque Markers
Medicare Statute 1833(T)

● **C1372** Stent, biliary, Smar Cord IS Nitinol Stent and Delivery System
Medicare Statute 1833(T)

● **C1375** Stent, coronary, Nir ON Ranger Stent Delivery System, Nir w/Sox Stent System, Nir Primo Premounted Stent System
Medicare Statute 1833(T)

● **C1376** Lead, neurostimulator, ANS Renew Spinal Cord Stimulation System Lead (with or without extension)
Medicare Statute 1833(T)

● **C1377** Lead, neurostimulator, Specify 3988 Lead
Medicare Statute 1833(T)

● **C1378** Lead, neurostimulator, Inerstim Therapy 3080 Lead, Interstim Therapy 3886 Lead
Medicare Statute 1833(T)

● **C1379** Lead, neurostimulator, Pisces-Quad Compact 3887 Lead
Medicare Statute 1833(T)

● **C1420** Anchor system, Stapletac2 Bone Anchor System with Dermis
Medicare Statute 1833(T)

● **C1421** Anchor System, Stapletac2 Bone Anchor System without Dermis
Medicare Statute 1833(T)

● **C1450** Orthosphere Spherical Interpositional Arthroplasty
Medicare Statute 1833(T)

● **C1451** Orthosphere Spherical Interpositional Arthroplasty Kit
Medicare Statute 1833(T)

● **C1500** Atherectomy system, peripheral, Rotablator Rotational Angioplasty System with Rotalink Exchangeable Catheter, Advancer, and Guide Wire
Medicare Statute 1833(T)

C1531 ~~Stent, colorectal, Bard Memotherm Colorectal Stent Model S30R060~~
This code was added and deleted in 2000.

● **C1700** Needle, brachytherapy needle, Authentic Mick TP Brachytherapy Needle
Medicare Statute 1833(T)

● **C1701** Needle, brachytherapy, Medtec MT-BT-5201-25 Brachytherapy Needle
Medicare Statute 1833(T)

● **C1702** Needle, brachytherapy, WMMT Brachytherapy Needle
Medicare Statute 1833(T)

● **C1703** Needle, brachytherapy, Mentor Prostate Brachytherapy Needle
Medicare Statute 1833(T)

C Codes

= Special Coverage Instructions Apply   = Carrier Discretion

= Noncovered by Medicare or Medicare Statute

● **C1704** Needle, brachytherapy, Medtec MT-BT-5001-25, MT-Bt-5051-25
Medicare Statute 1833(T)

● **C1705** Needle, brachytherapy, Best Industries Flexi Needle Brachytherapy Seed Implantation (13G, 14G, 15G, 16G, 17G, 18G), Best Industries Prostate Brachytherapy Needle *Medicare Statute 1833(T)*

● **C1706** Needle, brachytherapy, Indigo Prostate Seeding Needle
Medicare Statute 1833(T)

● **C1707** Needle, brachytherapy, Varisource Interstitial Implant Needle
Medicare Statute 1833(T)

● **C1708** Needle, brachytherapy, Uromed Prostate Seeding Needle
Medicare Statute 1833(T)

● **C1709** Needle, brachytherapy, Remington Medical Brachytherapy Needle
Medicare Statute 1833(T)

● **C1710** Needle, brachytherapy, US Biopsy Prostate Seeding Needle
Medicare Statute 1833(T)

● **C1711** Needle, brachytherapy, MD Tech P.S.S. Prostate Seeding Set (Needle)
Medicare Statute 1833(T)

● **C1712** Needle, brachytherapy, Imagyn Medical Technologies Isostar Prostate Brachytherapy Needle *Medicare Statute 1833(T)*

● **C1790** Brachytherapy seed, Nucletron Iridium 192 HDR *Medicare Statute 1833(T)*

● **C1791** Bracytherapy seed, Nycomed Amersham I-125 (Oncoseed, Rapid Strand) *Medicare Statute 1833(T)*

● **C1792** Brachytherapy seed, Uromed Symmetra I-125 *Medicare Statute 1833(T)*

● **C1793** Brachytherapy seed, Bard Intersource 103 Palladium Seed 1031I, 1031C *Medicare Statute 1833(T)*

● **C1794** Brachytherapy seed, Bard Isoseed 103 Palladium Seed PD3S111I, Pd3S111P *Medicare Statute 1833(T)*

● **C1795** Brachytherapy seed, Bard Brachysource 125 Iodine Seed 1251I, 1251C
Medicare Statute 1833(T)

● **C1796** Brachytherapy Seed, Source Tech Medical I-125 Seed Model STM 1251
Medicare Statute 1833(T)

● **C1797** Brachytherapy seed, Draximage I-125 Seed Model LS-1
Medicare Statute 1833(T)

● **C1798** Brachytherapy seed, Syncor I-125 Pharmaseed Model BT-125-1
Medicare Statute 1833(T)

● **C1799** Brachytherapy seed, I-Plant Iodine 125 Model 3500
Medicare Statute 1833(T)

● **C1800** Brachytherapy seed, Mentor PdGold Pd-103 *Medicare Statute 1833(T)*

● **C1801** Brachytherapy seed, Mentor IoGold I-125 *Medicare Statute 1833(T)*

● **C1802** Brachytherapy seed, Best Industries Iridium 192 *Medicare Statute 1833(T)*

● **C1803** Brachytherapy seed, Best Industries Iodine 125 *Medicare Statute 1833(T)*

= Invalid Medicare Code (no grace period)

= Code may require certificate of medical necessity (CMN) or DMERC information form (DIF)

● **C1804** Brachytherapy seed, Best Industries Palladium 103
Medicare Statute 1833(T)

● **C1805** Brachytherapy seed, Imagyn Isostar Iodine-125 Interstitial
Brachytherapy Seed *Medicare Statute 1833(T)*

● **C1806** Brachytherapy seed, Best Industries Gold 198 *Medicare Statute 1833(T)*

● **C1810** Catheter, balloon dilatation, D114S Over-the-Wire Balloon Dilatation
Catheter *Medicare Statute 1833(T)*

● **C1811** Anchor, Surgical Dynamics Anchorsew, Surgical Dynamics S.D. sorb EZ
TAC, Surgical Dynamics S.D. sorb Suture Anchor 2.0 mm, Surgical
Dynamics S.D. sorb Suture Anchor 3.0 mm *Medicare Statute 1833(T)*

● **C1812** Anchor, Obl 2.0 mm Mini TAC Achor, Obl 2.8 mm HS Anchor, OBL 2.8
mm S Anchor, OBL 3.5 mm TI Anchor, OBL RC5 Anchor, OBL PRC5
Anchor *Medicare Statute 1833(T)*

● **C1850** Repliform Tissue Regeneration Matrix, per 24 or 28 sq cm
Medicare Statute 1833(T)

● **C1851** Repliform Tissue Regeneration Matrix, per 24 or 28 sq cm
Medicare Statute 1833(T)

● **C1852** Transcyte, per 247 sq cm *Medicare Statute 1833(T)*

● **C1853** Suspend Tutoplast Processed Fascia Lata, per 8 or 14 sq cm
Medicare Statute 1833(T)

● **C1854** Suspend Tutoplast Processed Fascia Lata, per 24 or 28 sq cm
Medicare Statute 1833(T)

● **C1855** Suspend Tutoplast Processed Fascia Lata, per 36 sq cm
Medicare Statute 1833(T)

● **C1856** Suspend Tutoplast Processed Fascia Lata, per 48 sq cm
Medicare Statute 1833(T)

● **C1857** Suspend Tutoplast Processed Fascia Lata, per 84 sq cm
Medicare Statute 1833(T)

● **C1858** Duraderm Acellular Allograft, per 8 or 14 sq cm *Medicare Statute 1833(T)*

● **C1859** Duraderm Acellular Allograft, per 21, 24, or 28 sq cm
Medicare Statute 1833(T)

● **C1860** Duraderm Acellular Allograft, per 48 sq cm *Medicare Statute 1833(T)*

● **C1861** Duraderm Acellular Allograft, per 36 sq cm *Medicare Statute 1833(T)*

● **C1862** Duraderm Acellular Allograft, per 72 sq cm *Medicare Statute 1833(T)*

● **C1863** Duraderm Acellular Allograft, per 84 sq cm *Medicare Statute 1833(T)*

● **C1864** Bard Sperma Tex Mesh, per 13.44 sq cm *Medicare Statute 1833(T)*

● **C1865** Bard Faslata Allograft Tissue, per 8 or 14 sq cm *Medicare Statute 1833(T)*

● **C1866** Bard Faslata Allograft Tissue, per 24 or 28 sq cm *Medicare Statute 1833(T)*

● **C1867** Bard Faslata Allograft Tissue, per 36 or 48 sq cm *Medicare Statute 1833(T)*

● **C1868** Bard Faslata Allograft Tissue, per 96 sq cm *Medicare Statute 1833(T)*

C Codes

= Special Coverage Instructions Apply   = Carrier Discretion

= Noncovered by Medicare or Medicare Statute

● **C1869** Gore Thyroplasty Device, per 8, 12, 30, or 37.5 sq cm (0.6 mm)
Medicare Statute 1833(T)

● **C1870** Dermmatrix Surgical Mesh, per 16 sq cm *Medicare Statute 1833(T)*

● **C1871** Dermmatrix Surgical Mesh, per 32 or 64 sq cm *Medicare Statute 1833(T)*

● **C1872** Dermagraft, per 37.5 sq cm *Medicare Statute 1833(T)*

● **C1873** Bard 3DMax mesh, medium or large size *Medicare Statute 1833(T)*

● **C1929** Catheter, Maverick Monorail PTCA Catheter, Maverick Over-the-Wire
PTCA Catheter *Medicare Statute 1833(T)*

● **C1930** Catheter, percutaneous transluminal coronary angioplasty, Coyote
Dilatation Catheter 20 mm/30 mm/40 mm *Medicare Statute 1833(T)*

● **C1931** Catheter, Talon Balloon Dilatation Catheter *Medicare Statute 1833(T)*

● **C1932** Catheter, SciMed Remedy Coronary Balloon Dilatation Infusion
Catheter (20 mm) *Medicare Statute 1833(T)*

● **C1933** Catheter, Opti-Plast Centurion 5.5F PTA Catheter, shaft length 50 cm
To 120 cm, Opti-Plast Xl 5.5f PTA Catheter, shaft length 75 cm To 120
cm *Medicare Statute 1833(T)*

● **C1934** Catheter, Ultraverse 3.5F Balloon Dilatation Catheter
Medicare Statute 1833(T)

● **C1935** Catheter, WorkHorse PTA Balloon Catheter *Medicare Statute 1833(T)*

● **C1936** Catheter, Uromax Ultra High Pressure Balloon Dilatation Catheter with
Hydroplus Coating *Medicare Statute 1833(T)*

● **C1937** Catheter, Synergy Balloon Dilatation Catheter, Explorer St 6F
Medicare Statute 1833(T)

● **C1938** Catheter, Bard Uroforce Balloon Dilatation Catheter
Medicare Statute 1833(T)

● **C1939** Catheter, Ninja PTCA Dilatation Catheter, Raptor PTCA Dilatation
Catheter, NC Raptor PTCA Dilatation Catheter, Charger PTCA
Dilatation Catheter, Titan PTCA Dilatation Catheter, Titan Mega PTCA
Dilatation Catheter *Medicare Statute 1833(T)*

● **C1940** Catheter, Cordis Powerflex Extreme PTA Balloon Catheter, Cordis
Powerflex Plus PTA Balloon Catheter, Cordis OPTA LP PTA Balloon
Catheter, Cordis OPTA 5 PTA Balloon Catheter *Medicare Statute 1833(T)*

● **C1941** Catheter, Jupiter PTA Balloon Dilatation Catheter *Medicare Statute 1833(T)*

● **C1942** Catheter, Cordis Maxi LD PTA Balloon Catheter *Medicare Statute 1833(T)*

● **C1943** Catheter, RX CrossSail Coronary Dilatation Catheter, OTW OpenSail
Coronary Dilatation Catheter *Medicare Statute 1833(T)*

● **C1944** Catheter, Rapid Exchange Single-use Biliary Balloon Dilatation Catheter
Medicare Statute 1833(T)

● **C1945** Catheter, Cord Is Savvy PTA Dilatation Catheter *Medicare Statute 1833(T)*

● **C1946** Catheter, RLS Rapid Exchange Pre-Dilatation Balloon Catheter
Medicare Statute 1833(T)

= Invalid Medicare Code (no grace period)

= Code may require certificate of medical necessity (CMN) or DMERC information form (DIF)

● **C1947** Catheter, Gazelle Balloon Dilatation Catheter   *Medicare Statute 1833(T)*

● **C1948** Catheter, Pursuit Balloon Angioplasty Catheter   *Medicare Statute 1833(T)*

● **C1949** Catheter, Endosonics Oracle Megasonics Five-64 F/X PTCA Catheter
   Medicare Statute 1833(T)

● **C1979** Catheter, Endosonics Visions PV 8.2F Intravascular Ultrasound Imaging
Catheter, Endosonics Avanar F/X Intravascular Ultrasound Imaging
Catheter   *Medicare Statute 1833(T)*

● **C1980** Catheter, Atlantis SR coronary imaging catheter   *Medicare Statute 1833(T)*

● **C1981** Catheter, Coronary Angioplasty Balloon, Adante, Bonnie, Bonnie 15 mm, Bonnie Monorail 30 mm Or 40 mm, Bonnie Sliding Rail, Bypass Speedy, Chubby, Chubby Sliding Rail, Coyote 20 mm, Coyote 9/15/25 mm, Long Ranger 30 mm Or 40 mm, Maxxum, NC Ranger, NC Ranger 9 mm, NC Ranger 16/18 mm, NC Ranger 22/25/30 mm, NC Big Ranger, Ranger 20 mm, Quantum Ranger, Quantum Ranger 1/4 Sizes, Quantum Ranger 9/16/18 mm, Quantum Ranger 22/30 mm, Quantum Ranger 25 mm, Ranger LP 20/30/40, Viva/Long Viva
   Medicare Statute 1833(T)

● **C2000** Catheter, Orbiter ST Steerable Electrode CatheteR
   Medicare Statute 1833(T)

● **C2001** Catheter, Constellation Diagnostic Catheter   *Medicare Statute 1833(T)*

● **C2002** Catheter, Irvine Inquiry Steerable Electrophysiology 5F Catheter
   Medicare Statute 1833(T)

● **C2003** Catheter, Irvine Inquiry Steerable Electrophysiology 6F Catheter
   Medicare Statute 1833(T)

● **C2004** Catheter, electrophysiology, EP Deflectable Tip Catheter (Octapolar Small Anatomy Models Only)   *Medicare Statute 1833(T)*

● **C2005** Catheter, electrophysiology, EP Deflectable Tip Catheter (hexapolar small anatomy models only)   *Medicare Statute 1833(T)*

● **C2006** Catheter, electrophysiology, EP Deflectable Tip Catheter (decapolar small anatomy models only)   *Medicare Statute 1833(T)*

● **C2007** Catheter, electrophysiology, Irvine LUMA-Cath 6F Fixed Curve Electrophysiology Catheter   *Medicare Statute 1833(T)*

● **C2008** Catheter, electrophysiology, Irvine LUMA-Cath 7F Steerable Electrophysiology Catheter Model 81910, Model 81912, Model 81915
   Medicare Statute 1833(T)

● **C2009** Catheter, electrophysiology, Irvine LUMA-Cath 7F Steerable Electrophysiology Catheter Model 81920   *Medicare Statute 1833(T)*

● **C2010** Catheter, electrophysiology, Cord Is Fixed Curve Catheter (decapolar, hexapolar, octapolar, quadrapolar)   *Medicare Statute 1833(T)*

● **C2011** Catheter, electrophysiology, Deflectable Tip Catheter (Quadrapolar small anatomy models only)   *Medicare Statute 1833(T)*

C Codes

    = Special Coverage Instructions Apply   = Carrier Discretion

    = Noncovered by Medicare or Medicare Statute

● **C2012** Catheter, ablation, Biosense Webster Celsius Braided Tip Ablation Catheter, Biosense Webster Celsius 5 mm Temperature Ablation Catheter, Biosense Webster Celsius Temperature Sensing Diagnostic/Ablation Tip Catheter, Biosense Webster Celsius Long Reach Ablation Catheter *Medicare Statute 1833(T)*

● **C2013** Catheter, ablation, Biosense Webster Celsius Large Dome Ablation Catheter *Medicare Statute 1833(T)*

● **C2014** Catheter, ablation, Biosense Webster Celsius II Asymmetrical Ablation Catheter *Medicare Statute 1833(T)*

● **C2015** Catheter, ablation, Biosense Webster Celsius II Symmetrical Ablation Catheter *Medicare Statute 1833(T)*

● **C2016** Catheter, ablation, Navi-Star DS Diagnostic/Ablation Catheter, Navi-Star Thermo-Cool Temperature Diagnostic/Ablation Catheter *Medicare Statute 1833(T)*

● **C2017** Catheter, ablation, Navi-Star Diagnostic/Ablation Deflectable Tip Catheter *Medicare Statute 1833(T)*

● **C2018** Catheter, ablation, Polaris T Ablation Catheter *Medicare Statute 1833(T)*

● **C2019** Catheter, EP Medsystems Deflectable Electrophysiology Catheter *Medicare Statute 1833(T)*

● **C2020** Catheter, ablation, Blazer II Xp, Blazer II 6f, Blazer II High Torque *Medicare Statute 1833(T)*

● **C2021** Catheter, EP Medsystems SilverFlex Electrophysiology Catheter, non-deflectable *Medicare Statute 1833(T)*

● **C2022** Catheter, ablation, Cardiac Pathways Chilli Cooled Ablation Catheter Models 41422, 41442, 45422, 45442, 43422, 43442 *Medicare Statute 1833(T)*

● **C2023** Catheter, ablation, Cardiac Pathways Chilli Cooled Ablation Catheter, Standard Curve 3005 Or Large Curve 3006 *Medicare Statute 1833(T)*

● **C2100** Catheter, electrophysiology, Cardiac Pathways CS Reference Catheter *Medicare Statute 1833(T)*

● **C2101** Catheter, electrophysiology, Cardiac Pathways RV Reference Catheter *Medicare Statute 1833(T)*

● **C2102** Catheter, electrophysiology, Cardiac Pathways 7F Radii Catheter *Medicare Statute 1833(T)*

● **C2103** Catheter, electrophysiology, Cardiac Pathways 7F Radii Catheter with Tracking *Medicare Statute 1833(T)*

● **C2104** Catheter, electrophysiology, lasso deflectable circular tip mapping catheter *Medicare Statute 1833(T)*

● **C2151** Catheter, Veripath Peripheral Guiding Catheter *Medicare Statute 1833(T)*

● **C2152** Catheter, Cordis 5F, 6F, 7F, 8F, 9F, 10F Vista Brite Tip Guiding Catheter *Medicare Statute 1833(T)*

● **C2153** Catheter, electrophysiology, Bard Viking Fixed Curve Catheter (Bipolar, Quadrapolar, and ASP models only)   *Medicare Statute 1833(T)*

● **C2200** Catheter, Arrow-Trerotola Percutaneous Thrombolytic Device Catheter   *Medicare Statute 1833(T)*

● **C2300** Catheter, Varisource Standard Catheter   *Medicare Statute 1833(T)*

● **C2597** Catheter, Clinicath Peripherally Inserted Midline Catheter (PICC) Dual-Lumen Polyflow Polyurethane Catheter 18G/20G/24G (includes Catheter And Introducer), Clinicath Peripherally Inserted Central Catheter (PICC) Dual-Lumen Polyflow Polyurethane 16G/18G (includes Catheter and Introducer), Clinicath Peripherally Inserted Central Catheter (PICC) Single-lumen Polyflow Polyurethane 18G (includes Catheter and Introducer)   *Medicare Statute 1833(T)*

● **C2598** Catheter, Clinicath Peripherally Inserted Central Catheter (PICC) Single-lumen Polyflow Polyurethane Catheter 18G/20G/24G (Catheter And Introducer), Clinicath Peripherally Inserted Midline Catheter (PICC) Single-lumen Polyflow Polyurethane Catheter 20G/24G (Catheter and Introducer)   *Medicare Statute 1833(T)*

● **C2599** Catheter, Clinicath Peripherally Inserted Central Catheter (PICC) Dual-Lumen Polyflow Polyurethane Catheter 16G/18G (Catheter and Introducer)   *Medicare Statute 1833(T)*

● **C2600** Catheter, gold probe single-use electrohemostatis catheter   *Medicare Statute 1833(T)*

● **C2601** Catheter, Bard 10F Dual Lumen Ureteral Catheter *Medicare Statute 1833(T)*

● **C2602** Catheter, Spectranetics 1.4/1.7 mm Vitesse COS Concentric Laser Catheter   *Medicare Statute 1833(T)*

● **C2603** Catheter, Spectranetics 2.0 mm Vitesse COS Concentric Laser Catheter   *Medicare Statute 1833(T)*

● **C2604** Catheter, Spectranetics 2.0 mm Vitesse E Eccentric Laser Catheter   *Medicare Statute 1833(T)*

● **C2605** Catheter, Spectranetics Extreme Laser Catheter   *Medicare Statute 1833(T)*

● **C2606** Catheter, Oratec Spinecath XI Intradiscal Catheter *Medicare Statute 1833(T)*

● **C2607** Catheter, Oratec Spinecath Intradiscal Catheter   *Medicare Statute 1833(T)*

● **C2608** Catheter, Scimed 6F Wiseguide Guide Catheter   *Medicare Statute 1833(T)*

● **C2609** Catheter, Flexima Biliary Drainage Catheter with Locking Pigtail, Flexima Biliary Drainage Catheter with Twist Loc Hub, Flexima Bilary Drainage Catheters with Temp Tip   *Medicare Statute 1833(T)*

● **C2610** Catheter, Arrow Flex Tip Plus Intraspinal Catheter Kit   *Medicare Statute 1833(T)*

● **C2611** Catheter, Medtronic Ps Medical Algoline Intraspinal Catheter System/Kit 81102, 81192   *Medicare Statute 1833(T)*

● **C2612** Catheter, Indura Intraspinal Catheter   *Medicare Statute 1833(T)*

● **C2676** Catheter, Response CV Catheter   *Medicare Statute 1833(T)*

C Codes

= Special Coverage Instructions Apply   = Carrier Discretion

= Noncovered by Medicare or Medicare Statute

● **C2700** Defibrillator, single chamber, implantable, mycrophylax plus
Medicare Statute 1833(T)

● **C2701** Defibrillator, single chamber, implantable, Phylax XM
Medicare Statute 1833(T)

● **C2702** Defibrillator, single chamber, implantable, Ventak Prizm 2 VR 1860
Medicare Statute 1833(T)

● **C2703** Defibrillator, single chamber, implantable, Ventak Prizm VR HE 1857, 1858
Medicare Statute 1833(T)

● **C2704** Defibrillator, single chamber, implantable, Ventak Mini IV+ 1793, 1796
Medicare Statute 1833(T)

● **C2801** Defibrillator, dual chamber, implantable, ELA Medical Defender IV DR Model 612
Medicare Statute 1833(T)

● **C2802** Defibrillator, dual chamber, implantable, Phylax AV
Medicare Statute 1833(T)

● **C2803** Defibrillator, dual chamber, implantable, Ventak Prizm DR HE 1852, 1853
Medicare Statute 1833(T)

● **C2804** Defibrillator, dual chamber, implantable, Ventak Prizm 2 DR 1861
Medicare Statute 1833(T)

● **C2805** Defibrillator, dual chamber, implantable, Jewel AF 7250
Medicare Statute 1833(T)

● **C2806** Defibrillator, implantable, Gem VR 7227   *Medicare Statute 1833(T)*

● **C2807** Defibrillator, implantable, Contak CD 1823   *Medicare Statute 1833(T)*

● **C2808** Defibrillator, implantable, Contak TR 1241   *Medicare Statute 1833(T)*

● **C3001** Lead, defibrillator, implantable, Kainox SL, Kainox RV
Medicare Statute 1833(T)

● **C3002** Lead, defibrillator, implantable, Easytrak 4510, 4511, 4512, 4513
Medicare Statute 1833(T)

● **C3003** Lead, defibrillator, implantable, Endotak SQ Array XP 0085
Medicare Statute 1833(T)

● **C3004** Lead, defibrillator, implantable, Intervene 497-23, 497-24
Medicare Statute 1833(T)

● **C3400** Prosthesis, breast, Mentor Saline-filled Contour Profile, Mentor Siltex Spectrum Mammary Prosthesis   *Medicare Statute 1833(T)*

● **C3401** Prosthesis, breast, Mentor Saline-filled Spectrum *Medicare Statute 1833(T)*

● **C3500** Prosthesis, Mentor Alpha I Inflatable Penile Prosthesis, Mentor Alpha I Narrow-Base Inflatable Penile Prosthesis   *Medicare Statute 1833(T)*

● **C3510** Prosthesis, AMS Sphincter 800 Urinary Prosthesis *Medicare Statute 1833(T)*

● **C3551** Guide wire, percutaneous transluminal coronary angioplasty, Choice, Luge, Patriot, PT Graphix Intermediate, Trooper, Mailman 182/300 cm
Medicare Statute 1833(T)

● **C3552** Guide wire, coronary, Hi-Torque Whisper   *Medicare Statute 1833(T)*

▬▬ = Invalid Medicare Code (no grace period)

▬▬ = Code may require certificate of medical necessity (CMN) or DMERC information form (DIF)

● **C3553** Guide wire, Cordis Stabilizer Marker Wire Steerable Guidewire, Cordis Wizdom Marker Wire Steerable Guide wire, Cordis ATW Marker Wire Steerable Guidewire, Cordis Shinobi Steerable Guidewire
Medicare Statute 1833(T)

● **C3554** Guide wire, Jindo Tapered Peripheral Guidewire *Medicare Statute 1833(T)*

● **C3555** Guide wire, Wholey Hi-Torque Plus Guide Wire System, 145 cm, 190 cm, 300 cm *Medicare Statute 1833(T)*

● **C3556** Guide wire, Endosonics Cardiometrics Wavewire Pressure Guide Wire, Cardiometrics Flowire Doppler Guide Wire *Medicare Statute 1833(T)*

● **C3557** Guidewire, Hytek Guidewire *Medicare Statute 1833(T)*

● **C3800** Infusion pump, implantable, programmable, Synchromed EL Infusion Pump *Medicare Statute 1833(T)*

● **C3801** Infusion pump, Arrow/Microject PCA System *Medicare Statute 1833(T)*

● **C3851** Intraocular lens, Staar Elastic Ultraviolet-Absorbing Silicone Posterior Chamber Intraocular Lens with Toric Optic Model AA-4203T, Model AA-4203TF, Model AA-4203TL *Medicare Statute 1833(T)*

● **C4000** Pacemaker, single chamber, ELA Medical Opus G Model 4621, 4624
Medicare Statute 1833(T)

● **C4001** Pacemaker, single chamber, ELA Medical Opus G Model 4121, 4124
Medicare Statute 1833(T)

● **C4002** Pacemaker, single chamber, ELA Medical Talent Model 113
Medicare Statute 1833(T)

● **C4003** Pacemaker, single chamber, Kairos SR *Medicare Statute 1833(T)*

● **C4004** Pacemaker, single chamber, Actros SR+, Actros SR-B+
Medicare Statute 1833(T)

● **C4005** Pacemaker, single chamber, Philos SR, Philos SR-B *Medicare Statute 1833(T)*

● **C4006** Pacemaker, single chamber, Pulsar Max II SR 1180, 1181
Medicare Statute 1833(T)

● **C4007** Pacemaker, single chamber, Marathon SR 291-09, 292-09R, 292-09X
Medicare Statute 1833(T)

● **C4008** Pacemaker, single chamber, Discovery II SSI 481 *Medicare Statute 1833(T)*

● **C4009** Pacemaker, single chamber, Discovery II SR 1184, 1185, 1186, 1187
Medicare Statute 1833(T)

● **C4300** Pacemaker, dual chamber, Integrity AFX DR Model 5342
Medicare Statute 1833(T)

● **C4301** Pacemaker, dual chamber, Integrity AFX DR Model 5346
Medicare Statute 1833(T)

● **C4302** Pacemaker, dual chamber, Affinity VDR 5430 *Medicare Statute 1833(T)*

● **C4303** Pacemaker, dual chamber, ELA Brio Model 112 Pacemaker System
Medicare Statute 1833(T)

C Codes

= Special Coverage Instructions Apply   = Carrier Discretion

= Noncovered by Medicare or Medicare Statute

● C4304	Pacemaker, Dual Chamber, ELA Medical Brio Model 212, Talent Model 213, Talent Model 223	*Medicare Statute 1833(T)*
● C4305	Pacemaker, dual chamber, ELA Medical Brio Model 222	*Medicare Statute 1833(T)*
● C4306	Pacemaker, dual chamber, ELA Medical Brio Model 220	*Medicare Statute 1833(T)*
● C4307	Pacemaker, dual chamber, Kairos DR	*Medicare Statute 1833(T)*
● C4308	Pacemaker, dual chamber, Inos 2, Inos 2+	*Medicare Statute 1833(T)*
● C4309	Pacemaker, dual chamber, Actros DR+, Actros D+, Actros DR-A+, Actros SLR+	*Medicare Statute 1833(T)*
● C4310	Pacemaker, dual chamber, Actros DR-B+	*Medicare Statute 1833(T)*
● C4311	Pacemaker, dual chamber, Philos DR, Philos DR-B, Philor SLR	*Medicare Statute 1833(T)*
● C4312	Pacemaker, dual chamber, Pulsar Max II DR 1280	*Medicare Statute 1833(T)*
● C4313	Pacemaker, dual chamber, Marathon DR 293-09, 294-09, 294-09R, 294-10	*Medicare Statute 1833(T)*
● C4314	Pacemaker, dual chamber, Momentum DR 294-23	*Medicare Statute 1833(T)*
● C4315	Pacemaker, dual chamber, Selection AFM 902 SLC 902c	*Medicare Statute 1833(T)*
● C4316	Pacemaker, dual chamber, Discovery II DR 1283, 1284, 1285, 1286	*Medicare Statute 1833(T)*
● C4317	Pacemaker, dual chamber, Discovery II DDD 981	*Medicare Statute 1833(T)*
● C4600	Lead, Pacemaker, Synox, Polyrox, Elox, Retrox, SI-BP, ELC	*Medicare Statute 1833(T)*
● C4601	Lead, Pacemaker, Aescula LV 1055K	*Medicare Statute 1833(T)*
● C4602	Lead, pacemaker, Tendril SDX 1488k/46, Tendril SDX 1488K/52, Tendril SDX 1488K/58	*Medicare Statute 1833(T)*
● C4603	Lead, pacemaker, Oscor/Flexion 4015, 4016, 4017, 4018	*Medicare Statute 1833(T)*
● C4604	Lead, pacemaker, Crystalline ActFix ICD-09, CapSure Fix Novus 5076	*Medicare Statute 1833(T)*
● C4605	Lead, pacemaker, CapSure EPI 4968	*Medicare Statute 1833(T)*
● C4606	Lead, pacemaker, FlexTend 4080, 4081, 4082	*Medicare Statute 1833(T)*
● C4607	Lead, pacemaker, FineLine II 4452, 4453, 4454, 4455, 4477, 4478, FineLine II EZ 4463, 4464, 4465, 4466, 4467, 4468, ThinLine II 430-25, 430-35, 432-35, ThinLine II EZ 438-25, 438-35	*Medicare Statute 1833(T)*
● C5000	Stent, biliary, BX Velocity with Hepacoat on Raptor Stent System (28 or 33 mm in length)	*Medicare Statute 1833(T)*

= Invalid Medicare Code (no grace period)

= Code may require certificate of medical necessity (CMN) or DMERC information form (DIF)

● **C5001** Stent, biliary, Bard Memotherm-Flex Biliary Stent, small/medium diameter *Medicare Statute 1833(T)*

● **C5002** Stent, biliary, Bard Memotherm-Flex Biliary Stent, large diameter *Medicare Statute 1833(T)*

● **C5003** Stent, biliary, Bard Memotherm-Flex Biliary Stent, x-large diameter *Medicare Statute 1833(T)*

● **C5004** Stent, biliary, Cordis Palmaz Corinthian IQ Transhepatic Biliary Stent *Medicare Statute 1833(T)*

● **C5005** Stent, biliary, Cordis Palmaz Corinthian IQ Transhepatic Biliary Stent and Delivery System *Medicare Statute 1833(T)*

● **C5006** Stent, Biliary, Cordis Medium Palmaz Transhepatic Biliary Stent and Delivery System *Medicare Statute 1833(T)*

● **C5007** Stent, biliary, Cordis Palmaz XI Transhepatic Biliary Stent (40 mm length) *Medicare Statute 1833(T)*

● **C5008** Stent, biliary, Cordis Palmaz XI Transhepatic Biliary Stent (50 mm length) *Medicare Statute 1833(T)*

● **C5009** Stent, biliary, Biliary Vistaflex Stent *Medicare Statute 1833(T)*

● **C5010** Stent, biliary, Rapid Exchange Single-use Biliary Stent System *Medicare Statute 1833(T)*

● **C5011** Stent, biliary, Intrastent, Intrastent LP *Medicare Statute 1833(T)*

● **C5012** Stent, biliary, Intrastent Doublestrut LD *Medicare Statute 1833(T)*

● **C5013** Stent, Biliary, Intrastent Doublestrut, Intrastent Doublestrut XS *Medicare Statute 1833(T)*

● **C5014** Stent, biliary, Medtronic AVE Bridge Stent System--biliary indication (10 mm, 17 mm, 28 mm) *Medicare Statute 1833(T)*

● **C5015** Stent, biliary, Medtronic AVE Bridge Stent System--biliary indication (40-60 mm, 80-100 mm), Medtronic AVE Bridge X3 Biliary Stent System (17 mm) *Medicare Statute 1833(T)*

● **C5016** Stent, biliary, Wallstent Single-use Covered Biliary Endoprosthesis with Unistep Plus Delivery System *Medicare Statute 1833(T)*

● **C5017** Stent, biliary, Wallstent RP Biliary Endoprosthesis with Unistep Plus Delivery System (20/40/42/60/68 mm in length) *Medicare Statute 1833(T)*

● **C5018** Stent, biliary, Wallstent RP Biliary Endoprosthesis with Unistep Plus Delivery System (80/94 mm in length) *Medicare Statute 1833(T)*

● **C5019** Stent, biliary, Flexima Single-use Biliary Stent System *Medicare Statute 1833(T)*

● **C5020** Stent, biliary, Cordis Smart Nitinol Stent Transhepatic Biliary System (20 mm in length) *Medicare Statute 1833(T)*

● **C5021** Stent, biliary, Cordis Smart Nitinol Stent Transhepatic Biliary System (40 or 60 mm in length) *Medicare Statute 1833(T)*

C Codes

= Special Coverage Instructions Apply   = Carrier Discretion

= Noncovered by Medicare or Medicare Statute

● **C5022** Stent, biliary, Cordis Smart Nitinol Stent Transhepatic Biliary System (80 mm in length) *Medicare Statute 1833(T)*

● **C5023** Stent, biliary, BX Velocity Transhepatic Biliary Stent and Delivery System (8 or 13 mm in length) *Medicare Statute 1833(T)*

● **C5024** Stent, biliary, BX Velocity Transhepatic Biliary Stent and Delivery System (18 mm in length) *Medicare Statute 1833(T)*

● **C5025** Stent, biliary, BX Velocity Transhepatic Biliary Stent and Delivery System (23 mm in length) *Medicare Statute 1833(T)*

● **C5026** Stent, biliary, Bx Velocity Transhepatic Biliary Stent and Delivery System (28 0r 33 mm in length) *Medicare Statute 1833(T)*

● **C5027** Stent, biliary, BX Velocity with Hepacoat on Raptor Stent System (8 or 13 mm in length) *Medicare Statute 1833(T)*

● **C5028** Stent, biliary, BX Velocity with Hepacoat on Raptor Stent System (18 mm in length) *Medicare Statute 1833(T)*

● **C5029** Stent, biliary, BX Velocity with Hepacoat on Raptor Stent System (23 mm in length) *Medicare Statute 1833(T)*

● **C5030** Stent, coronary, S660 Discrete Technology Over-the-Wire Coronary Stent System 9 mm, 12 mm S660 with Discrete Technology Rapid Exchange Coronary Stent System 9 mm, 12 mm *Medicare Statute 1833(T)*

● **C5031** Stent, coronary, S660 Discrete Technology Over-the-Wire Coronary Stent System 15 mm, 18 mm S660 with Discrete Technology Rapid Exchange Coronary Stent System 15 mm, 18 mm *Medicare Statute 1833(T)*

● **C5032** Stent, coronary, S660 Discrete Technology Over-the-Wire Coronary Stent System 24 mm, 30 mm S660 with Discrete Technology Rapid Exchange Coronary Stent System 24 mm, 30 mm *Medicare Statute 1833(T)*

● **C5033** Stent, coronary, Niroyal Advance Premounted Stent System (9 mm) *Medicare Statute 1833(T)*

● **C5034** Stent, coronary, Niroyal Advance Premounted Stent System (12 mm/15 mm) *Medicare Statute 1833(T)*

● **C5035** Stent, coronary, Niroyal Advance Premounted Stent System (18 mm) *Medicare Statute 1833(T)*

● **C5036** Stent, coronary, Niroyal Advance Premounted Stent System (25 mm) *Medicare Statute 1833(T)*

● **C5037** Stent, coronary, Niroyal Advance Premounted Stent System (31 mm) *Medicare Statute 1833(T)*

● **C5038** Stent, coronary, BX Velocity Balloon-Expandable Stent with Raptor Over-the-Wire Delivery System *Medicare Statute 1833(T)*

● **C5039** Stent, peripheral, Intracoil Peripheral Stent (40 mm stent length) *Medicare Statute 1833(T)*

● **C5040** Stent, peripheral, Intracoil Peripheral Stent (60 mm stent length) *Medicare Statute 1833(T)*

= Invalid Medicare Code (no grace period)

= Code may require certificate of medical necessity (CMN) or DMERC information form (DIF)

● **C5041** Stent, coronary, Medtronic BeStent 2 Over-the-Wire Coronary Stent System (24 mm, 30 mm) *Medicare Statute 1833(T)*

● **C5042** Stent, coronary, Medtronic BeStent 2 Over-the-Wire Coronary Stent System (18 mm) *Medicare Statute 1833(T)*

● **C5043** Stent, coronary, Medtronic BeStent 2 Over-the-Wire Coronary Stent (15 mm) *Medicare Statute 1833(T)*

● **C5044** Stent, coronary, Medtronic BeStent 2 Over-the-Wire Coronary Stent System (9 mm, 12 mm) *Medicare Statute 1833(T)*

● **C5045** Stent, coronary, Multilink Tetra Coronary Stent System *Medicare Statute 1833(T)*

● **C5046** Stent, coronary, Radius 20 mm Self Expanding Stent with Over-the-Wire Delivery System *Medicare Statute 1833(T)*

● **C5047** Stent, coronary, Niroyal Elite Premounted Stent System 15 mm, 25 mm, or 31 mm *Medicare Statute 1833(T)*

● **C5048** Stent, coronary, GR II Coronary Stent *Medicare Statute 1833(T)*

● **C5130** Stent, Colorn Wilson-Cook Colonic Z-Stent *Medicare Statute 1833(T)*

● **C5131** Stent, colorectal, Bard Memotherm Colorectal Stent Model S30R060 *Medicare Statute 1833(T)*

● **C5132** Stent, colorectal, Bard Memotherm Colorectal Stent Model S30R080 *Medicare Statute 1833(T)*

● **C5133** Stent, colorectal, Bard Memotherm Colorectal Stent Model S30R100 *Medicare Statute 1833(T)*

● **C5134** Stent, Enteral, Wallstent Enteral Endoprosthesis and Unistep Delivery System (90 mm in length), Enteral Wallstent Endoprosthesis with Unistep Plus Delivery System (90 mm in length) *Medicare Statute 1833(T)*

● **C5279** Stent, Ureteral, Boston Scientific Contour Soft Percuflex Stent with Hydroplus Coating (Braided), Contour Soft Percuflex Stent with Hydroplus Coating, Contour VI Variable Length Percuflex Stent with Hydroplus Coating, Percuflex Plus Stent with Hydroplus Coating, Percuflex Stent (Braided), Contour Closed Soft Percuflex Stent with Hydroplus Coating, Contour Injection Soft Percuflex Stent with Hydroplus Coating, Soft Percuflex Stent, Percuflex Tail Plus Tapered Ureteral Stent *Medicare Statute 1833(T)*

● **C5280** Stent, ureteral, Bard Inlay Double Pigtail Ureteral Stent *Medicare Statute 1833(T)*

● **C5281** Stent, tracheobronchial, Wallgraft Tracheobronchial Endoprosthesis with Unistep Delivery System (70 mm in length) *Medicare Statute 1833(T)*

● **C5282** Stent, tracheobronchial, Wallgraft Tracheobronchial Endoprosthesis with Unistep Delivery System (20 mm, 30 mm, 50 mm in length) *Medicare Statute 1833(T)*

C Codes

= Special Coverage Instructions Apply   = Carrier Discretion

= Noncovered by Medicare or Medicare Statute

● **C5283** Stent, self-expandable for creation of intrahepatic shunts, Wallstent Transjugular Intrahepatic Protosystemic Shunt (TIPS) with Unistep Plus Delivery System (90/94 mm in length), Wallstent RP TIPS Endoprosthesis with Unistep Plus Delivery System (94 mm in length)
Medicare Statute 1833(T)

● **C5284** Stent, tracheobronchial, Ultraflex Tracheobronchial Endoprosthesis (covered and non-covered) *Medicare Statute 1833(T)*

● **C5600** Vascular closure device, Vasoseal ES (extravascular security) Device
Medicare Statute 1833(T)

● **C5601** Vascular closure device, Vascular Solutions Duett Sealing Device 1000
Medicare Statute 1833(T)

● **C6001** Mesh, hernia, Bard Composix Mesh, per 8 or 18 in
Medicare Statute 1833(T)

● **C6002** Mesh, hernia, Bard Composix Mesh, per 32 in *Medicare Statute 1833(T)*

● **C6003** Mesh, hernia, Bard Composix Mesh, per 48 in *Medicare Statute 1833(T)*

● **C6004** Mesh, hernia, Bard Composix Mesh, per 80 in *Medicare Statute 1833(T)*

● **C6005** Mesh, hernia, Bard Composix Mesh, per 140 in *Medicare Statute 1833(T)*

● **C6006** Mesh, hernia, Bard Composix Mesh, per 144 in *Medicare Statute 1833(T)*

● **C6012** Pelvicol Acellular Collagen Matrix, per 8 or 14 quare cm
Medicare Statute 1833(T)

● **C6013** Pelvicol Acellular Collagen Matrix, per 21, 24, or 28 sq cm
Medicare Statute 1833(T)

● **C6014** Pelvicol Acellular Collagen Matrix, per 40 sq cm *Medicare Statute 1833(T)*

● **C6015** Pelvicol Acellular Collagen Matrix, per 48 sq cm *Medicare Statute 1833(T)*

● **C6016** Pelvicol Acellular Collagen Matrix, per 96 sq cm *Medicare Statute 1833(T)*

● **C6017** Gore-Tex DualMesh Biomaterial, per 75 or 96 sq cm (1 mm thick)
Medicare Statute 1833(T)

● **C6018** Gore-Tex DualMesh Biomaterial, per 150 sq cm oval shaped (1 mm thick) *Medicare Statute 1833(T)*

● **C6019** Gore-Tex DualMesh Biomaterial, per 285 sq cm oval shaped (1 mm thick) *Medicare Statute 1833(T)*

● **C6020** Gore-Tex DualMesh Biomaterial, per 432 sq cm (1 mm thick)
Medicare Statute 1833(T)

● **C6021** Gore-Tex DualMesh Biomaterial, per 600 sq cm (1 mm thick)
Medicare Statute 1833(T)

● **C6022** Gore-Tex DualMesh Biomaterial, per 884 sq cm (1 mm thick)
Medicare Statute 1833(T)

● **C6023** Gore-Tex DualMesh Plus Biomaterial, per 75 or 96 sq cm (1 mm thick)
Medicare Statute 1833(T)

● **C6024** Gore-Tex DualMesh Plus Biomaterial, per 150 sq cm oval shaped (1 mm thick) *Medicare Statute 1833(T)*

= Invalid Medicare Code (no grace period)

= Code may require certificate of medical necessity (CMN) or DMERC information form (DIF)

● **C6025** Gore-Tex DualMesh Plus Biomaterial, per 285 sq cm oval shaped (1 mm thick) *Medicare Statute 1833(T)*

● **C6026** Gore-Tex DualMesh Plus Biomaterial, per 432 sq cm (1 mm thick) *Medicare Statute 1833(T)*

● **C6027** Gore-Tex DualMesh Plus Biomaterial, per 600 sq cm (1 mm thick) *Medicare Statute 1833(T)*

● **C6028** Gore-Tex DualMesh Plus Biomaterial, per 884 sq cm oval shaped (1 mm thick) *Medicare Statute 1833(T)*

● **C6029** Gore-Tex DualMesh Plus Biomaterial, per 150 sq cm oval shaped (2 mm thick) *Medicare Statute 1833(T)*

● **C6030** Gore-Tex DualMesh Plus Biomaterial, per 285 sq cm oval shaped (2 mm thick) *Medicare Statute 1833(T)*

● **C6031** Gore-Tex DualMesh Plus Biomaterial, per 432 sq cm (2 mm thick) *Medicare Statute 1833(T)*

● **C6032** Gore-Tex DualMesh Plus Biomaterial, per 600 sq cm (2 mm thick) *Medicare Statute 1833(T)*

● **C6033** Gore-Tex DualMesh Plus Biomaterial, per 884 sq cm (2 mm thick) *Medicare Statute 1833(T)*

● **C6034** Bard Reconix ePTFE Reconstruction Patch 150 sq cm (2 mm thick) *Medicare Statute 1833(T)*

● **C6035** Bard Reconix ePTFE Reconstruction Patch 150 sq cm (1 mm thick), 75 sq cm (2 mm thick) *Medicare Statute 1833(T)*

● **C6036** Bard Reconix ePTFE Reconstruction Patch 50/75 sq cm (1 mm thick), 50 sq cm (2 mm thick) *Medicare Statute 1833(T)*

● **C6037** Bard Reconix ePTFE Reconstruction Patch 300 sq cm (1 mm thick) *Medicare Statute 1833(T)*

● **C6038** Bard Reconix ePTFE Reconstruction Patch 600 sq cm (1 mm thick), 300 sq cm (2 mm thick) *Medicare Statute 1833(T)*

● **C6039** Bard Reconix ePTFE Reconstruction Patch 884 sq cm oval shaped (1 mm thick) *Medicare Statute 1833(T)*

● **C6040** Bard Reconix ePTFE Reconstruction Patch 600 sq cm (2 mm thick) *Medicare Statute 1833(T)*

● **C6041** Bard Reconix ePTFE Reconstruction Patch 884 sq cm oval shaped (2 mm thick) *Medicare Statute 1833(T)*

● **C6050** Sling fixation system for treatment of stress urinary incontinence, Female In-Fast Sling Fixation System with Electric Inserter with Sling Material, Female In-Fast Sling Fixation System with Electric Inserter without Sling Material *Medicare Statute 1833(T)*

● **C6051** Stratasis Urethral Sling, 20/40 cm *Medicare Statute 1833(T)*

● **C6052** Stratasis Urethral Sling, 60 cm *Medicare Statute 1833(T)*

● **C6053** Surgisis Soft Tissue Graft, per 70 cm, 105 cm, or 140 cm *Medicare Statute 1833(T)*

C Codes

= Special Coverage Instructions Apply   = Carrier Discretion

= Noncovered by Medicare or Medicare Statute

● **C6054** Surgisis Enhanced Strength Soft Tissue Graft, per 4.2 cm, 20 cm, 28 cm or 40 cm *Medicare Statute 1833(T)*

● **C6055** Surgisis Enhanced Strength Soft Tissue Graft, per 52.5 cm, 60 cm, or 70 cm *Medicare Statute 1833(T)*

● **C6056** Surgisis Enhanced Strength Soft Tissue Graft, per 105 cm, 140 cm *Medicare Statute 1833(T)*

● **C6057** Surgisis Hernia Graft, per 195 cm *Medicare Statute 1833(T)*

● **C6058** Sugipro Hernia Mate Plug, medium or large *Medicare Statute 1833(T)*

● **C6080** Sling fixation system for treatment of stress urinary incontinence, Male Straight-In Fixation System with Electric Inserter with Sling Material and Disposable Pressure Sensor, Male Straight-In Fixation System with Electric Inserter without Sling Material and Disposable Pressure Sensor *Medicare Statute 1833(T)*

● **C6200** Vascular graft, Exxcel Soft Eptfe vascular graft *Medicare Statute 1833(T)*

● **C6201** Vascular graft, Impra Venaflo Vascular Graft with Carbon, straight graft 10 cm or 20 cm in length *Medicare Statute 1833(T)*

● **C6202** Vascular graft, Impra Venaflo Vascular Graft with Carbon, Straight Graft 30 cm or 40 cm in length *Medicare Statute 1833(T)*

● **C6203** Vascular graft, Impra Venaflo Vascular Graft with Carbon, Straight Graft (50 cm in length) or Centerflex Venaflo Stepped Graft (45 cm in length) *Medicare Statute 1833(T)*

● **C6204** Vascular graft, Impra Venaflo Vascular Graft with Carbon, Stepped Graft 20 cm, 25 cm, 30 cm, 35 cm, 40 cm, or 45 cm in length *Medicare Statute 1833(T)*

● **C6205** Vascular graft, Impra Carboflo Vascular Graft, Straight Graft 10 cm in length *Medicare Statute 1833(T)*

● **C6206** Vascular graft, Impra Carboflo Vascular Graft, Straight Graft 20 cm in length *Medicare Statute 1833(T)*

● **C6207** Vascular graft, Impra Carboflo Vascular Graft, Straight Graft 30 cm, 35 cm or 40 cm in length *Medicare Statute 1833(T)*

● **C6208** Vascular graft, Impra Carboflo Vascular Graft, Straight Graft (50 cm in length), Access Tapered Graft (40 cm in length), or Stepped Graft (45 or 50 cm in length) *Medicare Statute 1833(T)*

● **C6209** Vascular graft, Impra Carboflo Vascular Graft, Centerflex Straight Graft (40 cm or 50 cm in length) or Centerflex Stepped Graft (40 cm, 45 cm, or 50 cm in length) *Medicare Statute 1833(T)*

● **C6210** Vascular graft, Exxcel ePTFE Vascular Graft, less than 6 mm in diameter *Medicare Statute 1833(T)*

● **C6300** Stent graft system, vanguard III bifurcated endovascular aortic graft *Medicare Statute 1833(T)*

● **C6500** Sheath, guiding, preface braided guiding sheath (anterior curve, multipurpose curve, posterior curve) *Medicare Statute 1833(T)*

● **C6501**　Sheath, soft-tip sheaths　　　　　*Medicare Statute 1833(T)*

● **C6525**　Spectranetics Laser Sheath 12F 500-001, 14F 500-012, 16F 500-013
　　　　　　　　　　　　　　　　　　　Medicare Statute 1833(T)

● **C6600**　Probe, Microvasive Swiss F/G Lithoclast Flexible Probe .89 mm,
　　　　　　　Microvasive Swiss F/G Lithoclast Flexible Probe II .89 mm
　　　　　　　　　　　　　　　　　　　Medicare Statute 1833(T)

● **C6650**　Introducer, guiding, Fast-Cath Two-Piece Guiding Introducer 406869,
　　　　　　　406892, 406893, 406904　　　*Medicare Statute 1833(T)*

● **C6651**　Introducer, guiding, Seal-Away CS Guiding Introducer 407508, 407510
　　　　　　　　　　　　　　　　　　　Medicare Statute 1833(T)

● **C6652**　Introducer, Bard Safety Excalibur Introducer　　*Medicare Statute 1833(T)*

● **C6700**　Synthetic absorbable sealant, Focal Seal-l　　*Medicare Statute 1833(T)*

● **C8099**　Spectranetics Lead Locking Device 518-018, 518-019, 518-020
　　　　　　　　　　　　　　　　　　　Medicare Statute 1833(T)

● **C8100**　Adhesion barrier, Adcon-l　　　*Medicare Statute 1833(T)*

● **C8102**　Surgi-Vision Esophageal Stylet Internal Coil　　*Medicare Statute 1833(T)*

● **C8103**　Capio Suture Capturing Device, standard or open access
　　　　　　　　　　　　　　　　　　　Medicare Statute 1833(T)

● **C8500**　Catheter, atherectomy, Aterocath-GTO atherectomy catheter
　　　　　　　　　　　　　　　　　　　Medicare Statute 1833(T)

● **C8501**　Pacemaker, single chamber, Vigor SSI　　*Medicare Statute 1833(T)*

● **C8502**　Catheter, diagnostic, electrophysiology, Livewire Steerable
　　　　　　　Electrophysiology Catheter　　*Medicare Statute 1833(T)*

● **C8503**　Catheter, Synchromed Vascular Catheter Model 8702
　　　　　　　　　　　　　　　　　　　Medicare Statute 1833(T)

● **C8504**　Closure device, Vasoseal Vascular Hemostasis Device
　　　　　　　　　　　　　　　　　　　Medicare Statute 1833(T)

● **C8505**　Infusion pump, implantable, programmable, Synchromed Infusion
　　　　　　　Pump　　　　　　　　　　　*Medicare Statute 1833(T)*

● **C8506**　Lead, pacemaker, 4057M, 4058M, 4557M, 4558M, 5058
　　　　　　　　　　　　　　　　　　　Medicare Statute 1833(T)

● **C8507**　Lead, pacemaker, 6721L, 6721M, 672LS, 6939 oval patch lead
　　　　　　　　　　　　　　　　　　　Medicare Statute 1833(T)

● **C8508**　Lead, defibrillator, CapSure 4965　　*Medicare Statute 1833(T)*

● **C8509**　Lead, defibrillator, Transvene 6933, Transvene 6937
　　　　　　　　　　　　　　　　　　　Medicare Statute 1833(T)

● **C8510**　Lead, defibrillator, DP-3238　　*Medicare Statute 1833(T)*

● **C8511**　Lead, defibrillator, Endotak DSP　　*Medicare Statute 1833(T)*

● **C8512**　Lead, neurostimulation, On-Point Model 3987, Pisces-Quad Plus Model
　　　　　　　3888, Resume Tl Model 3986　　*Medicare Statute 1833(T)*

C Codes

　　　= Special Coverage Instructions Apply　　　　　= Carrier Discretion

　　　= Noncovered by Medicare or Medicare Statute

● **C8513** Lead, Neurostimulation, Pisces-Quad Model 3487A, Resume II Model
3587A *Medicare Statute 1833(T)*

● **C8514** Prosthesis, penile, Dura II Penile Prosthesis *Medicare Statute 1833(T)*

~~**C8515**~~ ~~Prosthesis, Penile, Mentor Alpha I Narrow Base Inflatable Penile~~
~~Prosthesis~~ This code was added and deleted in 2000.

● **C8516** Prosthesis, penile, Mentor Acu-Form Malleable Penile Prosthesis,
Mentor Malleable Penile Prosthesis *Medicare Statute 1833(T)*

~~**C8517**~~ ~~Prosthesis, penile, Ambicor Penile Prosthesis~~ This code was added and
deleted in 2000.

● **C8518** Pacemaker, dual chamber, Vigor DDD *Medicare Statute 1833(T)*

● **C8519** Pacemaker, dual chamber, Vista DDD *Medicare Statute 1833(T)*

● **C8520** Pacemaker, single chamber, Legacy II S *Medicare Statute 1833(T)*

● **C8521** Receiver/transmitter, neurostimulator, Medtronic Mattrix
Medicare Statute 1833(T)

● **C8522** Stent, biliary, Palmaz Balloon Expandable Stent *Medicare Statute 1833(T)*

● **C8523** Stent, biliary, Wallstent Transhepatic Biliary Endoprosthesis
Medicare Statute 1833(T)

● **C8524** Stent, esophageal, Wallstent esophageal prosthesis
Medicare Statute 1833(T)

● **C8525** Stent, esophageal, Wallstent Esophageal Prosthesis (double)
Medicare Statute 1833(T)

● **C8526** Optiplast XT 5F Percutaneous Transluminal Angioplasty Catheter
(various sizes) *Medicare Statute 1833(T)*

● **C8528** MS Classique Balloon Dilatation Catheter *Medicare Statute 1833(T)*

● **C8529** Ismus Cath Deflectable 20-Pole Catheter/Crista Cath II Deflectable 20-
Pole Catheter *Medicare Statute 1833(T)*

● **C8530** Mentor Siltex Gel-Filled Mammary Prosthesis, Smooth-Surface Gel-
Filled Mammary Prosthesis *Medicare Statute 1833(T)*

● **C8531** Wilson-Cook Esophageal Z Metal Expandable Stent
Medicare Statute 1833(T)

● **C8532** Stent, esophageal, Ultraflex Esophageal Stent System
Medicare Statute 1833(T)

● **C8533** Catheter, Synchromed Vascular Catheter Model 8700A, Model 8700V
Medicare Statute 1833(T)

● **C8534** Prosthesis, penile, AMS Malleable 650 Penile Prosthesis
Medicare Statute 1833(T)

● **C8535** Stent, biliary, Spiral Z Biliary Metal Expandable Stent, ZA Biliary Metal
Expandable Stent *Medicare Statute 1833(T)*

● **C8536** Stent, esophageal, Esophageal Z Metal Expandable Stent with Dua
Anti-Reflux Valve, Esophageal Z Metal Expandable Stent with Uncoated
Flanges *Medicare Statute 1833(T)*

= Invalid Medicare Code (no grace period)

= Code may require certificate of medical necessity (CMN) or DMERC information form (DIF)

● **C8539** Wilson-Cook Quantum Dilatation Balloon *Medicare Statute 1833(T)*

● **C8540** Flex-EZ (Esophageal) Balloon Dilator 3302, 3304, 3306
Medicare Statute 1833(T)

● **C8541** Carson Zero Tip Balloon Dilatation Catheters with Hydroplus Coating Kit, Passport Balloon On A Wire Dilatation Catheters with Hydroplus Coating Kit *Medicare Statute 1833(T)*

● **C8542** Urethramax High Pressure Urethral Balloon Dilatation Catheter/Kit
Medicare Statute 1833(T)

● **C8543** Amplatz Renal Dilator Set *Medicare Statute 1833(T)*

● **C8550** Catheter, Livewire EP Catheter, 7F CSM 401935, 5F Decapolar 401938, 401939, 401940, 401941 *Medicare Statute 1833(T)*

● **C8551** Catheter, Livewire EP Catheter, 7F Duo-Decapolar 401932
Medicare Statute 1833(T)

● **C8552** Catheter, Santuro Fixed Curve Catheter *Medicare Statute 1833(T)*

● **C8597** Guide wire, Cordis Wisdom ST Steerable Guidewire 537-114, 537-114J, 537-114X, 537-114Y *Medicare Statute 1833(T)*

● **C8598** Guide Wire, Cordis Sv Guidewire 5 cm Distal Taper Configuration (Models 503-558, 503-558X), 8 cm Distal Taper Configuration (Models 503-658, 503-658X), 14 cm Distal Taper Configuration (Models 503-758, 503-758X) *Medicare Statute 1833(T)*

● **C8599** Guide Wire, Cordis Stabilizer XS Steerable Guidewire 527-914, 527-914J, 527-914X, 527-914Y *Medicare Statute 1833(T)*

● **C8600** Guide Wire, Cordis Shinobi Plus Steerable Guidewire 547-214, 547-214X *Medicare Statute 1833(T)*

● **C8650** Introducer, Cook Extra Large Check-Flo Introducer
Medicare Statute 1833(T)

● **C8724** Lead, neurostimulation, Octad Lead 3898-33/389861
Medicare Statute 1833(T)

● **C8725** Lead, neurostimulation, Symmix Lead 3982 *Medicare Statute 1833(T)*

● **C8748** Lead, defibrillator, Endotak sq patch 0047, 0063 *Medicare Statute 1833(T)*

● **C8749** Lead, defibrillator, Endotak sq array 0048, 0049 *Medicare Statute 1833(T)*

● **C8750** Pacemaker, dual chamber, Unity VDDR 292-07 *Medicare Statute 1833(T)*

● **C8775** Lead, pacemaker, 2188 Coronary Sinus Lead *Medicare Statute 1833(T)*

● **C8776** Lead, pacemaker, Innomedica Sutureless Myocardial 4045, 4058, 4046, 4047 *Medicare Statute 1833(T)*

● **C8777** Lead, pacemaker, Unipass 425-02, 425-04, 425-06
Medicare Statute 1833(T)

● **C8800** Stent, biliary, Large Palmaz Balloon Expandable Stent with Delivery System *Medicare Statute 1833(T)*

● **C8801** Stent, biliary, Cook Z Stent Gianturco-Rosch Biliary Design
Medicare Statute 1833(T)

C Codes

= Special Coverage Instructions Apply   = Carrier Discretion

= Noncovered by Medicare or Medicare Statute

● **C8802** Stent, biliary, Cook Oasis One Action Stent Introductory System
Medicare Statute 1833(T)

● **C8830** Stent, coronary, Cook Gianturco-Roubin Flex-Stent Coronary Stent
Medicare Statute 1833(T)

● **C8890** Perfluoron, per 2ml *Medicare Statute 1833(T)*

● **C8891** Perfluoron, per 5ml vial or 7ml vial *Medicare Statute 1833(T)*

● **C9000** Injection, sodium chromate Cr51, per 0.25 mCi *Medicare Statute 1833(T)*

● **C9001** Linezolid injection, per 200 mg *Medicare Statute 1833(T)*

● **C9002** Tenecteplase, per 50 mg/vial *Medicare Statute 1833(T)*

● **C9003** Palivizumab-rsv-igm, per 50 mg *Medicare Statute 1833(T)*

● **C9004** Injection, gemtuzumab ozogamicin, per 5 mg *Medicare Statute 1833(T)*

● **C9005** Injection, reteplase, 18.8 mg (one single-use vial) *Medicare Statute 1833(T)*

● **C9006** Injection, tacrolimus, per 5 mg (1 amp) *Medicare Statute 1833(T)*

● **C9007** Baclofen Intrathecal Screening Kit (1 amp) *Medicare Statute 1833(T)*

● **C9008** Baclofen Intrathecal Refill Kit, per 500 mcg *Medicare Statute 1833(T)*

● **C9009** Baclofen Refill Kit, per 2000 mcg *Medicare Statute 1833(T)*

● **C9010** Baclofen Intrathecal Refill Kit, per 4000 mcg *Medicare Statute 1833(T)*

● **C9011** Injection, caffeine citrate, per 1ml *Medicare Statute 1833(T)*

● **C9100** Supply of radiopharmaceutical diagnostic imaging agent, iodinated I-131 albumin, per mCi *Medicare Statute 1833(T)*

● **C9102** Supply of radiopharmaceutical diagnostic imaging agent, 51 sodium chromate, per 50 mCi *Medicare Statute 1833(T)*

● **C9103** Supply of radiopharmaceutical diagnostic imaging agent, sodium iothalamate I-125 injection, per 10 uCi *Medicare Statute 1833(T)*

● **C9104** Anti-thymocyte globulin, per 25 mg *Medicare Statute 1833(T)*

● **C9105** Injection, hepatitis B immune globulin, per 1 ml *Medicare Statute 1833(T)*

● **C9106** Sirolimus, per 1 mg/ml *Medicare Statute 1833(T)*

● **C9107** Injection, tinzaparin sodium, per 2ml vial *Medicare Statute 1833(T)*

● **C9500** Platelets, irradiated, each unit *Medicare Statute 1833(T)*

● **C9501** Platelets, pheresis, each unit *Medicare Statute 1833(T)*

● **C9502** Platelets, pheresis, irradiated, each unit *Medicare Statute 1833(T)*

● **C9503** Fresh frozen plasma, donor retested, each unit *Medicare Statute 1833(T)*

● **C9504** Red blood cells, deglycerolized, each unit *Medicare Statute 1833(T)*

● **C9505** Red blood cells, irradiated, each unit *Medicare Statute 1833(T)*

● **C9700** Water induced thermotherapy *Medicare Statute 1833(T)*

● **C9701** Stretta System *Medicare Statute 1833(T)*

● **C9702** Checkmate intravascular brachytherapy system *Medicare Statute 1833(T)*

= Invalid Medicare Code (no grace period)

= Code may require certificate of medical necessity (CMN) or DMERC information form (DIF)

Dental Procedures D0000–D9999

Items and services, in connection with the care, treatment, filling, removal, or replacement of teeth, or structures directly supporting the teeth, are not covered by Medicare. Prosthetic devices that replace the function of a permanently inoperative or malfunctioning internal body organ are, however, a covered service under the Prosthetic Devices guidelines.

The hospitalization or nonhospitalization of a patient has no direct bearing on the coverage or exclusion of a given dental procedure.

This section (codes D0100-D9999) incorporates numeric codes and descriptors from CDT-3, which is copyright American Dental Association.

Participants are authorized to use copies of CDT-3 material in HCPCS only for purposes directly related to participating in HCFA programs. Permission for any other use must be obtained from the American Dental Association.

Diagnostic D0100–D0999

Clinical Oral Evaluation

D0120 Periodic oral examination *CIM 50-26, Medicare Statute 1862A (12)*

D0140 Limited oral evaluation — problem focused *Medicare Statute 1862A (12)*

D0150 Comprehensive oral evaluation *CIM 50-26, MCM 2136, MCM 2336, ASC*

D0160 Detailed and extensive oral evaluation — problem focused, by report
Medicare Statute 1862A (12)

D0170 Re-evaluation — limited, problem focused (Established patient; not post-operative visit)

Radiographs

D0210 Intraoral — complete series (including bitewings). See also code 70320. *Cross-reference CPT 70320*

D0220 Intraoral — periapical, first film. See also code 70300. *Cross-reference CPT 70300*

D0230 Intraoral — periapical, each additional film. See also code 70310. *Cross-reference CPT 70310*

D0240 Intraoral — occlusal film *MCM 2136, MCM 2336, ASC*

D0250 Extraoral — first film *MCM 2136, MCM 2336, ASC*

D0260 Extraoral — each additional film *MCM 2136, MCM 2336, ASC*

D0270 Bitewing — single film *MCM 2136, MCM 2336, ASC*

D0272 Bitewings — two films *MCM 2136, MCM 2336, ASC*

D0274 Bitewings — four films *MCM 2136, MCM 2336, ASC*

D0277 Vertical bitewings — 7 to 8 films

D0290 Posterior-anterior or lateral skull and facial bone survey film. See also code 70150. *Cross-reference CPT 70150*

D Codes

███ = Special Coverage Instructions Apply   ███ = Carrier Discretion

███ = Noncovered by Medicare or Medicare Statute

D0310	Sialography. See also code 70390.	*Cross-reference CPT 70390*
D0320	Temporomandibular joint arthrogram, including injection. See also code 70332.	*Cross-reference CPT 70332*
D0321	Other temporomandibular joint films, by report. See also code 76499.	*Cross-reference 76499*
D0322	Tomographic survey. See also CPT.	*CIM 50-26*
D0330	Panoramic film. See also code 70320.	*Cross-reference CPT 70320*
D0340	Cephalometric film. See also code 70350.	*Cross-reference CPT 70350*
D0350	Oral/facial images (includes intra and extraoral images)	

Test and Laboratory Examinations

D0415	Bacteriologic studies for determination of pathologic agents	*CIM 50-26, Medicare Statute 1862A (12)*
D0425	Caries susceptibility tests	*CIM 50-26, Medicare Statute 1862A (12)*
D0460	Pulp vitality tests	*CIM 50-26, MCM 2136, MCM 2336, ASC*
D0470	Diagnostic casts	*Medicare Statute 1862A (12)*
D0472	Accession of tissue, gross examination, preparation and transmission of written report	
D0473	Accession of tissue, gross and microscopic examination, preparation and transmission of written report	
D0474	Accession of tissue, gross and microscopic examination, including assessment of surgical margins for presence of disease, preparation and transmission of written report	
D0480	Processing and interpretation of cytologic smears, including the preparation and transmission of written report	
D0501	Histopathologic examinations	*CIM 50-26, MCM 2136, MCM 2336, ASC*
D0502	Other oral pathology procedures, by report	*CIM 50-26, MCM 2136, MCM 2336, ASC*
D0999	Unspecified diagnostic procedure, by report	*CIM 50-26, MCM 2136, MCM 2336, ASC*

Preventive D1000–D1999

Dental Prophylaxis

D1110	Prophylaxis — adult	*Medicare Statute 1862A (12)*
D1120	Prophylaxis — child	*Medicare Statute 1862A (12)*

Topical Fluoride Treatment (Office Procedure)

D1201	Topical application of fluoride (including prophylaxis) — child	*Medicare Statute 1862A (12)*
D1203	Topical application of fluoride (prophylaxis not included) — child	*Medicare Statute 1862A (12)*

= Invalid Medicare Code (no grace period)

= Code may require certificate of medical necessity (CMN) or DMERC information form (DIF)

| **D1204** | Topical application of fluoride (prophylaxis not included) — adult |
| | *Medicare Statute 1862A (12)* |

| **D1205** | Topical application of fluoride (including prophylaxis) — adult |
| | *Medicare Statute 1862A (12)* |

Other Preventive Services

| **D1310** | Nutritional counseling for control of dental disease | *MCM 2300* |

| **D1320** | Tobacco counseling for the control and prevention of oral disease |
| | *MCM 2300* |

| **D1330** | Oral hygiene instructions | *MCM 2300* |

| **D1351** | Sealant — per tooth | *Medicare Statute 1862A (12)* |

Space Maintenance (Passive Appliances)

| **D1510** | Space maintainer — fixed-unilateral | *MCM 2336, ASC* |

| **D1515** | Space maintainer — fixed-bilateral | *MCM 2336, MCM 2136, ASC* |

| **D1520** | Space maintainer — removable-unilateral | *MCM 2336, MCM 2136, ASC* |

| **D1525** | Space maintainer — removable-bilateral | *MCM 2336, MCM 2136, ASC* |

| **D1550** | Recementation of space maintainer | *MCM 2336, MCM 2136, ASC* |

Restorative D2000–D2999

Amalgam Restorations (Including Polishing)

| **D2110** | Amalgam — one surface, primary | *Medicare Statute 1862A (12)* |

| **D2120** | Amalgam — two surfaces, primary | *Medicare Statute 1862A (12)* |

| **D2130** | Amalgam — three surfaces, primary | *Medicare Statute 1862A (12)* |

| **D2131** | Amalgam — four or more surfaces, primary | *Medicare Statute 1862A (12)* |

| **D2140** | Amalgam — one surface, permanent | *Medicare Statute 1862A (12)* |

| **D2150** | Amalgam — two surfaces, permanent | *Medicare Statute 1862A (12)* |

| **D2160** | Amalgam — three surfaces, permanent | *Medicare Statute 1862A (12)* |

| **D2161** | Amalgam — four or more surfaces, permanent | *Medicare Statute 1862A (12)* |

Resin Restorations

| **D2330** | Resin-based composite — one surface, anterior | *Medicare Statute 1862A (12)* |

| **D2331** | Resin-based composite — two surfaces, anterior |
| | *Medicare Statute 1862A (12)* |

| **D2332** | Resin-based composite — three surfaces, anterior |
| | *Medicare Statute 1862A (12)* |

| **D2335** | Resin-based composite — four or more surfaces or involving incisal angle (anterior) | *Medicare Statute 1862A (12)* |

| **D2336** | Resin-based composite crown, anterior — primary |
| | *Medicare Statute 1862A (12)* |

D Codes

= Special Coverage Instructions Apply   = Carrier Discretion

= Noncovered by Medicare or Medicare Statute

D2337	Resin-based composite crown, anterior — permanent	
D2380	Resin-based composite — one surface, posterior — primary	*Medicare Statute 1862A (12)*
D2381	Resin-based composite — two surfaces, posterior — primary	*Medicare Statute 1862A (12)*
D2382	Resin-based composite — three or more surfaces, posterior — primary	*Medicare Statute 1862A (12)*
D2385	Resin-based composite — one surface, posterior — permanent	*Medicare Statute 1862A (12)*
D2386	Resin-based composite — two surfaces, posterior — permanent	*Medicare Statute 1862A (12)*
D2387	Resin-based composite — three surfaces, posterior — permanent	*Medicare Statute 1862A (12)*
D2388	Resin-based composite — four or more surfaces, posterior — permanent	

Gold Foil Restorations

D2410	Gold foil — one surface	*Medicare Statute 1862A (12)*
D2420	Gold foil — two surfaces	*Medicare Statute 1862A (12)*
D2430	Gold foil — three surfaces	*Medicare Statute 1862A (12)*

Inlay/Onlay Restorations

D2510	Inlay — metallic — one surface	*Medicare Statute 1862A (12)*
D2520	Inlay — metallic — two surfaces	*Medicare Statute 1862A (12)*
D2530	Inlay — metallic — three or more surfaces	*Medicare Statute 1862A (12)*
D2542	Onlay — metallic — two surfaces	
D2543	Onlay — metallic — three surfaces	*Medicare Statute 1862A (12)*
D2544	Onlay — metallic — four or more surfaces	*Medicare Statute 1862A (12)*
D2610	Inlay — porcelain/ceramic — one surface	*Medicare Statute 1862A (12)*
D2620	Inlay — porcelain/ceramic — two surfaces	*Medicare Statute 1862A (12)*
D2630	Inlay — porcelain/ceramic — three or more surfaces	*Medicare Statute 1862A (12)*
D2642	Onlay — porcelain/ceramic — two surfaces	*Medicare Statute 1862A (12)*
D2643	Onlay — porcelain/ceramic — three surfaces	*Medicare Statute 1862A (12)*
D2644	Onlay — porcelain/ceramic — four or more surfaces	*Medicare Statute 1862A (12)*
D2650	Inlay — resin-based composite composite/resin — one surface	*Medicare Statute 1862A (12)*
D2651	Inlay — resin-based composite composite/resin — two surfaces	*Medicare Statute 1862A (12)*

= Invalid Medicare Code (no grace period)

= Code may require certificate of medical necessity (CMN) or DMERC information form (DIF)

D2652	Inlay — resin-based composite composite/resin — three or more surfaces	
		Medicare Statute 1862A (12)

D2662	Onlay — resin-based composite composite/resin — two surfaces
	Medicare Statute 1862A (12)

D2663	Onlay — resin-based composite composite/resin — three surfaces
	Medicare Statute 1862A (12)

D2664	Onlay — resin-based composite composite/resin — four or more surfaces
	Medicare Statute 1862A (12)

Crowns — Single Restoration Only

D2710	Crown — resin (laboratory)	*Medicare Statute 1862A (12)*
D2720	Crown — resin with high noble metal	*Medicare Statute 1862A (12)*
D2721	Crown — resin with predominantly base metal	*Medicare Statute 1862A (12)*
D2722	Crown — resin with noble metal	*Medicare Statute 1862A (12)*
D2740	Crown — porcelain/ceramic substrate	*Medicare Statute 1862A (12)*
D2750	Crown — porcelain fused to high noble metal	*Medicare Statute 1862A (12)*
D2751	Crown — porcelain fused to predominantly base metal	*Medicare Statute 1862A (12)*
D2752	Crown — porcelain fused to noble metal	*Medicare Statute 1862A (12)*
D2780	Crown — 3/4 cast high noble metal	
D2781	Crown — 3/4 cast predominately base metal	
D2782	Crown — 3/4 cast noble metal	
D2783	Crown — 3/4 porcelain/ceramic	
D2790	Crown — full cast high noble metal	*Medicare Statute 1862A (12)*
D2791	Crown — full cast predominantly base metal	*Medicare Statute 1862A (12)*
D2792	Crown — full cast noble metal	*Medicare Statute 1862A (12)*
D2799	Provisional crown	

Other Restorative Services

D2910	Recement inlay	*Medicare Statute 1862A (12)*
D2920	Recement crown	*Medicare Statute 1862A (12)*
D2930	Prefabricated stainless steel crown — primary tooth	*Medicare Statute 1862A (12)*
D2931	Prefabricated stainless steel crown — permanent tooth	*Medicare Statute 1862A (12)*
D2932	Prefabricated resin crown	*Medicare Statute 1862A (12)*
D2933	Prefabricated stainless steel crown with resin window	*Medicare Statute 1862A (12)*
D2940	Sedative filling	*Medicare Statute 1862A (12)*
D2950	Core buildup, including any pins	*Medicare Statute 1862A (12)*

D Codes

= Special Coverage Instructions Apply   = Carrier Discretion

= Noncovered by Medicare or Medicare Statute

D2951	Pin retention — per tooth, in addition to restoration
	Medicare Statute 1862A (12)

D2952	Cast post and core in addition to crown	*Medicare Statute 1862A (12)*

D2953	Each additional cast post — same tooth

D2954	Prefabricated post and core in addition to crown
	Medicare Statute 1862A (12)

D2955	Post removal (not in conjunction with endodontic therapy)

D2957	Each additional prefabricated post — same tooth

D2960	Labial veneer (resin laminate) — chairside	*Medicare Statute 1862A (12)*

D2961	Labial veneer (resin laminate) — laboratory	*Medicare Statute 1862A (12)*

D2962	Labial veneer (porcelain laminate) — laboratory
	Medicare Statute 1862A (12)

D2970	Temporary crown (fractured tooth)	*MCM 2336, MCM 2136, ASC*

D2980	Crown repair, by report	*Medicare Statute 1862A (12)*

D2999	Unspecified restorative procedure, by report	*MCM 2336, MCM 2136, ASC*

Endodontics D3000–D3999

Pulp Capping

D3110	Pulp cap — direct (excluding final restoration) *Medicare Statute 1862A (12)*

D3120	Pulp cap — indirect (excluding final restoration)
	Medicare Statute 1862A (12)

Pulpotomy

D3220	Therapeutic pulpotomy (excluding final restoration) — removal of pulp coronal to the dentinocemental junction and application of medicament
	Medicare Statute 1862A (12)

D3221	Gross pulpal debridement, primary and permanent teeth

Pulpal Therapy on Primary Teeth (Includes Primary Teeth with Succedaneous Teeth and Placement of Resorbable Filling)

D3230	Pulpal therapy (resorbable filling) — anterior, primary tooth (excluding final restoration)
	Medicare Statute 1862A (12)

D3240	Pulpal therapy (resorbable filling) — posterior, primary tooth (excluding final restoration)
	Medicare Statute 1862A (12)

Root Canal Therapy (Including Treatment Plan, Clinical Procedures, and Follow-up Care, Includes Primary Teeth without Succedaneous Teeth and Permanent Teeth)

D3310	Anterior (excluding final restoration)	*Medicare Statute 1862A (12)*

D3320	Bicuspid (excluding final restoration)	*Medicare Statute 1862A (12)*

D3330	Molar (excluding final restoration)	*Medicare Statute 1862A (12)*

D3331	Treatment of root canal obstruction; non-surgical access

= Invalid Medicare Code (no grace period)

= Code may require certificate of medical necessity (CMN) or DMERC information form (DIF)

D3332   Incomplete endodontic therapy; inoperable or fractured tooth

D3333   Internal root repair of perforation defects

D3346   Retreatment of previous root canal therapy — anterior
Medicare Statute 1862A (12)

D3347   Retreatment of previous root canal therapy — bicuspid
Medicare Statute 1862A (12)

D3348   Retreatment of previous root canal therapy — molar
Medicare Statute 1862A (12)

D3351   Apexification/recalcification — initial visit (apical closure/calcific repair of perforations, root resorption, etc.)   *Medicare Statute 1862A (12)*

D3352   Apexification/recalcification — interim medication replacement (apical closure/calcific repair of perforations, root resorption, etc.)
Medicare Statute 1862A (12)

D3353   Apexification/recalcification – final visit (includes completed root canal therapy — apical closure/calcific repair of perforations, root resorption, etc.)   *Medicare Statute 1862A (12)*

Apicoectomy/Periradicular Services

D3410   Apicoectomy/periradicular surgery — anterior
Medicare Statute 1862A (12)

D3421   Apicoectomy/periradicular surgery — bicuspid (first root)
Medicare Statute 1862A (12)

D3425   Apicoectomy/periradicular surgery — molar (first root)
Medicare Statute 1862A (12)

D3426   Apicoectomy/periradicular surgery (each additional root)
Medicare Statute 1862A (12)

D3430   Retrograde filling — per root   *Medicare Statute 1862A (12)*

D3450   Root amputation — per root   *Medicare Statute 1862A (12)*

D3460   Endodontic endosseous implant   *Medicare Statute 1862A (12), ASC*

D3470   Intentional reimplantation (including necessary splinting)
Medicare Statute 1862A (12)

Other Endodontic Procedures

D3910   Surgical procedure for isolation of tooth with rubber dam
Medicare Statute 1862A (12)

D3920   Hemisection (including any root removal), not including root canal therapy   *Medicare Statute 1862A (12)*

D3950   Canal preparation and fitting of preformed dowel or post
Medicare Statute 1862A (12)

D3999   Unspecified endodontic procedure, by report
MCM 2336, MCM 2136, ASC

D Codes

= Special Coverage Instructions Apply   = Carrier Discretion

= Noncovered by Medicare or Medicare Statute

Periodontics D4000–D4999

Surgical Services (Including Usual Postoperative Services)

D4210 Gingivectomy or gingivoplasty — per quadrant. See also code 41820.
Cross-reference CPT 41820

D4211 Gingivectomy or gingivoplasty — per tooth. See also code 41820 or 41872. *Cross-reference CPT*

D4220 Gingival curettage, surgical — per quadrant, by report
Medicare Statute 1862A (12)

D4240 Gingival flap procedure, including root planing — per quadrant
Medicare Statute 1862A (12)

D4245 Apically positioned flap

D4249 Clinical crown lengthening — hard tissue   *Medicare Statute 1862A (12)*

D4260 Osseous surgery (including flap entry and closure) — per quadrant
MCM 2336, MCM 2136, ASC

D4263 Bone replacement graft — first site in quadrant
CIM 50-26, MCM 2336, MCM 2136, ASC

D4264 Bone replacement graft — each additional site in quadrant (use if performed on same date of service as D4263)
CIM 50-26, MCM 2336, MCM 2136, ASC

D4266 Guided tissue regeneration — resorbable barrier, per site
Medicare Statute 1862A (12)

D4267 Guided tissue regeneration — nonresorbable barrier, per site (includes membrane removal) *Medicare Statute 1862A (12)*

D4268 Surgical revision procedure, per tooth

D4270 Pedicle soft tissue graft procedure   *MCM 2336, MCM 2136, ASC*

D4271 Free soft tissue graft procedure (including donor site surgery)
MCM 2336, MCM 2136, ASC

D4273 Subepithelial connective tissue graft procedure (including donor site surgery) *CIM 50-26, MCM 2336, MCM 2136, ASC*

D4274 Distal or proximal wedge procedure (when not performed in conjunction with surgical procedures in the same anatomical area)

Adjunctive Periodontal Services

D4320 Provisional splinting — intracoronal   *Medicare Statute 1862A (12)*

D4321 Provisional splinting — extracoronal   *Medicare Statute 1862A (12)*

D4341 Periodontal scaling and root planing, per quadrant
Medicare Statute 1862A (12)

D4355 Full mouth debridement to enable comprehensive periodontal evaluation and diagnosis   *Medicare Statute 1862A (12), ASC*

D4381 Localized delivery of chemotherapeutic agents via a controlled release vehicle into diseased crevicular tissue, per tooth, by report
CIM 50-26, MCM 2336, MCM 2136, ASC

Other Periodontal Services

D4910 Periodontal maintenance procedures (following active therapy)
Medicare Statute 1862A (12)

D4920 Unscheduled dressing change (by someone other than treating dentist)
Medicare Statute 1862A (12)

D4999 Unspecified periodontal procedure, by report *Medicare Statute 1862A (12)*

Prosthodontics (Removable) D5000–D5899

Complete Dentures (Including Routine Post Delivery Care)

D5110 Complete denture — maxillary *Medicare Statute 1862A (12)*

D5120 Complete denture — mandibular *Medicare Statute 1862A (12)*

D5130 Immediate denture — maxillary *Medicare Statute 1862A (12)*

D5140 Immediate denture — mandibular *Medicare Statute 1862A (12)*

Partial Dentures (Including Routine Post Delivery Care)

D5211 Maxillary partial denture — resin base (including any conventional clasps, rests and teeth) *Medicare Statute 1862A (12)*

D5212 Mandibular partial denture — resin base (including any conventional clasps, rests and teeth) *Medicare Statute 1862A (12)*

D5213 Maxillary partial denture — cast metal framework with resin denture bases (including any conventional clasps, rests and teeth)
Medicare Statute 1862A (12)

D5214 Mandibular partial denture— cast metal framework with resin denture bases (including any conventional clasps, rests and teeth)
Medicare Statute 1862A (12)

D5281 Removable unilateral partial denture — one piece cast metal (including clasps and teeth) *Medicare Statute 1862A (12)*

Adjustments to Removable Prostheses

D5410 Adjust complete denture — maxillary *Medicare Statute 1862A (12)*

D5411 Adjust complete denture — mandibular *Medicare Statute 1862A (12)*

D5421 Adjust partial denture — maxillary *Medicare Statute 1862A (12)*

D5422 Adjust partial denture — mandibular *Medicare Statute 1862A (12)*

Repairs to Complete Dentures

D5510 Repair broken complete denture base *Medicare Statute 1862A (12)*

D5520 Replace missing or broken teeth — complete denture (each tooth)
Medicare Statute 1862A (12)

D Codes

= Special Coverage Instructions Apply   = Carrier Discretion

= Noncovered by Medicare or Medicare Statute

Repairs to Partial Dentures

D5610	Repair resin denture base	*Medicare Statute 1862A (12)*
D5620	Repair cast framework	*Medicare Statute 1862A (12)*
D5630	Repair or replace broken clasp	*Medicare Statute 1862A (12)*
D5640	Replace broken teeth — per tooth	*Medicare Statute 1862A (12)*
D5650	Add tooth to existing partial denture	*Medicare Statute 1862A (12)*
D5660	Add clasp to existing partial denture	*Medicare Statute 1862A (12)*

Denture Rebase Procedures

D5710	Rebase complete maxillary denture	*Medicare Statute 1862A (12)*
D5711	Rebase complete mandibular denture	*Medicare Statute 1862A (12)*
D5720	Rebase maxillary partial denture	*Medicare Statute 1862A (12)*
D5721	Rebase mandibular partial denture	*Medicare Statute 1862A (12)*

Denture Reline Procedures

D5730	Reline complete maxillary denture (chairside)	*Medicare Statute 1862A (12)*
D5731	Reline complete mandibular denture (chairside)	*Medicare Statute 1862A (12)*
D5740	Reline maxillary partial denture (chairside)	*Medicare Statute 1862A (12)*
D5741	Reline mandibular partial denture (chairside)	*Medicare Statute 1862A (12)*
D5750	Reline complete maxillary denture (laboratory)	*Medicare Statute 1862A (12)*
D5751	Reline complete mandibular denture (laboratory)	*Medicare Statute 1862A (12)*
D5760	Reline maxillary partial denture (laboratory)	*Medicare Statute 1862A (12)*
D5761	Reline mandibular partial denture (laboratory)	*Medicare Statute 1862A (12)*

Other Removable Prosthetic Services

D5810	Interim complete denture (maxillary)	*Medicare Statute 1862A (12)*
D5811	Interim complete denture (mandibular)	*Medicare Statute 1862A (12)*
D5820	Interim partial denture (maxillary)	*Medicare Statute 1862A (12)*
D5821	Interim partial denture (mandibular)	*Medicare Statute 1862A (12)*
D5850	Tissue conditioning, maxillary	*Medicare Statute 1862A (12)*
D5851	Tissue conditioning, mandibular	*Medicare Statute 1862A (12)*
D5860	Overdenture — complete, by report	*Medicare Statute 1862A (12)*
D5861	Overdenture — partial, by report	*Medicare Statute 1862A (12)*
D5862	Precision attachment, by report	*Medicare Statute 1862A (12)*
D5867	Replacement of replaceable part of semi-precision or precision attachment (male or female component)	
D5875	Modification of removable prosthesis following implant surgery	

= Invalid Medicare Code (no grace period)

= Code may require certificate of medical necessity (CMN) or DMERC information form (DIF)

D5899	Unspecified removable prosthodontic procedure, by report
	Medicare Statute 1862A (12)

Maxillofacial Prosthetics D5900–D5999

D5911	Facial moulage (sectional)	*MCM 2136, MCM 2130A, ASC*
D5912	Facial moulage (complete)	*MCM 2130A, ASC*
D5913	Nasal prosthesis. See also code 21087.	*Cross-reference CPT 21087*
D5914	Auricular prosthesis. See also code 21086.	*Cross-reference CPT 21086*
D5915	Orbital prosthesis. See also code L8611.	*Cross-reference L8611*
D5916	Ocular prosthesis. See also code V2623, V2629 and CPT.	*Cross-reference V2623, V2629*
D5919	Facial prosthesis. See also code 21088.	*Cross-reference CPT 21088*
D5922	Nasal septal prosthesis. See also code 30220.	*Cross-reference CPT 30220*
D5923	Ocular prosthesis, interim. See also code 92330.	*Cross-reference CPT 92330*
D5924	Cranial prosthesis. See also code 62143.	*Cross-reference CPT 62143*
D5925	Facial augmentation implant prosthesis. See also code 21208.	*Cross-reference CPT 21208*
D5926	Nasal prosthesis, replacement. See also code 21087.	*Cross-reference CPT 21087*
D5927	Auricular prosthesis, replacement. See also code 21086.	*Cross-reference CPT 21086*
D5928	Orbital prosthesis, replacement. See also code 67550.	*Cross-reference CPT 67550*
D5929	Facial prosthesis, replacement. See also code 21088.	*Cross-reference CPT 21088*
D5931	Obturator prosthesis, surgical. See also code 21079.	*Cross-reference CPT 21079*
D5932	Obturator prosthesis, definitive. See also code 21080.	*Cross-reference CPT 21080*
D5933	Obturator prosthesis, modification. See also code 21080.	*Cross-reference CPT 21080*
D5934	Mandibular resection prosthesis with guide flange. See also code 21081.	*Cross-reference CPT 21081*
D5935	Mandibular resection prosthesis without guide flange. See also code 21081.	*Cross-reference CPT 21081*
D5936	Obturator/prosthesis, interim. See also code 21079.	*Cross-reference CPT 21079*
D5937	Trismus appliance (not for TMD treatment)	*MCM 2130*
D5951	Feeding aid	*MCM 2336, MCM 2130, ASC*

D Codes

	= Special Coverage Instructions Apply		= Carrier Discretion
	= Noncovered by Medicare or Medicare Statute		

D5952 Speech aid prosthesis, pediatric. See also code 21084.

Cross-reference CPT 21084

D5953 Speech aid prosthesis, adult. See also code 21084.

Cross-reference CPT 21084

D5954 Palatal augmentation prosthesis. See also code 21082.

Cross-reference CPT 21082

D5955 Palatal lift prosthesis, definitive. See also code 21083.

Cross-reference CPT 21083

D5958 Palatal lift prosthesis, interim. See also code 21083.

Cross-reference CPT 21083

D5959 Palatal lift prosthesis, modification. See also code 21083.

Cross-reference CPT 21083

D5960 Speech aid prosthesis, modification. See also code 21084.

Cross-reference CPT 21084

D5982 Surgical stent. See also code 21085.   *Cross-reference CPT 21085*

D5983 Radiation carrier   *MCM 2336, MCM 2136, ASC*

D5984 Radiation shield   *MCM 2336, MCM 2136, ASC*

D5985 Radiation cone locator   *MCM 2336, MCM 2136, ASC*

D5986 Fluoride gel carrier   *MCM 2336, MCM 2136*

D5987 Commissure splint   *MCM 2336, MCM 2136, ASC*

D5988 Surgical splint. See also CPT.   *Cross-reference CPT*

D5999 Unspecified maxillofacial prosthesis, by report. See also CPT.

Cross-reference CPT

Implant Services D6000–D6199

D6010 Surgical placement of implant body: endosteal implant. See also code 21248.   *Cross-reference CPT 21248*

D6020 Abutment placement or substitution: endosteal implant. See also code 21248.   *Cross-reference CPT 21248*

D6040 Surgical placement: eposteal implant. See also code 21245.

Cross-reference CPT 21245

D6050 Surgical placement: transosteal implant. See also code 21244.

Cross-reference CPT 21244

D6055 Dental implant supported connecting bar   *MCM 2136*

D6056 Prefabricated abutment

D6057 Custom abutment

D6058 Abutment supported porcelain/ceramic crown

D6059 Abutment supported porcelain fused to metal crown (high noble metal)

= Invalid Medicare Code (no grace period)

= Code may require certificate of medical necessity (CMN) or DMERC information form (DIF)

D6060	Abutment supported porcelain fused to metal crown (predominantly base metal)
D6061	Abutment supported porcelain fused to metal crown (noble metal)
D6062	Abutment supported cast metal crown (high noble metal)
D6063	Abutment supported cast metal crown (predominantly base metal)
D6064	Abutment supported cast metal crown (noble metal)
D6065	Implant supported porcelain/ceramic crown
D6066	Implant supported porcelain fused to metal crown (titanium, titanium alloy, high noble metal)
D6067	Implant supported metal crown (titanium, titanium alloy, high noble metal)
D6068	Abutment supported retainer for porcelain/ceramic FPD
D6069	Abutment supported retainer for porcelain fused to metal FPD (high noble metal)
D6070	Abutment supported retainer for porcelain fused to metal FPD (predominately base metal)
D6071	Abutment supported retainer for porcelain fused to metal FPD (noble metal)
D6072	Abutment supported retainer for cast metal FPD (high noble metal)
D6073	Abutment supported retainer for cast metal FPD (predominately base metal)
D6074	Abutment supported retainer for cast metal FPD (noble metal)
D6075	Implant supported retainer for ceramic FPD
D6076	Implant supported retainer for porcelain fused to metal FPD (titanium, titanium alloy, or high noble metal)
D6077	Implant supported retainer for cast metal FPD (titanium, titanium alloy, or high noble metal)
D6078	Implant/abutment supported fixed denture for completely edentulous arch
D6079	Implant/abutment supported fixed denture for partially edentulous arch
D6080	Implant maintenance procedures, including removal of prosthesis, cleansing of prosthesis and abutments, reinsertion of prosthesis *MCM 2136*
D6090	Repair implant supported prosthesis, by report. See also code 21299. *Cross-reference CPT 21299*
D6095	Repair implant abutment, by report. See also code 21299.
D6100	Implant removal, by report. See also code 21299. *Cross-reference CPT 21299*
D6199	Unspecified implant procedure, by report. See also code 21299. *Cross-reference CPT 21299*

D Codes

= Special Coverage Instructions Apply   = Carrier Discretion

= Noncovered by Medicare or Medicare Statute

Prosthodontics (Fixed) D6200–D6999

Fixed Partial Denture Pontics

D6210	Pontic — cast high noble metal	*Medicare Statute 1862A (12)*
D6211	Pontic — cast predominantly base metal	*Medicare Statute 1862A (12)*
D6212	Pontic — cast noble metal	*Medicare Statute 1862A (12)*
D6240	Pontic — porcelain fused to high noble metal	*Medicare Statute 1862A (12)*
D6241	Pontic — porcelain fused to predominantly base metal	
		Medicare Statute 1862A (12)
D6242	Pontic — porcelain fused to noble metal	*Medicare Statute 1862A (12)*
D6245	Pontic — porcelain/ceramic	
D6250	Pontic — resin with high noble metal	*Medicare Statute 1862A (12)*
D6251	Pontic — resin with predominantly base metal	*Medicare Statute 1862A (12)*
D6252	Pontic — resin with noble metal	*Medicare Statute 1862A (12)*
D6519	Inlay/onlay — porcelain/ceramic	

Fixed Partial Denture Retainers — Inlays/Onlays

D6520	Inlay — metallic — two surfaces	*Medicare Statute 1862A (12)*
D6530	Inlay — metallic — three or more surfaces	*Medicare Statute 1862A (12)*
D6543	Onlay — metallic — three surfaces	*Medicare Statute 1862A (12)*
D6544	Onlay — metallic — four or more surfaces	*Medicare Statute 1862A (12)*
D6545	Retainer — cast metal for resin bonded fixed prosthesis	
		Medicare Statute 1862A (12)
D6548	Retainer — porcelain/ceramic for resin bonded fixed prosthesis	

Fixed Partial Denture Retainers — Crowns

D6720	Crown — resin with high noble metal	*Medicare Statute 1862A (12)*
D6721	Crown — resin with predominantly base metal	*Medicare Statute 1862A (12)*
D6722	Crown — resin with noble metal	*Medicare Statute 1862A (12)*
D6740	Crown — porcelain/ceramic	
D6750	Crown — porcelain fused to high noble metal	*Medicare Statute 1862A (12)*
D6751	Crown — porcelain fused to predominantly base metal	
		Medicare Statute 1862A (12)
D6752	Crown — porcelain fused to noble metal	*Medicare Statute 1862A (12)*
D6780	Crown — 3⁄4 cast high noble metal	*Medicare Statute 1862A (12)*
D6781	Crown — 3/4 cast predominately based metal	
D6782	Crown — 3/4 cast noble metal	
D6783	Crown — 3/4 porcelain/ceramic	
D6790	Crown — full cast high noble metal	*Medicare Statute 1862A (12)*
D6791	Crown — full cast predominantly base metal	*Medicare Statute 1862A (12)*

	= Invalid Medicare Code (no grace period)
	= Code may require certificate of medical necessity (CMN) or DMERC information form (DIF)

| D6792 | Crown — full cast noble metal | Medicare Statute 1862A (12) |

Other Fixed Partial Denture Services

D6920	Connector bar	CIM 50-26, MCM 2136, MCM 2336, ASC
D6930	Recement fixed partial denture	Medicare Statute 1862A (12)
D6940	Stress breaker	Medicare Statute 1862A (12)
D6950	Precision attachment	Medicare Statute 1862A (12)
D6970	Cast post and core in addition to fixed partial denture retainer
		Medicare Statute 1862A (12)
D6971	Cast post as part of fixed partial denture retainer
		Medicare Statute 1862A (12)
D6972	Prefabricated post and core in addition to fixed partial denture retainer
		Medicare Statute 1862A (12)
D6973	Core build up for retainer, including any pins	Medicare Statute 1862A (12)
D6975	Coping — metal	Medicare Statute 1862A (12)
D6976	Each additional cast post — same tooth
D6977	Each additional prefabricated post — same tooth
D6980	Fixed partial denture repair, by report	Medicare Statute 1862A (12)
D6999	Unspecified, fixed prosthodontic procedure, by report
		Medicare Statute 1862A (12)

Oral and Maxillofacial Surgery D7000–D7999

Extraction (Includes Local Anesthesia and Routine Postoperative Care)

D7110	Extraction — single tooth	MCM 2336, MCM 2136, ASC
D7120	Extraction — each additional tooth	MCM 2336, MCM 2136, ASC
D7130	Root removal — exposed roots	MCM 2336, MCM 2136, ASC

Surgical Extractions (Includes Local Anesthesia and Routine Postoperative Care)

D7210	Surgical removal of erupted tooth requiring elevation of mucoperiosteal flap and removal of bone and/or section of tooth
		MCM 2336, MCM 2136, ASC
D7220	Removal of impacted tooth — soft tissue	MCM 2336, MCM 2136, ASC
D7230	Removal of impacted tooth — partially bony	ASC
D7240	Removal of impacted tooth — completely bony
		MCM 2336, MCM 2136, ASC
D7241	Removal of impacted tooth — completely bony, with unusual surgical complications	MCM 2336, MCM 2136, ASC
D7250	Surgical removal of residual tooth roots (cutting procedure)
		MCM 2336, MCM 2136, ASC

D Codes

= Special Coverage Instructions Apply   = Carrier Discretion

= Noncovered by Medicare or Medicare Statute

Other Surgical Procedures

D7260 Orolantral fistula closure *MCM 2336, MCM 2136, ASC*

D7270 Tooth reimplantation and/or stabilization of accidentally evulsed or displaced tooth and/or alveolus *MCM 2336, MCM 2136*

D7272 Tooth transplantation (includes reimplantation from one site to another and splinting and/or stabilization) *Medicare Statute 1862A (12)*

D7280 Surgical exposure of impacted or unerupted tooth for orthodontic reasons (including orthodontic attachments) *Medicare Statute 1862A (12)*

D7281 Surgical exposure of impacted or unerupted tooth to aid eruption *Medicare Statute 1862A (12)*

D7285 Biopsy of oral tissue — hard (bone, tooth) See also codes 20220, 20225, 20240, 20245. *Cross-reference CPT 20220, 20225, 20240, 20245*

D7286 Biopsy of oral tissue — soft (all others) See also code 40808. *Cross-reference CPT 40808*

D7290 Surgical repositioning of teeth *Medicare Statute 1862A (12)*

D7291 Transseptal fiberotomy, by report *MCM 2336, MCM 2136, ASC*

Alveoloplasty — Surgical Preparation of Ridge for Dentures

D7310 Alveoloplasty in conjunction with extractions — per quadrant. See also code 41874. *Cross-reference CPT 41874*

D7320 Alveoloplasty not in conjunction with extractions — per quadrant. See also code 41870. *Cross-reference CPT 41870*

Vestibuloplasty

D7340 Vestibuloplasty — ridge extension (second epithelialization), See also codes 40840, 40842, 40843, 40844. *Cross-reference CPT 40840, 40842, 40843, 40844*

D7350 Vestibuloplasty — ridge extension (including soft tissue grafts, muscle reattachments, revision of soft tissue attachment and management of hypertrophied and hyperplastic tissue). See also code 40845. *Cross-reference CPT 40845*

Surgical Excision of Reactive Inflammatory Lesions (Scar Tissue or Localized Congenital Lesions)

D7410 Radical excision — lesion diameter up to 1.25 cm. See also CPT. *Cross-reference CPT*

D7420 Radical excision — lesion diameter greater than 1.25 cm. See also CPT. *Cross-reference CPT*

Removal of Tumors, Cysts, and Neoplasms

D7430 Excision of benign tumor – lesion diameter up to 1.25 cm. See also CPT. *Cross-reference CPT*

D7431 Excision of benign tumor – lesion diameter greater than 1.25 cm. See also CPT. *Cross-reference CPT*

= Invalid Medicare Code (no grace period)

= Code may require certificate of medical necessity (CMN) or DMERC information form (DIF)

D7440	Excision of malignant tumor – lesion diameter up to 1.25 cm. See also CPT. *Cross-reference CPT*
D7441	Excision of malignant tumor – lesion diameter greater than 1.25 cm. See also CPT. *Cross-reference CPT*
D7450	Removal of odontogenic cyst or tumor – lesion diameter up to 1.25 cm. See also CPT. *Cross-reference CPT*
D7451	Removal of odontogenic cyst or tumor – lesion diameter greater than 1.25 cm. See also CPT. *Cross-reference CPT*
D7460	Removal of nonodontogenic cyst or tumor – lesion diameter up to 1.25 cm. See also CPT. *Cross-reference CPT*
D7461	Removal of nonodontogenic cyst or tumor – lesion diameter greater than 1.25 cm. See also CPT. *Cross-reference CPT*
D7465	Destruction of lesion(s) by physical or chemical method, by report. See also code 41850. *Cross-reference CPT 41850*
D7471	Removal of exostosis — per site
D7480	Partial ostectomy (guttering or saucerization). See also code 21025. *Cross-reference CPT 21025*
D7490	Radical resection of mandible with bone graft. See also code 21095. *Cross-reference CPT 21095*

Surgical Incision

D7510	Incision and drainage of abscess – intraoral soft tissue. See also code 41800. *Cross-reference CPT 41800*
D7520	Incision and drainage of abscess – extraoral soft tissue. See also code 40800. *Cross-reference CPT 40800*
D7530	Removal of foreign body, skin, or subcutaneous alveolar tissue. See also codes 41805, 41828. *Cross-reference CPT 41805, 41828*
D7540	Removal of reaction-producing foreign bodies, musculoskeletal system. See also codes 20520, 41800, 41806. *Cross-reference CPT 20520, 41800, 41806*
D7550	Sequestrectomy for osteomyelitis. See also code 20999. *Cross-reference CPT 20999*
D7560	Maxillary sinusotomy for removal of tooth fragment or foreign body. See also code 31020. *Cross-reference CPT 31020*

Treatment of Fractures — Simple

D7610	Maxilla — open reduction (teeth immobilized, if present). See also CPT. *Cross-reference CPT*
D7620	Maxilla — closed reduction (teeth immobilized, if present). See also CPT. *Cross-reference CPT*
D7630	Mandible — open reduction (teeth immobilized, if present). See also CPT. *Cross-reference CPT*

D Codes

= Special Coverage Instructions Apply   = Carrier Discretion

= Noncovered by Medicare or Medicare Statute

D7640 Mandible — closed reduction (teeth immobilized, if present). See also CPT. *Cross-reference CPT*

D7650 Malar and/or zygomatic arch — open reduction. See also CPT. *Cross-reference CPT*

D7660 Malar and/or zygomatic arch — closed reduction. See also CPT. *Cross-reference CPT*

D7670 Alveolus — stabilization of teeth, closed reduction splinting. See also CPT. *Cross-reference CPT*

D7680 Facial bones — complicated reduction with fixation and multiple surgical approaches. See also CPT. *Cross-reference CPT*

Treatment of Fractures — Compound

D7710 Maxilla — open reduction. See also code 21346. *Cross-reference CPT 21346*

D7720 Maxilla — closed reduction. See also code 21345. *Cross-reference CPT 21345*

D7730 Mandible — open reduction. See also codes 21461, 21462. *Cross-reference CPT 21461, 21462*

D7740 Mandible — closed reduction. See also code 21455. *Cross-reference CPT 21455*

D7750 Malar and/or zygomatic arch — open reduction. See also codes 21360, 21365. *Cross-reference CPT 21360, 21365*

D7760 Malar and/or zygomatic arch — closed reduction. See also code 21355. *Cross-reference CPT 21355*

D7770 Alveolus — stabilization of teeth, open reduction splinting. See also code 21422. *Cross-reference CPT 21422*

D7780 Facial bones — complicated reduction with fixation and multiple surgical approaches. See also codes 21433, 21435, 21436. *Cross-reference CPT 21433, 21435*

Reduction of Dislocation and Management of Other Temporomandibular Joint Dysfunctions

Procedures which are an integral part of a primary procedure should not be reported separately.

D7810 Open reduction of dislocation. See also code 21490. *Cross-reference CPT 21490*

D7820 Closed reduction of dislocation. See also code 21480. *Cross-reference CPT 21480*

D7830 Manipulation under anesthesia. See also code 00190. *Cross-reference CPT 00190*

D7840 Condylectomy. See also code 21050. *Cross-reference CPT 21050*

D7850 Surgical discectomy, with/without implant. See also code 21060. *Cross-reference CPT 21060*

D7852 Disc repair. See also code 21299. *Cross-reference CPT 21299*

= Invalid Medicare Code (no grace period)

= Code may require certificate of medical necessity (CMN) or DMERC information form (DIF)

D7854	Synovectomy. See also code 21299.	*Cross-reference CPT 21299*
D7856	Myotomy. See also code 21299.	*Cross-reference CPT 21299*
D7858	Joint reconstruction. See also codes 21242, 21243.	
		Cross-reference CPT 21242, 21243
D7860	Arthrotomy	*MCM 2336, MCM 2136*
D7865	Arthroplasty. See also code 21240.	*Cross-reference CPT 21240*
D7870	Arthrocentesis. See also code 21060.	*Cross-reference CPT 21060*
D7871	Non-arthroscopic lysis and lavage	
D7872	Arthroscopy — diagnosis, with or without biopsy. See also code 29800.	
	Cross-reference CPT 29800	
D7873	Arthroscopy — surgical: lavage and lysis of adhesions. See also code 29804.	*Cross-reference CPT 29804*
D7874	Arthroscopy — surgical: disc repositioning and stabilization. See also code 29804.	*Cross-reference CPT 29804*
D7875	Arthroscopy — surgical: synovectomy. See also code 29804.	*Cross-reference CPT 29804*
D7876	Arthroscopy — surgical: discectomy. See also code 29804. *Cross-reference CPT 29804*	
D7877	Arthroscopy — surgical: debridement. See also code 29804.	*Cross-reference CPT 29804*
D7880	Occlusal orthotic device, by report. See also code 21499.	*Cross-reference CPT 21499*
D7899	Unspecified TMD therapy, by report. See also code 21499.	*Cross-reference CPT 21499*

D Codes

Repair of Traumatic Wounds

D7910	Suture of recent small wounds up to 5 cm. See also codes 12011, 12013.	*Cross-reference CPT 12011, 12012*

Complicated Suturing (Reconstruction Requiring Delicate Handling of Tissues and Wide Undermining for Meticulous Closure)

D7911	Complicated suture — up to 5 cm. See also codes 12051, 12052.	*Cross-reference CPT 12051, 12052*
D7912	Complicated suture — greater than 5 cm. See also code 13132.	*Cross-reference CPT 13132*

Other Repair Procedures

D7920	Skin graft (identify defect covered, location and type of graft). See also CPT.	*Cross-reference CPT*
D7940	Osteoplasty — for orthognathic deformities	*MCM 2336, MCM 2136, ASC*
D7941	Osteotomy — mandibular rami. See also codes 21193, 21195, 21196.	*Cross-reference CPT 21193, 21195, 21196*

= Special Coverage Instructions Apply	= Carrier Discretion
= Noncovered by Medicare or Medicare Statute	

D7943 Osteotomy — mandibular rami with bone graft; includes obtaining the graft. See also code 21194. *Cross-reference CPT 21194*

D7944 Osteotomy — segmented or subapical — per sextant or quadrant. See also codes 21198, 21206. *Cross-reference CPT 21198, 21206*

D7945 Osteotomy — body of mandible. See also codes 21193, 21194, 21195, 21196. *Cross-reference CPT 21193, 21194, 21195, 21196*

D7946 LeFort I (maxilla — total). See also code 21147. *Cross-reference CPT 21147*

D7947 LeFort I (maxilla — segmented). See also codes 21145, 21146. *Cross-reference CPT 21145, 21146*

D7948 LeFort II or LeFort III (osteoplasty of facial bones for midface hypoplasia or retrusion) — without bone graft. See also code 21150. *Cross-reference CPT 21150*

D7949 LeFort II or LeFort III — with bone graft. See also CPT. *Cross-reference CPT*

D7950 Osseous, osteoperiosteal, or cartilage graft of the mandible or facial bones— autogenous or nonautogenous, by report. See also code 21247. *Cross-reference CPT 21247*

D7955 Repair of maxillofacial soft and hard tissue defect. See also code 21299. *Cross-reference CPT 21299*

D7960 Frenulectomy (frenectomy or frenotomy) — separate procedure. See also codes 40819, 41010, 41115. *Cross-reference CPT 40819, 41010, 41115*

D7970 Excision of hyperplastic tissue — per arch. See also CPT. *Cross-reference CPT*

D7971 Excision of pericoronal gingiva. See also code 41821. *Cross-reference CPT 41821*

D7980 Sialolithotomy. See also codes 42330, 42335, 42340. *Cross-reference CPT 42330, 42335, 42340*

D7981 Excision of salivary gland, by report. See also code 42408. *Cross-reference CPT 42408*

D7982 Sialodochoplasty. See also code 42500. *Cross-reference CPT 42500*

D7983 Closure of salivary fistula. See also code 42600. *Cross-reference CPT 42600*

D7990 Emergency tracheotomy. See also codes 31603, 31605. *Cross-reference CPT 31605*

D7991 Coronoidectomy. See also code 21070. *Cross-reference CPT 21070*

D7995 Synthetic graft — mandible or facial bones, by report. See also code 21299. *Cross-reference CPT 21299*

D7996 Implant — mandible for augmentation purposes (excluding alveolar ridge), by report. See also code 21299. *Cross-reference CPT 21299*

D7997 Appliance removal (not by dentist who placed appliance), includes removal of archbar

D7999 Unspecified oral surgery procedure, by report. See also code 21299. *Cross-reference CPT 21299*

= Invalid Medicare Code (no grace period)

= Code may require certificate of medical necessity (CMN) or DMERC information form (DIF)

Orthodontics D8000–D8999

D8010	Limited orthodontic treatment of the primary dentition	
		Medicare Statute 1862A (12)
D8020	Limited orthodontic treatment of the transitional dentition	
		Medicare Statute 1862A (12)
D8030	Limited orthodontic treatment of the adolescent dentition	
		Medicare Statute 1862A (12)
D8040	Limited orthodontic treatment of the adult dentition	
		Medicare Statute 1862A (12)
D8050	Interceptive orthodontic treatment of the primary dentition	
		Medicare Statute 1862A (12)
D8060	Interceptive orthodontic treatment of the transitional dentition	
		Medicare Statute 1862A (12)
D8070	Comprehensive orthodontic treatment of the transitional dentition	
		Medicare Statute 1862A (12)
D8080	Comprehensive orthodontic treatment of the adolescent dentition	
		Medicare Statute 1862A (12)
D8090	Comprehensive orthodontic treatment of the adult dentition	
		Medicare Statute 1862A (12)

Minor Treatment to Control Harmful Habits

D8210	Removable appliance therapy	*Medicare Statute 1862A (12)*
D8220	Fixed appliance therapy	*Medicare Statute 1862A (12)*

Other Orthodontic Services

D8660	Pre-orthodontic treatment visit	*Medicare Statute 1862A (12)*
D8670	Periodic orthodontic treatment visit (as part of contract) *Medicare Statute 1862A (12)*	
D8680	Orthodontic retention (removal of appliances, construction and placement of retainer(s))	*Medicare Statute 1862A (12)*
D8690	Orthodontic treatment (alternative billing to a contract fee)	
		Medicare Statute 1862A (12)
D8691	Repair of orthodontic appliance	
D8692	Replacement of lost or broken retainer	
D8999	Unspecified orthodontic procedure, by report *Medicare Statute 1862A (12)*	

Adjunctive General Services D9110–D9999

Unclassified Treatment

D9110	Palliative (emergency) treatment of dental pain — minor procedure	
		MCM 2336, MCM 2136, ASC

D Codes

▨ = Special Coverage Instructions Apply	▨ = Carrier Discretion
■ = Noncovered by Medicare or Medicare Statute	

Anesthesia

D9210 Local anesthesia not in conjunction with operative or surgical procedures. See also code 90784. *Cross-reference CPT 90784*

D9211 Regional block anesthesia. See also code 01995. *Cross-reference CPT 01995*

D9212 Trigeminal division block anesthesia. See also code 64400.
Cross-reference CPT 64400

D9215 Local anesthesia. See also code 90784. *Cross-reference CPT 90784*

D9220 General anesthesia — first 30 minutes. See also CPT. *Cross-reference CPT*

D9221 General anesthesia — each additional 15 minutes *MCM 2336, MCM 2136*

D9230 Analgesia, anxiolysis, inhalation of nitrous oxide
MCM 2336, MCM 2136, ASC

D9241 Intravenous sedation/analgesia — first 30 minutes

D9242 Intravenous sedation/analgesia — each additional 15 minutes

D9248 Non-intravenous conscious sedation

Professional Consultation

D9310 Consultation (diagnostic service provided by dentist or physician other than practitioner providing treatment). See also CPT. *Cross-reference CPT*

Professional Visits

D9410 House/extended care facility call. See also CPT. *Cross-reference CPT*

D9420 Hospital call. See also CPT. *Cross-reference CPT*

D9430 Office visit for observation (during regularly scheduled hours) — no other services performed. See also CPT. *Cross-reference CPT*

D9440 Office visit — after regularly scheduled hours. See also code 99050.
Cross-reference CPT 99050

Drugs

D9610 Therapeutic drug injection, by report. See also codes 90784, 90788.
Cross-reference CPT 90784, 90788

D9630 Other drugs and/or medicaments, by report *MCM 2336, MCM 2136, ASC*

Miscellaneous Services

D9910 Application of desensitizing medicament *Medicare Statute 1862A (12)*

D9911 Application of desensitizing resin for cervical and/or root surface, per tooth

D9920 Behavior management, by report *Medicare Statute 1862A (12)*

D9930 Treatment of complications (post-surgical) — unusual circumstances, by report *MCM 2336, MCM 2136, ASC*

D9940 Occlusal guard, by report *MCM 2336, MCM 2136, ASC*

D9941 Fabrication of athletic mouthguard. See also code 21089.
Medicare Statute 1862A (12); Cross-reference CPT 21089

D9950 Occlusion analysis — mounted case *MCM 2336, MCM 2136, ASC*

= Invalid Medicare Code (no grace period)

= Code may require certificate of medical necessity (CMN) or DMERC information form (DIF)

Code	Description	
D9951	Occlusal adjustment — limited	*MCM 2336, MCM 2136, ASC*
D9952	Occlusal adjustment — complete	*MCM 2336, MCM 2136, ASC*
D9970	Enamel microabrasion	*Medicare Statute 1862A (12)*
D9971	Odontoplasty 1–2 teeth; includes removal of enamel projections	
D9972	External bleaching — per arch	
D9973	External bleaching — per tooth	
D9974	Internal bleaching — per tooth	
D9999	Unspecified adjunctive procedure, by report	*Cross-reference CPT 21499*

D Codes

= Special Coverage Instructions Apply   = Carrier Discretion

= Noncovered by Medicare or Medicare Statute

Durable Medical Equipment E0100–E9999

Before an item can be considered to be durable medical equipment, it must meet all the following requirements: it must be able to withstand repeated use; be primarily and customarily used to serve a medical purpose; generally not useful to a person in the absence of an illness or injury; and appropriate for use in the home.

Canes

E0100 Cane, includes canes of all materials, adjustable or fixed, with tip
CIM 60-3, CIM 60-9, MCM 2100.1, ASC

E0105 Cane, quad or three-prong, includes canes of all materials, adjustable or fixed, with tips
CIM 60-15, CIM 60-9, MCM 2100.1, ASC

Crutches

E0110 Crutches, forearm, includes crutches of various materials, adjustable or fixed, pair, complete with tips and handgrips *CIM 60-9, MCM 2100.1, ASC*

E0111 Crutch, forearm, includes crutches of various materials, adjustable or fixed, each, with tip and handgrip *CIM 60-9, MCM 2100.1, ASC*

E0112 Crutches, underarm, wood, adjustable or fixed, pair, with pads, tips and handgrips *CIM 60-9, MCM 2100.1, ASC*

E0113 Crutch, underarm, wood, adjustable or fixed, each, with pad, tip and handgrip *CIM 60-9, MCM 2100.1, ASC*

E0114 Crutches, underarm, other than wood, adjustable or fixed, pair, with pads, tips and handgrips *CIM 60-9, MCM 2100.1, ASC*

E0116 Crutch, underarm, other than wood, adjustable or fixed, each, with pad, tip and handgrip *CIM 60-9, MCM 2100.1, ASC*

Walkers

E0130 Walker, rigid (pickup), adjustable or fixed height
CIM 60-9, MCM 2100.1, ASC

E0135 Walker, folding (pickup), adjustable or fixed height
CIM 60-9, MCM 2100.1, ASC

E0141 Rigid walker, wheeled, without seat *CIM 60-9, MCM 2100.1, ASC*

E0142 Rigid walker, wheeled, with seat *CIM 60-9, MCM 2100.1, ASC*

E0143 Folding walker, wheeled, without seat *CIM 60-9, MCM 2100.1, ASC*

E0144 Enclosed, framed folding walker, wheeled, with posterior seat
CIM 60-9, MCM 2100.1

E0145 Walker, wheeled, with seat and crutch attachments
CIM 60-9, MCM 2100.1, ASC

E0146 Folding walker, wheeled, with seat *CIM 60-9, MCM 2100.1, ASC*

E0147 Heavy duty, multiple breaking system, variable wheel resistance walker
CIM 60-15, MCM 2100.1, ASC

E Codes

▨ = Special Coverage Instructions Apply ▨ = Carrier Discretion

▨ = Noncovered by Medicare or Medicare Statute

- **E0148** Walker, heavy duty, without wheels, rigid or folding, any type, each
- **E0149** Walker, heavy duty, wheeled, rigid or folding, any type, each

E0153 Platform attachment, forearm crutch, each *ASC*

E0154 Platform attachment, walker, each *ASC*

E0155 Wheel attachment, rigid pick-up walker, per pair seat attachment, walker

Attachments

E0156 Seat attachment, walker *ASC*

E0157 Crutch attachment, walker, each *ASC*

E0158 Leg extensions for walker, per set of four (4)

E0159 Brake attachment for wheeled walker, replacement, each *ASC*

Commodes

E0160 Sitz type bath or equipment, portable, used with or without commode
CIM 60-9, ASC

E0161 Sitz type bath or equipment, portable, used with or without commode, with faucet attachment/s *CIM 60-9, ASC*

E0162 Sitz bath chair *CIM 60-9, ASC*

E0163 Commode chair, stationary, with fixed arms *CIM 60-9, MCM 2100.1, ASC*

E0164 Commode chair, mobile, with fixed arms *CIM 60-9, MCM 2100.1, ASC*

E0165 Commode chair, stationary, with detachable arms
CIM 60-9, MCM 2100.1, ASC

E0166 Commode chair, mobile, with detachable arms
CIM 60-9, MCM 2100.1, ASC

E0167 Pail or pan for use with commode chair *CIM 60-9, ASC*

- **E0168** Commode chair, extra wide and/or heavy duty, stationary or mobile, with or without arms, any type, each

E0175 Foot rest, for use with commode chair, each *ASC*

E0176 Air pressure pad or cushion, nonpositioning *CIM 60-9, ASC*

E0177 Water pressure pad or cushion, nonpositioning *CIM 60-9, ASC*

E0178 Gel or gel-like pressure pad or cushion, nonpositioning *CIM 60-9, ASC*

E0179 Dry pressure pad or cushion, nonpositioning *CIM 60-9, ASC*

Decubitis Care Equipment

E0180 Pressure pad, alternating with pump *CIM 60-9, MCM 4107.6, ASC*

E0181 Pressure pad, alternating with pump, heavy duty
CIM 60-9, MCM 4107.6, ASC

E0182 Pump for alternating pressure pad *CIM 60-9, MCM 4107.6, ASC*

E0184 Dry pressure mattress *CIM 60-9, MCM 4107.6, ASC*

= Invalid Medicare Code (no grace period)

= Code may require certificate of medical necessity (CMN) or DMERC information form (DIF)

E0185	Gel or gel-like pressure pad for mattress, standard mattress length and width	CIM 60-9, MCM 4107.6, ASC
E0186	Air pressure mattress	CIM 60-9, ASC
E0187	Water pressure mattress	CIM 60-9, ASC
E0188	Synthetic sheepskin pad	CIM 60-9, MCM 4107.6, ASC
E0189	Lambswool sheepskin pad, any size	CIM 60-9, MCM 4107.6, ASC
E0191	Heel or elbow protector, each	ASC
E0192	Low pressure and positioning equalization pad, for wheelchair	CIM 60-9, MCM 4107.6, ASC
E0193	Powered air flotation bed (low air loss therapy)	ASC
E0194	Air fluidized bed	CIM 60-9, ASC
E0196	Gel pressure mattress	CIM 60-9, ASC
E0197	Air pressure pad for mattress, standard mattress length and width	CIM 60-9, ASC
E0198	Water pressure pad for mattress, standard mattress length and width	CIM 60-9, ASC
E0199	Dry pressure pad for mattress, standard mattress length and width	CIM 60-9, ASC

Heat/Cold Application

E0200	Heat lamp, without stand (table model), includes bulb, or infrared element	CIM 60-9, MCM 2100.1, ASC
E0202	Phototherapy (bilirubin) light with photometer	ASC
E0205	Heat lamp, with stand, includes bulb, or infrared element	CIM 60-9, MCM 2100.1, ASC
E0210	Electric heat pad, standard	CIM 60-9, ASC
E0215	Electric heat pad, moist	CIM 60-9, ASC
E0217	Water circulating heat pad with pump	CIM 60-9, ASC
E0218	Water circulating cold pad with pump	CIM 60-9, ASC
E0220	Hot water bottle	ASC
E0225	Hydrocollator unit, includes pads	CIM 60-9, MCM 2210.3, ASC
E0230	Ice cap or collar	ASC
E0235	Paraffin bath unit, portable (see medical supply code A4265 for paraffin)	CIM 60-9, MCM 2210.3, ASC
E0236	Pump for water circulating pad	CIM 60-9, ASC
E0238	Nonelectric heat pad, moist	CIM 60-9, ASC
E0239	Hydrocollator unit, portable	CIM 60-9 MCM 2210.3, ASC

Bath and Toilet Aids

E0241	Bathtub wall rail, each	CIM 60-9, MCM 2100.1, ASC

E Codes

= Special Coverage Instructions Apply   = Carrier Discretion

= Noncovered by Medicare or Medicare Statute

E0242	Bathtub rail, floor base	CIM 60-9, MCM 2100.1, ASC
E0243	Toilet rail, each	CIM 60-9, MCM 2100.1, ASC
E0244	Raised toilet seat	CIM 60-9, ASC
E0245	Tub stool or bench	CIM 60-9, ASC
E0246	Transfer tub rail attachment	ASC
E0249	Pad for water circulating heat unit	CIM 60-9, ASC

Hospital Beds and Accessories

E0250	Hospital bed, fixed height, with any type side rails, with mattress	CIM 60-18, MCM 2100.1, ASC
E0251	Hospital bed, fixed height, with any type side rails, without mattress	CIM 60-18 MCM 2100.1, ASC
E0255	Hospital bed, variable height, hi-lo, with any type side rails, with mattress	CIM 60-18, MCM 2100.1, ASC
E0256	Hospital bed, variable height, hi-lo, with any type side rails, without mattress	CIM 60-18, MCM 2100.1, ASC
E0260	Hospital bed, semi-electric (head and foot adjustment), with any type side rails, with mattress	CIM 60-18, MCM 2100.1, ASC
E0261	Hospital bed, semi-electric (head and foot adjustment), with any type side rails, without mattress	CIM 60-18 MCM 2100.1, ASC
E0265	Hospital bed, total electric (head, foot, and height adjustments), with any type side rails, with mattress	CIM 60-18 MCM 2100.1, ASC
E0266	Hospital bed, total electric (head, foot, and height adjustments), with any type side rails, without mattress	CIM 60-18, MCM 2100.1, ASC
E0270	Hospital bed, institutional type includes: oscillating, circulating and stryker frame, with mattress	CIM 60-9, ASC
E0271	Mattress, inner spring	CIM 60-18, CIM 60-9, ASC
E0272	Mattress, foam rubber	CIM 60-18, CIM 60-9, ASC
E0273	Bed board	CIM 60-9, ASC
E0274	Over-bed table	CIM 60-9, ASC
E0275	Bed pan, standard, metal or plastic	CIM 60-9, ASC
E0276	Bed pan, fracture, metal or plastic	CIM 60-9, ASC
E0277	Powered pressure-reducing air mattress	CIM 60-9, ASC
E0280	Bed cradle, any type	ASC
E0290	Hospital bed, fixed height, without side rails, with mattress	CIM 60-18, MCM 2100.1, ASC
E0291	Hospital bed, fixed height, without side rails, without mattress	CIM 60-18, MCM 2100.1, ASC
E0292	Hospital bed, variable height, hi-lo, without side rails, with mattress	CIM 60-18, MCM 2100.1, ASC

= Invalid Medicare Code (no grace period)

= Code may require certificate of medical necessity (CMN) or DMERC information form (DIF)

E0293	Hospital bed, variable height, hi-lo, without side rails, without mattress	*CIM 60-18, MCM 2100.1, ASC*
E0294	Hospital bed, semi-electric (head and foot adjustment), without side rails, with mattress	*CIM 60-18, MCM 2100.1, ASC*
E0295	Hospital bed, semi-electric (head and foot adjustment), without side rails, without mattress	*CIM 60-18, MCM 2100.1, ASC*
E0296	Hospital bed, total electric (head, foot, and height adjustments), without side rails, with mattress	*CIM 60-18, MCM 2100.1, ASC*
E0297	Hospital bed, total electric (head, foot, and height adjustments), without side rails, without mattress	*CIM 60-18, MCM 2100.1, ASC*
● **E0298**	Hospital bed, heavy duty, extra wide, with any type side rails, with mattress	
E0305	Bedside rails, half-length	*CIM 60-18, ASC*
E0310	Bedside rails, full-length	*CIM 60-18, ASC*
E0315	Bed accessory: board, table, or support device, any type	*CIM 60-9, ASC*
E0325	Urinal; male, jug-type, any material	*CIM 60-9, ASC*
E0326	Urinal; female, jug-type, any material	*CIM 60-9, ASC*
E0350	Control unit for electronic bowel irrigation/evacuation system	*ASC*
E0352	Disposable pack (water reservoir bag, speculum, valving mechanism and collection bag/box) for use with the electronic bowel irrigation/evacuation system	*ASC*
E0370	Air pressure elevator for heel	*ASC*
E0371	Nonpowered advanced pressure reducing overlay for mattress, standard mattress length and width	*ASC*
E0372	Powered air overlay for mattress, standard mattress length and width	*ASC*
E0373	Nonpowered advanced pressure reducing mattress	*ASC*

Oxygen and Related Respiratory Equipment

▲ **E0424**	Stationary compressed gaseous oxygen system, rental; includes container, contents, regulator, flowmeter, humidifier, nebulizer, cannula or mask, and tubing	*CIM 60-4, MCM 4107.9*
E0425	Stationary compressed gas system, purchase; includes regulator, flowmeter, humidifier, nebulizer, cannula or mask, and tubing	*CIM 60-4, MCM 4107.9, ASC*
E0430	Portable gaseous oxygen system, purchase; includes regulator, flowmeter, humidifier, cannula or mask, and tubing	*CIM 60-4, MCM 4107.9, ASC*
▲ **E0431**	Portable gaseous oxygen system, rental; includes portable container, regulator, flowmeter, humidifier, cannula or mask, and tubing	*CIM 60-4, MCM 4107.9, ASC*

E Codes

	= Special Coverage Instructions Apply		= Carrier Discretion
	= Noncovered by Medicare or Medicare Statute		

E0434	Portable liquid oxygen system, rental; includes portable container, supply reservoir, humidifier, flowmeter, refill adaptor, contents gauge, cannula or mask, and tubing *CIM 60-4, MCM 4107.9, ASC*
E0435	Portable liquid oxygen system, purchase; includes portable container, supply reservoir, flowmeter, humidifier, contents gauge, cannula or mask, tubing, and refill adapter *CIM 60-4, MCM 4107.9, ASC*
▲ E0439	Stationary liquid oxygen system, rental; includes container, contents, regulator, flowmeter, humidifier, nebulizer, cannula or mask, and tubing *CIM 60-4, MCM 4107.9*
E0440	Stationary liquid oxygen system, purchase; includes use of reservoir, contents indicator, regulator, flowmeter, humidifier, nebulizer, cannula or mask, and tubing *CIM 60-4, MCM 4107.9, ASC*
▲ E0441	Oxygen contents, gaseous (for use with owned gaseous stationary systems or when both a stationary and portable gaseous system are owned) *CIM 60-4, MCM 4107.9*
▲ E0442	Oxygen contents, liquid (for use with owned liquid stationary systems or when both a stationary and portable liquid system are owned) *CIM 60-4, MCM 4107.9*
▲ E0443	Portable oxygen contents, gaseous (for use only with portable gaseous systems when no stationary gas or liquid system is used) *CIM 60-4, MCM 4107.9*
▲ E0444	Portable oxygen contents, liquid (for use only with portable liquid systems when no stationary gas or liquid system is used) *CIM 60-4, MCM 4107.9*
E0450	Volume ventilator, stationary or portable, with backup rate feature, used with invasive interface (e.g., tracheostomy tube) *CIM 60-9*
E0455	Oxygen tent, excluding croup or pediatric tents *CIM 60-4, MCM 4107.9, ASC*
E0457	Chest shell (cuirass) *ASC*
E0459	Chest wrap *ASC*
E0460	Negative pressure ventilator; portable or stationary *CIM 60-9, ASC*
E0462	Rocking bed, with or without side rails *ASC*
E0480	Percussor, electric or pneumatic, home model *CIM 60-9, ASC*

IPPB Machines

| E0500 | IPPB machine, all types, with built-in nebulization; manual or automatic valves; internal or external power source *CIM 60-9, ASC* |

Humidifiers/Compressors/Nebulizers for Use with Oxygen IPPB Equipment

| E0550 | Humidifier, durable for extensive supplemental humidification during IPPB treatments or oxygen delivery *CIM 60-9, ASC* |
| E0555 | Humidifier, durable, glass or autoclavable plastic bottle type, for use with regulator or flowmeter *CIM 60-9, ASC* |

▨ = Invalid Medicare Code (no grace period)

▨ = Code may require certificate of medical necessity (CMN) or DMERC information form (DIF)

| E0560 | Humidifier, durable for supplemental humidification during IPPB treatment or oxygen delivery | CIM 60-9, ASC |

| E0565 | Compressor, air power source for equipment which is not self-contained or cylinder driven | ASC |

| E0570 | Nebulizer, with compressor | CIM 60-9, MCM 4107.9, ASC |

● | E0571 | Aerosol compressor, battery powered, for use with small volume nebulizer | CIM 60-9 |

● | E0572 | Aerosol compressor, adjustable pressure, light duty for intermittent use |

● | E0574 | Ultrasonic generator with small volume ultrasonic nebulizer |

▲ | E0575 | Nebulizer, ultrasonic, large volume | CIM 60-9, ASC |

| E0580 | Nebulizer, durable, glass or autoclavable plastic, bottle type, for use with regulator or flowmeter | CIM 60-9, MCM 4107.9, ASC |

| E0585 | Nebulizer, with compressor and heater | CIM 60-9, MCM 4107.9, ASC |

| E0590 | Dispensing fee covered drug administered through DME nebulizer suction pump, home model, portable |

Suction Pump/Room Vaporizers

| E0600 | Suction pump, home model, portable | CIM 60-9, ASC |

| E0601 | Continuous airway pressure (CPAP) device | CIM 60-17, ASC |

| E0602 | Breast pump, all types |

| E0605 | Vaporizer, room type | CIM 60-9, ASC |

| E0606 | Postural drainage board | CIM 60-9, ASC |

Monitoring Equipment

| E0607 | Home blood glucose monitor | CIM 60-11, ASC |

| E0608 | Apnea monitor | CIM 60-17, ASC |

| E0609 | Blood glucose monitor with special features (e.g., voice synthesizers, automatic timers, etc.) | CIM 60-11, ASC |

Pacemaker Monitor

| E0610 | Pacemaker monitor, self-contained, checks battery depletion, includes audible and visible check systems | CIM 50-1, CIM 60-7, ASC |

| E0615 | Pacemaker monitor, self-contained, checks battery depletion and other pacemaker components, includes digital/visible check systems | CIM 50-1, CIM 60-7, ASC |

| E0616 | Implantable cardiac event recorder with memory, activator and programmer |

● | E0617 | External defibrillator with integrated electrocardiogram analysis |

Patient Lifts

| E0621 | Sling or seat, patient lift, canvas or nylon | CIM 60-9, ASC |

| E0625 | Patient lift, Kartop, bathroom or toilet | CIM 60-9, ASC |

E Codes

= Special Coverage Instructions Apply   = Carrier Discretion

= Noncovered by Medicare or Medicare Statute

E0627	Seat lift mechanism incorporated into a combination lift-chair mechanism *CIM 60-8, MCM 4107.8, ASC*
E0628	Separate seat lift mechanism for use with patient owned furniture — electric *CIM 60-9, MCM 4107.8, ASC*
E0629	Separate seat lift mechanism for use with patient owned furniture — nonelectric *MCM 4107.8, ASC*
E0630	Patient lift, hydraulic, with seat or sling *CIM 60-9, ASC*
E0635	Patient lift, electric, with seat or sling *CIM 60-9, ASC*

Pneumatic Compressor and Appliances

E0650	Pneumatic compressor, nonsegmental home model *CIM 60-16, ASC*
E0651	Pneumatic compressor, segmental home model without calibrated gradient pressure *CIM 60-16, ASC*
E0652	Pneumatic compressor, segmental home model with calibrated gradient pressure *CIM 60-16, ASC*
E0655	Nonsegmental pneumatic appliance for use with pneumatic compressor, half arm *CIM 60-16, ASC*
E0660	Nonsegmental pneumatic appliance for use with pneumatic compressor, full leg *CIM 60-16, ASC*
E0665	Nonsegmental pneumatic appliance for use with pneumatic compressor, full arm *CIM 60-16, ASC*
E0666	Nonsegmental pneumatic appliance for use with pneumatic compressor, half leg *CIM 60-16, ASC*
E0667	Segmental pneumatic appliance for use with pneumatic compressor, full leg *CIM 60-16, ASC*
E0668	Segmental pneumatic appliance for use with pneumatic compressor, full arm *CIM 60-16, ASC*
E0669	Segmental pneumatic appliance for use with pneumatic compressor, half leg *CIM 60-16, ASC*
E0671	Segmental gradient pressure pneumatic appliance, full leg *CIM 60-16, ASC*
E0672	Segmental gradient pressure pneumatic appliance, full arm *CIM 60-16, ASC*
E0673	Segmental gradient pressure pneumatic appliance, half leg *CIM 60-16, ASC*

Ultraviolet Cabinet

E0690	Ultraviolet cabinet, appropriate for home use *CIM 60-9, ASC*

Safety Equipment

E0700	Safety equipment (e.g., belt, harness or vest) *ASC*

= Invalid Medicare Code (no grace period)

= Code may require certificate of medical necessity (CMN) or DMERC information form (DIF)

Restraints

E0710 Restraint, any type (body, chest, wrist or ankle) *ASC*

Transcutaneous and/or Neuromuscular Electrical Nerve Stimulators — TENS

E0720 TENS, two lead, localized stimulation
CIM 35-20, CIM 35-46, MCM 4107.6, ASC

E0730 TENS, four lead, larger area/multiple nerve stimulation
CIM 35-20, CIM 35-46, MCM 4107.6, ASC

E0731 Form-fitting conductive garment for delivery of TENS or NMES (with conductive fibers separated from the patient's skin by layers of fabric)
CIM 45-25, ASC

E0740 Incontinence treatment system, pelvic floor stimulator, monitor, sensor and/or trainer *CIM 65-11, ASC*

E0744 Neuromuscular stimulator for scoliosis *ASC*

E0745 Neuromuscular stimulator, electronic shock unit *CIM 35-77, ASC*

E0746 Electromyography (EMG), biofeedback device *CIM 35-27, ASC*

E0747 Osteogenesis stimulator, electrical, noninvasive, other than spinal applications *CIM 35-48, ASC*

E0748 Osteogenesis stimulator, electrical, noninvasive, spinal applications
CIM 35-48, ASC

E0749 Osteogenesis stimulator, electrical, surgically implanted *CIM 35-48, ASC*

E0751 ~~Implantable neurostimulator pulse generator or combination of external transmitter with implantable receiver (includes extension)~~ This code has been deleted in 2001.

E0753 Implantable neurostimulator electrodes, per group of four *CIM 65-8, ASC*

E0755 Electronic salivary reflex stimulator (intraoral/noninvasive) *ASC*

● **E0756** Implantable neurostimulator pulse generator *CIM 65-8*

● **E0757** Implantable neurostimulator radiofrequency receiver *CIM 65-8*

● **E0758** Radiofrequency transmitter (external) for use with implantable neurostimulator radiofrequency receiver *CIM 65-8*

E0760 Osteogenesis stimulator, low intensity ultrasound, non-invasive
CIM 35-48, ASC

● **E0765** FDA approved nerve stimulator, with replaceable batteries, for treatment of nausea and vomiting

Infusion Supplies

E0776 IV pole *ASC*

E0779 Ambulatory infusion pump, mechanical, reusable, for infusion 8 hours or greater

E0780 Ambulatory infusion pump, mechanical, reusable, for infusion less than 8 hours

E Codes

= Special Coverage Instructions Apply   = Carrier Discretion

= Noncovered by Medicare or Medicare Statute

E0781	Ambulatory infusion pump, single or multiple channels, electric or battery operated, with administrative equipment, worn by patient _CIM 60-14_
E0782	Infusion pump, implantable, non-programmable _CIM 60-14, ASC_
E0783	Infusion pump system, implantable, programmable (includes all components, e.g., pump, catheter, connectors, etc.) _CIM 60-14, ASC_
E0784	External ambulatory infusion pump, insulin _CIM 60-14, ASC_
E0785	Implantable intraspinal (epidural/intrathecal) catheter used with implantable infusion pump, replacement _CIM 60-14_
● E0786	Implantable programmable infusion pump, replacement (excludes implantable intraspinal catheter) _CIM 60-14_
E0791	Parenteral infusion pump, stationary, single or multichannel _CIM 65-10, MCM 2130, MCM 4450, ASC_
● E0830	Ambulatory traction device, all types, each _CIM 60-9_

Traction — Cervical

E0840	Traction frame, attached to headboard, cervical traction _CIM 60-9, ASC_
E0850	Traction stand, freestanding, cervical traction _CIM 60-9, ASC_
E0855	Cervical traction equipment not requiring additional stand or frame _ASC_

Traction — Overdoor

E0860	Traction equipment, overdoor, cervical _CIM 60-9, ASC_

Traction — Extremity

E0870	Traction frame, attached to footboard, extremity traction (e.g., Buck's) _CIM 60-9, ASC_
E0880	Traction stand, freestanding, extremity traction (e.g., Buck's) _CIM 60-9, ASC_

Traction — Pelvic

E0890	Traction frame, attached to footboard, pelvic traction _CIM 60-9, ASC_
E0900	Traction stand, freestanding, pelvic traction (e.g., Buck's) _CIM 60-9, ASC_

Trapeze Equipment, Fracture Frame, and Other Orthopedic Devices

E0910	Trapeze bars, also known as Patient Helper, attached to bed, with grab bar _CIM 60-9, ASC_
E0920	Fracture frame, attached to bed, includes weights _CIM 60-9, ASC_
E0930	Fracture frame, freestanding, includes weights _CIM 60-9, ASC_
E0935	Passive motion exercise device _CIM 60-9, ASC_
E0940	Trapeze bar, freestanding, complete with grab bar _CIM 60-9, ASC_
E0941	Gravity assisted traction device, any type _CIM 60-9, ASC_

| **E0942** | Cervical head harness/halter | *ASC* |

| **E0943** | Cervical pillow | *ASC* |

| **E0944** | Pelvic belt/harness/boot | *ASC* |

| **E0945** | Extremity belt/harness | *ASC* |

| **E0946** | Fracture, frame, dual with cross bars, attached to bed (e.g., Balken, Four Poster) | *CIM 60-9, ASC* |

| **E0947** | Fracture frame, attachments for complex pelvic traction | *CIM 60-9, ASC* |

| **E0948** | Fracture frame, attachments for complex cervical traction | *CIM 60-9, ASC* |

Wheelchairs
Note: See also K0001–K0109.

| **E0950** | Tray | *ASC* |

| **E0951** | Loop heel, each | *ASC* |

| **E0952** | Loop toe, each | *ASC* |

| **E0953** | Pneumatic tire, each | *CIM 60-9, ASC* |

| **E0954** | Semi-pneumatic caster, each | *CIM 60-9, ASC* |

Wheelchair Accessories

| **E0958** | Wheelchair attachment to convert any wheelchair to one arm drive | *CIM 60-9, ASC* |

| **E0959** | Amputee adapter (device used to compensate for transfer of weight due to lost limbs to maintain proper balance) | *CIM 60-9, ASC* |

| **E0961** | Brake extension, for wheelchair | *CIM 60-9, ASC* |

| **E0962** | One-inch cushion, for wheelchair | *CIM 60-9, ASC* |

| **E0963** | Two-inch cushion, for wheelchair | *CIM 60-9, ASC* |

| **E0964** | Three-inch cushion, for wheelchair | *CIM 60-9, ASC* |

| **E0965** | Four-inch cushion, for wheelchair | *CIM 60-9, ASC* |

| **E0966** | Hook on headrest extension | *CIM 60-9, ASC* |

| **E0967** | Wheelchair hand rims with eight vertical rubber-tipped projections, pair | *CIM 60-9, ASC* |

| **E0968** | Commode seat, wheelchair | *CIM 60-9, ASC* |

| **E0969** | Narrowing device, wheelchair | *CIM 60-9, ASC* |

| **E0970** | No. 2 footplates, except for elevating legrest | *CIM 60-9, ASC* |

| **E0971** | Anti-tipping device, wheelchair | *CIM 60-9, ASC* |

| **E0972** | Transfer board or device | *ASC* |

| **E0973** | Adjustable height detachable arms, desk or full-length, wheelchair | *CIM 60-9, ASC* |

| **E0974** | "Grade-aid" (device to prevent rolling back on an incline) for wheelchair | *ASC* |

E Codes

= Special Coverage Instructions Apply   = Carrier Discretion

= Noncovered by Medicare or Medicare Statute

E0975	Reinforced seat upholstery, wheelchair	CIM 60-9, ASC
E0976	Reinforced back, wheelchair, upholstery or other material	CIM 60-9, ASC
E0977	Wedge cushion, wheelchair	ASC
E0978	Belt, safety with airplane buckle, wheelchair	ASC
E0979	Belt, safety with Velcro closure, wheelchair	ASC
E0980	Safety vest, wheelchair	ASC
E0990	Elevating leg rest, each	CIM 60-9, ASC
E0991	Upholstery seat	CIM 60-9, ASC
E0992	Solid seat insert	CIM 60-9, ASC
E0993	Back, upholstery	CIM 60-9, ASC
E0994	Armrest, each	CIM 60-9, ASC
E0995	Calf rest, each	CIM 60-9, ASC
E0996	Tire, solid, each	CIM 60-9, ASC
E0997	Caster with fork	CIM 60-9, ASC
E0998	Caster without fork	CIM 60-9, ASC
E0999	Pneumatic tire with wheel	CIM 60-9, ASC
E1000	Tire, pneumatic caster	CIM 60-9, ASC
E1001	Wheel, single	CIM 60-9, ASC

Rollabout Chair

E1031	Rollabout chair, any and all types with casters five inches or greater	CIM 60-9, ASC
● E1035	Multi-positional patient transfer system, with integrated seat, operated by care giver	MCM 2100

Wheelchairs — Fully Reclining

E1050	Fully reclining wheelchair; fixed full-length arms, swing-away, detachable, elevating legrests	CIM 60-9, ASC
E1060	Fully reclining wheelchair; detachable arms, desk or full-length, swing-away, detachable, elevating legrests	CIM 60-9, ASC
E1065	Power attachment (to convert any wheelchair to motorized wheelchair, e.g., Solo)	CIM 60-9, ASC
E1066	Battery charger	CIM 60-9, ASC
E1069	Deep cycle battery	CIM 60-9, ASC
E1070	Fully reclining wheelchair; detachable arms, desk or full-length, swing-away, detachable footrests	CIM 60-9, ASC
E1083	Hemi-wheelchair; fixed full-length arms, swing-away, detachable, elevating legrests	CIM 60-9, ASC
E1084	Hemi-wheelchair; detachable arms, desk or full-length, swing-away, detachable, elevating legrests	CIM 60-9, ASC

= Invalid Medicare Code (no grace period)

= Code may require certificate of medical necessity (CMN) or DMERC information form (DIF)

E1085	Hemi-wheelchair; fixed full-length arms, swing-away, detachable footrests	*CIM 60-9, ASC*
E1086	Hemi-wheelchair; detachable arms, desk or full-length, swing-away, detachable footrests	*CIM 60-9, ASC*
E1087	High-strength lightweight wheelchair; fixed full-length arms, swing-away, detachable, elevating legrests	*CIM 60-9, ASC*
E1088	High-strength lightweight wheelchair; detachable arms, desk or full-length, swing-away, detachable, elevating legrests	*CIM 60-9, ASC*
E1089	High-strength lightweight wheelchair; fixed-length arms, swing-away, detachable footrests	*CIM 60-9, ASC*
E1090	High-strength lightweight wheelchair; detachable arms, desk or full-length, swing-away, detachable footrests	*CIM 60-9, ASC*
E1091	Youth wheelchair; any type	*CIM 60-9, ASC*
E1092	Wide, heavy-duty wheelchair; detachable arms, desk or full-length, swing-away, detachable, elevating legrests	*CIM 60-9, ASC*
E1093	Wide, heavy-duty wheelchair; detachable arms, desk or full-length arms, swing-away, detachable footrests	*CIM 60-9, ASC*

Wheelchair — Semi-reclining

E1100	Semi-reclining wheelchair; fixed full-length arms, swing-away, detachable, elevating legrests	*CIM 60-9, ASC*
E1110	Semi-reclining wheelchair; detachable arms, desk or full-length, elevating legrest	*CIM 60-9, ASC*

Wheelchair — Standard

E1130	Standard wheelchair; fixed full-length arms, fixed or swing-away, detachable footrests	*CIM 60-9, ASC*
E1140	Wheelchair; detachable arms, desk or full-length, swing-away, detachable footrests	*CIM 60-9, ASC*
E1150	Wheelchair; detachable arms, desk or full-length, swing-away, detachable, elevating legrests	*CIM 60-9, ASC*
E1160	Wheelchair; fixed full-length arms, swing-away, detachable, elevating legrests	*CIM 60-9, ASC*

Wheelchair — Amputee

E1170	Amputee wheelchair; fixed full-length arms, swing-away, detachable, elevating legrests	*CIM 60-9, ASC*
E1171	Amputee wheelchair; fixed full-length arms, without footrests or legrests	*CIM 60-9, ASC*
E1172	Amputee wheelchair; detachable arms, desk or full-length, without footrests or legrests	*CIM 60-9, ASC*
E1180	Amputee wheelchair; detachable arms, desk or full-length, swing-away, detachable footrests	*CIM 60-9, ASC*

E Codes

= Special Coverage Instructions Apply

= Carrier Discretion

= Noncovered by Medicare or Medicare Statute

E1190	Amputee wheelchair; detachable arms, desk or full-length, swing-away, detachable, elevating legrests *CIM 60-9, ASC*
E1195	Heavy duty wheelchair; fixed full-length arms, swing-away, detachable, elevating legrests *CIM 60-9, ASC*
E1200	Amputee wheelchair; fixed full-length arms, swing-away, detachable footrests *CIM 60-9, ASC*

Wheelchair — Power

E1210	Motorized wheelchair; fixed full-length arms, swing-away, detachable, elevating legrests *CIM 60-5, CIM 60-9, ASC*
E1211	Motorized wheelchair; detachable arms, desk or full-length, swing-away, detachable, elevating legrests *CIM 60-5, CIM 60-9, ASC*
E1212	Motorized wheelchair; fixed full-length arms, swing-away, detachable footrests *CIM 60-5, CIM 60-9, ASC*
E1213	Motorized wheelchair; detachable arms, desk or full-length, swing-away, detachable footrests *CIM 60-5, CIM 60-9, ASC*

Wheelchair — Special Size

E1220	Wheelchair; specially sized or constructed (indicate brand name, model number, if any, and justification) *Medicaid suspend for medical review, CIM 60-6, ASC*
E1221	Wheelchair with fixed arm, footrests *CIM 60-6, ASC*
E1222	Wheelchair with fixed arm, elevating legrests *CIM 60-6, ASC*
E1223	Wheelchair with detachable arms, footrests *CIM 60-6, ASC*
E1224	Wheelchair with detachable arms, elevating legrests *CIM 60-6, ASC*
E1225	Semi-reclining back for customized wheelchair *CIM 60-6, ASC*
E1226	Full reclining back for customized wheelchair *CIM 60-6, ASC*
E1227	Special height arms for wheelchair *CIM 60-6, ASC*
E1228	Special back height for wheelchair *CIM 60-6, ASC*
E1230	Power operated vehicle (three- or four-wheel nonhighway), specify brand name and model number *Medicaid suspend for medical review, CIM 60-5, MCM 4107.6, ASC*

Wheelchair — Lightweight

E1240	Lightweight wheelchair; detachable arms, desk or full-length, swing-away, detachable, elevating legrest *CIM 60-9, ASC*
E1250	Lightweight wheelchair; fixed full-length arms, swing-away, detachable footrests *CIM 60-9, ASC*
E1260	Lightweight wheelchair; detachable arms, desk or full-length, swing-away, detachable footrests *CIM 60-9, ASC*
E1270	Lightweight wheelchair; fixed full-length arms, swing-away, detachable elevating legrests *CIM 60-9, ASC*

= Invalid Medicare Code (no grace period)

= Code may require certificate of medical necessity (CMN) or DMERC information form (DIF)

Wheelchair — Heavy-duty

E1280 Heavy-duty wheelchair; detachable arms, desk or full-length, elevating
legrests
CIM 60-9, ASC

E1285 Heavy-duty wheelchair; fixed full-length arms, swing-away, detachable
footrests
CIM 60-9, ASC

E1290 Heavy-duty wheelchair; detachable arms, desk or full-length, swing-
away, detachable footrests
CIM 60-9, ASC

E1295 Heavy-duty wheelchair; fixed full-length arms, elevating legrests
CIM 60-9, ASC

E1296 Special wheelchair seat height from floor   *CIM 60-6, ASC*

E1297 Special wheelchair seat depth, by upholstery   *CIM 60-6, ASC*

E1298 Special wheelchair seat depth and/or width, by construction
CIM 60-6, ASC

Whirlpool — Equipment

E1300 Whirlpool, portable (overtub type)   *CIM 60-9, ASC*

E1310 Whirlpool, nonportable (built-in type)   *CIM 60-9, ASC*

Repairs and Replacement Supplies

E1340 Repair or nonroutine service for durable medical equipment requiring
the skill of a technician, labor component, per 15 minutes
MCM 2100.4, ASC

Additional Oxygen Related Equipment

E1353 Regulator   *CIM 60-4, MCM 4107.9, ASC*

E1355 Stand/rack   *CIM 60-4, ASC*

E1372 Immersion external heater for nebulizer   *CIM 60-4, ASC*

E1375 ~~Nebulizer portable with small compressor, with limited flow~~ This code
has been deleted in 2001. See E0570.

E1377 ~~Oxygen concentrator, high humidity system equiv. to 244 cu. ft.~~ This
code has been deleted in 2001. See Q0036.

E1378 ~~Oxygen concentrator, high humidity system equiv. to 488 cu. ft.~~ This
code has been deleted in 2001. See Q0036.

E1379 ~~Oxygen concentrator, high humidity system equiv. to 732 cu. ft.~~ This
code has been deleted in 2001. See Q0036.

E1380 ~~Oxygen concentrator, high humidity system equiv. to 976 cu. ft.~~ This
code has been deleted in 2001. See Q0036.

E1381 ~~Oxygen concentrator, high humidity system equiv. to 1220 cu. ft.~~ This
code has been deleted in 2001. See Q0036.

E1382 ~~Oxygen concentrator, high humidity system equiv. to 1464 cu. ft.~~ This
code has been deleted in 2001. See Q0036.

E1383 ~~Oxygen concentrator, high humidity system equiv. to 1708 cu. ft.~~ This
code has been deleted in 2001. See Q0036.

E Codes

= Special Coverage Instructions Apply   = Carrier Discretion

= Noncovered by Medicare or Medicare Statute

E1384	~~Oxygen concentrator, high humidity system equiv. to 1952 cu. ft.~~ This code has been deleted in 2001. See Q0036.
E1385	~~Oxygen concentrator, high humidity system equiv. to over 1952 cu. ft.~~ This code has been deleted in 2001. See Q0036.
E1390	Oxygen concentrator, capable of delivering 85 percent or greater oxygen concentration at the prescribed flow rate *CIM 60-4*
E1399	Durable medical equipment, miscellaneous *ASC*
E1405	Oxygen and water vapor enriching system with heated delivery *CIM 60-4, MCM 4107, ASC*
E1406	Oxygen and water vapor enriching system without heated delivery *CIM 60-4, MCM 4107, ASC*

Artificial Kidney Machines and Accessories

For suppplies for ESRD, see procedure codes A4650–A4999.

E1510	Kidney, dialysate delivery system kidney machine, pump recirculating, air removal system, flowrate meter, power off, heater and temp control with alarm, IV poles, pressure gauge, concentrate container *ASC*
E1520	Heparin infusion pump for dialysis *ASC*
E1530	Air bubble detector for dialysis *ASC*
E1540	Pressure alarm for dialysis *ASC*
E1550	Bath conductivity meter for dialysis *ASC*
E1560	Blood leak detector for dialysis *ASC*
E1570	Adjustable chair, for ESRD patients *ASC*
E1575	Transducer protector/fluid barrier, any size, each *ASC*
E1580	Unipuncture control system for dialysis *ASC*
E1590	Hemodialysis machine *ASC*
E1592	Automatic intermittent peritoneal dialysis system *ASC*
E1594	Cycler dialysis machine for peritoneal dialysis *ASC*
E1600	Delivery and/or installation charges for renal dialysis equipment *Medicaid suspend for medical review, ASC*
E1610	Reverse osmosis water purification system *CIM 55-1 A, ASC*
E1615	Deionizer water purification system *CIM 55-1 A, ASC*
E1620	Blood pump for dialysis *ASC*
E1625	Water softening system *CIM 55-1 B, ASC*
E1630	Reciprocating peritoneal dialysis system *ASC*
E1632	Wearable artificial kidney *ASC*
E1635	Compact (portable) travel hemodialyzer system *Medicaid suspend for medical review, ASC*
E1636	Sorbent cartridges, per case *ASC*

= Invalid Medicare Code (no grace period)

= Code may require certificate of medical necessity (CMN) or DMERC information form (DIF)

| **E1640** | Replacement components for hemodialysis and/or peritoneal dialysis machines that are owned or being purchased by the patient | *ASC* |
| **E1699** | Dialysis equipment, unspecified, by report | *ASC* |

Jaw Motion Rehabilitation System and Accessories

E1700	Jaw motion rehabilitation system	*ASC*
E1701	Replacement cushions for jaw motion rehabilitation system, package of six	*ASC*
E1702	Replacement measuring scales for jaw motion rehabilitation system, package of 200	*ASC*

Other Orthopedic Devices

▲ **E1800**	Dynamic adjustable elbow extension/flexion device, or equal	*ASC*
▲ **E1805**	Dynamic adjustable wrist extension/flexion device, or equal	*ASC*
▲ **E1810**	Dynamic adjustable knee extension/flexion device, or equal	*ASC*
▲ **E1815**	Dynamic adjustable ankle extension/flexion device, or equal	*ASC*
E1820	Soft interface material, dynamic adjustable extension/flexion device	*ASC*
▲ **E1825**	Dynamic adjustable finger extension/flexion device, or equal	*ASC*
▲ **E1830**	Dynamic adjustable toe extension/flexion device, or equal	*ASC*
E1900	Synthesized speech augmentative communication device with dynamic display	*CIM 60-9*

E Codes

| | = Special Coverage Instructions Apply | | = Carrier Discretion |
| | = Noncovered by Medicare or Medicare Statute | | |

Procedures/Professional Services (Temporary) G0000–G9999

HCFA assigns temporary G codes to procedures and services which are being reviewed prior to inclusion in the American Medical Association's Current Procedural Terminology (CPT). Once CPT codes for these services and procedures are assigned, the G codes are removed from this section.

PET Scan Modifiers
Use the following single digit alpha characters, in combination as two-character modifiers to indicate the results of a current PET scan and a previous test.

N Negative

E Equivocal

P Positive, but not suggestive of extensive ischemia

S Positive and suggestive of extensive ischemia (greater than 20 percent of the left ventricle)

G0001	Routine venipuncture for collection of specimen(s)
G0002	Office procedure, insertion of temporary indwelling catheter, Foley type (separate procedure)
G0004	Patient demand single or multiple event recording with presymptom memory loop and 24-hour attended monitoring, per 30-day period; includes transmission, physician review and interpretation *CIM 50-15*
G0005	Patient demand single or multiple event recording with presymptom memory loop and 24-hour attended monitoring, per 30-day period; recording (includes hookup, recording and disconnection) *CIM 50-15*
G0006	Patient demand single or multiple event recording with presymptom memory loop and 24-hour attended monitoring, per 30-day period; 24-hour attended monitoring, receipt of transmissions, and analysis *CIM 50-15*
G0007	Patient demand single or multiple event recording with presymptom memory loop and 24-hour attended monitoring, per 30-day period; physician review and interpretation only *CIM 50-15*
G0008	Administration of influenza virus vaccine when no physician fee schedule service on the same day *ASC*
G0009	Administration of pneumococcal vaccine when no physician fee schedule service on the same day *ASC*
G0010	Administration of hepatitis B vaccine when no physician fee schedule service on the same day *ASC*
G0015	Post-symptom telephonic transmission of electrocardiogram rhythm strip(s) and 24-hour attended monitoring, per 30-day period: Tracing only *CIM 50-15*

G Codes

= Special Coverage Instructions Apply   = Carrier Discretion

= Noncovered by Medicare or Medicare Statute

G0016 Post-symptom telephonic transmission of electrocardiogram rhythm strip(s) and 24-hour attended monitoring, per 30-day period: Physician review and interpretation only   *CIM 50-15*

G0025 Collagen skin test kit   *CIM 65-9*

G0026 Fecal leukocyte examination   *ASC*

G0027 Semen analysis; presence and/or motility of sperm excluding Huhner test   *ASC*

G0030 PET myocardial perfusion imaging, (following previous PET, G0030–G0047); single study, rest or stress (exercise and/or pharmacologic)   *CIM 50-36, ASC*

G0031 PET myocardial perfusion imaging, (following previous PET, G0030–G0047); multiple studies, rest or stress (exercise and/or pharmacologic)   *CIM 50-36, ASC*

G0032 PET myocardial perfusion imaging, (following rest SPECT, 78464); single study, rest or stress (exercise and/or pharmacologic)   *CIM 50-36, ASC*

G0033 PET myocardial perfusion imaging, (following rest SPECT, 78464); multiple studies, rest or stress (exercise and/or pharmacologic)   *CIM 50-36, ASC*

G0034 PET myocardial perfusion imaging, (following stress SPECT, 78465); single study, rest or stress (exercise and/or pharmacologic)   *CIM 50-36, ASC*

G0035 PET myocardial perfusion imaging, (following stress SPECT, 78465); multiple studies, rest or stress (exercise and/or pharmacologic)   *CIM 50-36, ASC*

G0036 PET myocardial perfusion imaging, (following coronary angiography, 93510–93529); single study, rest or stress (exercise and/or pharmacologic)   *CIM 50-36, ASC*

G0037 PET myocardial perfusion imaging, (following coronary angiography, 93510–93529); multiple studies, rest or stress (exercise and/or pharmacologic)   *CIM 50-36, ASC*

G0038 PET myocardial perfusion imaging, (following stress planar myocardial perfusion, 78460); single study, rest or stress (exercise and/or pharmacologic)   *CIM 50-36, ASC*

G0039 PET myocardial perfusion imaging, (following stress planar myocardial perfusion, 78460); multiple studies, rest or stress (exercise and/or pharmacologic)   *CIM 50-36, ASC*

G0040 PET myocardial perfusion imaging, (following stress echocardiogram, 93350); single study, rest or stress (exercise and/or pharmacologic)   *CIM 50-36, ASC*

G0041 PET myocardial perfusion imaging, (following stress echocardiogram, 93350); multiple studies, rest or stress (exercise and/or pharmacologic)   *CIM 50-36, ASC*

G0042	PET myocardial perfusion imaging, (following stress nuclear ventriculogram, 78481 or 78483); single study, rest or stress (exercise and/or pharmacologic) *CIM 50-36, ASC*
G0043	PET myocardial perfusion imaging, (following stress nuclear ventriculogram, 78481 or 78483); multiple studies, rest or stress (exercise and/or pharmacologic) *CIM 50-36, ASC*
G0044	PET myocardial perfusion imaging, (following rest ECG, 93000); single study, rest or stress (exercise and/or pharmacologic) *CIM 50-36, ASC*
G0045	PET myocardial perfusion imaging, (following rest ECG, 93000); multiple studies, rest or stress (exercise and/or pharmacologic) *CIM 50-36, ASC*
G0046	PET myocardial perfusion imaging, (following stress ECG, 93015); single study, rest or stress (exercise and/or pharmacologic) *CIM 50-36, ASC*
G0047	PET myocardial perfusion imaging, (following stress ECG, 93015); multiple studies, rest or stress (exercise and/or pharmacologic) *CIM 50-36, ASC*
G0050	Measurement of post-voiding residual urine and/or bladder capacity by ultrasound
G0101	Cervical or vaginal cancer screening; pelvic and clinical breast examination *ASC*
G0102	Prostate cancer screening; digital rectal examination *CIM 50-55, MCM 4182*
G0103	Prostate cancer screening; prostate specific antigen test (PSA), total *CIM 50-55, MCM 4182*
G0104	Colorectal cancer screening; flexible sigmoidoscopy
G0105	Colorectal cancer screening; colonoscopy on individual at high risk
G0106	Colorectal cancer screening; alternative to G0104, screening sigmoidoscopy, barium enema *ASC*
G0107	Colorectal cancer screening; fecal-occult blood test, 1-3 simultaneous determinations *ASC*
▲ **G0108**	Diabetes outpatient self-management training services, individual, per 30 minutes
▲ **G0109**	Diabetes self-management training services, group session (2 or more), per 30 minutes
G0110	NETT pulmonary rehabilitation; education/skills training, individual *CIM 35-93, ASC*
G0111	NETT pulmonary rehabilitation; education/skills, group *CIM 35-93, ASC*
G0112	NETT pulmonary rehabilitation; nutritional guidance, initial *CIM 35-93, ASC*
G0113	NETT pulmonary rehabilitation; nutritional guidance, subsequent *CIM 35-93, ASC*

G Codes

 = Special Coverage Instructions Apply   = Carrier Discretion

 = Noncovered by Medicare or Medicare Statute

G0114	NETT pulmonary rehabilitation; psychosocial consultation *CIM 35-93, ASC*
G0115	NETT pulmonary rehabilitation; psychological testing *CIM 35-93, ASC*
G0116	NETT pulmonary rehabilitation; psychosocial counselling *CIM 35-93, ASC*
G0120	Colorectal cancer screening; alternative to G0105, screening colonoscopy, barium enema *ASC*
G0121	Colorectal cancer screening; colonoscopy on individual not meeting criteria for high risk
G0122	Colorectal cancer screening; barium enema
G0123	Screening cytopathology, cervical or vaginal (any reporting system), collected in preservative fluid, automated thin layer preparation, screening by cytotechnologist under physician supervision *CIM 50-20*
G0124	Screening cytopathology, cervical or vaginal (any reporting system), collected in preservative fluid, automated thin layer preparation, requiring interpretation by physician *CIM 50-20*
G0125	PET lung imaging of solitary pulmonary nodules, using 2-(fluorine-18)-fluoro-2-deoxy-d-glucose (FDG), following CT (71250/71260 or 71270) *CIM 50-36, MCM 4173*
G0126	PET lung imaging of solitary pulmonary nodules, using 2-(fluorine-18)-fluoro-2-deoxy-d-glucose (FDG), following CT (71250/71260 or 71270); initial staging of pathologically diagnosed non-small cell lung cancer *CIM 50-36, MCM 4173*
G0127	Trimming of dystrophic nails, any number *MCM 2323, MCM 4120*
G0128	Direct (face-to-face with patient) skilled nursing services of a registered nurse provided in a comprehensive outpatient rehabilitation facility, each 10 minutes beyond the first 5 minutes *Medicare Statute 1833(a)*
G0129	Occupational therapy requiring the skills of a qualified occupational therapist, furnished as a component of a partial hospitalization treatment program, per day
G0130	Single energy x-ray absorptiometry (SEXA) bone density study, one or more sites; appendicular skeleton (peripheral) (e.g., radius, wrist, heel) *CIM 50-44*
G0131	Computerized tomography bone mineral density study, one or more sites; axial skeleton (e.g., hips, pelvis, spine) *CIM 50-44*
G0132	Computerized tomography bone mineral density study, one or more sites; appendicular skeleton (peripheral) (e.g., radius, wrist, heel) *CIM 50-44*
G0141	Screening cytopathology smears, cervical or vaginal, performed by automated system, with manual rescreening, requiring interpretation by physician
G0143	Screening cytopathology, cervical or vaginal (any reporting system), collected in preservative fluid, automated thin layer preparation, with manual screening and rescreening by cytotechnologist under physician supervision

= Invalid Medicare Code (no grace period)

= Code may require certificate of medical necessity (CMN) or DMERC information form (DIF)

G0144 Screening cytopathology, cervical or vaginal (any reporting system), collected in preservative fluid, automated thin layer preparation, with manual screening and computer-assisted rescreening by cytotechnologist under physician supervision

G0145 Screening cytopathology, cervical or vaginal (any reporting system), collected in preservative fluid, automated thin layer preparation, with manual screening and computer-assisted rescreening using cell selection and review under physician supervision

G0147 Screening cytopathology smears, cervical or vaginal, performed by automated system under physician supervision

G0148 Screening cytopathology smears, cervical or vaginal, performed by automated system with manual rescreening

G0151 Services of physical therapist in home health setting, each 15 minutes

G0152 Services of occupational therapist in home health setting, each 15 minutes

G0153 Services of speech and language pathologist in home health setting, each 15 minutes

G0154 Services of skilled nurse in home health setting, each 15 minutes

G0155 Services of clinical social worker in home health setting, each 15 minutes

G0156 Services of home health aide in home health setting, each 15 minutes

G0159 ~~Percutaneous thrombectomy and/or revision, arteriovenous fistula, autogenous or nonautogenous dialysis graft~~ This code has been deleted in 2001.

G0160 ~~Cryosurgical ablation of localized prostate cancer, primary treatment only (post-operative irrigations and aspiration of sloughing tissue included)~~ This code has been deleted in 2001.

G0161 ~~Ultrasonic guidance for interstitial placement of cryosurgical probes~~ This code has been deleted in 2001.

G0163 Positron emission tomography (PET), whole body, for recurrence of colorectal metastatic cancer *CIM 50-36, MCM 4173*

G0164 Positron emission tomography (PET), whole body, for staging and characterization of lymphoma *CIM 50-36, MCM 4173*

G0165 Positron emission tomography (PET), whole body, for recurrence of melanoma or melanoma metastatic cancer *CIM 50-36, MCM 4173*

G0166 External counterpulsation, per treatment session *CIM 35-74*

G0167 Hyperbaric oxygen treatment not requiring physician attendance, per treatment session *CIM 35-10*

G0168 Wound closure utilizing tissue adhesive(s) only

G0169 ~~Removal of devitalized tissue, without use of anesthesia (conscious sedation, local, regional, general)~~ This code has been deleted in 2001.

G Codes

= Special Coverage Instructions Apply   = Carrier Discretion

= Noncovered by Medicare or Medicare Statute

G0170 ~~Application of tissue-cultured skin grafts, including bilaminate skin substitutes or neodermis, including site preparation, initial 25 sq cm~~ This code has been deleted in 2001.

G0171 ~~Application of tissue-cultured skin grafts, including bilaminate skin substitutes or neodermis, including site preparation, each additional 25 sq cm~~ This code has been deleted in 2001.

G0172 ~~Training and educational services furnished as a component of a partial hospitalization treatment program, per day~~ This code has been deleted in 2001. See G0177.

● **G0173** Stereotactic radiosurgery, complete course of therapy in one session

● **G0174** Intensity modulated radiation therapy (IMRT) plan, per session

● **G0175** Scheduled interdisciplinary team conference (minimum of three exclusive of patient care nursing staff) with patient present

● **G0176** Activity therapy, such as music, dance, art or play therapies not for recreation, related to the care and treatment of patient's disabling mental health problems, per session (45 minutes or more)

● **G0177** Training and educational services related to the care and treatment of patient's disabling mental health problems per session (45 minutes or more)

● **G0178** Intensity modulated radiation therapy (IMRT) delivery to multiple areas with treatment setup and verification images

● **G0179** Intensity modulated radiation therapy (IMRT) planning, includes dose volume nistograms, inverse plan optimization, plan positional accuracy and dose verification

● **G0180** Physician certification services for Medicare-covered services provided by a participating home health agency (patient not present), including review of initial or subsequent reports of patient status, review of patient's responses to the Oasis assessment instrument, contact with the home health agency to ascertain the initial implementation plan of care, and documentation in the patient's office record, per certification period

● **G0181** Physician supervision of a patient receiving Medicare-covered services provided by a participatient home health agency (patient not present) requiring complex and multidisciplinary care modalities involving regular physician development and/or revision of care plans, review of subsequent reports of patient status, review of laboratory and other studies, communication (including telephone calls) with other health care professionals involved in the patient's care, integration of new information into the medical treatment plan and/or adjustment of medical therapy, within a calendar month, 30 minutes or more

● **G0182** Physician supervision of a patient under a Medicare-approved hospice (patient not present) requiring complex and multidisciplinary care modalities involving regular physician development and/or revision of care plans, review of subsequent reports of patient status, review of laboratory and other studies, communication (including telephone calls) with other health care professionals involved in the patient's care, integration of new information into the medical treatment plan and/or adjustment of medical therapy, within a calendar month, 30 minutes or more

G0183 ~~Destruction of localized lesion of choroid (for example, choroidal neovascularization); ocular photodynamic therapy (includes intravenous infusion)~~ This code has been deleted in 2001.

● **G0184** Destruction of localized lesion of choroid (for example, choroidal neovascularization); photocoagulation, (for example by laser) one or more sessions

● **G0185** Destruction of localized lesion of choroid (for example, choroidal neovascularization); transpupillary thermotherapy (one or more sessions)

● **G0186** Destruction of localized lesion of choroid (for example, choroidal neovascularization); photocoagulation, feeder vessel technique (one or more sessions)

● **G0187** Destruction of macular drusen, photocoagulation (one or more sessions)

● **G0188** Full length radiography of lower extremity, which includes hip, knee, and ankle

● **G0190** Immunization administration (includes percutaneous, intradermal, subcutaneous, intramuscular and jet injections; each additional vaccine (single or combination vaccine/toxoid)

● **G0191** Immunization administration (includes percutaneous, intradermal, subcutaneous, intramuscular and jet injections); each additional vaccine (single or combination vaccine/toxoid); list separately in addition to code for primary procedure

● **G0192** Intranasal or oral administration; one vaccine (single or combination vaccine/toxoid)   *MCM 2320, 2049.4*

● **G0193** Endoscopic study of swallowing function (also fiberoptic endoscopic evaluation of swallowing) (FEES)

● **G0194** Sensory testing during endoscopic study of swallowing (add on code) referred to as fiberoptic endoscopic evaluation of swallowing with sensory testing (FEEST)

● **G0195** Clinical evaluation of swallowing function (not involving interpretation of dynamic radiological studies or endoscopic study of swallowing)

● **G0196** Evaluation of swallowing involving swallowing of radio-opaque materials

● **G0197** Evaluation of patient for prescription of speech generating devices

G Codes

- **G0198** Patient adaptation and training for use of speech generating devices
- **G0199** Re-evaluation of patient using speech generating devices
- **G0200** Evaluation of patient for prescription of voice prosthetic
- **G0201** Modification or training in use of voice prosthetic
- **G9001** Coordinated care fee, initial rate
- **G9002** Coordinated care fee, maintenance rate
- **G9003** Coordinated care fee, risk adjusted high, initial
- **G9004** Coordinated care fee, risk adjusted low, initial
- **G9005** Coordinated care fee, risk adjusted maintenance
- **G9006** Coordinated care fee, home monitoring
- **G9007** Coordinated care fee, schedule team conference
- **G9008** Coordinated care fee, physician coordinated care oversight services
- **G9016** Smoking cessation counseling, individual, in the absence of or in addition to any other evaluation and management service, per session (6-10 minutes) [demo project code only]

H Codes — Alcohol and Drug Abuse Treatment Services

H Codes are temporary codes established based on requests from state and federal agencies other than Medicare and Medicaid.

● **H0001** Alcohol and/or drug assessment

● **H0002** Alcohol and/or drug screening to determine eligibility for admission to treatment program

● **H0003** Alcohol and/or drug screening; laboratory analysis of specimens for presence of alcohol and/or drugs

● **H0004** Alcohol and/or drug services; individual counseling by a clinician

● **H0005** Alcohol and/or drug services; group counseling by a clinician

● **H0006** Alcohol and/or drug services; case management

● **H0007** Alcohol and/or drug services; crisis intervention (outpatient)

● **H0008** Alcohol and/or drug services; sub-acute detoxification (hospital inpatient)

● **H0009** Alcohol and/or drug services; acute detoxification (hospital inpatient)

● **H0010** Alcohol and/or drug services; sub-acute detoxification (residential addiction program inpatient)

● **H0011** Alcohol and/or drug services; acute detoxification (residential addiction program inpatient)

● **H0012** Alcohol and/or drug services; sub-acute detoxification (residential addiction program outpatient)

● **H0013** Alcohol and/or drug services; acute detoxification (residential addiction program outpatient)

● **H0014** Alcohol and/or drug services; ambulatory detoxification

● **H0015** Alcohol and/or drug services; intensive outpatient (treatment program that operates at least 3 hours/day and at least 3 days/week and is based on an individualized treatment plan), including assessment, counseling; crisis intervention, and activity therapies or education

● **H0016** Alcohol and/or drug services; medical/somatic (medical intervention in ambulatory setting)

● **H0017** Alcohol and/or drug services; residential (hospital residential treatment program)

● **H0018** Alcohol and/or drug services; short-term residential (non-hospital residential treatment program)

● **H0019** Alcohol and/or drug services; long-term residential (non-medical, non-acute care in residential treatment program where stay is typically longer than 30 days)

● **H0020** Alcohol and/or drug services; methadone administration and/or service (provision of the drug by a licensed program)

H Codes

= Special Coverage Instructions Apply   = Carrier Discretion

= Noncovered by Medicare or Medicare Statute

● **H0021** Alcohol and/or drug training service (for staff and personnel not employed by providers)

● **H0022** Alcohol and/or drug intervention service (planned facilitation)

● **H0023** Alcohol and/or drug outreach service (planned approach to reach a target population)

● **H0024** Alcohol and/or drug prevention information dissemination service (one-way direct or non-direct contact with service audiences to affect knowledge or attitude)

● **H0025** Alcohol and/or drug prevention education service (delivery of services with target population to affect knowledge, attitude and/or behavior)

● **H0026** Alcohol and/or drug prevention process service, community-based (delivery of services to develop skills of impactors)

● **H0027** Alcohol and/or drug prevention environmental service (broad range of external activities geared toward modifying systems in order to mainstream prevention through policy and law)

● **H0028** Alcohol and/or drug prevention problem identification and referral service (e.g., student assistance and employee assistance programs), does not include assessment

● **H0029** Alcohol and/or drug prevention alternatives service (services for populations that exclude alcohol and other drug use e.g., alcohol free social events)

● **H0030** Alcohol and/or drug hotline service

Drugs Administered Other Than Oral Method J0000–J8999

Drugs and biologicals are usually covered by Medicare if: they are of the type that cannot be self-administered; they are not excluded by being immunizations; they are reasonable and necessary for the diagnosis or treatment of the illness or injury for which they are administered; and they have not been determined by the FDA to be less than effective. In addition they must meet all the general requirements for coverage of items as incident to a physician's services. Generally, prescription and nonprescription drugs and biologicals purchased by or dispensed to a patient are not covered.

The following list of drugs can be injected either subcutaneously, intramuscularly, or intravenously. Third-party payers may wish to determine a threshold and pay up to a certain dollar limit before developing for the drug.

Exception: Oral Immunosuppressive Drugs

J0120	Injection, tetracycline, up to 250 mg	*MCM 2049*
J0130	Injection abciximab, 10 mg	*MCM 2049*
J0150	Injection, adenosine, 6 mg (not to be used to report any adenosine phosphate compounds; instead use A9270)	*MCM 2049*
J0151	Injection, adenosine, 90 mg (not to be used to report any adenosine phosphate compounds; instead use A9270)	*MCM 2049*
J0170	Injection, adrenalin, epinephrine, up to 1 ml ampule	*MCM 2049*
J0190	Injection, biperiden lactate, per 5 mg	*MCM 2049*
J0200	Injection, alatrofloxacin mesylate, 100 mg	*MCM 2049.5*
J0205	Injection, alglucerase, per 10 units	*MCM 2049*
J0207	Injection, amifostine, 500 mg	*MCM 2049*
J0210	Injection, methyldopate HCl, up to 250 mg	*MCM 2049*
J0256	Injection, alpha 1-proteinase inhibitor — human, 10 mg	*MCM 2049*
J0270	Injection, alprostadil, 1.25 mcg (code may be used for Medicare when drug administered under direct supervision of a physician, not for use when drug is self-administered)	
J0275	Alprostadil urethral suppository (code may be used for Medicare when drug administered under direct supervision of a physician, not for use when drug is self-administered)	
J0280	Injection, aminophyllin, up to 250 mg	*MCM 2049*
● J0282	Injection, amiodarone hydrochloride, 30 mg	
J0285	Injection, amphotericin B, 50 mg	*MCM 2049*
J0286	Injection, amphotericin B, any lipid formulation, 50 mg	*MCM 2049*
J0290	Injection, ampicillin sodium, 500 mg	*MCM 2049*
J0295	Injection, ampicillin sodium/sulbactam sodium, per 1.5 g	*MCM 2049*

     = Special Coverage Instructions Apply   = Carrier Discretion

     = Noncovered by Medicare or Medicare Statute

J0300	Injection, amobarbital, up to 125 mg	*MCM 2049*
J0330	Injection, succinylcholine chloride, up to 20 mg	*MCM 2049*
J0340	Injection, nandrolone phenpropionate, up to 50 mg	*MCM 2049*
J0350	Injection, anistreplase, per 30 units	*MCM 2049*
J0360	Injection, hydralazine HCl, up to 20 mg	*MCM 2049*
J0380	Injection, metaraminol bitartrate, per 10 mg	*MCM 2049*
J0390	Injection, chloroquine HCl, up to 250 mg	*MCM 2049*
J0395	Injection, arbutamine HCl, 1 mg	*MCM 2049*
J0400	Injection, trimethaphan camsylate, up to 500 mg	*MCM 2049*
J0456	Injection, azithromycin, 500 mg	*MCM 2049.5*
J0460	Injection, atropine sulfate, up to 0.3 mg	*MCM 2049*
J0470	Injection, dimercaprol, per 100 mg	*MCM 2049*
J0475	Injection, baclofen, 10 mg	*MCM 2049*
J0476	Injection, baclofen, 50 mcg for intrathecal trial	*MCM 2049*
J0500	Injection, dicyclomine HCl, up to 20 mg	*MCM 2049*
J0510	Injection, benzquinamide HCl, up to 50 mg	*MCM 2049*
J0515	Injection, benztropine mesylate, per 1 mg	*MCM 2049*
J0520	Injection, bethanechol chloride, mytonachol or urecholine, up to 5 mg *MCM 2049*	
J0530	Injection, penicillin G benzathine and penicillin G procaine, up to 600,000 units	*MCM 2049*
J0540	Injection, penicillin G benzathine and penicillin G procaine, up to 1,200,000 units	*MCM 2049*
J0550	Injection, penicillin G benzathine and penicillin G procaine, up to 2,400,000 units	*MCM 2049*
J0560	Injection, penicillin G benzathine, up to 600,000 units	*MCM 2049*
J0570	Injection, penicillin G benzathine, up to 1,200,000 units	*MCM 2049*
J0580	Injection, penicillin G benzathine, up to 2,400,000 units	*MCM 2049*
J0585	Botulinum toxin type A, per unit	*MCM 2049*
J0590	Injection, ethylnorepinephrine HCl, 1 ml	*MCM 2049*
J0600	Injection, edetate calcium disodium, up to 1000 mg	*MCM 2049*
J0610	Injection, calcium gluconate, per 10 ml	*MCM 2049*
J0620	Injection, calcium glycerophosphate and calcium lactate, per 10 ml *MCM 2049*	
J0630	Injection, calcitonin-salmon, up to 400 units	*MCM 2049*
J0635	Injection, calcitriol, 1 mcg ampule	*MCM 2049*
J0640	Injection, leucovorin calcium, per 50 mg	*MCM 2049*
J0670	Injection, mepivacaine HCl, per 10 ml	*MCM 2049*

▓ = Invalid Medicare Code (no grace period)

▓ = Code may require certificate of medical necessity (CMN) or DMERC information form (DIF)

J0690	Injection, cefazolin sodium, 500 mg	
J0694	Injection, cefoxitin sodium, 1 g	MCM 2049
J0695	Injection, cefonicid sodium, 1 g	MCM 2049
J0696	Injection, ceftriaxone sodium, per 250 mg	MCM 2049
J0697	Injection, sterile cefuroxime sodium, per 750 mg	MCM 2049
J0698	Cefotaxime sodium, per g	MCM 2049
J0702	Injection, betamethasone acetate and betamethasone sodium phosphate, per 3 mg	MCM 2049
J0704	Injection, betamethasone sodium phosphate, per 4 mg	MCM 2049
J0710	Injection, cephapirin sodium, up to 1 g	MCM 2049
J0713	Injection, ceftazidime, per 500 mg	MCM 2049
J0715	Injection, ceftizoxime sodium, per 500 mg	MCM 2049
J0720	Injection, chloramphenicol sodium succinate, up to 1 g	MCM 2049
J0725	Injection, chorionic gonadotropin, per 1,000 USP units	MCM 2049
J0730	Injection, chlorpheniramine maleate, per 10 mg	MCM 2049
J0735	Injection, clonidine hydrochloride, 1 mg	MCM 2049
J0740	Injection, cidofovir, 375 mg	MCM 2049
J0743	Injection, cilastatin sodium imipenem, per 250 mg	MCM 2049
J0745	Injection, codeine phosphate, per 30 mg	MCM 2049
J0760	Injection, colchicine, per 1 mg	MCM 2049
J0770	Injection, colistimethate sodium, up to 150 mg	MCM 2049
J0780	Injection, prochlorperazine, up to 10 mg	MCM 2049
J0800	Injection, corticotropin, up to 40 units	MCM 2049
J0810	Injection, cortisone, up to 50 mg	MCM 2049
J0835	Injection, cosyntropin, per 0.25 mg	MCM 2049
J0850	Injection, cytomegalovirus immune globulin intravenous (human), per vial	MCM 2049
▲ J0895	Injection, deferoxamine mesylate, 500 mg	MCM 2049
J0900	Injection, testosterone enanthate and estradiol valerate, up to 1 cc	MCM 2049
J0945	Injection, brompheniramine maleate, per 10 mg	MCM 2049
J0970	Injection, estradiol valerate, up to 40 mg	MCM 2049
J1000	Injection, depo-estradiol cypionate, up to 5 mg	MCM 2049
J1020	Injection, methylprednisolone acetate, 20 mg	MCM 2049
J1030	Injection, methylprednisolone acetate, 40 mg	MCM 2049
J1040	Injection, methylprednisolone acetate, 80 mg	MCM 2049
J1050	Injection, medroxyprogesterone acetate, 100 mg	MCM 2049

= Special Coverage Instructions Apply   = Carrier Discretion

= Noncovered by Medicare or Medicare Statute

J1055	Injection, medroxyprogesterone acetate for contraceptive use, 150 mg	
		Medicare Statute 1862.A1
J1060	Injection, testosterone cypionate and estradiol cypionate, up to 1 ml	
		MCM 2049
J1070	Injection, testosterone cypionate, up to 100 mg	*MCM 2049*
J1080	Injection, testosterone cypionate, 1 cc, 200 mg	*MCM 2049*
J1090	Injection, testosterone cypionate, 1 cc, 50 mg	*MCM 2049*
J1095	Injection, dexamethasone acetate, per 8 mg	*MCM 2049*
▲ **J1100**	Injection, dexamethosone sodium phosphate, 1 mg	*MCM 2049*
J1110	Injection, dihydroergotamine mesylate, per 1 mg	*MCM 2049*
J1120	Injection, acetazolamide sodium, up to 500 mg	*MCM 2049*
J1160	Injection, digoxin, up to 0.5 mg	*MCM 2049*
J1165	Injection, phenytoin sodium, per 50 mg	*MCM 2049*
J1170	Injection, hydromorphone, up to 4 mg	*MCM 2049*
J1180	Injection, dyphylline, up to 500 mg	*MCM 2049*
J1190	Injection, dexrazoxane hydrochloride, per 250 mg	*MCM 2049*
J1200	Injection, diphenhydramine HCl, up to 50 mg	*MCM 2049*
J1205	Injection, chlorothiazide sodium, per 500 mg	*MCM 2049*
J1212	Injection, DMSO, dimethyl sulfoxide, 50%, 50 ml	*MCM 2049*
J1230	Injection, methadone HCl, up to 10 mg	*MCM 2049*
J1240	Injection, dimenhydrinate, up to 50 mg	*MCM 2049*
J1245	Injection, dipyridamole, per 10 mg	*MCM 2049, 15030*
J1250	Injection, dobutamine HCl, per 250 mg	*MCM 2049*
J1260	Injection, dolasetron mesylate, 10 mg	*MCM 2049*
J1320	Injection, amitriptyline HCl, up to 20 mg	*MCM 2049*
J1325	Injection, epoprostenol, 0.5 mg	*MCM 2049*
J1327	Injection, eptifibatide, 5 mg	*MCM 2049*
J1330	Injection, ergonovine maleate, up to 0.2 mg	*MCM 2049*
J1362	Injection, erythromycin gluceptate, per 250 mg	*MCM 2049*
J1364	Injection, erythromycin lactobionate, per 500 mg	*MCM 2049*
J1380	Injection, estradiol valerate, up to 10 mg	*MCM 2049*
J1390	Injection, estradiol valerate, up to 20 mg	*MCM 2049*
J1410	Injection, estrogen conjugated, per 25 mg	*MCM 2049*
J1435	Injection, estrone, per 1 mg	*MCM 2049*
J1436	Injection, etidronate disodium, per 300 mg	*MCM 2049*

= Invalid Medicare Code (no grace period)

= Code may require certificate of medical necessity (CMN) or DMERC information form (DIF)

J1438	Injection, etanercept, 25 mg (code may be used for Medicare when drug administered under the direct supervision of a physician, not for use when drug is self-administered)	*MCM 2049*
J1440	Injection, filgrastim (G-CSF), 300 mcg	*MCM 2049*
J1441	Injection, filgrastim (G-CSF), 480 mcg	*MCM 2049*
J1450	Injection, fluconazole, 200 mg	*MCM 2049.5*
● **J1452**	Injection, fomivirsen sodium, intraocular, 1.65 mg	*MCM 2049.3*
J1455	Injection, foscarnet sodium, per 1,000 mg	*MCM 2049*
J1460	Injection, gamma globulin, intramuscular, 1 cc	*MCM 2049*
J1470	Injection, gamma globulin, intramuscular, 2 cc	*MCM 2049*
J1480	Injection, gamma globulin, intramuscular, 3 cc	*MCM 2049*
J1490	Injection, gamma globulin, intramuscular, 4 cc	*MCM 2049*
J1500	Injection, gamma globulin, intramuscular, 5 cc	*MCM 2049*
J1510	Injection, gamma globulin, intramuscular, 6 cc	*MCM 2049*
J1520	Injection, gamma globulin, intramuscular, 7 cc	*MCM 2049*
J1530	Injection, gamma globulin, intramuscular, 8 cc	*MCM 2049*
J1540	Injection, gamma globulin, intramuscular, 9 cc	*MCM 2049*
J1550	Injection, gamma globulin, intramuscular, 10 cc	*MCM 2049*
J1560	Injection, gamma globulin, intramuscular, over 10 cc	*MCM 2049*
J1561	Injection, immune globulin, intravenous, 500 mg	*MCM 2049*
J1562	~~Injection, immune globulin, intravenous 5 g~~ This code has been deleted in 2001.	
● **J1563**	Injection, immune globulin, intravenous, 1 g	*MCM 2049*
J1565	Injection, respiratory syncytial virus immune globulin, intravenous, 50 mg	*MCM 2049*
J1570	Injection, ganciclovir sodium, 500 mg	*MCM 2049*
J1580	Injection, Garamycin, gentamicin, up to 80 mg	*MCM 2049*
J1600	Injection, gold sodium thiomalate, up to 50 mg	*MCM 2049*
J1610	Injection, glucagon hydrochloride, per 1 mg	*MCM 2049*
J1620	Injection, gonadorelin hydrochloride, per 100 mcg	*MCM 2049*
J1626	Injection, granisetron hydrochloride, 100 mcg	*MCM 2049*
J1630	Injection, haloperidol, up to 5 mg	*MCM 2049*
J1631	Injection, haloperidol decanoate, per 50 mg	*MCM 2049*
J1642	Injection, heparin sodium, (Heparin Lock Flush), per 10 units	*MCM 2049*
J1644	Injection, heparin sodium, per 1,000 units	*MCM 2049*
J1645	Injection, dalteparin sodium, per 2500 IU	*MCM 2049*
J1650	Injection, enoxaparin sodium, 10 mg	*MCM 2049*

= Special Coverage Instructions Apply   = Carrier Discretion

= Noncovered by Medicare or Medicare Statute

J1670	Injection, tetanus immune globulin, human, up to 250 units	*MCM 2049*
J1690	Injection, prednisolone tebutate, up to 20 mg	*MCM 2049*
J1700	Injection, hydrocortisone acetate, up to 25 mg	*MCM 2049*
J1710	Injection, hydrocortisone sodium phosphate, up to 50 mg	*MCM 2049*
J1720	Injection, hydrocortisone sodium succinate, up to 100 mg	*MCM 2049*
J1730	Injection, diazoxide, up to 300 mg	*MCM 2049*
J1739	Injection, hydroxyprogesterone caproate, 125 mg/ml	*MCM 2049*
J1741	Injection, hydroxyprogesterone caproate, 250 mg/ml	*MCM 2049*
J1742	Injection, ibutilide fumarate, 1 mg	*MCM 2049*
J1745	Injection, infliximab, 10 mg	*MCM 2049*
J1750	Injection, iron dextran, 50 mg	*MCM 2049.5*
J1785	Injection, imiglucerase, per unit	*MCM 2049*
J1790	Injection, droperidol, up to 5 mg	*MCM 2049*
J1800	Injection, propranolol HCl, up to 1 mg	*MCM 2049*
J1810	Injection, droperidol and fentanyl citrate, up to 2 ml ampule	*MCM 2049*
J1820	Injection, insulin, up to 100 units	*CIM 60-14, MCM 2049*
J1825	Injection, interferon beta-1a, 33 mcg (code may be used for Medicare when drug administered under direct supervision of a physician, not for use when drug is self-administered)	*MCM 2049*
J1830	Injection interferon beta-1b, 0.25 mg (code may be used for Medicare when drug administered under direct supervision of a physician, not for use when drug is self-administered)	*MCM 2049*
J1840	Injection, kanamycin sulfate, up to 500 mg	*MCM 2049*
J1850	Injection, kanamycin sulfate, up to 75 mg	*MCM 2049*
J1885	Injection, ketorolac tromethamine, per 15 mg	*MCM 2049*
J1890	Injection, cephalothin sodium, up to 1 g	*MCM 2049*
J1910	Injection, kutapressin, up to 2 ml	*MCM 2049*
J1930	Injection, propiomazine HCl, up to 20 mg	*MCM 2049*
J1940	Injection, furosemide, up to 20 mg	*MCM 2049*
J1950	Injection, leuprolide acetate (for depot suspension), per 3.75 mg	*MCM 2049*
J1955	Injection, levocarnitine, per 1 g	*MCM 2049*
J1956	Injection, levofloxacin, 250 mg	*MCM 2049*
J1960	Injection, levorphanol tartrate, up to 2 mg	*MCM 2049*
J1970	Injection, methotrimeprazine, up to 20 mg	*MCM 2049*
J1980	Injection, hyoscyamine sulfate, up to 0.25 mg	*MCM 2049*
J1990	Injection, chlordiazepoxide HCl, up to 100 mg	*MCM 2049*
J2000	Injection, lidocaine HCl, 50 cc	*MCM 2049*

= Invalid Medicare Code (no grace period)

= Code may require certificate of medical necessity (CMN) or DMERC information form (DIF)

J Codes

J2010	Injection, lincomycin HCl, up to 300 mg	*MCM 2049*
J2060	Injection, lorazepam, 2 mg	*MCM 2049*
J2150	Injection, mannitol, 25% in 50 ml	*MCM 2049*
J2175	Injection, meperidine HCl, per 100 mg	*MCM 2050.5*
J2180	Injection, meperidine and promethazine HCl, up to 50 mg	*MCM 2049*
J2210	Injection, methylergonovine maleate, up to 0.2 mg	*MCM 2049*
J2240	Injection, metocurine iodide, up to 2 mg	*MCM 2049*
J2250	Injection, midazolam HCl, per 1 mg	*MCM 2049*
J2260	Injection, milrinone lactate, per 5 ml	*MCM 2049*
J2270	Injection, morphine sulfate, up to 10 mg	*MCM 2049*
J2271	Injection, morphine sulfate, 100 mg	*CIM 60-14a, MCM 2049*
J2275	Injection, morphine sulfate (preservative-free sterile solution), per 10 mg	*MCM 2049, CIM 60-14b*
J2300	Injection, nalbuphine HCl, per 10 mg	*MCM 2049*
J2310	Injection, naloxone HCl, per 1 mg	*MCM 2049*
J2320	Injection, nandrolone decanoate, up to 50 mg	*MCM 2049*
J2321	Injection, nandrolone decanoate, up to 100 mg	*MCM 2049*
J2322	Injection, nandrolone decanoate, up to 200 mg	*MCM 2049*
J2330	Injection, thiothixene, up to 4 mg	*MCM 2049*
J2350	Injection, niacinamide, niacin, up to 100 mg	*MCM 2049*
J2352	Injection, octreotide acetate, 1 mg	
J2355	Injection, oprelvekin, 5 mg	*MCM 2049*
J2360	Injection, orphenadrine citrate, up to 60 mg	*MCM 2049*
J2370	Injection, phenylephrine HCl, up to 1 ml	*MCM 2049*
J2400	Injection, chloroprocaine HCl, per 30 ml	*MCM 2049*
J2405	Injection, ondansetron HCl, per 1 mg	*MCM 2049*
J2410	Injection, oxymorphone HCl, up to 1 mg	*MCM 2049*
J2430	Injection, pamidronate disodium, per 30 mg	*MCM 2049*
J2440	Injection, papaverine HCl, up to 60 mg	*MCM 2049*
J2460	Injection, oxytetracycline HCl, up to 50 mg	*MCM 2049*
J2480	Injection, hydrochlorides of opium alkaloids, up to 20 mg	*MCM 2049*
J2500	Injection, paricalcitol, 5 mcg	*MCM 2049*
J2510	Injection, penicillin G procaine, aqueous, up to 600,000 units	*MCM 2049*
J2512	Injection, pentagastrin, per 2 ml	*MCM 2049*
J2515	Injection, pentobarbital sodium, per 50 mg	*MCM 2049*
J2540	Injection, penicillin G potassium, up to 600,000 units	*MCM 2049*

= Special Coverage Instructions Apply   = Carrier Discretion

= Noncovered by Medicare or Medicare Statute

▲ **J2543** Injection, piperacillin sodium/tazobactam sodium, 1 gram/0.125 grams (1.125 grams) *MCM 2049*

J2545 Pentamidine isethionate, inhalation solution, per 300 mg, administered through a DME *MCM 2049*

J2550 Injection, promethazine HCl, up to 50 mg *MCM 2049*

J2560 Injection, phenobarbital sodium, up to 120 mg *MCM 2049*

J2590 Injection, oxytocin, up to 10 units *MCM 2049*

J2597 Injection, desmopressin acetate, per 1 mcg *MCM 2049*

J2640 Injection, prednisolone sodium phosphate, up to 20 mg *MCM 2049*

J2650 Injection, prednisolone acetate, up to 1 ml *MCM 2049*

J2670 Injection, tolazoline HCl, up to 25 mg *MCM 2049*

J2675 Injection, progesterone, per 50 mg *MCM 2049*

J2680 Injection, fluphenazine decanoate, up to 25 mg *MCM 2049*

J2690 Injection, procainamide HCl, up to 1 g *MCM 2049*

J2700 Injection, oxacillin sodium, up to 250 mg *MCM 2049*

J2710 Injection, neostigmine methylsulfate, up to 0.5 mg *MCM 2049*

J2720 Injection, protamine sulfate, per 10 mg *MCM 2049*

J2725 Injection, protirelin, per 250 mcg *MCM 2049*

J2730 Injection, pralidoxime chloride, up to 1 g *MCM 2049*

J2760 Injection, phentolamine mesylate, up to 5 mg *MCM 2049*

J2765 Injection, metoclopramide HCl, up to 10 mg *MCM 2049*

● **J2770** Injection, quinupristin/dalfopristin, 500 mg (150/350) *MCM 2090*

J2780 Injection, ranitidine hydrochloride, 25 mg *MCM 2049*

J2790 Injection, Rho (D) immune globulin, human, one dose package *MCM 2049*

J2792 Injection, rho D immune globulin, intravenous, human, solvent detergent, 100 I.U. *MCM 2049*

● **J2795** Injection, ropivacaine hydrochloride, 1 mg

J2800 Injection, methocarbamol, up to 10 ml *MCM 2050.5*

J2810 Injection, theophylline, per 40 mg *MCM 2050.5*

J2820 Injection, sargramostim (GM-CSF), 50 mcg *MCM 2049*

J2860 Injection, secobarbital sodium, up to 250 mg *MCM 2049*

J2910 Injection, aurothioglucose, up to 50 mg *MCM 2049*

J2912 Injection, sodium chloride, 0.9%, per 2 ml *MCM 2049*

● **J2915** Injection, sodium ferric gluconate complex in sucrose injection, 62.5 mg *MCM 2049.2, 2049.4*

J2920 Injection, methylprednisolone sodium succinate, up to 40 mg *MCM 2049*

= Invalid Medicare Code (no grace period)

= Code may require certificate of medical necessity (CMN) or DMERC information form (DIF)

J Codes

J2930	Injection, methylprednisolone sodium succinate, up to 125 mg	
		MCM 2049
J2950	Injection, promazine HCl, up to 25 mg	*MCM 2049*
J2970	Injection, methicillin sodium, up to 1 g	*MCM 2049*
● **J2993**	Reteplase, 18.1 mg	*MCM 2049* ~~049~~
J2994	~~Injection reteplase, 37.6 mg (two single use vials)~~ This code has been deleted in 2001.	
J2995	Injection, streptokinase, per 250,000 IU	
J2996	~~Injection, alteplase recombinant, per 10 mg~~ This code was deleted in 2001.	
● **J2997**	Injection, alteplase recombinant, 1 mg	*MCM 2049*
J3000	Injection, streptomycin, up to 1 g	*MCM 2049*
▲ **J3010**	Injection, fentanyl citrate, 0.1 mg	*MCM 2049*
J3030	Injection, sumatriptan succinate, 6 mg (code may not be used for Medicare when drug administered under direct supervision of a physician, not for use when drug is self-administered)	
J3070	Injection, pentazocine HCl, up to 30 mg	*MCM 2049*
J3080	Injection, chlorprothixene, up to 50 mg	*MCM 2049*
J3105	Injection, terbutaline sulfate, up to 1 mg	*MCM 2049*
J3120	Injection, testosterone enanthate, up to 100 mg	*MCM 2049*
J3130	Injection, testosterone enanthate, up to 200 mg	*MCM 2049*
J3140	Injection, testosterone suspension, up to 50 mg	*MCM 2049*
J3150	Injection, testosterone propionate, up to 100 mg	*MCM 2049*
J3230	Injection, chlorpromazine HCl, up to 50 mg	*MCM 2049*
J3240	Injection, thyrotropin alpha, 0.9 mg	*MCM 2049*
J3245	Injection, tirofiban hydrochloride, 12.5 mg	*MCM 2049*
J3250	Injection, trimethobenzamide HCl, up to 200 mg	*MCM 2049*
J3260	Injection, tobramycin sulfate, up to 80 mg	*MCM 2049*
J3265	Injection, torsemide, 10 mg/ml	*MCM 2049*
J3270	Injection, imipramine HCl, up to 25 mg	*MCM 2049*
J3280	Injection, thiethylperazine maleate, up to 10 mg	*MCM 2049*
J3301	Injection, triamcinolone acetonide, per 10 mg	*MCM 2049*
J3302	Injection, triamcinolone diacetate, per 5 mg	*MCM 2049*
J3303	Injection, triamcinolone hexacetonide, per 5 mg	*MCM 2049*
J3305	Injection, trimetrexate glucoronate, per 25 mg	*MCM 2049*
J3310	Injection, perphenazine, up to 5 mg	*MCM 2049*
J3320	Injection, spectinomycin dihydrochloride, up to 2 g	*MCM 2049*

= Special Coverage Instructions Apply		= Carrier Discretion
= Noncovered by Medicare or Medicare Statute		

J3350	Injection, urea, up to 40 g	MCM 2049
J3360	Injection, diazepam, up to 5 mg	MCM 2049
J3364	Injection, urokinase, 5,000 IU vial	MCM 2049
J3365	Injection, IV, urokinase, 250,000 IU vial	MCM 2049
J3370	Injection, vancomycin HCl, 500 mg	CIM 60-14, MCM 2049
J3390	Injection, methoxamine HCl, up to 20 mg	MCM 2049
J3400	Injection, triflupromazine HCl, up to 20 mg	MCM 2049
J3410	Injection, hydroxyzine HCl, up to 25 mg	MCM 2049
J3420	Injection, vitamin B-12 cyanocobalamin, up to 1,000 mcg	CIM 45-4, MCM 2049
J3430	Injection, phytonadione (vitamin K), per 1 mg	MCM 2049
J3450	Injection, mephentermine sulfate, up to 30 mg	MCM 2049
J3470	Injection, hyaluronidase, up to 150 units	MCM 2049
J3475	Injection, magnesium sulphate, per 500 mg	MCM 2049
J3480	Injection, potassium chloride, per 2 mEq	MCM 2049
● J3485	Injection, zidovudine, 10 mg	MCM 2049
J3490	Unclassified drugs	MCM 2049
J3520	Edetate disodium, per 150 mg	Medicaid suspend for medical review, CIM 35-64, 45-20
J3530	Nasal vaccine inhalation	MCM 2049
J3535	Drug administered through a metered dose inhaler	MCM 2050.5
J3570	Laetrile, amygdalin, vitamin B-17	CIM 45-10

Miscellaneous Drugs and Solutions

J7030	Infusion, normal saline solution, 1,000 cc	MCM 2049
J7040	Infusion, normal saline solution, sterile (500 ml = 1 unit)	MCM 2049
J7042	5% dextrose/normal saline (500 ml = 1 unit)	MCM 2049
J7050	Infusion, normal saline solution, 250 cc	MCM 2049
J7051	Sterile saline or water, up to 5 cc	MCM 2049
J7060	5% dextrose/water (500 ml = 1 unit)	MCM 2049
J7070	Infusion, D-5-W, 1,000 cc	MCM 2049
J7100	Infusion, dextran 40, 500 ml	MCM 2049
J7110	Infusion, dextran 75, 500 ml	MCM 2049
J7120	Ringer's lactate infusion, up to 1,000 cc	MCM 2049
J7130	Hypertonic saline solution, 50 or 100 mEq, 20 cc vial	MCM 2049
J7190	Factor VIII (antihemophilic factor, human) per I.U.	MCM 2049, ASC
J7191	Factor VIII (anti-hemophilic factor (porcine)), per I.U.	ASC
J7192	Factor VIII (antihemophilic factor, recombinant) per I.U.	MCM 2049, ASC

= Invalid Medicare Code (no grace period)

= Code may require certificate of medical necessity (CMN) or DMERC information form (DIF)

J7194	Factor IX complex, per IU	*MCM 2049, ASC*
J7197	Antithrombin III (human), per IU	*MCM 2049, ASC*
J7198	Anti-inhibitor, per i.u.	*CIM 45-24, MCM 2049*
J7199	Hemophilia clotting factor, not otherwise classified	*CIM 45-24, MCM 2049*
J7300	Intrauterine copper contraceptive	*Medicare Statute 1862.A1*
J7310	Ganciclovir, 4.5 mg, long-acting implant	*MCM 2049*
J7315	Sodium hyaluronate, 20 mg, for intra-articular injection	
J7320	Hylan G-F 20, 16 mg, for intra-articular injection	
● **J7330**	Autologous cultured chondrocytes, implant	
J7500	Azathioprine, oral, 50 mg	*MCM 2049.5*
J7501	Azathioprine, parenteral,100 mg	*MCM 2049*
J7502	Cyclosporine, oral, 100 mg	*MCM 2049.5*
J7504	Lymphocyte immune globulin, antithymocyte globulin, parenteral, 250 mg	*CIM 45-22, MCM 2049*
▲ **J7505**	Muromonab-CD3, parenteral, 5 mg	*MCM 2049, ASC*
J7506	Prednisone, oral, per 5 mg	*MCM 2049.5, ASC*
J7507	Tacrolimus, oral, per 1 mg	*MCM 2049.5*
J7508	Tacrolimus, oral, per 5 mg	*MCM 2049.5*
J7509	Methylprednisolone, oral, per 4 mg	*MCM 2049.5, ASC*
J7510	Prednisolone, oral, per 5 mg	*MCM 2049.5, ASC*
J7513	Daclizumab, parenteral, 25 mg	*MCM 2049.5*
J7515	Cyclosporine, oral, 25 mg	
J7516	Cyclosporine, parenteral, 250 mg	
J7517	Mycophenolate mofetil, oral, 250 mg	
● **J7520**	Sirolimus, oral, 1 mg	*MCM 2049.5*
● **J7525**	Tacrolimus, parenteral, 5 mg	*MCM 2049.5*
J7599	Immunosuppressive drug, not otherwise classified	*MCM 2049.5, ASC*
J7608	Acetylcysteine, inhalation solution administered through DME, unit dose form, per gram	*MCM 2100.5*

Inhalation Solutions

J7610 ~~Acetylcysteine, 10%, per ml, inhalation solution administered through DME~~ This code has been deleted in 2001.

J7615 ~~Acetylcysteine, 20%, per ml, inhalation solution administered through DME~~ This code has been deleted in 2001.

▲ **J7618** Albuterol, all formulations including separated isomers, inhalation solution administered through DME, concentrated form, per 1 mg
MCM 2100.5

▲ **J7619** Albuterol, all formulations including separated isomers, inhalation solution administered through DME, unit dose form, per 1 mg
MCM 2100.5

J7620 ~~Albuterol sulfate, 0.083%, per ml, inhalation solution administered through DME~~ This code has been deleted in 2001.

J7625 ~~Albuterol sulfate, 0.5%, per ml, inhalation solution administered through DME~~ This code has been deleted in 2001.

J7627 ~~Bitolterol mesylate, 0.2%, per 10 ml, inhalation solution administered through DME~~ This code has been deleted in 2001.

J7628 Bitolterol mesylate, inhalation solution administered through DME, concentrated form, per milligram
MCM 2100.5

J7629 Bitolterol mesylate, inhalation solution administered through DME, unit dose form, per milligram
MCM 2100.5

J7630 ~~Cromolyn sodium, per 20 mg, inhalation solution administered through DME~~ This code has been deleted in 2001.

J7631 Cromolyn sodium, inhalation solution administered through DME, unit dose form, per 10 milligrams
MCM 2100.5

J7635 Atropine, inhalation solution administered through DME, concentrated form, per milligram
MCM 2100.5

J7636 Atropine, inhalation solution administered through DME, unit dose form, per milligram
MCM 2100.5

J7637 Dexamethasone, inhalation solution administered through DME, concentrated form, per milligram
MCM 2100.5

J7638 Dexamethasone, inhalation solution administered through DME, unit dose form, per milligram
MCM 2100.5

J7639 Dornase alpha, inhalation solution administered through DME, unit dose form, per milligram
MCM 2100.5

J7640 ~~Epinephrine, 2.25%, per ml, inhalation solution administered through DME~~ This code has been deleted in 2001.

J7642 Glycopyrrolate, inhalation solution administered through DME, concentrated form, per milligram
MCM 2100.5

J7643 Glycopyrrolate, inhalation solution administered through DME, unit dose form, per milligram
MCM 2100.5

J7644 Ipratropium bromide, inhalation solution administered through DME, unit dose form, per milligram
MCM 2100.5

J7645 ~~Ipratropium bromide 0.02%, per ml, inhalation solution, administered through a DME~~ This code has been deleted in 2001.

J7648 Isoetharine HCl, inhalation solution administered through DME, concentrated form, per milligram
MCM 2100.5

J7649 Isoetharine HCl, inhalation solution administered through DME, unit dose form, per milligram
MCM 2100.5

= Invalid Medicare Code (no grace period)

= Code may require certificate of medical necessity (CMN) or DMERC information form (DIF)

J7650 ~~Isoetharine HCl, 0.1%, per ml, inhalation solution administered through DME~~ This code has been deleted in 2001.

J7651 ~~Isoetharine HCl, 0.125%, per ml, inhalation solution administered through DME~~ This code has been deleted in 2001.

J7652 ~~Isoetharine HCl, 0.167%, per ml, inhalation solution administered through DME~~ This code has been deleted in 2001.

J7653 ~~Isoetharine HCl, 0.2%, per ml, inhalation solution administered through DME~~ This code has been deleted in 2001.

J7654 ~~Isoetharine HCl, 0.25%, per ml, inhalation solution administered through DME~~ This code has been deleted in 2001.

J7655 ~~Isoetharine HCl, 1.0%, per ml, inhalation solution administered through DME~~ This code has been deleted in 2001.

J7658 Isoproterenol HCl, inhalation solution administered through DME, concentrated form, per milligram   *MCM 2100.5*

J7659 Isoproterenol HCl, inhalation solution administered through DME, unit dose form, per milligram   *MCM 2100.5*

J7660 ~~Isoproterenol HCl, 0.5%, per ml, inhalation solution administered through DME~~ This code has been deleted in 2001.

J7665 ~~Isoproterenol HCl, 1.0%, per ml, inhalation solution administered through DME~~ This code has been deleted in 2001.

J7668 Metaproterenol sulfate, inhalation solution administered through DME, concentrated form, per 10 milligrams   *MCM 2100.5*

J7669 Metaproterenol sulfate, inhalation solution administered through DME, unit dose form, per 10 milligrams   *MCM 2100.5*

J7670 ~~Metaproterenol sulfate, 0.4%, per 2.5 ml, inhalation solution administered through DME~~ This code has been deleted in 2001.

J7672 ~~Metaproterenol sulfate, 0.6%, per 2.5 ml, inhalation solution administered through DME~~ This code has been deleted in 2001.

J7675 ~~Metaproterenol sulfate, 5.0%, per ml, inhalation solution administered through DME~~ This code has been deleted in 2001.

J7680 Terbutaline sulfate, inhalation solution administered through DME, concentrated form, per milligram   *MCM 2100.5*

J7681 Terbutaline sulfate, inhalation solution administered through DME, unit dose form, per milligram   *MCM 2100.5*

J7682 Tobramycin, unit dose form, 300 mg, inhalation solution, administered through DME   *MCM 2100.5*

J7683 Triamcinolone, inhalation solution administered through DME, concentrated form, per milligram   *MCM 2100.5*

J7684 Triamcinolone, inhalation solution administered through DME, unit dose form, per milligram   *MCM 2100.5*

J7699 NOC drugs, inhalation solution administered through DME *MCM 2100.5*

= Special Coverage Instructions Apply   = Carrier Discretion

= Noncovered by Medicare or Medicare Statute

J7799	NOC drugs, other than inhalation drugs, administered through DME	
		MCM 2100.5
J8499	Prescription drug, oral, nonchemotherapeutic, not otherwise specified	
		MCM 2049
J8510	Bulsulfan; oral, 2 mg	*MCM 2049.5*
J8520	Capecitabine, oral, 150 mg	*MCM 2049.5*
J8521	Capecitabine, oral, 500 mg	*MCM 2049.5*
J8530	Cyclophosphamide, oral, 25 mg	*MCM 2049.5*
J8560	Etoposide, oral, 50 mg	*MCM 2049.5*
J8600	Melphalan, oral 2 mg	*MCM 2049.5*
J8610	Methotrexate, oral, 2.5 mg	*MCM 2049.5*
● **J8700**	Temozolomide, oral, 5 mg	*MCM 2049*
J8999	Prescription drug, oral, chemotherapeutic, not otherwise specified	
		MCM 2049.5

Chemotherapy Drugs J9000–J9999

These codes cover the cost of the chemotherapy drug only, not the administration. See also J8999.

J9000	Doxorubicin HCl, 10 mg	*MCM 2049*
J9001	Doxorubicin hydrochloride, all lipid formulations, 10 mg	*MCM 2049*
J9015	Aldesleukin, per single use vial	*MCM 2049*
J9020	Asparaginase, 10,000 units	*MCM 2049*
J9031	BCG live (intravesical), per installation	*MCM 2049*
J9040	Bleomycin sulfate, 15 units	*MCM 2049*
J9045	Carboplatin, 50 mg	*MCM 2049*
J9050	Carmustine, 100 mg	*MCM 2049*
J9060	Cisplatin, powder or solution, per 10 mg	*MCM 2049*
J9062	Cisplatin, 50 mg	*MCM 2049*
J9065	Injection, cladribine, per 1 mg	*MCM 2049*
J9070	Cyclophosphamide, 100 mg	*MCM 2049*
J9080	Cyclophosphamide, 200 mg	*MCM 2049*
J9090	Cyclophosphamide, 500 mg	*MCM 2049*
J9091	Cyclophosphamide, 1 g	*MCM 2049*
J9092	Cyclophosphamide, 2 g	*MCM 2049*
J9093	Cyclophosphamide, lyophilized, 100 mg	*MCM 2049*
J9094	Cyclophosphamide, lyophilized, 200 mg	*MCM 2049*
J9095	Cyclophosphamide, lyophilized, 500 mg	*MCM 2049*

J9096	Cyclophosphamide, lyophilized, 1 g	MCM 2049
J9097	Cyclophosphamide, lyophilized, 2 g	MCM 2049
J9100	Cytarabine, 100 mg	MCM 2049
J9110	Cytarabine, 500 mg	MCM 2049
J9120	Dactinomycin, 0.5 mg	MCM 2049
J9130	Dacarbazine, 100 mg	MCM 2049
J9140	Dacarbazine, 200 mg	MCM 2049
J9150	Daunorubicin HCl, 10 mg	MCM 2049
J9151	Daunorubicin citrate, liposomal formulation, 10 mg	MCM 2049
● J9160	Denileukin diftitox, 300 mcg	
J9165	Diethylstilbestrol diphosphate, 250 mg	MCM 2049
J9170	Docetaxel, 20 mg	MCM 2049
● J9180	Epirubicin hydrochloride, 50 mg	MCM 2049
J9181	Etoposide, 10 mg	MCM 2049
J9182	Etoposide, 100 mg	MCM 2049
J9185	Fludarabine phosphate, 50 mg	MCM 2049
J9190	Fluorouracil, 500 mg	MCM 2049
J9200	Floxuridine, 500 mg	MCM 2049
J9201	Gemcitabine HCl, 200 mg	MCM 2049
J9202	Goserelin acetate implant, per 3.6 mg	MCM 2049
J9206	Irinotecan, 20 mg	MCM 2049
J9208	Ifosfamide, per 1 g	MCM 2049
J9209	Mesna, 200 mg	MCM 2049
J9211	Idarubicin HCl, 5 mg	MCM 2049
J9212	Injection, interferon Alfacon-1, recombinant, 1 mcg	MCM 2049
J9213	Interferon alfa-2A, recombinant, 3 million units	MCM 2049
J9214	Interferon alfa-2B, recombinant, 1 million units	MCM 2049
J9215	Interferon alfa-N3, (human leukocyte derived), 250,000 IU	MCM 2049
J9216	Interferon gamma-1B, 3 million units	MCM 2049
J9217	Leuprolide acetate (for depot suspension), 7.5 mg	MCM 2049
J9218	Leuprolide acetate, per 1 mg	MCM 2049
● J9219	Leuprolide acetate implant, 65 mg	MCM 2049
J9230	Mechlorethamine HCl, (nitrogen mustard), 10 mg	MCM 2049
J9245	Injection, melphalan HCl, 50 mg	MCM 2049
J9250	Methotrexate sodium, 5 mg	MCM 2049
J9260	Methotrexate sodium, 50 mg	MCM 2049
J9265	Paclitaxel, 30 mg	MCM 2049

= Special Coverage Instructions Apply   = Carrier Discretion

= Noncovered by Medicare or Medicare Statute

J9266	Pegaspargase, per single dose vial	*MCM 2049*
J9268	Pentostatin, per 10 mg	*MCM 2049*
J9270	Plicamycin, 2.5 mg	*MCM 2049*
J9280	Mitomycin, 5 mg	*MCM 2049*
J9290	Mitomycin, 20 mg	*MCM 2049*
J9291	Mitomycin, 40 mg	*MCM 2049*
J9293	Injection, mitoxantrone HCl, per 5 mg	*MCM 2049*
J9310	Rituximab, 100 mg	*MCM 2049*
J9320	Streptozocin, 1 g	*MCM 2049*
J9340	Thiotepa, 15 mg	*MCM 2049*
J9350	Topotecan, 4 mg	*MCM 2049*
J9355	Trastuzumab, 10 mg	
J9357	Valrubicin, intravesical, 200 mg	*MCM 2049*
J9360	Vinblastine sulfate, 1 mg	*MCM 2049*
J9370	Vincristine sulfate, 1 mg	*MCM 2049*
J9375	Vincristine sulfate, 2 mg	*MCM 2049*
J9380	Vincristine sulfate, 5 mg	*MCM 2049*
J9390	Vinorelbine tartrate, per 10 mg	*MCM 2049*
J9600	Porfimer sodium, 75 mg	*MCM 2049*
J9999	Not otherwise classified, antineoplastic drug	*CIM 45-16, MCM 2049*

K Codes (Temporary) K0000–K9999

K Codes Assigned to Durable Medical Equipment Regional Carriers (DMERC)

Wheelchair and Wheelchair Accessories

Code	Description	
K0001	Standard wheelchair	*ASC*
K0002	Standard hemi (low seat) wheelchair	*ASC*
K0003	Lightweight wheelchair	*ASC*
K0004	High strength, lightweight wheelchair	*ASC*
K0005	Ultralightweight wheelchair	*ASC*
K0006	Heavy-duty wheelchair	*ASC*
K0007	Extra heavy-duty wheelchair	*ASC*
K0008	Custom manual wheelchair/base	*ASC*
K0009	Other manual wheelchair/base	*ASC*
K0010	Standard-weight frame motorized/power wheelchair	*ASC*
K0011	Standard-weight frame motorized/power wheelchair with programmable control parameters for speed adjustment, tremor dampening, acceleration control and braking	*ASC*
K0012	Lightweight portable motorized/power wheelchair	*ASC*
K0013	Custom motorized/power wheelchair base	*ASC*
K0014	Other motorized/power wheelchair base	*ASC*
K0015	Detachable, nonadjustable height armrest, each	*ASC*
K0016	Detachable, adjustable height armrest, complete assembly, each	*ASC*
K0017	Detachable, adjustable height armrest, base, each	*ASC*
K0018	Detachable, adjustable height armrest, upper portion, each	*ASC*
K0019	Arm pad, each	*ASC*
K0020	Fixed, adjustable height armrest, pair	*ASC*
K0021	Antitipping device, each	*ASC*
K0022	Reinforced back upholstery	*ASC*
K0023	Solid back insert, planar back, single density foam, attached with straps	*ASC*
K0024	Solid back insert, planar back, single density foam, with adjustable hook-on hardware	*ASC*
K0025	Hook-on headrest extension	*ASC*
K0026	Back upholstery for ultralightweight or high-strength lightweight wheelchair	*ASC*
K0027	Back upholstery for wheelchair type other than ultralightweight or high-strength lightweight wheelchair	*ASC*

K Codes

= Special Coverage Instructions Apply   = Carrier Discretion

= Noncovered by Medicare or Medicare Statute

K0028	Fully reclining back	*ASC*
K0029	Reinforced seat upholstery	*ASC*
K0030	Solid seat insert, planar seat, single density foam	*ASC*
K0031	Safety belt/pelvic strap, each	
K0032	Seat upholstery for ultralightweight or high-strength lightweight wheelchair	*ASC*
K0033	Seat upholstery for wheelchair type other than ultralightweight or high-strength lightweight wheelchair	*ASC*
K0034	Heel loop, each	*ASC*
K0035	Heel loop with ankle strap, each	*ASC*
K0036	Toe loop, each	*ASC*
K0037	High mount flip-up footrest, each	*ASC*
K0038	Leg strap, each	*ASC*
K0039	Leg strap, H style, each	*ASC*
K0040	Adjustable angle footplate, each	*ASC*
K0041	Large size footplate, each	*ASC*
K0042	Standard size footplate, each	*ASC*
K0043	Footrest, lower extension tube, each	*ASC*
K0044	Footrest, upper hanger bracket, each	*ASC*
K0045	Footrest, complete assembly	*ASC*
K0046	Elevating legrest, lower extension tube, each	*ASC*
K0047	Elevating legrest, upper hanger bracket, each	*ASC*
K0048	Elevating legrest, complete assembly	*ASC*
K0049	Calf pad, each	*ASC*
K0050	Ratchet assembly	*ASC*
K0051	Cam release assembly, footrest or legrest, each	*ASC*
K0052	Swingaway, detachable footrests, each	*ASC*
K0053	Elevating footrests, articulating (telescoping), each	*ASC*
K0054	Seat width of 10, 11, 12, 15, 17, or 20 inches for a high-strength, lightweight or ultralightweight wheelchair	*ASC*
K0055	Seat depth of 15, 17, or 18 inches for a high strength, lightweight or ultralightweight wheelchair	*ASC*
K0056	Seat height less than 17 inches or equal to or greater than 21 inches for a high strength, lightweight, or ultralightweight wheelchair	*ASC*
K0057	Seat width 19 or 20 inches for heavy duty or extra heavy-duty chair	*ASC*
K0058	Seat depth 17 or 18 inches for a motorized/power wheelchair	*ASC*
K0059	Plastic coated handrim, each	*ASC*
K0060	Steel handrim, each	*ASC*

= Invalid Medicare Code (no grace period)

= Code may require certificate of medical necessity (CMN) or DMERC information form (DIF)

K0061	Aluminum handrim, each	ASC
K0062	Handrim with 8 to 10 vertical or oblique projections, each	ASC
K0063	Handrim with 12 to 16 vertical or oblique projections, each	ASC
K0064	Zero pressure tube (flat free insert), any size, each	ASC
K0065	Spoke protectors, each	
K0066	Solid tire, any size, each	ASC
K0067	Pneumatic tire, any size, each	ASC
K0068	Pneumatic tire tube, each	ASC
K0069	Rear wheel assembly, complete, with solid tire, spokes or molded, each	ASC
K0070	Rear wheel assembly, complete with pneumatic tire, spokes or molded, each	ASC
K0071	Front caster assembly, complete, with pneumatic tire, each	ASC
K0072	Front caster assembly, complete, with semipneumatic tire, each	ASC
K0073	Caster pin lock, each	ASC
K0074	Pneumatic caster tire, any size, each	ASC
K0075	Semipneumatic caster tire, any size, each	ASC
K0076	Solid caster tire, any size, each	ASC
K0077	Front caster assembly, complete, with solid tire, each	ASC
K0078	Pneumatic caster tire tube, each	ASC
K0079	Wheel lock extension, pair	ASC
K0080	Antirollback device, pair	ASC
K0081	Wheel lock assembly, complete, each	ASC
K0082	22 NF deep cycle lead acid battery, each	ASC
K0083	22 NF gel cell battery, each	ASC
K0084	Group 24 deep cycle lead acid battery, each	ASC
K0085	Group 24 gel cell battery, each	ASC
K0086	U-1 lead acid battery, each	ASC
K0087	U-1 gel cell battery, each	ASC
K0088	Battery charger, lead acid or gel cell	ASC
K0089	Battery charger, dual mode	ASC
K0090	Rear wheel tire for power wheelchair, any size, each	ASC
K0091	Rear wheel tire tube other than zero pressure for power wheelchair, any size, each	ASC
K0092	Rear wheel assembly for power wheelchair, complete, each	ASC
K0093	Rear wheel zero pressure tire tube (flat free insert) for power wheelchair, any size, each	ASC

K Codes

= Special Coverage Instructions Apply   = Carrier Discretion

= Noncovered by Medicare or Medicare Statute

K0094	Wheel tire for power base, any size, each	ASC
K0095	Wheel tire tube other than zero pressure for each base, any size, each	ASC
K0096	Wheel assembly for power base, complete, each	ASC
K0097	Wheel zero-pressure tire tube (flat free insert) for power base, any size, each	ASC
K0098	Drive belt for power wheelchair	ASC
K0099	Front caster for power wheelchair	ASC
K0100	Wheelchair adapter for amputee, pair	
K0101	One-arm drive attachment, each	
K0102	Crutch and cane holder, each	
K0103	Transfer board, less than 25 inches	ASC
K0104	Cylinder tank carrier, each	
K0105	IV hanger, each	
K0106	Arm trough, each	ASC
K0107	Wheelchair tray	ASC
K0108	Other accessories	ASC

Spinal Orthotics

K0112	Trunk support device, vest type, with inner frame, prefabricated	ASC
K0113	Trunk support device, vest type, without inner frame, prefabricated	ASC
K0114	Back support system for use with a wheelchair, with inner frame, prefabricated	ASC
K0115	Seating system, back module, posterior-lateral control, with or without lateral supports, custom fabricated for attachment to wheelchair base ASC	
K0116	Seating system, combined back and seat module, custom fabricated for attachment to wheelchair base	ASC
K0182	~~Water, distilled, used with large volume nebulizer 1000 ml~~ This code has been deleted in 2001. See A7018.	
K0183	Nasal application device used with positive airway pressure device	ASC
K0184	Nasal pillows/seals, replacement for nasal application device, pair	ASC
K0185	Headgear used with positive airway pressure device	ASC
K0186	Chin strap used with positive airway pressure device	ASC
K0187	Tubing used with positive airway pressure device	ASC
K0188	Filter, disposable, used with positive airway pressure device	ASC
K0189	Filter, nondisposable, used with positive airway pressure device	ASC
K0195	Elevating legrest, pair (for use with capped rental wheelchair base)	CIM 60-9, ASC

= Invalid Medicare Code (no grace period)

= Code may require certificate of medical necessity (CMN) or DMERC information form (DIF)

Miscellaneous

K0268 Humidifier, nonheated, used with positive airway pressure device *ASC*

K0269 ~~Aerosol compressor, adjustable pressure, light duty for intermittent use~~ This code has been deleted in 2001. See E0572.

K0270 ~~Ultrasonic generator with small volume ultrasonic nebulizer~~ This code has been deleted in 2001. See E0574.

K0280 ~~Extension drainage tubing, any type, any length, with connector/adaptor, for use with urinary leg bag or urostomy pouch, each~~ This code has been deleted in 2001. See A4331.

K0281 ~~Lubricant, individual sterile packet, for insertion of urinary catheter, each~~ This code has been deleted in 2001. See A4332.

K0283 ~~Saline solution, per 10 ml, metered dose dispenser, for use with inhalation drugs~~ This code has been deleted in 2001. See A7019.

K0407 ~~Urinary catheter anchoring device, adhesive skin attachment~~ This code has been deleted in 2001. See A4333.

K0408 ~~Urinary catheter anchoring device, leg strap~~ This code has been deleted in 2001. See A4334.

K0409 ~~Sterile water irrigation solution, 1000 ml~~ This code has been deleted in 2001. See A4319.

K0410 ~~Male external catheter, with adhesive coating, each~~ This code has been deleted in 2001. See A4324.

K0411 ~~Male external catheter, with adhesive strip, each~~ This code has been deleted in 2001. See A4325.

K0415 Prescription antiemetic drug, oral, per 1 mg, for use in conjunction with oral anti-cancer drug, not otherwise specified *MCM 2049.5c, ASC*

K0416 Prescription antiemetic drug, rectal, per 1 mg, for use in conjunction with oral anti-cancer drug, not otherwise specified *MCM 2049.5c, ASC*

K0440 ~~Nasal prosthesis, provided by a non-physician~~ This code has been deleted in 2001. See L8040.

K0441 ~~Midfacial prosthesis, provided by a non-physician~~ This code has been deleted in 2001. See L8041.

K0442 ~~Orbital prosthesis, provided by a non-physician~~ This code has been deleted in 2001. See L8042.

K0443 ~~Upper facial prosthesis, provided by a non-physician~~ This code has been deleted in 2001. See L8043.

K0444 ~~Hemi-facial prosthesis, provided by a non-physician~~ This code has been deleted in 2001. See L8044.

K0445 ~~Auricular prosthesis, provided by a non-physician~~ This code has been deleted in 2001. See L8045.

K0446 ~~Partial facial prosthesis, provided by a non-physician~~ This code has been deleted in 2001. See L8046.

K Codes

= Special Coverage Instructions Apply   = Carrier Discretion

= Noncovered by Medicare or Medicare Statute

K0447 ~~Nasal septal prosthesis, provided by a non-physician~~ This code has been deleted in 2001. See L8047.

K0448 ~~Unspecified maxillofacial prosthesis, by report, provided by a non-physician~~ This code has been deleted in 2001. See L8048.

K0449 ~~Repair or modification of maxillofacial prosthesis, labor component, 15 minute increments, provided by a non-physician~~ This code has been deleted in 2001. See L8049.

K0450 ~~Adhesive liquid, for use with facial prosthesis only, per ounce~~ This code has been deleted in 2001. See A4364.

K0451 ~~Adhesive remover, wipes, for use with facial prosthesis, per box of 50~~ This code has been deleted in 2001. See A4365.

K0452 Wheelchair bearings, any type   *ASC*

K0455 Infusion pump used for uninterrupted administration of epoprostenol
CIM 60-14, ASC

K0456 ~~Hospital bed, heavy duty, extra wide, with any type side rails, with mattress~~ This code has been deleted in 2001. See E0298.

K0457 ~~Extra wide/heavy duty commode chair, each~~ This code has been deleted in 2001. See E0168.

K0458 ~~Heavy duty walker, without wheels, each~~ This code has been deleted in 2001. See E0148.

K0459 ~~Heavy duty wheeled walker, each~~ This code has been deleted in 2001. See E0149.

K0460 Power add-on, to convert manual wheelchair to motorized wheelchair, joystick control

K0461 Power add-on, to convert manual wheelchair to power operated vehicle, tiller control

K0462 Temporary replacement for patient owned equipment being repaired, any type   *MCM 5102.3*

K0501 ~~Aerosol compressor, battery powered, for use with small volume nebulizer~~ This code has been deleted in 2001. See E0571.

K0529 ~~Sterile water or sterile saline, 1,000 ml, used with large volume nebulizer~~ This code has been deleted in 2001. See A7020.

K0531 Humidifier, heated, used with positive airway pressure device   *CIM 60-9*

K0532 Respiratory assist device, bi-level pressure capability, without backup rate feature, used with noninvasive interface, e.g., nasal or facial mask (intermittent assist device with continuous positive airway pressure device)
CIM 60-9

K0533 Respiratory assist device, bi-level pressure capability, with backup rate feature, used with noninvasive interface, e.g., nasal or facial mask (intermittent assist device with continuous positive airway pressure device)
CIM 60-9

= Invalid Medicare Code (no grace period)

= Code may require certificate of medical necessity (CMN) or DMERC information form (DIF)

K0534 Respiratory assist device, bi-level pressure capacity, with backup rate feature, used with invasive interface, e.g., tracheostomy tube (intermittent assist device with continuous positive airway pressure device) *CIM 60-9*

K0535 ~~Gauze, impregnated, hydrogel, for direct wound contact pad size 16 sq. in. or less, without adhesive border, each dressing~~ This code was added and deleted in 2000. See A6231.

K0536 ~~Gauze, impregnated, hydrogel, for direct wound contact pad size more than 16 sq. in., but less than or equal to 48 sq in, without adhesive border, each dressing~~ This code was added and deleted in 2000. See A6232.

K0537 ~~Gauze, impregnated, hydrogel, for direct wound contact, pad size more than 48 sq. in., without adhesive border, each dressing~~ This code was added and deleted in 2000. See A6233.

● **K0538** Negative pressure wound therapy electrical pump, stationary or portable

● **K0539** Dressing set for negative pressure wound therapy electrical pump, stationary or portable, each

● **K0540** Canister set for negative pressure wound therapy electrical pump, stationary or portable, each

● **K0541** Speech generating device, digitized speech using pre-recorded messages, less than or equal to 8 minutes recording time *CIM 60-23*

● **K0542** Speech generating device, digitized speech, using pre-recorded messages, greater than 8 minutes recording time *CIM 60-23*

● **K0543** Speech generating device, synthesized speech, requiring message formulation by spelling and access by physical contact with the device *CIM 60-23*

● **K0544** Speech generating device, synthesized speech, permitting multiple methods of message formulation and multiple methods of device access *CIM 60-23*

● **K0545** Speech generating software program, for personal computer or personal digital assistant *CIM 60-23*

● **K0546** Accessory for speech generating device, mounting system *CIM 60-23*

● **K0547** Accessory for speech generating device, not otherwise classified *CIM 60-23*

K Codes

= Special Coverage Instructions Apply   = Carrier Discretion

= Noncovered by Medicare or Medicare Statute

Orthotic Procedures L0000–L4999

Braces, trusses, and artificial legs, arms, and eyes are covered when furnished incident to physicians' services or on a physician's order. A brace includes rigid and semi-rigid devices used for the purpose of supporting a weak or deformed body member or restricting or eliminating motion in a diseased or injured part of the body. Back braces include, but are not limited to, sacroiliac, sacrolumbar, dorsolumbar corsets and belts. Stump stockings and harnesses (including replacements) are also covered when these appliances are essential to the effective use of an artificial limb. Adjustments to an artificial limb or other appliance required by wear or by a change in the patient's condition are covered when ordered by a physician. Adjustments, repairs and replacements are covered so long as the device continues to be medically required.

Orthotic Devices — Spinal

Cervical

L0100	Cervical, craniostenosis, helmet molded to patient model	*ASC*
L0110	Cervical, craniostenosis, helmet, nonmolded	*ASC*
L0120	Cervical, flexible, nonadjustable (foam collar)	*ASC*
L0130	Cervical, flexible, thermoplastic collar, molded to patient	*ASC*
L0140	Cervical, semi-rigid, adjustable (plastic collar)	*ASC*
L0150	Cervical, semi-rigid, adjustable molded chin cup (plastic collar with mandibular/occipital piece)	*ASC*
L0160	Cervical, semi-rigid, wire frame occipital/mandibular support	*ASC*
L0170	Cervical, collar, molded to patient model	*ASC*
L0172	Cervical, collar, semi-rigid thermoplastic foam, two piece	*ASC*
L0174	Cervical, collar, semi-rigid, thermoplastic foam, two piece with thoracic extension	*ASC*

Multiple Post Collar

L0180	Cervical, multiple post collar, occipital/mandibular supports, adjustable	*ASC*
L0190	Cervical, multiple post collar, occipital/mandibular supports, adjustable cervical bars (Somi, Guilford, Taylor types)	*ASC*
L0200	Cervical, multiple post collar, occipital/mandibular supports, adjustable cervical bars, and thoracic extension	*ASC*

Thoracic

L0210	Thoracic, rib belt	*ASC*
L0220	Thoracic, rib belt, custom fabricated	*ASC*

Thoracic-Lumbar-Sacral Orthosis (TLSO)

Flexible

L0300	TLSO, flexible (dorso-lumbar surgical support)	*ASC*

= Special Coverage Instructions Apply	= Carrier Discretion
= Noncovered by Medicare or Medicare Statute	

L0310	TLSO, flexible (dorso-lumbar surgical support), custom fabricated	*ASC*
L0315	TLSO, flexible (dorso-lumbar surgical support), elastic type, with rigid posterior panel	*ASC*
L0317	TLSO, flexible (dorso-lumbar surgical support), hyperextension, elastic type, with rigid posterior panel	*ASC*

Anterior-Posterior Control

| **L0320** | TLSO, anterior-posterior control (Taylor type), with apron front | *ASC* |
| **L0330** | TLSO, anterior-posterior-lateral control (Knight-Taylor type), with apron front | *ASC* |

Anterior-Posterior-Lateral-Rotary Control

L0340	TLSO, anterior-posterior-lateral-rotary control (Arnold, Magnuson, Steindler types), with apron front	*ASC*
L0350	TLSO, anterior-posterior-lateral-rotary control, flexion compression jacket, custom fitted	*ASC*
L0360	TLSO, anterior-posterior-lateral-rotary control, flexion compression jacket molded to patient model	*ASC*
L0370	TLSO, anterior-posterior-lateral-rotary control, hyperextension (Jewett, Lennox, Baker, Cash types)	*ASC*
L0380	TLSO, anterior-posterior-lateral-rotary control, with extensions	*ASC*
L0390	TLSO, anterior-posterior-lateral control molded to patient model	*ASC*
L0400	TLSO, anterior-posterior-lateral control molded to patient model, with interface material	*ASC*
L0410	TLSO, anterior-posterior-lateral control, two-piece construction, molded to patient model	*ASC*
L0420	TLSO, anterior-posterior-lateral control, two-piece construction, molded to patient model, with interface material	*ASC*
L0430	TLSO, anterior-posterior-lateral control, with interface material, custom fitted	*ASC*
L0440	TLSO, anterior-posterior-lateral control, with overlapping front section, spring steel front, custom fitted	*ASC*

Lumbar-Sacral Orthosis (LSO)

Flexible

L0500	LSO, flexible (lumbo-sacral surgical support)	*ASC*
L0510	LSO, flexible (lumbo-sacral surgical support), custom fabricated	*ASC*
L0515	LSO, flexible (lumbo-sacral surgical support) elastic type, with rigid posterior panel	*ASC*

Anterior-Posterior-Lateral Control

| **L0520** | LSO, anterior-posterior-lateral control (Knight, Wilcox types), with apron front | *ASC* |

= Invalid Medicare Code (no grace period)

= Code may require certificate of medical necessity (CMN) or DMERC information form (DIF)

Anterior-Posterior Control
L0530 LSO, anterior-posterior control (Macausland type), with apron front *ASC*

Lumbar Flexion
L0540 LSO, lumbar flexion (Williams flexion type) *ASC*

L0550 LSO, anterior-posterior-lateral control, molded to patient model *ASC*

L0560 LSO, anterior-posterior-lateral control, molded to patient model, with interface material *ASC*

L0565 LSO, anterior-posterior-lateral control, custom fitted *ASC*

Sacroiliac

Flexible
L0600 Sacroiliac, flexible (sacroiliac surgical support) *ASC*

L0610 Sacroiliac, flexible (sacroiliac surgical support), custom fabricated *ASC*

Semi-Rigid
L0620 Sacroiliac, semi-rigid (Goldthwaite, Osgood types), with apron front *ASC*

Cervical-Thoracic-Lumbar-Sacral Orthosis (CTLSO)

Anterior-Posterior-Lateral Control
L0700 CTLSO, anterior-posterior-lateral control, molded to patient model (Minerva type) *ASC*

L0710 CTLSO, anterior-posterior-lateral control, molded to patient model, with interface material (Minerva type) *ASC*

Halo Procedure
L0810 Halo procedure, cervical halo incorporated into jacket vest *ASC*

L0820 Halo procedure, cervical halo incorporated into plaster body jacket *ASC*

L0830 Halo procedure, cervical halo incorporated into Milwaukee type orthosis *ASC*

L0860 Addition to halo procedure, magnetic resonance image compatible system *ASC*

Torso Supports

Ptosis Supports
L0900 Torso support, ptosis support *ASC*

L0910 Torso support, ptosis support, custom fabricated *ASC*

Pendulous Abdomen Supports
L0920 Torso support, pendulous abdomen support *ASC*

L0930 Torso support, pendulous abdomen support, custom fabricated *ASC*

Postsurgical Supports

L0940	Torso support, postsurgical support	ASC
L0950	Torso support, postsurgical support, custom fabricated	ASC
L0960	Torso support, postsurgical support, pads for postsurgical support	ASC

Additions to Spinal Orthosis

L0970	TLSO, corset front	ASC
L0972	LSO, corset front	ASC
L0974	TLSO, full corset	ASC
L0976	LSO, full corset	ASC
L0978	Axillary crutch extension	ASC
L0980	Peroneal straps, pair	ASC
L0982	Stocking supporter grips, set of four (4)	ASC
L0984	Protective body sock, each	ASC
L0999	Addition to spinal orthosis, not otherwise specified	ASC

Orthotic Devices — Scoliosis Procedures

The orthotic care of scoliosis differs from other orthotic care in that the treatment is more dynamic in nature and uses ongoing continual modification of the orthosis to the patient's changing condition. This coding structure uses the proper names - or eponyms - of the procedures because they have historic and universal acceptance in the profession. It should be recognized that variations to the basic procedures described by the founders/ developers are accepted in various medical and orthotic practices throughout the country. All procedures include model of patient when indicated.

Cervical-Thoracic-Lumbar-Sacral Orthosis (CTLSO) (Milwaukee)

L1000	CTLSO (Milwaukee), inclusive of furnishing initial orthosis, including model	ASC
L1010	Addition to CTLSO or scoliosis orthosis, axilla sling	ASC
L1020	Addition to CTLSO or scoliosis orthosis, kyphosis pad	ASC
L1025	Addition to CTLSO or scoliosis orthosis, kyphosis pad, floating	ASC
L1030	Addition to CTLSO or scoliosis orthosis, lumbar bolster pad	ASC
L1040	Addition to CTLSO or scoliosis orthosis, lumbar or lumbar rib pad	ASC
L1050	Addition to CTLSO or scoliosis orthosis, sternal pad	ASC
L1060	Addition to CTLSO or scoliosis orthosis, thoracic pad	ASC
L1070	Addition to CTLSO or scoliosis orthosis, trapezius sling	ASC
L1080	Addition to CTLSO or scoliosis orthosis, outrigger	ASC
L1085	Addition to CTLSO or scoliosis orthosis, outrigger, bilateral with vertical extensions	ASC
L1090	Addition to CTLSO or scoliosis orthosis, lumbar sling	ASC

= Invalid Medicare Code (no grace period)

= Code may require certificate of medical necessity (CMN) or DMERC information form (DIF)

L1100	Addition to CTLSO or scoliosis orthosis, ring flange, plastic or leather	
		ASC

L1110	Addition to CTLSO or scoliosis orthosis, ring flange, plastic or leather, molded to patient model	*ASC*

L1120	Addition to CTLSO, scoliosis orthosis, cover for upright, each	*ASC*

Thoracic-Lumbar-Sacral Orthosis (TLSO) (Low Profile)

L1200	TLSO, inclusive of furnishing initial orthosis only	*ASC*
L1210	Addition to TLSO, (low profile), lateral thoracic extension	*ASC*
L1220	Addition to TLSO, (low profile), anterior thoracic extension	*ASC*
L1230	Addition to TLSO, (low profile), Milwaukee type superstructure	*ASC*
L1240	Addition to TLSO, (low profile), lumbar derotation pad	*ASC*
L1250	Addition to TLSO, (low profile), anterior ASIS pad	*ASC*
L1260	Addition to TLSO, (low profile), anterior thoracic derotation pad	*ASC*
L1270	Addition to TLSO, (low profile), abdominal pad	*ASC*
L1280	Addition to TLSO, (low profile), rib gusset (elastic), each	*ASC*
L1290	Addition to TLSO, (low profile), lateral trochanteric pad	*ASC*

Other Scoliosis Procedures

L1300	Other scoliosis procedure, body jacket molded to patient model	*ASC*
L1310	Other scoliosis procedure, postoperative body jacket	*ASC*
L1499	Spinal orthosis, not otherwise specified	*ASC*

Thoracic-Hip-Knee-Ankle Orthosis (THKAO)

L1500	THKAO, mobility frame (Newington, Parapodium types)	*ASC*
L1510	THKAO, standing frame	*ASC*
L1520	THKAO, swivel walker	*ASC*

Orthotic Devices — Lower Limb

The procedures in L1600-L2999 are considered as "base" or "basic procedures" and may be modified by listing procedure from the "additions" sections and adding them to the base procedures.

Hip Orthosis (HO) — Flexible

▲ L1600	HO, abduction control of hip joints, flexible, Frejka type with cover, prefabricated, includes fitting and adjustment	*ASC*
▲ L1610	HO, abduction control of hip joints, flexible, (Frejka cover only), prefabricated, includes fitting and adjustment	*ASC*
▲ L1620	HO, abduction control of hip joints, flexible, (Pavlik harness), prefabricated, includes fitting and adjustment	*ASC*
▲ L1630	HO, abduction control of hip joints, semi-flexible (Von Rosen type), custom fabricated	*ASC*

L Codes

■ = Special Coverage Instructions Apply   ■ = Carrier Discretion

■ = Noncovered by Medicare or Medicare Statute

▲ **L1640** HO, abduction control of hip joints, static, pelvic band or spreader bar, thigh cuffs, custom fabricated *ASC*

▲ **L1650** HO, abduction control of hip joints, static, adjustable (Ilfled type), prefabricated, includes fitting and adjustment *ASC*

▲ **L1660** HO, abduction control of hip joints, static, plastic, prefabricated, includes fitting and adjustment *ASC*

▲ **L1680** HO, abduction control of hip joints, dynamic, pelvic control, adjustable hip motion control, thigh cuffs (Rancho hip action type), custom fabricated *ASC*

▲ **L1685** HO, abduction control of hip joint, postoperative hip abduction type, custom fabricated *ASC*

▲ **L1686** HO, abduction control of hip joint, postoperative hip abduction type, prefabricated, includes fitting and adjustments *ASC*

▲ **L1690** Combination, bilateral, lumbo-sacral, hip, femur orthosis providing adduction and internal rotation control, prefabricated, includes fitting and adjustment

Legg Perthes

▲ **L1700** Legg Perthes orthosis, (Toronto type), custom fabricated *ASC*

▲ **L1710** Legg Perthes orthosis, (Newington type), custom fabricated *ASC*

▲ **L1720** Legg Perthes orthosis, trilateral, (Tachdijan type), custom fabricated *ASC*

▲ **L1730** Legg Perthes orthosis, (Scottish Rite type), custom fabricated *ASC*

▲ **L1750** Legg Perthes orthosis, Legg Perthes sling (Sam Brown type), prefabricated, includes fitting and adjustment *ASC*

▲ **L1755** Legg Perthes orthosis, (Patten bottom type), custom fabricated *ASC*

Knee Orthosis (KO)

▲ **L1800** KO, elastic with stays, prefabricated, includes fitting and adjustment *ASC*

▲ **L1810** KO, elastic with joints, prefabricated, includes fitting and adjustment *ASC*

▲ **L1815** KO, elastic or other elastic type material with condylar pad(s), prefabricated, includes fitting and adjustment *ASC*

▲ **L1820** KO, elastic with condylar pads and joints, prefabricated, includes fitting and adjustment *ASC*

▲ **L1825** KO, elastic knee cap, prefabricated, includes fitting and adjustment *ASC*

▲ **L1830** KO, immobilizer, canvas longitudinal, prefabricated, inlcudes fitting and adjustment *ASC*

▲ **L1832** KO, adjustable knee joints, positional orthosis, rigid support, prefabricated, includes fitting and adjustment *ASC*

▲ **L1834** KO, without knee joint, rigid, custom fabricated *ASC*

▲ **L1840** KO, derotation, medial-lateral, anterior cruciate ligament, custom fabricated *ASC*

= Invalid Medicare Code (no grace period)

= Code may require certificate of medical necessity (CMN) or DMERC information form (DIF)

▲ **L1843** KO, single upright, thigh and calf, with adjustable flexion and extension joint, medial-lateral and rotation control, prefabricated, includes fitting and adjustment *ASC*

▲ **L1844** KO, single upright, thigh and calf, with adjustable flexion and extension joint, medial-lateral and rotation control, custom fabricated *ASC*

▲ **L1845** KO, double upright, thigh and calf, with adjustable flexion and extension joint, medial-lateral and rotation control, prefabricated, includes fitting and adjustment *ASC*

▲ **L1846** KO, double upright, thigh and calf, with adjustable flexion and extension joint, medial-lateral and rotation control, custom fabricated *ASC*

▲ **L1847** KO, double upright with adjustable joint, with inflatable air support chamber(s), prefabricated, includes fitting and adjustment

▲ **L1850** KO, Swedish type, prefabricated, includes fitting and adjustment *ASC*

▲ **L1855** KO, molded plastic, thigh and calf sections, with double upright knee joints, custom fabricated *ASC*

▲ **L1858** KO, molded plastic, polycentric knee joints, pneumatic knee pads (CTI), custom fabricated *ASC*

▲ **L1860** KO, modification of supracondylar prosthetic socket, custom fabricated (SK) *ASC*

▲ **L1870** KO, double upright, thigh and calf lacers, with knee joints, custom fabricated *ASC*

▲ **L1880** KO, double upright, nonmolded thigh and calf cuffs/lacers with knee joints, custom fabricated *ASC*

▲ **L1885** KO, single or double upright, thigh and calf, with funtional active resistance control, prefabricated, includes fitting and adjustment *ASC*

Ankle-Foot Orthosis (AFO)

▲ **L1900** AFO, spring wire, dorsiflexion assist calf band, custom fabricated *ASC*

▲ **L1902** AFO, ankle gauntlet, prefabricated, includes fitting and adjustment *ASC*

▲ **L1904** AFO, molded ankle gauntlet, custom fabricated *ASC*

▲ **L1906** AFO, multiligamentus ankle support, prefabricated, includes fitting and adjustment *ASC*

▲ **L1910** AFO, posterior, single bar, clasp attachment to shoe counter, prefabricated, includes fitting and adjustment *ASC*

▲ **L1920** AFO, single upright with static or adjustable stop (Phelps or Perlstein type), custom fabricated *ASC*

▲ **L1930** AFO, plastic, prefabricated, includes fitting and adjustment *ASC*

▲ **L1940** AFO, plastic, custom fabricated *ASC*

▲ **L1945** AFO, molded to patient model, plastic, rigid anterior tibial section (floor reaction), custom fabricated *ASC*

L Codes

= Special Coverage Instructions Apply   = Carrier Discretion

= Noncovered by Medicare or Medicare Statute

▲ **L1950**	AFO, spiral, (IRM type), plastic, custom fabricated	ASC
▲ **L1960**	AFO, posterior solid ankle, plastic, custom fabricated	ASC
▲ **L1970**	AFO, plastic, with ankle joint, custom fabricated	ASC
▲ **L1980**	AFO, single upright free plantar dorsiflexion, solid stirrup, calf band/cuff (single bar "BK" orthosis), custom fabricated	ASC
▲ **L1990**	AFO, double upright free plantar dorsiflexion, solid stirrup, calf band/cuff (double bar "BK" orthosis), custom fabricated	ASC

Knee-Ankle-Foot Orthosis (KAFO) — Or Any Combination

L2000, L2020, L2036 are base procedures to be used with any knee joint, L2010 and L2030 are to be used only with no knee joint.

▲ **L2000**	KAFO, single upright, free knee, free ankle, solid stirrup, thigh and calf bands/cuffs (single bar "AK" orthosis), custom fabricated	ASC
▲ **L2010**	KAFO, single upright, free ankle, solid stirrup, thigh and calf bands/cuffs (single bar "AK" orthosis), without knee joint, custom fabricated	ASC
▲ **L2020**	KAFO, double upright, free knee, free ankle, solid stirrup, thigh and calf bands/cuffs (double bar "AK" orthosis), custom fabricated	ASC
▲ **L2030**	KAFO, double upright, free ankle, solid stirrup, thigh and calf bands/cuffs, (double bar "AK" orthosis), without knee joint, custom fabricated	ASC
▲ **L2035**	KAFO, full plastic, static, (pediatric size), prefabricated, includes fitting and adjustment	ASC
▲ **L2036**	KAFO, full plastic, double upright, free knee, custom fabricated	ASC
▲ **L2037**	KAFO, full plastic, single upright, free knee, custom fabricated	ASC
▲ **L2038**	KAFO, full plastic, without knee joint, multiaxis ankle, (Lively orthosis or equal), custom fabricated	ASC
▲ **L2039**	KAFO, full plastic, single upright, poly-axial hinge, medial lateral rotation control, custom fabricated	ASC

Torsion Control: Hip-Knee-Ankle-Foot Orthosis (HKAFO)

▲ **L2040**	HKAFO, torsion control, bilateral rotation straps, pelvic band/belt, custom fabricated	ASC
▲ **L2050**	HKAFO, torsion control, bilateral torsion cables, hip joint, pelvic band/belt, custom fabricated	ASC
▲ **L2060**	HKAFO, torsion control, bilateral torsion cables, ball bearing hip joint, pelvic band/ belt, custom fabricated	ASC
▲ **L2070**	HKAFO, torsion control, unilateral rotation straps, pelvic band/belt, custom fabricated	ASC
▲ **L2080**	HKAFO, torsion control, unilateral torsion cable, hip joint, pelvic band/belt, custom fabricated	ASC

= Invalid Medicare Code (no grace period)

= Code may require certificate of medical necessity (CMN) or DMERC information form (DIF)

▲ **L2090**   HKAFO, torsion control, unilateral torsion cable, ball bearing hip joint, pelvic band/belt, custom fabricated   *ASC*

Fracture Orthosis

▲ **L2102**   AFO, fracture orthosis, tibial fracture cast orthosis, plaster type casting material, custom fabricated   *ASC*

▲ **L2104**   AFO, fracture orthosis, tibial fracture cast orthosis, synthetic type casting material, custom fabricated   *ASC*

▲ **L2106**   AFO, fracture orthosis, tibial fracture cast orthosis, thermoplastic type casting material, custom fabricated   *ASC*

▲ **L2108**   AFO, fracture orthosis, tibial fracture cast orthosis, custom fabricated   *ASC*

▲ **L2112**   AFO, fracture orthosis, tibial fracture orthosis, soft, prefabricated, includes fitting and adjustment   *ASC*

▲ **L2114**   AFO, fracture orthosis, tibial fracture orthosis, semi-rigid, prefabricated, includes fitting and adjustment   *ASC*

▲ **L2116**   AFO, fracture orthosis, tibial fracture orthosis, rigid, prefabricated, includes fitting and adjustment   *ASC*

▲ **L2122**   KAFO, fracture orthosis, femoral fracture cast orthosis, plaster type casting material, custom fabricated   *ASC*

▲ **L2124**   KAFO, fracture orthosis, femoral fracture cast orthosis, synthetic type casting material, custom fabricated   *ASC*

▲ **L2126**   KAFO, fracture orthosis, femoral fracture cast orthosis, thermoplastic type casting material, custom fabricated   *ASC*

▲ **L2128**   KAFO, fracture orthosis, femoral fracture cast orthosis, custom fabricated   *ASC*

▲ **L2132**   KAFO, fracture orthosis, femoral fracture cast orthosis, soft, prefabricated, includes fitting and adjustment   *ASC*

▲ **L2134**   KAFO, fracture orthosis, femoral fracture cast orthosis, semi-rigid, prefabricated, includes fitting and adjustment   *ASC*

▲ **L2136**   KAFO, fracture orthosis, femoral fracture cast orthosis, rigid, prefabricated, includes fitting and adjustment   *ASC*

Additions to Fracture Orthosis

L2180   Addition to lower extremity fracture orthosis, plastic shoe insert with ankle joints   *ASC*

L2182   Addition to lower extremity fracture orthosis, drop lock knee joint   *ASC*

L2184   Addition to lower extremity fracture orthosis, limited motion knee joint   *ASC*

L2186   Addition to lower extremity fracture orthosis, adjustable motion knee joint, Lerman type   *ASC*

L2188   Addition to lower extremity fracture orthosis, quadrilateral brim   *ASC*

L2190   Addition to lower extremity fracture orthosis, waist belt   *ASC*

L Codes

L2192 Addition to lower extremity fracture orthosis, hip joint, pelvic band, thigh flange, and pelvic belt *ASC*

Additions to Lower Extremity Orthosis: Shoe-Ankle-Shin-Knee

L2200 Addition to lower extremity, limited ankle motion, each joint *ASC*

L2210 Addition to lower extremity, dorsiflexion assist (plantar flexion resist), each joint *ASC*

L2220 Addition to lower extremity, dorsiflexion and plantar flexion assist/resist, each joint *ASC*

L2230 Addition to lower extremity, split flat caliper stirrups and plate attachment *ASC*

L2240 Addition to lower extremity, round caliper and plate attachment *ASC*

L2250 Addition to lower extremity, foot plate, molded to patient model, stirrup attachment *ASC*

L2260 Addition to lower extremity, reinforced solid stirrup (Scott-Craig type) *ASC*

L2265 Addition to lower extremity, long tongue stirrup *ASC*

L2270 Addition to lower extremity, varus/valgus correction ("T") strap, padded/lined or malleolus pad *ASC*

L2275 Addition to lower extremity, varus/vulgus correction, plastic modification, padded/lined *ASC*

L2280 Addition to lower extremity, molded inner boot *ASC*

L2300 Addition to lower extremity, abduction bar (bilateral hip involvement), jointed, adjustable *ASC*

L2310 Addition to lower extremity, abduction bar, straight *ASC*

L2320 Addition to lower extremity, nonmolded lacer *ASC*

L2330 Addition to lower extremity, lacer molded to patient model *ASC*

L2335 Addition to lower extremity, anterior swing band *ASC*

L2340 Addition to lower extremity, pretibial shell, molded to patient model *ASC*

L2350 Addition to lower extremity, prosthetic type, (BK) socket, molded to patient model, (used for "PTB," "AFO" orthoses) *ASC*

L2360 Addition to lower extremity, extended steel shank *ASC*

L2370 Addition to lower extremity, Patten bottom *ASC*

L2375 Addition to lower extremity, torsion control, ankle joint and half solid stirrup *ASC*

L2380 Addition to lower extremity, torsion control, straight knee joint, each joint *ASC*

L2385 Addition to lower extremity, straight knee joint, heavy duty, each joint *ASC*

L2390 Addition to lower extremity, offset knee joint, each joint *ASC*

= Invalid Medicare Code (no grace period)

= Code may require certificate of medical necessity (CMN) or DMERC information form (DIF)

| **L2395** | Addition to lower extremity, offset knee joint, heavy duty, each joint *ASC* |
| **L2397** | Addition to lower extremity orthosis, suspension sleeve *ASC* |

Additions to Straight Knee or Offset Knee Joints

L2405	Addition to knee joint, drop lock, each joint *ASC*
L2415	Addition to knee joint, cam lock (Swiss, French, bail types) each joint *ASC*
L2425	Addition to knee joint, disc or dial lock for adjustable knee flexion, each joint *ASC*
L2430	Addition to knee joint, ratchet lock for active and progressive knee extension, each joint *ASC*
L2435	Addition to knee joint, polycentric joint, each joint *ASC*
L2492	Addition to knee joint, lift loop for drop lock ring *ASC*

Additions: Thigh/Weight Bearing — Gluteal/Ischial Weight Bearing

L2500	Addition to lower extremity, thigh/weight bearing, gluteal/ischial weight bearing, ring *ASC*
L2510	Addition to lower extremity, thigh/weight bearing, quadri-lateral brim, molded to patient model *ASC*
L2520	Addition to lower extremity, thigh/weight bearing, quadri-lateral brim, custom fitted *ASC*
L2525	Addition to lower extremity, thigh/weight bearing, ischial containment/narrow M-L brim molded to patient model *ASC*
L2526	Addition to lower extremity, thigh/weight bearing, ischial containment/narrow M-L brim, custom fitted *ASC*
L2530	Addition to lower extremity, thigh/weight bearing, lacer, nonmolded *ASC*
L2540	Addition to lower extremity, thigh/weight bearing, lacer, molded to patient model *ASC*
L2550	Addition to lower extremity, thigh/weight bearing, high roll cuff *ASC*

Additions: Pelvic and Thoracic Control

L2570	Addition to lower extremity, pelvic control, hip joint, Clevis type, two position joint, each *ASC*
L2580	Addition to lower extremity, pelvic control, pelvic sling *ASC*
L2600	Addition to lower extremity, pelvic control, hip joint, Clevis type, or thrust bearing, free, each *ASC*
L2610	Addition to lower extremity, pelvic control, hip joint, Clevis or thrust bearing, lock, each *ASC*
L2620	Addition to lower extremity, pelvic control, hip joint, heavy-duty, each *ASC*

L Codes

= Special Coverage Instructions Apply   = Carrier Discretion

= Noncovered by Medicare or Medicare Statute

L2622	Addition to lower extremity, pelvic control, hip joint, adjustable flexion, each ASC
L2624	Addition to lower extremity, pelvic control, hip joint, adjustable flexion, extension, abduction control, each ASC
L2627	Addition to lower extremity, pelvic control, plastic, molded to patient model, reciprocating hip joint and cables ASC
L2628	Addition to lower extremity, pelvic control, metal frame, reciprocating hip joint and cables ASC
L2630	Addition to lower extremity, pelvic control, band and belt, unilateral ASC
L2640	Addition to lower extremity, pelvic control, band and belt, bilateral ASC
L2650	Addition to lower extremity, pelvic and thoracic control, gluteal pad, each ASC
L2660	Addition to lower extremity, thoracic control, thoracic band ASC
L2670	Addition to lower extremity, thoracic control, paraspinal uprights ASC
L2680	Addition to lower extremity, thoracic control, lateral support uprights ASC

Additions: General

L2750	Addition to lower extremity orthosis, plating chrome or nickel, per bar ASC
L2755	Addition to lower extremity orthosis, carbon graphite lamination ASC
L2760	Addition to lower extremity orthosis, extension, per extension, per bar (for lineal adjustment for growth) ASC
L2770	Addition to lower extremity orthosis, any material, per bar or joint ASC
L2780	Addition to lower extremity orthosis, noncorrosive finish, per bar ASC
L2785	Addition to lower extremity orthosis, drop lock retainer, each ASC
L2795	Addition to lower extremity orthosis, knee control, full kneecap ASC
L2800	Addition to lower extremity orthosis, knee control, kneecap, medial or lateral pull ASC
L2810	Addition to lower extremity orthosis, knee control, condylar pad ASC
L2820	Addition to lower extremity orthosis, soft interface for molded plastic, below knee section ASC
L2830	Addition to lower extremity orthosis, soft interface for molded plastic, above knee section ASC
L2840	Addition to lower extremity orthosis, tibial length sock, fracture or equal, each ASC
L2850	Addition to lower extremity orthosis, femoral length sock, fracture or equal, each ASC
L2860	Addition to lower extremity joint, knee or ankle, concentric adjustable torsion style mechanism, each ASC
L2999	Lower extremity orthoses, not otherwise specified ASC

= Invalid Medicare Code (no grace period)

= Code may require certificate of medical necessity (CMN) or DMERC information form (DIF)

Orthopedic Shoes

Inserts

L3000   Foot insert, removable, molded to patient model, "UCB" type, Berkeley shell, each   *MCM 2323, ASC*

L3001   Foot insert, removable, molded to patient model, Spenco, each   *MCM 2323, ASC*

L3002   Foot insert, removable, molded to patient model, Plastazote or equal, each   *MCM 2323, ASC*

L3003   Foot insert, removable, molded to patient model, silicone gel, each   *MCM 2323, ASC*

L3010   Foot insert, removable, molded to patient model, longitudinal arch support, each   *MCM 2323, ASC*

L3020   Foot insert, removable, molded to patient model, longitudinal/metatarsal support, each   *MCM 2323, ASC*

L3030   Foot insert, removable, formed to patient foot, each   *MCM 2323, ASC*

Arch Support, Removable, Premolded

L3040   Foot, arch support, removable, premolded, longitudinal, each   *MCM 2323, ASC*

L3050   Foot, arch support, removable, premolded, metatarsal, each   *MCM 2323, ASC*

L3060   Foot, arch support, removable, premolded, longitudinal/metatarsal, each   *MCM 2323, ASC*

Arch Support, Nonremovable, Attached to Shoe

L3070   Foot, arch support, nonremovable, attached to shoe, longitudinal, each   *MCM 2323, ASC*

L3080   Foot, arch support, nonremovable, attached to shoe, metatarsal, each   *MCM 2323, ASC*

L3090   Foot, arch support, nonremovable, attached to shoe, longitudinal/metatarsal, each   *MCM 2323, ASC*

L3100   Hallus-Valgus night dynamic splint   *MCM 2323, ASC*

Abduction and Rotation Bars

L3140   Foot, abduction rotation bar, including shoes   *MCM 2323, ASC*

L3150   Foot, abduction rotation bar, without shoes   *MCM 2323, ASC*

L3160   Foot, adjustable shoe-styled positioning device   *ASC*

L3170   Foot, plastic heel stabilizer   *MCM 2323, ASC*

Orthopedic Footwear

L3201   Orthopedic shoe, oxford with supinator or pronator, infant   *MCM 2323, ASC*

L Codes

L3202	Orthopedic shoe, oxford with supinator or pronator, child
	MCM 2323, ASC
L3203	Orthopedic shoe, oxford with supinator or pronator, junior
	MCM 2323, ASC
L3204	Orthopedic shoe, hightop with supinator or pronator, infant
	MCM 2323, ASC
L3206	Orthopedic shoe, hightop with supinator or pronator, child
	MCM 2323, ASC
L3207	Orthopedic shoe, hightop with supinator or pronator, junior
	MCM 2323, ASC
L3208	Surgical boot, each, infant MCM 2079, ASC
L3209	Surgical boot, each, child MCM 2079, ASC
L3211	Surgical boot, each, junior MCM 2079, ASC
L3212	Benesch boot, pair, infant MCM 2079, ASC
L3213	Benesch boot, pair, child MCM 2079, ASC
L3214	Benesch boot, pair, junior MCM 2079, ASC
L3215	Orthopedic footwear, woman's shoes, oxford
	Medicare Statute 1862.A8, ASC
L3216	Orthopedic footwear, woman's shoes, depth inlay
	Medicare Statute 1862.A8, ASC
L3217	Orthopedic footwear, woman's shoes, hightop, depth inlay
	Medicare Statute 1862.A8, ASC
L3218	Orthopedic footwear, woman's surgical boot, each MCM 2323, ASC
L3219	Orthopedic footwear, man's shoes, oxford Medicare Statute 1862.A8, ASC
L3221	Orthopedic footwear, man's shoes, depth inlay
	Medicare Statute 1862.A8, ASC
L3222	Orthopedic footwear, man's shoes, hightop, depth inlay
	Medicare Statute 1862.A8, ASC
L3223	Orthopedic footwear, man's surgical boot, each MCM 2323, ASC
L3224	Orthopedic footwear, woman's shoe, oxford, used as an integral part of a brace (orthosis) MCM 2323D, ASC
L3225	Orthopedic footwear, man's shoe, oxford, used as an integral part of a brace (orthosis) MCM 2323D, ASC
L3230	Orthopedic footwear, custom shoes, depth inlay MCM 2323, ASC
L3250	Orthopedic footwear, custom molded shoe, removable inner mold, prosthetic shoe, each MCM 2323, ASC
L3251	Foot, shoe molded to patient model, silicone shoe, each MCM 2323, ASC
L3252	Foot, shoe molded to patient model, Plastazote (or similar), custom fabricated, each MCM 2323, ASC

= Invalid Medicare Code (no grace period)

= Code may require certificate of medical necessity (CMN) or DMERC information form (DIF)

L3253	Foot, molded shoe Plastazote (or similar), custom fitted, each	
		MCM 2323, ASC
L3254	Nonstandard size or width	*MCM 2323, ASC*
L3255	Nonstandard size or length	*MCM 2323, ASC*
L3257	Orthopedic footwear, additional charge for split size	*MCM 2323, ASC*
L3260	Ambulatory surgical boot, each	*MCM 2079, ASC*
L3265	Plastazote sandal, each	*ASC*

Shoe Modification — Lifts

L3300	Lift, elevation, heel, tapered to metatarsals, per inch	*MCM 2323, ASC*
L3310	Lift, elevation, heel and sole, neoprene, per inch	*MCM 2323, ASC*
L3320	Lift, elevation, heel and sole, cork, per inch	*MCM 2323, ASC*
L3330	Lift, elevation, metal extension (skate)	*MCM 2323, ASC*
L3332	Lift, elevation, inside shoe, tapered, up to one-half inch	*MCM 2323, ASC*
L3334	Lift, elevation, heel, per inch	*MCM 2323, ASC*

Shoe Modification — Wedges

L3340	Heel wedge, SACH	*MCM 2323, ASC*
L3350	Heel wedge	*MCM 2323, ASC*
L3360	Sole wedge, outside sole	*MCM 2323, ASC*
L3370	Sole wedge, between sole	*MCM 2323, ASC*
L3380	Clubfoot wedge	*MCM 2323, ASC*
L3390	Outflare wedge	*MCM 2323, ASC*
L3400	Metatarsal bar wedge, rocker	*MCM 2323, ASC*
L3410	Metatarsal bar wedge, between sole	*MCM 2323, ASC*
L3420	Full sole and heel wedge, between sole	*MCM 2323, ASC*

Shoe Modifications — Heels

L3430	Heel, counter, plastic reinforced	*MCM 2323, ASC*
L3440	Heel, counter, leather reinforced	*MCM 2323, ASC*
L3450	Heel, SACH cushion type	*MCM 2323, ASC*
L3455	Heel, new leather, standard	*MCM 2323, ASC*
L3460	Heel, new rubber, standard	*MCM 2323, ASC*
L3465	Heel, Thomas with wedge	*MCM 2323, ASC*
L3470	Heel, Thomas extended to ball	*MCM 2323, ASC*
L3480	Heel, pad and depression for spur	*MCM 2323, ASC*
L3485	Heel, pad, removable for spur	*MCM 2323, ASC*

L Codes

= Special Coverage Instructions Apply　　　= Carrier Discretion

= Noncovered by Medicare or Medicare Statute

Miscellaneous Shoe Additions

L3500	Orthopedic shoe addition, insole, leather	*MCM 2323, ASC*
L3510	Orthopedic shoe addition, insole, rubber	*MCM 2323, ASC*
L3520	Orthopedic shoe addition, insole, felt covered with leather	*MCM 2323, ASC*
L3530	Orthopedic shoe addition, sole, half	*MCM 2323, ASC*
L3540	Orthopedic shoe addition, sole, full	*MCM 2323, ASC*
L3550	Orthopedic shoe addition, toe tap, standard	*MCM 2323, ASC*
L3560	Orthopedic shoe addition, toe tap, horseshoe	*MCM 2323, ASC*
L3570	Orthopedic shoe addition, special extension to instep (leather with eyelets)	*MCM 2323, ASC*
L3580	Orthopedic shoe addition, convert instep to velcro closure	*MCM 2323, ASC*
L3590	Orthopedic shoe addition, convert firm shoe counter to soft counter	*MCM 2323, ASC*
L3595	Orthopedic shoe addition, March bar	*MCM 2323, ASC*

Transfer or Replacement

L3600	Transfer of an orthosis from one shoe to another, caliper plate, existing	*MCM 2323, ASC*
L3610	Transfer of an orthosis from one shoe to another, caliper plate, new	*MCM 2323, ASC*
L3620	Transfer of an orthosis from one shoe to another, solid stirrup, existing	*MCM 2323, ASC*
L3630	Transfer of an orthosis from one shoe to another, solid stirrup, new	*MCM 2323, ASC*
L3640	Transfer of an orthosis from one shoe to another, Dennis Browne splint (Riveton), both shoes	*MCM 2323, ASC*
L3649	Orthopedic shoe, modification, addition or transfer, not otherwise specified	*MCM 2323, ASC*

Orthotic Devices — Upper Limb

The procedures in this section are considered as "base" or "basic procedures" and may be modified by listing procedures from the "additions" sections and adding them to the base procedure.

Shoulder Orthosis (SO)

▲ **L3650**	SO, figure of eight design abduction re- strainer, prefabricated, includes fitting and adjustment	
▲ **L3660**	SO, figure of eight design abduction restrainer, canvas and webbing, prefabricated, includes fitting and adjustment	*ASC*
▲ **L3670**	SO, acromio/clavicular (canvas and webbing type), prefabricated, includes fitting and adjustment	*ASC*

▲ **L3675** SO, vest type abduction restrainer, canvas webbing type, or equal, prefabricated, includes fitting and adjustment

Elbow Orthosis (EO)

▲ **L3700** EO, elastic with stays, prefabricated, includes fitting and adjustment
ASC

▲ **L3710** EO, elastic with metal joints, prefabricated, includes fitting and adjustment
ASC

▲ **L3720** EO, double upright with forearm/arm cuffs, free motion, custom fabricated
ASC

▲ **L3730** EO, double upright with forearm/arm cuffs, extension/flexion assist, custom fabricated
ASC

▲ **L3740** EO, double upright with forearm/arm cuffs, adjustable position lock with active control, custom fabricated
ASC

● **L3760** Elbow orthosis, with adjustable position locking joint(s), prefabricated, includes fitting and adjustments, any type

Wrist-Hand-Finger Orthosis (WHFO)

▲ **L3800** WHFO, short opponens, no attachments, custom fabricated
ASC

▲ **L3805** WHFO, long opponens, no attachment, custom fabricated
ASC

▲ **L3807** WHFO, without joint(s), prefabricated, includes fitting and adjustments, any type

Additions

L3810 WHFO, addition to short and long opponens, thumb abduction ("C") bar
ASC

L3815 WHFO, addition to short and long opponens, second M.P. abduction assist
ASC

L3820 WHFO, addition to short and long opponens, I.P. extension assist, with M.P. extension stop
ASC

L3825 WHFO, addition to short and long opponens, M.P. extension stop *ASC*

L3830 WHFO, addition to short and long opponens, M.P. extension assist *ASC*

L3835 WHFO, addition to short and long opponens, M.P. spring extension assist
ASC

L3840 WHFO, addition to short and long opponens, spring swivel thumb *ASC*

L3845 WHFO, addition to short and long opponens, thumb I.P. extension assist, with M.P. stop
ASC

L3850 WHO, addition to short and long opponens, action wrist, with dorsiflexion assist
ASC

L3855 WHFO, addition to short and long opponens, adjustable M.P. flexion control
ASC

L3860 WHFO, addition to short and long opponens, adjustable M.P. flexion control and I.P.
ASC

L Codes

= Special Coverage Instructions Apply   = Carrier Discretion

= Noncovered by Medicare or Medicare Statute

L3890 Addition to upper extremity joint, wrist or elbow, concentric adjustable torsion style mechanism, each *ASC*

Dynamic Flexor Hinge, Reciprocal Wrist Extension/Flexion, Finger Flexion/Extension

▲ **L3900** WHFO, dynamic flexor hinge, reciprocal wrist extension/flexion, finger flexion/extension, wrist or finger driven, custom fabricated *ASC*

▲ **L3901** WHFO, dynamic flexor hinge, reciprocal wrist extension/flexion, finger flexion/extension, cable driven, custom fabricated *ASC*

External Power

▲ **L3902** WHFO, external powered, compressed gas, custom fabricated *ASC*

▲ **L3904** WHFO, external powered, electric, custom fabricated *ASC*

Other WHFOs — Custom Fitted

▲ **L3906** WHO, wrist gauntlet, molded to patient model, custom fabricated *ASC*

▲ **L3907** WHFO, wrist gauntlet with thumb spica, molded to patient model, custom fabricated *ASC*

▲ **L3908** WHO, wrist extension control cock-up, nonmolded, prefabricated, includes fitting and adjustment *ASC*

▲ **L3910** WHFO, Swanson design, prefabricated, includes fitting and adjustment *ASC*

▲ **L3912** HFO, flexion glove with elastic finger control, prefabricated, includes fitting and adjustment *ASC*

▲ **L3914** WHO, wrist extension cock-up, prefabricated, includes fitting and adjustment *ASC*

▲ **L3916** WHFO, wrist extension cock-up, with outrigger, prefabricated, includes fitting and adjustment *ASC*

▲ **L3918** HFO, knuckle bender, prefabricated, includes fitting and adjustment *ASC*

▲ **L3920** HFO, knuckle bender, with outrigger, prefabricated, includes fitting and adjustment *ASC*

▲ **L3922** HFO, knuckle bender, two segment to flex joints, prefabricated, includes fitting and adjustment *ASC*

● **L3923** Hand finger orthosis, without joint(s), prefabricated, includes fitting and adjustments, any type

▲ **L3924** WHFO, Oppenheimer, prefabricated, includes fitting and adjustment *ASC*

▲ **L3926** WHFO, Thomas suspension, prefabricated, includes fitting and adjustment *ASC*

▲ **L3928** HFO, finger extension, with clock spring, prefabricated, includes fitting and adjustment *ASC*

▲ **L3930** WHFO, finger extension, with wrist support, prefabricated, includes fitting and adjustment *ASC*

= Invalid Medicare Code (no grace period)

= Code may require certificate of medical necessity (CMN) or DMERC information form (DIF)

▲ **L3932** FO, safety pin, spring wire, prefabricated, includes fitting and adjustment *ASC*

▲ **L3934** FO, safety pin, modified, prefabricated, includes fitting and adjustment *ASC*

▲ **L3936** WHFO, Palmer, prefabricated, includes fitting and adjustment *ASC*

▲ **L3938** WHFO, dorsal wrist, prefabricated, includes fitting and adjustment *ASC*

▲ **L3940** WHFO, dorsal wrist, with outrigger attachment, prefabricated, includes fitting and adjustment *ASC*

▲ **L3942** HFO, reverse knuckle bender, prefabricated, includes fitting and adjustment *ASC*

▲ **L3944** HFO, reverse knuckle bender, with outrigger, prefabricated, includes fitting and adjustment *ASC*

▲ **L3946** HFO, composite elastic, prefabricated, includes fitting and adjustment *ASC*

▲ **L3948** FO, finger knuckle bender, prefabricated, includes fitting and adjustment *ASC*

▲ **L3950** WHFO, combination Oppenheimer, with knuckle bender and two attachments, prefabricated, includes fitting and adjustment *ASC*

▲ **L3952** WHFO, combination Oppenheimer, with reverse knuckle and two attachments, prefabricated, includes fitting and adjustment *ASC*

▲ **L3954** HFO, spreading hand, prefabricated, includes fitting and adjustment *ASC*

L3956 Addition of joint to upper extremity orthosis, any material; per joint *ASC*

Shoulder-Elbow-Wrist-Hand Orthosis (SEWHO)

Abduction Position, Custom Fitted

▲ **L3960** SEWHO, abduction positioning, airplane design, prefabricated, includes fitting and adjustment *ASC*

▲ **L3962** SEWHO, abduction positioning, Erb's palsey design, prefabricated, includes fitting and adjustment *ASC*

▲ **L3963** SEWHO, molded shoulder, arm, forearm, and wrist, with articulating elbow joint, custom fabricated *ASC*

▲ **L3964** SEO, mobile arm support attached to wheelchair, balanced, adjustable, prefabricated, includes fitting and adjustment *ASC*

▲ **L3965** SEO, mobile arm support attached to wheelchair, balanced, adjustable Rancho type, prefabricated, includes fitting and adjustment *ASC*

▲ **L3966** SEO, mobile arm support attached to wheelchair, balanced, reclining, prefabricated, includes fitting and adjustment *ASC*

▲ **L3968** SEO, mobile arm support attached to wheelchair, balanced, friction arm support (friction dampening to proximal and distal joints), prefabricated, includes fitting and adjustment *ASC*

L Codes

= Special Coverage Instructions Apply   = Carrier Discretion

= Noncovered by Medicare or Medicare Statute

▲ **L3969** SEO, mobile arm support, monosuspension arm and hand support, overhead elbow forearm hand sling support, yoke type arm suspension support, prefabricated, includes fitting and adjustment *ASC*

Additions to Mobile Arm Supports

L3970 SEO, addition to mobile arm support, elevating proximal arm *ASC*

L3972 SEO, addition to mobile arm support, offset or lateral rocker arm with elastic balance control *ASC*

L3974 SEO, addition to mobile arm support, supinator *ASC*

Fracture Orthosis

▲ **L3980** Upper extremity fracture orthosis, humeral, prefabricated, includes fitting and adjustment *ASC*

▲ **L3982** Upper extremity fracture orthosis, radius/ulnar, prefabricated, includes fitting and adjustment *ASC*

▲ **L3984** Upper extremity fracture orthosis, wrist, prefabricated, includes fitting and adjustment *ASC*

▲ **L3985** Upper extremity fracture orthosis, forearm, hand with wrist hinge, custom fabricated *ASC*

▲ **L3986** Upper extremity fracture orthosis, combination of humeral, radius/ulnar, wrist (example: Colles' fracture), custom fabricated *ASC*

L3995 Addition to upper extremity orthosis, sock, fracture or equal, each *ASC*

L3999 Upper limb orthosis, not otherwise specified *ASC*

Specific Repair

L4000 Replace girdle for Milwaukee orthosis *ASC*

L4010 Replace trilateral socket brim *ASC*

L4020 Replace quadrilateral socket brim, molded to patient model *ASC*

L4030 Replace quadrilateral socket brim, custom fitted *ASC*

L4040 Replace molded thigh lacer *ASC*

L4045 Replace nonmolded thigh lacer *ASC*

L4050 Replace molded calf lacer *ASC*

L4055 Replace nonmolded calf lacer *ASC*

L4060 Replace high roll cuff *ASC*

L4070 Replace proximal and distal upright for KAFO *ASC*

L4080 Replace metal bands KAFO, proximal thigh *ASC*

L4090 Replace metal bands KAFO-AFO, calf or distal thigh *ASC*

L4100 Replace leather cuff KAFO, proximal thigh *ASC*

L4110 Replace leather cuff KAFO-AFO, calf or distal thigh *ASC*

L4130 Replace pretibial shell *ASC*

Repairs

L4205 Repair of orthotic device, labor component, per 15 minutes
MCM 2100.4, ASC

L4210 Repair of orthotic device, repair or replace minor parts
MCM 2100.4, MCM 2130D, MCM 2133, ASC

▲ **L4350** Pneumatic ankle control splint (e.g., aircast), prefabricated, includes fitting and adjustment *ASC*

▲ **L4360** Pneumatic walking splint (e.g., aircast), prefabricated, includes fitting and adjustment *ASC*

▲ **L4370** Pneumatic full leg splint (e.g., aircast), prefabricated, includes fitting and adjustment *ASC*

▲ **L4380** Pneumatic knee splint (e.g., aircast), prefabricated, includes fitting and adjustment *ASC*

▲ **L4392** Replacement soft interface material, static AFO

L4394 Replace soft interface material, foot drop splint *ASC*

▲ **L4396** Static AFO, including soft interface material, for positioning, pressure reduction, may be used for minimal ambulation

▲ **L4398** Foot drop splint, recumbent positioning device, prefabricated, includes fitting and adjustment *ASC*

L Codes

Prosthetic Procedures L5000–L9999

Lower Limb
The procedures in this section are considered as "base" or "basic procedures" and may be modified by listing items/procedures or special materials from the "additions" sections and adding them to the base procedure.

Partial Foot

L5000 Partial foot, shoe insert with longitudinal arch, toe filler *MCM 2323, ASC*

L5010 Partial foot, molded socket, ankle height, with toe filler *MCM 2323, ASC*

L5020 Partial foot, molded socket, tibial tubercle height, with toe filler
MCM 2323, ASC

Ankle

L5050 Ankle, Symes, molded socket, SACH foot *ASC*

L5060 Ankle, Symes, metal frame, molded leather socket, articulated ankle/foot *ASC*

Below Knee

L5100 Below knee, molded socket, shin, SACH foot *ASC*

L5105 Below knee, plastic socket, joints and thigh lacer, SACH foot *ASC*

= Special Coverage Instructions Apply   = Carrier Discretion

= Noncovered by Medicare or Medicare Statute

Knee Disarticulation

L5150 Knee disarticulation (or through knee), molded socket, external knee joints, shin, SACH foot
ASC

L5160 Knee disarticulation (or through knee), molded socket, bent knee configuration, external knee joints, shin, SACH foot
ASC

Above Knee

L5200 Above knee, molded socket, single axis constant friction knee, shin, SACH foot
ASC

L5210 Above knee, short prosthesis, no knee joint ("stubbies"), with foot blocks, no ankle joints, each
ASC

L5220 Above knee, short prosthesis, no knee joint ("stubbies"), with articulated ankle/foot, dynamically aligned, each
ASC

L5230 Above knee, for proximal femoral focal deficiency, constant friction knee, shin, SACH foot
ASC

Hip Disarticulation

L5250 Hip disarticulation, Canadian type; molded socket, hip joint, single axis constant friction knee, shin, SACH foot
ASC

L5270 Hip disarticulation, tilt table type; molded socket, locking hip joint, single axis constant friction knee, shin, SACH foot
ASC

Hemipelvectomy

L5280 Hemipelvectomy, Canadian type; molded socket, hip joint, single axis constant friction knee, shin, SACH foot
ASC

Endoskeletal: Below Knee

L5300 Below knee, molded socket, SACH foot, endoskeletal system, including soft cover and finishing
ASC

Endoskeletal: Knee Disarticulation

L5310 Knee disarticulation (or through knee), molded socket, SACH foot endoskeletal system, including soft cover and finishing
ASC

Endoskeletal: Above Knee

L5320 Above knee, molded socket, open end, SACH foot, endoskeletal system, single axis knee, including soft cover and finishing
ASC

Endoskeletal: Hip Disarticulation

L5330 Hip disarticulation, Canadian type; molded socket, endo-skeletal system, hip joint, single axis knee, SACH foot, including soft cover and finishing
ASC

Endoskeletal: Hemipelvectomy

L5340 Hemipelvectomy, Canadian type; molded socket, endoskeletal system, hip joint, single axis knee, SACH foot, including soft cover and finishing
ASC

= Invalid Medicare Code (no grace period)

= Code may require certificate of medical necessity (CMN) or DMERC information form (DIF)

Immediate Postsurgical or Early Fitting Procedures

L5400 Immediate postsurgical or early fitting, application of initial rigid dressing, including fitting, alignment, suspension, and one cast change, below knee *ASC*

L5410 Immediate postsurgical or early fitting, application of initial rigid dressing, including fitting, alignment and suspension, below knee, each additional cast change and realignment *ASC*

L5420 Immediate postsurgical or early fitting, application of initial rigid dressing, including fitting, alignment and suspension and one cast change "AK" or knee disarticulation *ASC*

L5430 Immediate postsurgical or early fitting, application of initial rigid dressing, including fitting, alignment and suspension, "AK" or knee disarticulation, each additional cast change and realignment *ASC*

L5450 Immediate postsurgical or early fitting, application of nonweight bearing rigid dressing, below knee *ASC*

L5460 Immediate postsurgical or early fitting, application of nonweight bearing rigid dressing, above knee *ASC*

Initial Prosthesis

L5500 Initial, below knee "PTB" type socket, non-alignable system, pylon, no cover, SACH foot, plaster socket, direct formed *ASC*

L5505 Initial, above knee — knee disarticulation, ischial level socket, non-alignable system, pylon, no cover, SACH foot plaster socket, direct formed *ASC*

Preparatory Prosthesis

L5510 Preparatory, below knee "PTB" type socket, non-alignable system, pylon, no cover, SACH foot, plaster socket, molded to model *ASC*

L5520 Preparatory, below knee "PTB" type socket, non-alignable system, pylon, no cover, SACH foot, thermoplastic or equal, direct formed *ASC*

L5530 Preparatory, below knee "PTB" type socket, non-alignable system, pylon, no cover, SACH foot, thermoplastic or equal, molded to model *ASC*

L5535 Preparatory, below knee "PTB" type socket, non-alignable system, pylon, no cover, SACH foot, prefabricated, adjustable open end socket *ASC*

L5540 Preparatory, below knee "PTB" type socket, non-alignable system, pylon, no cover, SACH foot, laminated socket, molded to model *ASC*

L5560 Preparatory, above knee — knee disarticulation, ischial level socket, non-alignable system, pylon, no cover, SACH foot, plaster socket, molded to model *ASC*

L5570 Preparatory, above knee — knee disarticulation, ischial level socket, non-alignable system, pylon, no cover, SACH foot, thermoplastic or equal, direct formed *ASC*

L Codes

= Special Coverage Instructions Apply   = Carrier Discretion

= Noncovered by Medicare or Medicare Statute

L5580	Preparatory, above knee — knee disarticulation, ischial level socket, non-alignable system, pylon, no cover, SACH foot, thermoplastic or equal, molded to model	*ASC*
L5585	Preparatory, above knee — knee disarticulation, ischial level socket, non-alignable system, pylon, no cover, SACH foot, prefabricated adjustable open end socket	*ASC*
L5590	Preparatory, above knee — knee disarticulation, ischial level socket, non-alignable system, pylon, no cover, SACH foot, laminated socket, molded to model	*ASC*
L5595	Preparatory, hip disarticulation — hemipelvectomy, pylon, no cover, SACH foot, thermoplastic or equal, molded to patient model	*ASC*

Additions: Lower Extremity

L5600	Preparatory, hip disarticulation — hemipelvectomy, pylon, no cover, SACH foot, laminated socket, molded to patient model	*ASC*
L5610	Addition to lower extremity, endoskeletal system, above knee, hydracadence system	*ASC*
L5611	Addition to lower extremity, endoskeletal system, above knee — knee disarticulation, 4-bar linkage, with friction swing phase control	*ASC*
L5613	Addition to lower extremity, endoskeletal system, above knee — knee disarticulation, 4-bar linkage, with hydraulic swing phase control	*ASC*
L5614	Addition to lower extremity, endoskeletal system, above knee — knee disarticulation, 4-bar linkage, with pneumatic swing phase control	*ASC*
L5616	Addition to lower extremity, endoskeletal system, above knee, universal multiplex system, friction swing phase control	*ASC*
L5617	Addition to lower extremity, quick change self-aligning unit, above or below knee, each	*ASC*

Additions: Test Sockets

L5618	Addition to lower extremity, test socket, Symes	*ASC*
L5620	Addition to lower extremity, test socket, below knee	*ASC*
L5622	Addition to lower extremity, test socket, knee disarticulation	*ASC*
L5624	Addition to lower extremity, test socket, above knee	*ASC*
L5626	Addition to lower extremity, test socket, hip disarticulation	*ASC*
L5628	Addition to lower extremity, test socket, hemipelvectomy	*ASC*
L5629	Addition to lower extremity, below knee, acrylic socket	*ASC*

Additions: Socket Variations

L5630	Addition to lower extremity, Symes type, expandable wall socket	*ASC*
L5631	Addition to lower extremity, above knee or knee disarticulation, acrylic socket	*ASC*
L5632	Addition to lower extremity, Symes type, "PTB" brim design socket	*ASC*

L5634	Addition to lower extremity, Symes type, posterior opening (Canadian) socket *ASC*
L5636	Addition to lower extremity, Symes type, medial opening socket *ASC*
L5637	Addition to lower extremity, below knee, total contact *ASC*
L5638	Addition to lower extremity, below knee, leather socket *ASC*
L5639	Addition to lower extremity, below knee, wood socket *ASC*
L5640	Addition to lower extremity, knee disarticulation, leather socket *ASC*
L5642	Addition to lower extremity, above knee, leather socket *ASC*
L5643	Addition to lower extremity, hip disarticulation, flexible inner socket, external frame *ASC*
L5644	Addition to lower extremity, above knee, wood socket *ASC*
L5645	Addition to lower extremity, below knee, flexible inner socket, external frame *ASC*
L5646	Addition to lower extremity, below knee, air cushion socket *ASC*
L5647	Addition to lower extremity, below knee, suction socket *ASC*
L5648	Addition to lower extremity, above knee, air cushion socket *ASC*
L5649	Addition to lower extremity, ischial containment/narrow M-L socket *ASC*
L5650	Addition to lower extremity, total contact, above knee or knee disarticulation socket *ASC*
L5651	Addition to lower extremity, above knee, flexible inner socket, external frame *ASC*
L5652	Addition to lower extremity, suction suspension, above knee or knee disarticulation socket *ASC*
L5653	Addition to lower extremity, knee disarticulation, expandable wall socket *ASC*

Additions: Socket Insert and Suspension

L5654	Addition to lower extremity, socket insert, Symes (Kemblo, Pelite, Aliplast, Plastazote or equal) *ASC*
L5655	Addition to lower extremity, socket insert, below knee (Kemblo, Pelite, Aliplast, Plastazote or equal) *ASC*
L5656	Addition to lower extremity, socket insert, knee disarticulation (Kemblo, Pelite, Aliplast, Plastazote or equal) *ASC*
L5658	Addition to lower extremity, socket insert, above knee (Kemblo, Pelite, Aliplast, Plastazote or equal) *ASC*
L5660	Addition to lower extremity, socket insert, Symes, silicone gel or equal *ASC*
L5661	Addition to lower extremity, socket insert, multidurometer, Symes *ASC*
L5662	Addition to lower extremity, socket insert, below knee, silicone gel or equal *ASC*

L Codes

= Special Coverage Instructions Apply   = Carrier Discretion

= Noncovered by Medicare or Medicare Statute

L5663	Addition to lower extremity, socket insert, knee disarticulation, silicone gel or equal	*ASC*
L5664	Addition to lower extremity, socket insert, above knee, silicone gel or equal	*ASC*
L5665	Addition to lower extremity, socket insert, multidurometer, below knee	*ASC*
L5666	Addition to lower extremity, below knee, cuff suspension	*ASC*
L5667	Addition to lower extremity, below knee/above knee, socket insert, suction suspension with locking mechanism	*ASC*
L5668	Addition to lower extremity, below knee, molded distal cushion	*ASC*
L5669	Addition to lower extremity, below knee/above knee, socket insert, suction suspension without locking mechanism	*ASC*
L5670	Addition to lower extremity, below knee, molded supracondylar suspension ("PTS" or similar)	*ASC*
L5672	Addition to lower extremity, below knee, removable medial brim suspension	*ASC*
▲ **L5674**	Addition to lower extremity, below knee, suspension sleeve, any material, each	*ASC*
▲ **L5675**	Addition to lower extremity, below knee, suspension sleeve, heavy duty, any material, each	*ASC*
L5676	Addition to lower extremity, below knee, knee joints, single axis, pair	*ASC*
L5677	Addition to lower extremity, below knee, knee joints, polycentric, pair	*ASC*
L5678	Addition to lower extremity, below knee joint covers, pair	*ASC*
L5680	Addition to lower extremity, below knee, thigh lacer, nonmolded	*ASC*
L5682	Addition to lower extremity, below knee, thigh lacer, gluteal/ischial, molded	*ASC*
L5684	Addition to lower extremity, below knee, fork strap	*ASC*
L5686	Addition to lower extremity, below knee, back check (extension control)	*ASC*
L5688	Addition to lower extremity, below knee, waist belt, webbing	*ASC*
L5690	Addition to lower extremity, below knee, waist belt, padded and lined	*ASC*
L5692	Addition to lower extremity, above knee, pelvic control belt, light	*ASC*
L5694	Addition to lower extremity, above knee, pelvic control belt, padded and lined	*ASC*
L5695	Addition to lower extremity, above knee, pelvic control, sleeve suspension, neoprene or equal, each	*ASC*
L5696	Addition to lower extremity, above knee or knee disarticulation, pelvic joint	*ASC*

= Invalid Medicare Code (no grace period)

= Code may require certificate of medical necessity (CMN) or DMERC information form (DIF)

L5697	Addition to lower extremity, above knee or knee disarticulation, pelvic band	*ASC*
L5698	Addition to lower extremity, above knee or knee disarticulation, Silesian bandage	*ASC*
L5699	All lower extremity prostheses, shoulder harness	*ASC*

Replacements

L5700	Replacement, socket, below knee, molded to patient model	*ASC*
L5701	Replacement, socket, above knee/knee disarticulation, including attachment plate, molded to patient model	*ASC*
L5702	Replacement, socket, hip disarticulation, including hip joint, molded to patient model	*ASC*
L5704	Replacement, custom shaped protective cover, below knee	*ASC*
L5705	Replacement, custom shaped protective cover, above knee	*ASC*
L5706	Replacement, custom shaped protective cover, knee disarticulation	*ASC*
L5707	Replacement, custom shaped protective cover, hip disarticulation	*ASC*

Additions: Exoskeletal Knee-Shin System

L5710	Addition, exoskeletal knee-shin system, single axis, manual lock	*ASC*
L5711	Addition, exoskeletal knee-shin system, single axis, manual lock, ultra-light material	*ASC*
L5712	Addition, exoskeletal knee-shin system, single axis, friction swing and stance phase control (safety knee)	*ASC*
L5714	Addition, exoskeletal knee-shin system, single axis, variable friction swing phase control	*ASC*
L5716	Addition, exoskeletal knee-shin system, polycentric, mechanical stance phase lock	*ASC*
L5718	Addition, exoskeletal knee-shin system, polycentric, friction swing and stance phase control	*ASC*
L5722	Addition, exoskeletal knee-shin system, single axis, pneumatic swing, friction stance phase control	*ASC*
L5724	Addition, exoskeletal knee-shin system, single axis, fluid swing phase control	*ASC*
L5726	Addition, exoskeletal knee-shin system, single axis, external joints, fluid swing phase control	*ASC*
L5728	Addition, exoskeletal knee-shin system, single axis, fluid swing and stance phase control	*ASC*
L5780	Addition, exoskeletal knee-shin system, single axis, pneumatic/hydra pneumatic swing phase control	*ASC*

L Codes

| | = Special Coverage Instructions Apply | | = Carrier Discretion |

| | = Noncovered by Medicare or Medicare Statute |

Component Modification

L5785 Addition, exoskeletal system, below knee, ultra-light material (titanium, carbon fiber or equal) *ASC*

L5790 Addition, exoskeletal system, above knee, ultra-light material (titanium, carbon fiber or equal) *ASC*

L5795 Addition, exoskeletal system, hip disarticulation, ultra-light material (titanium, carbon fiber or equal) *ASC*

Additions: Endoskeletal Knee-Shin System

L5810 Addition, endoskeletal knee-shin system, single axis, manual lock *ASC*

L5811 Addition, endoskeletal knee-shin system, single axis, manual lock, ultra-light material *ASC*

L5812 Addition, endoskeletal knee-shin system, single axis, friction swing and stance phase control (safety knee) *ASC*

L5814 Addition, endoskeletal knee-shin system, polycentric, hydraulic swing phase control, mechanical stance phase lock *ASC*

L5816 Addition, endoskeletal knee-shin system, polycentric, mechanical stance phase lock *ASC*

L5818 Addition, endoskeletal knee-shin system, polycentric, friction swing and stance phase control *ASC*

L5822 Addition, endoskeletal knee-shin system, single axis, pneumatic swing, friction stance phase control *ASC*

L5824 Addition, endoskeletal knee-shin system, single axis, fluid swing phase control *ASC*

L5826 Addition, endoskeletal knee-shin system, single axis, hydraulic swing phase control, with miniature high activity frame *ASC*

L5828 Addition, endoskeletal knee-shin system, single axis, fluid swing and stance phase control *ASC*

L5830 Addition, endoskeletal knee-shin system, single axis, pneumatic/swing phase control *ASC*

L5840 Addition, endoskeletal knee-shin system, 4-bar linkage or multiaxial, pneumatic swing phase control *ASC*

L5845 Addition, endoskeletal knee-shin system, stance flexion feature, adjustable *ASC*

L5846 Addition, endoskeletal knee-shin system, microprocessor control feature, swing phase only *ASC*

L5850 Addition, endoskeletal system, above knee or hip disarticulation, knee extension assist *ASC*

L5855 Addition, endoskeletal system, hip disarticulation, mechanical hip extension assist *ASC*

L5910 Addition, endoskeletal system, below knee, alignable system *ASC*

▓ = Invalid Medicare Code (no grace period)

▓ = Code may require certificate of medical necessity (CMN) or DMERC information form (DIF)

L5920 Addition, endoskeletal system, above knee or hip disarticulation, alignable system *ASC*

L5925 Addition, endoskeletal system, above knee, knee disarticulation or hip disarticulation, manual lock

L5930 Addition, endoskeletal system, high activity knee control frame *ASC*

L5940 Addition, endoskeletal system, below knee, ultra-light material (titanium, carbon fiber or equal) *ASC*

L5950 Addition, endoskeletal system, above knee, ultra-light material (titanium, carbon fiber or equal) *ASC*

L5960 Addition, endoskeletal system, hip disarticulation, ultra-light material (titanium, carbon fiber or equal) *ASC*

L5962 Addition, endoskeletal system, below knee, flexible protective outer surface covering system *ASC*

L5964 Addition, endoskeletal system, above knee, flexible protective outer surface covering system *ASC*

L5966 Addition, endoskeletal system, hip disarticulation, flexible protective outer surface covering system *ASC*

L5968 Addition to lower limb prosthesis, multiaxial ankle with swing phase active dorsiflexion feature

L5970 All lower extremity prostheses, foot, external keel, SACH foot *ASC*

L5972 All lower extremity prostheses, flexible keel foot (Safe, Sten, Bock Dynamic or equal) *ASC*

L5974 All lower extremity prostheses, foot, single axis ankle/foot *ASC*

L5975 All lower extremity prosthesis, combination single axis ankle and flexible keel foot

L5976 All lower extremity prostheses, energy storing foot (Seattle Carbon Copy II or equal) *ASC*

L5978 All lower extremity prostheses, foot, multi-axial ankle/foot *ASC*

▲ **L5979** All lower extremity prostheses, multi-axial ankle, dynamic response foot, one piece system *ASC*

L5980 All lower extremity prostheses, flex-foot system *ASC*

L5981 All lower extremity prostheses, flex-walk system or equal *ASC*

L5982 All exoskeletal lower extremity prostheses, axial rotation unit *ASC*

L5984 All endoskeletal lower extremity prostheses, axial rotation unit *ASC*

L5985 All endoskeletal lower extremity prostheses, dynamic prosthetic pylon *ASC*

L5986 All lower extremity prostheses, multi-axial rotation unit ("MCP" or equal) *ASC*

L5987 All lower extremity prosthesis, shank foot system with vertical loading pylon *ASC*

L Codes

= Special Coverage Instructions Apply   = Carrier Discretion

= Noncovered by Medicare or Medicare Statute

| **L5988** | Addition to lower limb prosthesis, vertical shock reducing pylon feature |
| **L5999** | Lower extremity prosthesis, not otherwise specified | *ASC* |

Upper Limb

The procedures in L6000-L6599 are considered as "base" or "basic procedures" and may be modified by listing procedures from the "addition" sections. The base procedures include only standard friction wrist and control cable system unless otherwise specified.

Partial Hand

L6000	Partial hand, Robin-Aids, thumb remaining (or equal)	*ASC*
L6010	Partial hand, Robin-Aids, little and/or ring finger remaining (or equal)	*ASC*
L6020	Partial hand, Robin-Aids, no finger remaining (or equal)	*ASC*

Wrist Disarticulation

| **L6050** | Wrist disarticulation, molded socket, flexible elbow hinges, triceps pad | *ASC* |
| **L6055** | Wrist disarticulation, molded socket with expandable interface, flexible elbow hinges, triceps pad | *ASC* |

Below Elbow

L6100	Below elbow, molded socket, flexible elbow hinge, triceps pad	*ASC*
L6110	Below elbow, molded socket (Muenster or Northwestern suspension types)	*ASC*
L6120	Below elbow, molded double wall split socket, step-up hinges, half cuff	*ASC*
L6130	Below elbow, molded double wall split socket, stump activated locking hinge, half cuff	*ASC*

Elbow Disarticulation

| **L6200** | Elbow disarticulation, molded socket, outside locking hinge, forearm | *ASC* |
| **L6205** | Elbow disarticulation, molded socket with expandable interface, outside locking hinges, forearm | *ASC* |

Above Elbow

| **L6250** | Above elbow, molded double wall socket, internal locking elbow, forearm | *ASC* |

Shoulder Disarticulation

L6300	Shoulder disarticulation, molded socket, shoulder bulkhead, humeral section, internal locking elbow, forearm	*ASC*
L6310	Shoulder disarticulation, passive restoration (complete prosthesis)	*ASC*
L6320	Shoulder disarticulation, passive restoration (shoulder cap only)	*ASC*

= Invalid Medicare Code (no grace period)

= Code may require certificate of medical necessity (CMN) or DMERC information form (DIF)

Interscapular Thoracic

L6350 Interscapular thoracic, molded socket, shoulder bulkhead, humeral section, internal locking elbow, forearm *ASC*

L6360 Interscapular thoracic, passive restoration (complete prosthesis) *ASC*

L6370 Interscapular thoracic, passive restoration (shoulder cap only) *ASC*

Immediate and Early Postsurgical Procedures

L6380 Immediate postsurgical or early fitting, application of initial rigid dressing, including fitting alignment and suspension of components, and one cast change, wrist disarticulation or below elbow *ASC*

L6382 Immediate postsurgical or early fitting, application of initial rigid dressing including fitting alignment and suspension of components, and one cast change, elbow disarticulation or above elbow *ASC*

L6384 Immediate postsurgical or early fitting, application of initial rigid dressing including fitting alignment and suspension of components, and one cast change, shoulder disarticulation or interscapular thoracic *ASC*

L6386 Immediate postsurgical or early fitting, each additional cast change and realignment *ASC*

L6388 Immediate postsurgical or early fitting, application of rigid dressing only *ASC*

Endoskeletal: Below Elbow

L6400 Below elbow, molded socket, endoskeletal system, including soft prosthetic tissue shaping *ASC*

Endoskeletal: Elbow Disarticulation

L6450 Elbow disarticulation, molded socket, endoskeletal system, including soft prosthetic tissue shaping *ASC*

Endoskeletal: Above Elbow

L6500 Above elbow, molded socket, endoskeletal system, including soft prosthetic tissue shaping *ASC*

Endoskeletal: Shoulder Disarticulation

L6550 Shoulder disarticulation, molded socket, endoskeletal system, including soft prosthetic tissue shaping *ASC*

Endoskeletal: Interscapular Thoracic

L6570 Interscapular thoracic, molded socket, endoskeletal system, including soft prosthetic tissue shaping *ASC*

L6580 Preparatory, wrist disarticulation or below elbow, single wall plastic socket, friction wrist, flexible elbow hinges, figure of eight harness, humeral cuff, Bowden cable control, "USMC" or equal pylon, no cover, molded to patient model *ASC*

L Codes

= Special Coverage Instructions Apply   = Carrier Discretion

= Noncovered by Medicare or Medicare Statute

L6582	Preparatory, wrist disarticulation or below elbow, single wall socket, friction wrist, flexible elbow hinges, figure of eight harness, humeral cuff, Bowden cable control, "USMC" or equal pylon, no cover, direct formed *ASC*
L6584	Preparatory, elbow disarticulation or above elbow, single wall plastic socket, friction wrist, locking elbow, figure of eight harness, fair lead cable control, "USMC" or equal pylon, no cover, molded to patient model *ASC*
L6586	Preparatory, elbow disarticulation or above elbow, single wall socket, friction wrist, locking elbow, figure of eight harness, fair lead cable control, "USMC" or equal pylon, no cover, direct formed *ASC*
L6588	Preparatory, shoulder disarticulation or interscapular thoracic, single wall plastic socket, shoulder joint, locking elbow, friction wrist, chest strap, fair lead cable control, "USMC" or equal pylon, no cover, molded to patient model *ASC*
L6590	Preparatory, shoulder disarticulation or interscapular thoracic, single wall socket, shoulder joint, locking elbow, friction wrist, chest strap, fair lead cable control, "USMC" or equal pylon, no cover, direct formed *ASC*

Additions: Upper Limb

The following procedures/modifications/ components may be added to other base procedures. The items in this section should reflect the additional complexity of each modification procedrue, in addition to the base procedure, at the time of the original order.

L6600	Upper extremity additions, polycentric hinge, pair *ASC*
L6605	Upper extremity additions, single pivot hinge, pair *ASC*
L6610	Upper extremity additions, flexible metal hinge, pair *ASC*
L6615	Upper extremity addition, disconnect locking wrist unit *ASC*
L6616	Upper extremity addition, additional disconnect insert for locking wrist unit, each *ASC*
L6620	Upper extremity addition, flexion-friction wrist unit *ASC*
L6623	Upper extremity addition, spring assisted rotational wrist unit with latch release *ASC*
L6625	Upper extremity addition, rotation wrist unit with cable lock *ASC*
L6628	Upper extremity addition, quick disconnect hook adapter, Otto Bock or equal *ASC*
L6629	Upper extremity addition, quick disconnect lamination collar with coupling piece, Otto Bock or equal *ASC*
L6630	Upper extremity addition, stainless steel, any wrist *ASC*
L6632	Upper extremity addition, latex suspension sleeve, each *ASC*
L6635	Upper extremity addition, lift assist for elbow *ASC*
L6637	Upper extremity addition, nudge control elbow lock *ASC*

L6640	Upper extremity additions, shoulder abduction joint, pair	*ASC*
L6641	Upper extremity addition, excursion amplifier, pulley type	*ASC*
L6642	Upper extremity addition, excursion amplifier, lever type	*ASC*
L6645	Upper extremity addition, shoulder flexion-abduction joint, each	*ASC*
L6650	Upper extremity addition, shoulder universal joint, each	*ASC*
L6655	Upper extremity addition, standard control cable, extra	*ASC*
L6660	Upper extremity addition, heavy duty control cable	*ASC*
L6665	Upper extremity addition, Teflon, or equal, cable lining	*ASC*
L6670	Upper extremity addition, hook to hand, cable adapter	*ASC*
L6672	Upper extremity addition, harness, chest or shoulder, saddle type	*ASC*
L6675	Upper extremity addition, harness, figure of eight type, for single control	*ASC*
L6676	Upper extremity addition, harness, figure of eight type, for dual control	*ASC*
L6680	Upper extremity addition, test socket, wrist disarticulation or below elbow	*ASC*
L6682	Upper extremity addition, test socket, elbow disarticulation or above elbow	*ASC*
L6684	Upper extremity addition, test socket, shoulder disarticulation or interscapular thoracic	*ASC*
L6686	Upper extremity addition, suction socket	*ASC*
L6687	Upper extremity addition, frame type socket, below elbow or wrist disarticulation	*ASC*
L6688	Upper extremity addition, frame type socket, above elbow or elbow disarticulation	*ASC*
L6689	Upper extremity addition, frame type socket, shoulder disarticulation	*ASC*
L6690	Upper extremity addition, frame type socket, interscapular-thoracic	*ASC*
L6691	Upper extremity addition, removable insert, each	*ASC*
L6692	Upper extremity addition, silicone gel insert or equal, each	*ASC*
L6693	Upper extremity addition, locking elbow, forearm counterbalance	

Terminal Devices

Hooks

L6700	Terminal device, hook, Dorrance or equal, model #3	*MCM 2133, ASC*
L6705	Terminal device, hook, Dorrance or equal, model #5	*MCM 2133, ASC*
L6710	Terminal device, hook, Dorrance or equal, model #5X	*MCM 2133, ASC*
L6715	Terminal device, hook, Dorrance or equal, model #5XA	*MCM 2133, ASC*
L6720	Terminal device, hook, Dorrance or equal, model #6	*MCM 2133, ASC*

L Codes

= Special Coverage Instructions Apply   = Carrier Discretion

= Noncovered by Medicare or Medicare Statute

L6725	Terminal device, hook, Dorrance or equal, model #7	*MCM 2133, ASC*
L6730	Terminal device, hook, Dorrance or equal, model #7LO	*MCM 2133, ASC*
L6735	Terminal device, hook, Dorrance or equal, model #8	*MCM 2133, ASC*
L6740	Terminal device, hook, Dorrance or equal, model #8X	*MCM 2133, ASC*
L6745	Terminal device, hook, Dorrance or equal, model #88X	*MCM 2133, ASC*
L6750	Terminal device, hook, Dorrance or equal, model #10P	*MCM 2133, ASC*
L6755	Terminal device, hook, Dorrance or equal, model #10X	*MCM 2133, ASC*
L6765	Terminal device, hook, Dorrance or equal, model #12P	*MCM 2133, ASC*
L6770	Terminal device, hook, Dorrance or equal, model #99X	*MCM 2133, ASC*
L6775	Terminal device, hook, Dorrance or equal, model #555	*MCM 2133, ASC*
L6780	Terminal device, hook, Dorrance or equal, model #SS555	*MCM 2133, ASC*
L6790	Terminal device, hook, Accu hook or equal	*MCM 2133, ASC*
L6795	Terminal device, hook, 2 load or equal	*MCM 2133, ASC*
L6800	Terminal device, hook, APRL VC or equal	*MCM 2133, ASC*
L6805	Terminal device, modifier wrist flexion unit	*MCM 2133, ASC*
L6806	Terminal device, hook, TRS Grip, Grip III, VC, or equal	*MCM 2133, ASC*
L6807	Terminal device, hook, Grip I, Grip II, VC, or equal	*MCM 2133, ASC*
L6808	Terminal device, hook, TRS Adept, infant or child, VC, or equal	*MCM 2133, ASC*
L6809	Terminal device, hook, TRS Super Sport, passive	*MCM 2133, ASC*
L6810	Terminal device, pincher tool, Otto Bock or equal	*MCM 2133, ASC*

Hands

L6825	Terminal device, hand, Dorrance, VO	*MCM 2133, ASC*
L6830	Terminal device, hand, APRL, VC	*MCM 2133, ASC*
L6835	Terminal device, hand, Sierra, VO	*MCM 2133, ASC*
L6840	Terminal device, hand, Becker Imperial	*MCM 2133, ASC*
L6845	Terminal device, hand, Becker Lock Grip	*MCM 2133, ASC*
L6850	Terminal device, hand, Becker Plylite	*MCM 2133, ASC*
L6855	Terminal device, hand, Robin-Aids, VO	*MCM 2133, ASC*
L6860	Terminal device, hand, Robin-Aids, VO soft	*MCM 2133, ASC*
L6865	Terminal device, hand, passive hand	*MCM 2133, ASC*
L6867	Terminal device, hand, Detroit Infant Hand (mechanical)	*MCM 2133, ASC*
L6868	Terminal device, hand, passive infant hand, Steeper, Hosmer or equal	*MCM 2133, ASC*
L6870	Terminal device, hand, child mitt	*MCM 2133, ASC*
L6872	Terminal device, hand, NYU child hand	*MCM 2133, ASC*

= Invalid Medicare Code (no grace period)

= Code may require certificate of medical necessity (CMN) or DMERC information form (DIF)

L6873	Terminal device, hand, mechanical infant hand, Steeper or equal	
		MCM 2133, ASC
L6875	Terminal device, hand, Bock, VC	*MCM 2133, ASC*
L6880	Terminal device, hand, Bock, VO	*MCM 2133, ASC*

Gloves for Above Hands

L6890	Terminal device, glove for above hands, production glove	*ASC*
L6895	Terminal device, glove for above hands, custom glove	*ASC*

Hand Restoration

L6900	Hand restoration (casts, shading and measurements included), partial hand, with glove, thumb or one finger remaining	*ASC*
L6905	Hand restoration (casts, shading and measurements included), partial hand, with glove, multiple fingers remaining	*ASC*
L6910	Hand restoration (casts, shading and measurements included), partial hand, with glove, no fingers remaining	*ASC*
L6915	Hand restoration (shading and measurements included), replacement glove for above	*ASC*

External Power

Base Devices

L6920	Wrist disarticulation, external power, self-suspended inner socket, removable forearm shell, Otto Bock or equal switch, cables, two batteries and one charger, switch control of terminal device	*ASC*
L6925	Wrist disarticulation, external power, self-suspended inner socket, removable forearm shell, Otto Bock or equal electrodes, cables, two batteries and one charger, myoelectronic control of terminal device	*ASC*
L6930	Below elbow, external power, self-suspended inner socket, removable forearm shell, Otto Bock or equal switch, cables, two batteries and one charger, switch control of terminal device	*ASC*
L6935	Below elbow, external power, self-suspended inner socket, removable forearm shell, Otto Bock or equal electrodes, cables, two batteries and one charger, myoelectronic control of terminal device	*ASC*
L6940	Elbow disarticulation, external power, molded inner socket, removable humeral shell, outside locking hinges, forearm, Otto Bock or equal switch, cables, two batteries and one charger, switch control of terminal device	*ASC*
L6945	Elbow disarticulation, external power, molded inner socket, removable humeral shell, outside locking hinges, forearm, Otto Bock or equal electrodes, cables, two batteries and one charger, myoelectronic control of terminal device	*ASC*

L Codes

= Special Coverage Instructions Apply   = Carrier Discretion

= Noncovered by Medicare or Medicare Statute

L6950	Above elbow, external power, molded inner socket, removable humeral shell, internal locking elbow, forearm, Otto Bock or equal switch, cables, two batteries and one charger, switch control of terminal device *ASC*
L6955	Above elbow, external power, molded inner socket, removable humeral shell, internal locking elbow, forearm, Otto Bock or equal electrodes, cables, two batteries and one charger, myoelectronic control of terminal device *ASC*
L6960	Shoulder disarticulation, external power, molded inner socket, removable shoulder shell, shoulder bulkhead, humeral section, mechanical elbow, forearm, Otto Bock or equal switch, cables, two batteries and one charger, switch control of terminal device *ASC*
L6965	Shoulder disarticulation, external power, molded inner socket, removable shoulder shell, shoulder bulkhead, humeral section, mechanical elbow, forearm, Otto Bock or equal electrodes, cables, two batteries and one charger, myoelectronic control of terminal device *ASC*
L6970	Interscapular-thoracic, external power, molded inner socket, removable shoulder shell, shoulder bulkhead, humeral section, mechanical elbow, forearm, Otto Bock or equal switch, cables, two batteries and one charger, switch control of terminal device *ASC*
L6975	Interscapular-thoracic, external power, molded inner socket, removable shoulder shell, shoulder bulkhead, humeral section, mechanical elbow, forearm, Otto Bock or equal electrodes, cables, two batteries and one charger, myoelectronic control of terminal device *ASC*
L7010	Electronic hand, Otto Bock, Steeper or equal, switch controlled *ASC*
L7015	Electronic hand, System Teknik, Variety Village or equal, switch controlled *ASC*
L7020	Electronic greifer, Otto Bock or equal, switch controlled *ASC*
L7025	Electronic hand, Otto Bock or equal, myoelectronically controlled *ASC*
L7030	Electronic hand, System Teknik, Variety Village or equal, myoelectronically controlled *ASC*
L7035	Electronic greifer, Otto Bock or equal, myoelectronically controlled *ASC*
L7040	Prehensile actuator, Hosmer or equal, switch controlled *ASC*
L7045	Electronic hook, child, Michigan or equal, switch controlled *ASC*

Elbow

L7170	Electronic elbow, Hosmer or equal, switch controlled *ASC*
L7180	Electronic elbow, Boston, Utah or equal, myoelectronically controlled *ASC*
L7185	Electronic elbow, adolescent, Variety Village or equal, switch controlled *ASC*
L7186	Electronic elbow, child, Variety Village or equal, switch controlled *ASC*

= Invalid Medicare Code (no grace period)

= Code may require certificate of medical necessity (CMN) or DMERC information form (DIF)

L7190	Electronic elbow, adolescent, Variety Village or equal, myoelectronically controlled	
L7191	Electronic elbow, child, Variety Village or equal, myoelectronically controlled	*ASC*
L7260	Electronic wrist rotator, Otto Bock or equal	*ASC*
L7261	Electronic wrist rotator, for Utah arm	*ASC*
L7266	Servo control, Steeper or equal	*ASC*
L7272	Analogue control, UNB or equal	*ASC*
L7274	Proportional control, 6-12 volt, Liberty, Utah or equal	*ASC*

Battery Components

L7360	Six volt battery, Otto Bock or equal, each	*ASC*
L7362	Battery charger, six volt, Otto Bock or equal	*ASC*
L7364	Twelve volt battery, Utah or equal, each	*ASC*
L7366	Battery charger, twelve volt, Utah or equal	*ASC*
L7499	Upper extremity prosthesis, not otherwise specified	*ASC*

Repairs

L7500	Repair of prosthetic device, hourly rate	
	MCM 2100.4, MCM 2130D, MCM 2133, ASC	
L7510	Repair of prosthetic device, repair or replace minor parts	
	MCM 2100.4, MCM 2130D, MCM 2133, ASC	
L7520	Repair prosthetic device, labor component, per 15 minutes	*ASC*
L7900	Vacuum erection system	*ASC*

General

Prosthesis

L8000	Breast prosthesis, mastectomy bra	*MCM 2130A, ASC*
L8010	Breast prosthesis, mastectomy sleeve	*MCM 2130A, ASC*
L8015	External breast prosthesis garment, with mastectomy form, post-mastectomy	*MCM 2130*
L8020	Breast prosthesis, mastectomy form	*MCM 2130A, ASC*
L8030	Breast prosthesis, silicone or equal	*MCM 2130A, ASC*
L8035	Custom breast prosthesis, post mastectomy, molded to patient model	*MCM 2130*
L8039	Breast prosthesis, not otherwise specified	*ASC*
● **L8040**	Nasal prosthesis, provided by a non-physician	
● **L8041**	Midfacial prosthesis, provided by a non-physician	
● **L8042**	Orbital prosthesis, provided by a non-physician	
● **L8043**	Upper facial prosthesis, provided by a non-physician	

L Codes

= Special Coverage Instructions Apply   = Carrier Discretion

= Noncovered by Medicare or Medicare Statute

● **L8044** Hemi-facial prosthesis, provided by a non-physician

● **L8045** Auricular prosthesis, provided by a non-physician

● **L8046** Partial facial prosthesis, provided by a non-physician

● **L8047** Nasal septal prosthesis, provided by a non-physician

● **L8048** Unspecified maxillofacial prosthesis, by report, provided by a non-physician

● **L8049** Repair or modification of maxillofacial prosthesis, labor component, 15 minute increments, provided by a non-physician

Elastic Supports

L8100 Gradient compression stocking, below knee, 18-30 mmhg, each
CIM 60-9, MCM 2133, ASC

L8110 Gradient compression stocking, below knee, 30-40 mmhg, each
CIM 60-9, MCM 2133, ASC

L8120 Gradient compression stocking, below knee, 40-50 mmhg, each
CIM 60-9, MCM 2133, ASC

L8130 Gradient compression stocking, thigh length, 18-30 mmhg, each
CIM 60-9, MCM 2133, ASC

L8140 Gradient compression stocking, thigh length, 30-40 mmhg, each
CIM 60-9, MCM 2133, ASC

L8150 Gradient compression stocking, thigh length, 40-50 mmhg, each
CIM 60-9, MCM 2133, ASC

L8160 Gradient compression stocking, full length/chap style, 18-30 mmhg, each
CIM 60-9, MCM 2133, ASC

L8170 Gradient compression stocking, full length/chap style, 30-40 mmhg, each
CIM 60-9, MCM 2133, ASC

L8180 Gradient compression stocking, full length/chap style, 40-50 mmhg, each
CIM 60-9, MCM 2133, ASC

L8190 Gradient compression stocking, waist length, 18-30 mmhg, each
CIM 60-9, MCM 2133, ASC

L8195 Gradient compression stocking, waist length, 30-40 mmhg, each
CIM 60-9, MCM 2133

L8200 Gradient compression stocking, waist length, 40-50 mmhg, each
CIM 60-9, MCM 2133, ASC

L8210 Gradient compression stocking, custom made   *CIM 60-9, MCM 2133, ASC*

L8220 Gradient compression stocking, lymphedema   *CIM 60-9, MCM 2133, ASC*

L8230 Gradient compression stocking, garter belt   *CIM 60-9, MCM 2133, ASC*

L8239 Gradient compression stocking, not otherwise specified   *ASC*

Trusses

L8300 Truss, single with standard pad   *CIM 70-1, CIM 70-2, MCM 2133, ASC*

= Invalid Medicare Code (no grace period)

= Code may require certificate of medical necessity (CMN) or DMERC information form (DIF)

| L8310 | Truss, double with standard pads | CIM 70-1, CIM 70-2, MCM 2133, ASC |

| L8320 | Truss, addition to standard pad, water pad |
| | | CIM 70-1, CIM 70-2, MCM 2133, ASC |

| L8330 | Truss, addition to standard pad, scrotal pad |
| | | CIM 70-1, CIM 70-2, MCM 2133, ASC |

Prosthetic Socks

L8400	Prosthetic sheath, below knee, each	MCM 2133, ASC
L8410	Prosthetic sheath, above knee, each	MCM 2133, ASC
L8415	Prosthetic sheath, upper limb, each	MCM 2133, ASC
L8417	Prosthetic sheath/sock, including a gel cushion layer, below knee or above knee, each	ASC
L8420	Prosthetic sock, multiple ply, below knee, each	MCM 2133, ASC
L8430	Prosthetic sock, multiple ply, above knee, each	MCM 2133, ASC
L8435	Prosthetic sock, multiple ply, upper limb, each	MCM 2133
L8440	Prosthetic shrinker, below knee, each	MCM 2133, ASC
L8460	Prosthetic shrinker, above knee, each	MCM 2133, ASC
L8465	Prosthetic shrinker, upper limb, each	MCM 2133, ASC
L8470	Prosthetic sock, single ply, fitting, below knee, each	MCM 2133, ASC
L8480	Prosthetic sock, single ply, fitting, above knee, each	MCM 2133, ASC
L8485	Prosthetic sock, single ply, fitting, upper limb, each	MCM 2133, ASC
L8490	Addition to prosthetic sheath/sock, air seal suction retention system	ASC
L8499	Unlisted procedure for miscellaneous prosthetic services	ASC

Prosthetic Implants

Integumentary System

L8500	Artificial larynx, any type	CIM 65-5, MCM 2130, ASC
L8501	Tracheostomy speaking valve	CIM 65-16, ASC
L8600	Implantable breast prosthesis, silicone or equal	CIM 35-47, MCM 2130, ASC
▲ L8603	Injectable bulking agent, collagen implant, urinary tract, 2.5 ml syringe, includes shipping and necessary supplies	CIM 65-9, ASC
● L8606	Injectable bulking agent, synthetic implant, urinary tract, 1 ml syringe, includes shipping and necessary supplies	CIM 65-9

Head: Skull, Facial Bones, and Temporomandibular Joint

L8610	Ocular implant	MCM 2130, ASC
L8612	Aqueous shunt	MCM 2130, ASC
L8613	Ossicular implant	MCM 2130, ASC
L8614	Cochlear device/system	CIM 65-14, MCM 2130, ASC
L8619	Cochlear implant external speech processor, replacement	CIM 65-14, ASC

L Codes

Upper Extremity
L8630   Metacarpophalangeal joint implant   *MCM 2130, ASC*

Lower Extremity — Joint: Knee, Ankle, Toe
L8641   Metatarsal joint implant   *MCM 2130, ASC*

L8642   Hallux implant   *MCM 2130, ASC*

Miscellaneous Muscular-Skeletal
L8658   Interphalangeal joint implant   *MCM 2130, ASC*

Cardiovascular System
L8670   Vascular graft material, synthetic, implant   *MCM 2130, ASC*

Genital
L8699   Prosthetic implant, not otherwise specified   *ASC*

L9900   Orthotic and prosthetic supply, accessory, and/or service component of another HCPCS L code

---

= Invalid Medicare Code (no grace period)

= Code may require certificate of medical necessity (CMN) or DMERC information form (DIF)

Medical Services M0000–M0302

Other Medical Services

M0064 Brief office visit for the sole purpose of monitoring or changing drug prescriptions used in the treatment of mental psychoneurotic and personality disorders *MCM 2476.3, ASC*

M0075 Cellular therapy *CIM 35-5*

M0076 Prolotherapy *CIM 35-13*

M0100 Intragastric hypothermia using gastric freezing (MNP) *CIM 35-65*

Cardiovascular Services

M0300 IV chelation therapy (chemical endarterectomy) *CIM 35-64*

M0301 Fabric wrapping of abdominal aneurysm (MNP) *CIM 35-34*

M0302 Assessment of cardiac output by electrical bioimpedance *CIM 50-54*

M Codes

= Special Coverage Instructions Apply   = Carrier Discretion

= Noncovered by Medicare or Medicare Statute

Pathology and Laboratory Services
P0000–P9999

Under certain circumstances, Medicare allows physicians and laboratories a fee for drawing or collecting test specimens. If the test specimen is collected from a homebound patient, physicians and laboratories may also bill for a travel allowance.

Chemistry and Toxicology Tests

P2028	Cephalin floculation, blood	*CIM 50-34, ASC*
P2029	Congo red, blood	*CIM 50-34, ASC*
P2031	Hair analysis (excluding arsenic)	*CIM 50-24*
P2033	Thymol turbidity, blood	*CIM 50-34, ASC*
P2038	Mucoprotein, blood (seromucoid) (medical necessity procedure) *CIM 50-34, ASC*

Pathology Screening Tests

P3000	Screening Papanicolaou smear, cervical or vaginal, up to three smears, by technician under physician supervision	*CIM 50-20, ASC*
P3001	Screening Papanicolaou smear, cervical or vaginal, up to three smears, requiring interpretation by physician	*CIM 50-20, ASC*

Microbiology Tests

P7001	Culture, bacterial, urine; quantitative, sensitivity study *Cross-reference CPT*

Miscellaneous

P9010	Blood (whole), for transfusion, per unit	*MCM 2455A*
P9011	Blood (split unit), specify amount	*MCM 2455A*
P9012	Cryoprecipitate, each unit	*MCM 2455B*
~~**P9013**~~	~~Fibrinogen unit~~ This code has been deleted in 2001.	
▲ **P9016**	Red blood cells, leukocytes reduced, each unit	*MCM 2049, 2455B*
▲ **P9017**	Fresh frozen plasma (single donor), each unit	*MCM 2455B*
~~**P9018**~~	~~Plasma protein fraction, each unit~~ This code has been deleted in 2001.	
▲ **P9019**	Platelets, each unit	*MCM 2455B*
P9020	Platelet rich plasma, each unit	*MCM 2455B*
P9021	Red blood cells, each unit	*MCM 2455A*
▲ **P9022**	Red blood cells, washed, each unit	*MCM 2455A*
P9023	Plasma, pooled multiple donor, solvent/detergent treated, frozen, each unit	*MCM 2455B*
● **P9031**	Platelets, leukocytes reduced, each unit	*MCM 2455*
● **P9032**	Platelets, irradiated, each unit	*MCM 2455*
● **P9033**	Platelets, leukocytes reduced, irradiated, each unit	*MCM 2455*

P Codes

= Special Coverage Instructions Apply   = Carrier Discretion

= Noncovered by Medicare or Medicare Statute

● **P9034**	Platelets, pheresis, each unit	*MCM 2455*
● **P9035**	Platelets, pheresis, leukocytes reduced, each unit	*MCM 2455*
● **P9036**	Platelets, pheresis, irradiated, each unit	*MCM 2455*
● **P9037**	Platelets, pheresis, leukocytes reduced, irradiated, each unit	*MCM 2455*
● **P9038**	Red blood cells, irradiated, each unit	*MCM 2455*
● **P9039**	Red blood cells, deglycerolized, each unit	*MCM 2455*
● **P9040**	Red blood cells, leukocytes reduced, irradiated, each unit	*MCM 2455*
● **P9041**	Infusion, albumin (human), 5%, 50 ml	
● **P9042**	Infusion, albumin (human), 25%, 10 ml	
● **P9043**	Infusion, plasma protein fraction (human), 5%, 50 ml	*MCM 2455B*
● **P9044**	Plasma, cryoprecipitate reduced, each unit	*MCM 2455B*
P9603	Travel allowance one way in connection with medically necessary laboratory specimen collection drawn from homebound or nursing home bound patient; prorated miles actually travelled	
		MCM 5114.1K, ASC
P9604	Travel allowance one way in connection with medically necessary laboratory specimen collection drawn from homebound or nursing home bound patient; prorated trip charge	*MCM 5114.1K, ASC*
P9612	Catheterization for collection of specimen, single patient, all places of service	*MCM 5114.1D*
P9615	Catheterization for collection of specimen(s) (multiple patients)	*MCM 5114.1D, ASC*

Q Codes (Temporary) Q0000–Q9999

HCFA assigns Q codes to procedures, services and supplies on a temporary basis. When a permanent code is assigned, the Q code is deleted and cross-referenced.

This section contains national codes assigned by HCFA on a temporary basis. The list contains current codes.

Q0034 ~~Administration of influenza vaccine to Medicare beneficiaries by participating demonstration sites~~ This code has been deleted in 2001.

Q0035 Cardiokymography *CIM 50-50, ASC*

Q0081 Infusion therapy, using other than chemotherapeutic drugs, per visit
CIM 60-14, ASC

Q0082 ~~Activity therapy furnished in connection with partial hospitalization (e.g., music, dance, art or play therapies that are not primarily recreational), per visit~~ This code has been deleted in 2001.

Q0083 Chemotherapy administration by other than infusion technique only (e.g., subcutaneous, intramuscular, push), per visit *ASC*

Q0084 Chemotherapy administration by infusion technique only, per visit
CIM 60-14, ASC

Q0085 Chemotherapy administration by both infusion technique and other technique(s) (e.g., subcutaneous, intramuscular, push), per visit *ASC*

Q0086 Physical therapy evaluation/treatment, per visit *MCM 2210, ASC*

Q0091 Screening Papanicolaou smear; obtaining, preparing and conveyance of cervical or vaginal smear to laboratory *CIM 50-20, ASC*

Q0092 Set-up portable x-ray equipment *MCM 2070.4, ASC*

Q0111 Wet mounts, including preparations of vaginal, cervical or skin specimens *ASC*

Q0112 All potassium hydroxide (KOH) preparations *Lab Certification - Mycology, ASC*

Q0113 Pinworm examination *Lab Certification - Parasitology, ASC*

Q0114 Fern test *Lab Certification - Routine Chemistry, ASC*

Q0115 Post-coital direct, qualitative examinations of vaginal or cervical mucous *Lab Certification - Hematology, ASC*

Q0136 Injection, epoetin alpha, (for non ESRD use), per 1,000 units
MCM 2049, ASC

Q0144 Azithromycin dihydrate, oral, capsules/powder, 1 gram (Zithromax)

Q0156 ~~Infusion, albumin (human), 5%, 500 ml~~ This code has been deleted in 2001.

Q0157 ~~Infusion, albumin (human), 25%, 50 ml~~ This code has been deleted in 2001.

Q0160 Factor IX (antihemophilic factor, purified, non-recombinant) per I.U.
MCM 2049

Q Codes

= Special Coverage Instructions Apply   = Carrier Discretion

= Noncovered by Medicare or Medicare Statute

Q0161	Factor IX (antihemophilic factor, recombinant) per I.U.	*MCM 2049*
Q0163	Diphenhydramine hydrochloride, 50 mg, oral, FDA approved prescription anti-emetic, for use as a complete therapeutic substitute for an IV anti-emetic at time of chemotherapy treatment not to exceed a 48-hour dosage regimen	*Medicare Statute 4557*
Q0164	Prochlorperazine maleate, 5 mg, oral, FDA approved prescription anti-emetic, for use as a complete therapeutic substitute for an IV anti-emetic at the time of chemotherapy treatment, not to exceed a 48-hour dosage regimen	*Medicare Statute 4557*
Q0165	Prochlorperazine maleate, 10 mg, oral, FDA approved prescription anti-emetic, for use as a complete therapeutic substitute for an IV anti-emetic at the time of chemotherapy treatment, not to exceed a 48-hour dosage regimen	*Medicare Statute 4557*
Q0166	Granisetron hydrochloride, 1 mg, oral, FDA approved prescription anti-emetic, for use as a complete therapeutic substitute for an IV anti-emetic at the time of chemotherapy treatment, not to exceed a 24-hour dosage regimen	*Medicare Statute 4557*
Q0167	Dronabinol, 2.5 mg, oral, FDA approved prescription anti-emetic, for use as a complete therapeutic substitute for an IV anti-emetic at the time of chemotherapy treatment, not to exceed a 48-hour dosage regimen	*Medicare Statute 4557*
Q0168	Dronabinol, 5 mg, oral, FDA approved prescription anti-emetic, for use as a complete therapeutic substitute for an IV anti-emetic at the time of chemotherapy treatment, not to exceed a 48-hour dosage regimen	*Medicare Statute 4557*
Q0169	Promethazine hydrochloride, 12.5 mg, oral, FDA approved prescription anti-emetic, for use as a complete therapeutic substitute for an IV anti-emetic at the time of chemotherapy treatment, not to exceed a 48-hour dosage regimen	*Medicare Statute 4557*
Q0170	Promethazine hydrochloride, 25 mg, oral, FDA approved prescription anti-emetic, for use as a complete therapeutic substitute for an IV anti-emetic at the time of chemotherapy treatment, not to exceed a 48-hour dosage regimen	*Medicare Statute 4557*
Q0171	Chlorpromazine hydrochloride, 10 mg, oral, FDA approved prescription anti-emetic, for use as a complete therapeutic substitute for an IV anti-emetic at the time of chemotherapy treatment, not to exceed a 48-hour dosage regimen	*Medicare Statute 4557*
Q0172	Chlorpromazine hydrochloride, 25 mg, oral, FDA approved prescription anti-emetic, for use as a complete therapeutic substitute for an IV anti-emetic at the time of chemotherapy treatment, not to exceed a 48-hour dosage regimen	*Medicare Statute 4557*
Q0173	Trimethobenzamide hydrochloride, 250 mg, oral, FDA approved prescription anti-emetic, for use as a complete therapeutic substitute for an IV anti-emetic at the time of chemotherapy treatment, not to exceed a 48-hour dosage regimen	*Medicare Statute 4557*

= Invalid Medicare Code (no grace period)

= Code may require certificate of medical necessity (CMN) or DMERC information form (DIF)

Q0174   Thiethylperazine maleate, 10 mg, oral, FDA approved prescription anti-emetic, for use as a complete therapeutic substitute for an IV anti-emetic at the time of chemotherapy treatment, not to exceed a 48-hour dosage regimen   *Medicare Statute 4557*

Q0175   Perphenzaine, 4 mg, oral, FDA approved prescription anti-emetic, for use as a complete therapeutic substitute for an IV anti-emetic at the time of chemotherapy treatment, not to exceed a 48-hour dosage regimen   *Medicare Statute 4557*

Q0176   Perphenzaine, 8mg, oral, FDA approved prescription anti-emetic, for use as a complete therapeutic substitute for an IV anti-emetic at the time of chemotherapy treatment, not to exceed a 48-hour dosage regimen   *Medicare Statute 4557*

Q0177   Hydroxyzine pamoate, 25 mg, oral, FDA approved prescription anti-emetic, for use as a complete therapeutic substitute for an IV anti-emetic at the time of chemotherapy treatment, not to exceed a 48-hour dosage regimen   *Medicare Statute 4557*

Q0178   Hydroxyzine pamoate, 50 mg, oral, FDA approved prescription anti-emetic, for use as a complete therapeutic substitute for an IV anti-emetic at the time of chemotherapy treatment, not to exceed a 48-hour dosage regimen   *Medicare Statute 4557*

Q0179   Ondansetron hydrochloride 8 mg, oral, FDA approved prescription anti-emetic, for use as a complete therapeutic substitute for an IV anti-emetic at the time of chemotherapy treatment, not to exceed a 48-hour dosage regimen   *Medicare Statute 4557*

Q0180   Dolasetron mesylate, 100 mg, oral, FDA approved prescription anti-emetic, for use as a complete therapeutic substitute for an IV anti-emetic at the time of chemotherapy treatment, not to exceed a 24-hour dosage regimen   *Medicare Statute 4557*

Q0181   Unspecified oral dosage form, FDA approved prescription anti-emetic, for use as a complete therapeutic substitute for an IV anti-emetic at the time of chemotherapy treatment, not to exceed a 48-hour dosage regimen   *Medicare Statute 4557*

Q0183   Dermal tissue, of human origin, with and without other bioengineered or processed elements, but without metabolically active elements, per square centimeter

Q0184   Dermal tissue, of human origin, with or without other bioengineered or processed elements, with metabolically active elements, per square centimeter

Q0185   Dermal and epidermal tissue, of human origin, with or without bioengineered or processed elements, with metabolically active elements, per square centimeter

Q0186   ~~Paramedic intercept, rural area, transport furnished by a volunteer ambulance company which is prohibited by state law from billing third party payers~~ This code has been deleted in 2001. See A0432.

Q Codes

Q0187	Factor VIIa (coagulation factor, recombinant) per 1.2 mg	*MCM 2049*
~~**Q0188**~~	~~Supply of injectable contrast material for use in echocardiography, per study~~ This code was added and deleted in 2000. See A9700.	
▲ **Q1001**	New technology intraocular lens category 1 as defined in Federal Register notice, Vol. 65, date May 3, 2000	
Q1002	New technology intraocular lens category 2 as defined in Federal Register notice, Vol. 65, dated May 3, 2000	
Q1003	New technology intraocular lens category 3 as defined in Federal Register notice	
Q1004	New technology intraocular lens category 4 as defined in Federal Register notice	
Q1005	New technology intraocular lens category 5 as defined in Federal Register notice	
● **Q2001**	Oral, cabergoline, 0.5 mg	*MCM 2049.5*
● **Q2002**	Injection, Elliott's B solution, per ml	*Medicare Statute 1861S2B, MCM 2049*
● **Q2003**	Injection, aprotinin, 10,000 kiu	*Medicare Statute 1861S2B, MCM 2049*
● **Q2004**	Irrigation solution for treatment of bladder calculi, for example renacidin, per 500 ml	*Medicare Statute 1861S2B, MCM 2049*
● **Q2005**	Injection, corticorelin ovine triflutate, per dose	*Medicare Statute 1861S2B, MCM 2049*
● **Q2006**	Injection, digoxin immune fab (ovine), per vial	*Medicare Statute 1861S2B, MCM 2049*
● **Q2007**	Injection, ethanolamine oleate, 100 mg	*Medicare Statute 1861S2B, MCM 2049*
● **Q2008**	Injection, fomepizole, 1.5 mg	*Medicare Statute 1861S2B, MCM 2049*
● **Q2009**	Injection, fosphenytoin, 50 mg	*Medicare Statute 1861S2B, MCM 2049*
● **Q2010**	Injection, glatiramer acetate, per dose	*Medicare Statute 1861S2B, MCM 2049*
● **Q2011**	Injection, hemin, per 1 mg	*Medicare Statute 1861S2B, MCM 2049*
● **Q2012**	Injection, pegademase bovine, 25 iu	*Medicare Statute 1861S2B, MCM 2049*
● **Q2013**	Injection, pentastarch, 10% solution, per 100 ml	*Medicare Statute 1861S2B, MCM 2049*
● **Q2014**	Injection, sermorelin acetate, 0.5 mg	*Medicare Statute 1861S2B, MCM 2049*
● **Q2015**	Injection, somatrem, 5 mg	*Medicare Statute 1861S2B, MCM 2049*
● **Q2016**	Injection, somatropin, 1 mg	*Medicare Statute 1861S2B, MCM 2049*
● **Q2017**	Injection, teniposide, 50 mg	*Medicare Statute 1861S2B, MCM 2049*
● **Q2018**	Injection, urofollitropin, 75 iu	*Medicare Statute 1861S2B, MCM 2049*
● **Q2019**	Injection, basiliximab, 20 mg	*Medicare Statute 1861S2B, MCM 2049*
● **Q2020**	Injection, histrelin acetate, 10 mg	*Medicare Statute 1861S2B, MCM 2049*
● **Q2021**	Injection, lepirudin, 50 mg	*Medicare Statute 1861S2B, MCM 2049*

= Invalid Medicare Code (no grace period)

= Code may require certificate of medical necessity (CMN) or DMERC information form (DIF)

● **Q2022** von Willebrand factor complex, human, per iu   *CIM 35-3, MCM 2049.5*

● **Q3002** Supply of radiopharmaceutical diagnostic imaging agent, gallium GA 67, per mCi   *MCM 15022*

● **Q3003** Supply of radiopharmaceutical diagnostic imaging agent, technetium Tc 99m bicisate, per unit dose   *MCM 15022*

● **Q3004** Supply of radiopharmaceutical diagnostic imaging agent, xenon XE 133, per 10 mCi   *MCM 15022*

● **Q3005** Supply of radiopharmaceutical diagnostic imaging agent, technetium Tc 99m mertiatide, per mCi   *MCM 15022*

● **Q3006** Supply of radiopharmaceutical diagnostic imaging agent, technetium Tc 99m glucepatate, per 5 mCi   *MCM 15022*

● **Q3007** Supply of radiopharmaceutical diagnostic imaging agent, sodium phosphate P32, per mCi   *MCM 15022*

● **Q3008** Supply of radiopharmaceutical diagnostic imaging agent, indium 111 — in pentetreotide, per 3 mCi   *MCM 15022*

● **Q3009** Supply of radiopharmaceutical diagnostic imaging agent, technetium Tc 99m oxidronate, per mCi   *MCM 15022*

● **Q3010** Supply of radiopharmaceutical diagnostic imaging agent, technetium Tc 99m — labeled red blood cells, per mCi   *MCM 15022*

● **Q3011** Supply of radiopharmaceutical diagnostic imaging agent, chromic phosphate P32 suspension, per mCi   *MCM 15022*

● **Q3012** Supply of oral radiopharmaceutical diagnostic imaging agent, cyanocobalamin cobalt Co57, per 0.5 mCi   *MCM 15022*

Injection Codes for Epoetin Alpha (EPO)

Q9920 Injection of EPO, per 1000 units, at patient HCT of 20 or less   *MCM 4273.1*

Q9921 Injection of EPO, per 1000 units, at patient HCT of 21   *MCM 4273.1*

Q9922 Injection of EPO, per 1000 units, at patient HCT of 22   *MCM 4273.1*

Q9923 Injection of EPO, per 1000 units, at patient HCT of 23   *MCM 4273.1*

Q9924 Injection of EPO, per 1000 units, at patient HCT of 24   *MCM 4273.1*

Q9925 Injection of EPO, per 1000 units, at patient HCT of 25   *MCM 4273.1*

Q9926 Injection of EPO, per 1000 units, at patient HCT of 26   *MCM 4273.1*

Q9927 Injection of EPO, per 1000 units, at patient HCT of 27   *MCM 4273.1*

Q9928 Injection of EPO, per 1000 units, at patient HCT of 28   *MCM 4273.1*

Q9929 Injection of EPO, per 1000 units, at patient HCT of 29   *MCM 4273.1*

Q9930 Injection of EPO, per 1000 units, at patient HCT of 30   *MCM 4273.1*

Q9931 Injection of EPO, per 1000 units, at patient HCT of 31   *MCM 4273.1*

Q9932 Injection of EPO, per 1000 units, at patient HCT of 32   *MCM 4273.1*

Q9933 Injection of EPO, per 1000 units, at patient HCT of 33   *MCM 4273.1*

Q Codes

= Special Coverage Instructions Apply   = Carrier Discretion

= Noncovered by Medicare or Medicare Statute

Q9934	Injection of EPO, per 1000 units, at patient HCT of 34	*MCM 4273.1*
Q9935	Injection of EPO, per 1000 units, at patient HCT of 35	*MCM 4273.1*
Q9936	Injection of EPO, per 1000 units, at patient HCT of 36	*MCM 4273.1*
Q9937	Injection of EPO, per 1000 units, at patient HCT of 37	*MCM 4273.1*
Q9938	Injection of EPO, per 1000 units, at patient HCT of 38	*MCM 4273.1*
Q9939	Injection of EPO, per 1000 units, at patient HCT of 39	*MCM 4273.1*
Q9940	Injection of EPO, per 1000 units, at patient HCT of 40 or above	*MCM 4273.1*

Diagnostic Radiology Services
R0000–R5999

R0070 Transportation of portable x-ray equipment and personnel to home or nursing home, per trip to facility or location, one patient seen
MCM 5244B, MCM 2070.4, ASC

R0075 Transportation of portable x-ray equipment and personnel to home or nursing home, per trip to facility or location, more than one patient seen, per patient
MCM 5244B, MCM 2070.4, ASC

R0076 Transportation of portable EKG to facility or location, per patient
CIM 50-15, MCM 2070.1, MCM 2070.4, ASC

R Codes

= Special Coverage Instructions Apply   = Carrier Discretion

= Noncovered by Medicare or Medicare Statute

Temporary National Codes (Non-Medicare) (S0009–S9999)

S codes are developed by Blue Cross/Blue Shield and other commercial payers to report drugs, services, and supplies. They may not be used to bill services paid under any Medicare payment system.

Code	Description
S0009	Injection, butorphanol tartrate, 1mg
S0010	~~Injection, somatrem, 5 mg~~ This code has been deleted in 2001. See Q2015.
S0011	~~Injection, somatropin, 5 mg~~ This code has been deleted in 2001. See Q2016.
S0012	Butorphanol tartrate, nasal spray, 25 mg
S0014	Tacrine hydrochloride, 10 mg
S0016	Injection, amikacin sulfate, 500 mg
S0017	Injection, aminocaproic acid, 5 grams
S0020	Injection, bupivicaine hydrochloride, 30 ml
S0021	Injection, ceftoperazone sodium, 1 gram
S0023	Injection, cimetidine hydrochloride, 300 mg
S0024	Injection, ciprofloxacin, 200 mg
S0028	Injection, famotidine, 20 mg
S0029	Injection, fluconazole, 400 mg
S0030	Injection, metronidazole, 500 mg
S0032	Injection, nafcillin sodium, 2 grams
S0034	Injection, ofloxacin, 400 mg
S0039	Injection, sulfamethoxazole and trimethoprim, 10 ml
S0040	Injection, ticarcillin disodium and clavulanate potassium, 3.1 grams
S0071	Injection, acyclovir sodium, 50 mg
S0072	Injection, amikacin sulfate, 100 mg
S0073	Injection, aztreonam, 500 mg
S0074	Injection, cefotetan disodium, 500 mg
S0077	Injection, clindamycin phosphate, 300 mg
S0078	Injection, fosphenytoin sodium, 750 mg
S0080	Injection, pentamidine isethionate, 300 mg
S0081	Injection, piperacillin sodium, 500 mg
● **S0085**	Injection, gatifloxacin, 200 mg
● **S0086**	Injection, verteporfin, 15 mg
S0090	Sildenafil citrate, 25 mg
S0096	Injection, itraconazole, 200 mg

= Special Coverage Instructions Apply   = Carrier Discretion

= Noncovered by Medicare or Medicare Statute

S0097 ~~Injection, ibutilide fumarate, 1 mg~~ This code has been deleted in 2001. See J1742.

S0098 ~~Injection, sodium ferric gluconate complex in sucrose, 62.5 mg~~ This code has been deleted in 2001.

● **S0156** Exemestane, 25 mg

● **S0157** Becaplermin gel 0.01%, 0.5 gm

● **S0220** Medical conference by a physician with interdisciplinary team of health professionals or representatives of community agencies to coordinate activities of patient care (patient is present); approximately 30 minutes

● **S0221** Medical conference by a physician with interdisciplinary team of health professionals or representatives of community agencies to coordinate activities of patient care (patient is present); approximately 60 minutes

S0601 Screening proctoscopy

S0605 Digital rectal examination, annual

S0610 Annual gynecological examination; new patient

S0612 Annual gynecological examination; established patient

S0620 Routine ophthalmological examination including refraction; new patient

S0621 Routine ophthalmological examination including refraction; established patient

● **S0630** Removal of sutures by a physician other than the physician who originally closed the wound

S0800 Laser in situ keratomileusis (LASIK)

S0810 Photorefractive keratectomy (PRK)

● **S0820** Computerized corneal topography, unilateral

● **S0830** Ultrasound pacymetry to determine corneal thickness, with interpretation and report, unilateral

● **S1015** IV tubing extension set

● **S1016** Non-PVC (polyvinyl chloride) intravenous administration set, for use with drugs that are not stable in PVC e.g., paclitaxel

S2050 ~~Donor enterectomy, with preparation and maintenance of allograft; from cadaver donor~~ This code has been deleted in 2001. See CPT code 44132.

S2052 Transplantation of small intestine, allograft

S2053 Transplantation of small intestine, and liver allografts

S2054 Transplantation of multivisceral organs

S2055 Harvesting of donor multivisceral organs, with preparation and maintenance of allografts; from cadaver donor

● **S2060** Lobar lung transplantation

● **S2061** Donor lobectomy (lung) for transplantation, living donor

= Invalid Medicare Code (no grace period)

= Code may require certificate of medical necessity (CMN) or DMERC information form (DIF)

● **S2102** Islet cell tissue transplant from pancreas

● **S2103** Adrenal tissue transplant to brain

S2109 ~~Autologous chondrocyte transplantation (preparation of autologous cultured chondrocytes)~~ This code has been deleted in 2001. See J7330.

● **S2120** Low density lipoprotein (LDL) apheresis using heparin-induced extracorporeal LDL precipitation

● **S2140** Cord blood harvesting for transplantation, allogeneic

● **S2142** Cord blood-derived stem-cell transplantation, allogeneic

● **S2180** Donor leukocyte infusion (e.g., DLI, donor lymphocyte infusion, donor buffy coat cell transfusion, donor peripheral blood monocyte transfusion)

S2190 ~~Subcutaneous implantation of medication pellet(s)~~ This code has been deleted in 2001. See CPT code 11980.

● **S2202** Echosclerotherapy

S2204 ~~Transmyocardial laser revascularization~~ This code has been deleted in 2001. See CPT code 33140.

S2205 Minimally invasive direct coronary artery bypass surgery involving mini-thoracotomy or mini-sternotomy surgery, performed under direct vision; using arterial graft(s), single coronary arterial graft

S2206 Minimally invasive direct coronary artery bypass surgery involving mini-thoracotomy or mini-sternotomy surgery, performed under direct vision; using arterial graft(s), two coronary arterial grafts

S2207 Minimally invasive direct coronary artery bypass surgery involving mini-thoracotomy or mini-sternotomy surgery, performed under direct vision; using venous graft only, single coronary venous graft

S2208 Minimally invasive direct coronary artery bypass surgery involving mini-thoracotomy or mini-sternotomy surgery, performed under direct vision; using single arterial and venous graft(s), single venous graft

S2209 Minimally invasive direct coronary artery bypass surgery involving mini-thoracotomy or mini-sternotomy surgery, performed under direct vision; using two arterial grafts and single venous graft

S2210 Cryosurgical ablation (in situ destruction) of tumorous tissue, one or more lesions; liver

● **S2220** Thrombectomy, coronary; by mechanical means (e.g., using rheolytic catheter)

S2300 Arthroscopy, shoulder, surgical; with thermally-induced capsulorrhaphy

● **S2340** Chemodenervation of abductor muscle(s) of vocal cord

S2350 Diskectomy, anterior, with decompression of spinal cord and/or nerve root(s), including osteophytectomy; lumbar, single interspace

S2351 Diskectomy, anterior, with decompression of spinal cord and/or nerve root(s), including osteophytectomy; lumbar, each additional interspace (list separately in addition to code for primary procedure)

= Special Coverage Instructions Apply   = Carrier Discretion

= Noncovered by Medicare or Medicare Statute

Code	Description
● **S2370**	Intradiscal electrothermal therapy, single interspace
● **S2371**	Each additional interspace (list separately in addition to code for primary procedure)
● **S3620**	Newborn metabolic screening panel, includes test kit, postage and the following tests: hemoglobin, electrophoresis; hydroxyprogesterone; 17-d; phenalanine (PKU); and thyroxine, total
S3645	HIV-1 antibody testing of oral mucosal transudate
S3650	Saliva test, hormone level; during menopause
S3652	Saliva test, hormone level; to assess preterm labor risk
● **S3700**	Bladder tumor-associated antigen test
● **S3708**	Gastrointestinal fat absorption study
● **S3902**	Ballistocardiogram
● **S3904**	Masters two step
● **S3906**	Transfusion, direct, blood or blood components
● **S5000**	Prescription drug, generic
● **S5001**	Prescription drug, brand name
● **S5002**	Fat emulsion 10% in 250 ml, with administration set
● **S5003**	Fat emulsion 20% in 250 ml, with administration set
● **S5010**	5% dextrose and 45% normal saline, 1000 ml
● **S5011**	5% dextrose in lactated ringer's, 1000 ml
● **S5012**	5% dextrose with potassium chloride, 1000 ml
● **S5013**	5% dextrose/45% normal saline with potassium chloride and magnesium sulfate, 1000 ml
● **S5014**	5% dextrose/45% normal saline with potassium chloride and magnesium sulfate, 1500 ml
● **S5016**	Antibiotic administration supplies (with pump), per diem
● **S5017**	Antibiotic administration supplies (without pump), per diem
● **S5018**	Pain therapy administration supplies (PCA or continuous), per diem
● **S5019**	Chemotherapy administration supplies (with pump), per diem
● **S5020**	Chemotherapy administration supplies (without pump), per diem
● **S5021**	Hydration therapy administration supplies, per diem
● **S5022**	Growth hormone therapy (e.g., protropin, humatrope)
● **S5025**	Infusion pump rental, per diem
● **S5503**	Maintenance of implanted vascular access device, including supplies; per diem
● **S8001**	Radiofrequency stimulation of the thalamus for tremor accomplished by stereotactic method, including burr holes, localizing and recording techniques and placement of the electrode(s)

= Invalid Medicare Code (no grace period)

= Code may require certificate of medical necessity (CMN) or DMERC information form (DIF)

S8035	Magnetic source imaging
S8040	Topographic brain mapping
S8048	~~Isolated limb perfusion~~ This code has been deleted in 2001. See CPT code 36823.
S8049	Intraoperative radiation therapy (single administration)
S8060	~~Supply of contrast material for use in echocardiography (use in addition to echocardiography code)~~ This code has been deleted in 2001. See A9700.
● S8080	Scintimammography (radioimmunoscintigraphy of the breast), unilateral, including supply of radiopharmaceutical
● S8085	Fluorine-18 fluorodeoxyglucose (F-18 FDG) imaging using dual-head coincidence detection system (non-dedicated PET scan)
S8092	Electron beam computed tomography (also known as ultrafast CT, cine CT)
S8095	Wig (for medically-induced hair loss)
S8096	Portable peak flow meter
● S8105	Oximeter for measuring blood oxygen levels noninvasively
S8110	Peak expiratory flow rate (physician services)
S8200	Chest compression vest
S8205	Chest compression system generator and hoses (for use with chest compression vest — S8200)
● S8210	Mucus trap
S8260	Oral orthotic for treatment of sleep apnea, includes fitting, fabrication, and materials
S8300	~~Sacral nerve stimulation test lead kit~~ This code has been deleted in 2001.
● S8400	Incontinence pants, each
● S8402	Diapers, each
● S8405	Incontinence liners, each
S8950	Complex lymphedema therapy, each 15 minutes
● S8999	Resuscitation bag (for use by patient on artificial respiration during power failure or other catastropic event)
S9001	Home uterine monitor with or without associated nursing services
● S9007	Ultrafiltration monitor
● S9015	Automated EEG monitoring
S9022	Digital subtraction angiography (use in addition to CPT code for the procedure for further identification)
S9023	Xenon regional cerebral blood flow studies
S9024	Paranasal sinus ultrasound

= Special Coverage Instructions Apply   = Carrier Discretion

= Noncovered by Medicare or Medicare Statute

● **S9025** Omnicardiogram/cardiointegram

S9033 ~~Gait analysis~~ This code has been deleted in 2001. See CPT codes 95979 and 95986.

● **S9035** Medical equipment or supplies distributed by home care provider without professional nursing intervention, per diem

S9055 Procuren or other growth factor preparation to promote wound healing

S9056 Coma stimulation per diem

● **S9061** Medical supplies and equipment rental distributed by the home care provider; aerosolized drug therapy; per diem

S9075 Smoking cessation treatment

S9085 Meniscal allograft transplantation

● **S9088** Services provided in an urgent care center

S9090 Vertebral axial decompression, per session

S9122 Home health aide or certified nurse assistant, providing care in the home; per hour

S9123 Nursing care, in the home; by registered nurse, per hour

S9124 Nursing care, in the home; by licensed practical nurse, per hour

S9125 Respite care, in the home, per diem

S9126 Hospice care, in the home, per diem

S9127 Social work visit, in the home, per diem

S9128 Speech therapy, in the home, per diem

S9129 Occupational therapy, in the home, per diem

S9140 Diabetic management program, follow-up visit to non-MD provider

S9141 Diabetic management program, follow-up visit to MD provider

● **S9200** Nursing services and all necessary supplies (including PCA pump rental) for home administration of patient controlled analgesia (PCA) per diem (drugs not included)

● **S9210** Nursing services and all necessary equipment and supplies for continuous, uninterrupted infusion of epoprostenol (includes venous access device, infusion pump, back up pump, ice packs for cassettes, batteries, all related supplies, and all nursing services including follow-up visits, telephone monitoring, 24 hour/7 day a week availability, and all education to patient and care givers); per diem

● **S9220** Nursing services and all necessary equipment and supplies for home administration of controlled rate intravenous infusion (e.g. dobutamine) requiring prolonged attendance by the nurse, per diem (drugs not included)

● **S9225** Nursing services and all necessary equipment and supplies for home administration of intravenous tocolytic therapy, per diem

---

= Invalid Medicare Code (no grace period)

= Code may require certificate of medical necessity (CMN) or DMERC information form (DIF)

S Codes

- **S9230** Nursing services and all necessary equipment and supplies for home administration of heparin, per diem
- **S9300** Nursing services and all necessary supplies for home enteral feeding by gravity, per diem (enteral formula not included)
- **S9308** Nursing services and all necessary supplies for home enteral feeding by pump, including pump rental, per diem (enteral formula not included)
- **S9310** Nursing services and all necessary supplies for home parenteral nutrition without lipids, including pump rental, per diem (parenteral solutions not included)
- **S9395** Nursing services and all necessary supplies and additives for home IV hydration (via gravity or pump), per diem (hydration solution and drugs not included)
- **S9420** Nursing services and all necessary supplies for interim home maintenance of implanted vascular access port/catheter/reservoir, per diem (for interim maintenance of vascular access not currently in use)
- **S9423** Nursing services, patient assessment and education, follow-up visits, electronic programmer and equipment (use of computer), programming of the pump, all necessary supplies, products or services for intrathecal drug infusion, per diem
- **S9425** Nursing services and all necessary supplies and additives for home IV chemotherapy (via IV push, gravity drip, stationary pump, ambulatory belt pump), per diem (hydration solution and drugs not included)
- **S9435** Medical foods for inborn errors of metabolism
- **S9455** Diabetic management program, group session
- **S9460** Diabetic management program, nurse visit
- **S9465** Diabetic management program, dietitian visit
- **S9470** Nutritional counseling, dietitian visit
- **S9472** Cardiac rehabilitation program, non-physician provider, per diem
- **S9473** Pulmonary rehabilitation program, non-physician provider, per diem
- **S9474** Enterostomal therapy by a registered nurse certified in enterostomal therapy, per diem
- **S9475** Ambulatory setting substance abuse treatment or detoxification services, per diem
- **S9480** Intensive outpatient psychiatric services, per diem
- **S9485** Crisis intervention mental health services, per diem
- **S9524** Nursing services related to home iv therapy, per diem
- **S9526** Skilled nursing visits for blood product administration, including pump and all related supplies; per service
- **S9527** Insertion of a peripherally inserted central venous catheter (PICC), including nursing services and all supplies

= Special Coverage Instructions Apply   = Carrier Discretion
= Noncovered by Medicare or Medicare Statute

S9528	Insertion of midline central venous catheter, including nursing services and all supplies
● **S9533**	Pain management, intravenous, epidural or subcutaneous, including solution, equipment rental, nursing care, and supplies; per diem (drugs not included)
● **S9535**	Administration of hematopoietic hormones (e.g. erythropoietin, G-CSF, GM-CSF) or platelets, intravenously, in the home setting, including all nursing care, equipment, and supplies; per diem
● **S9539**	Administration of antibiotics, intravenously, in the home setting, including all nursing care, equipment, and supplies; per diem
S9543	Administration of medication, intramuscularly, epidurally or subcutaneously, in the home setting, including all nursing care, equipment, and supplies; per diem
● **S9545**	Administration of immune globulin, intravenously, in the home setting, including all nursing care, equipment, and supplies; per diem
● **S9550**	Home IV therapy, hydration fluids and electrolytes, including all nursing care, equipment, and supplies; per diem
● **S9555**	Additional home infusion therapy, including all nursing care, equipment, and supplies; each therapy, per diem (S9555 should be used in addition to the code for the primary therapy)
S9990	Services provided as part of a phase II clinical trial
S9991	Services provided as part of a phase III clinical trial
S9992	Transportation costs to and from trial location and local transportation costs (e.g., fares for taxicab or bus) for clinical trial participant and one caregiver/companion
S9994	Lodging costs (e.g., hotel charges) for clinical trial participant and one caregiver/companion
S9996	Meals for clinical trial participant and one caregiver/companion
S9999	Sales tax

Vision Services V0000–V2999

Frames

V2020	Frames, purchases	MCM 2130, ASC
V2025	Deluxe frame	MCM 3045.4

Spectacle Lenses

If procedure code 92390 or 92395 is reported, recode with the specific lens type listed below. For aphakic temporary spectacle correction, see 92358.

Single Vision, Glass, or Plastic

V2100	Sphere, single vision, plano to plus or minus 4.00, per lens	ASC
V2101	Sphere, single vision, plus or minus 4.12 to plus or minus 7.00d, per lens	ASC
V2102	Sphere, single vision, plus or minus 7.12 to plus or minus 20.00d, per lens	ASC
V2103	Spherocylinder, single vision, plano to plus or minus 4.00d sphere, 0.12 to 2.00d cylinder, per lens	ASC
V2104	Spherocylinder, single vision, plano to plus or minus 4.00d sphere, 2.12 to 4.00d cylinder, per lens	ASC
V2105	Spherocylinder, single vision, plano to plus or minus 4.00d sphere, 4.25 to 6.00d cylinder, per lens	ASC
V2106	Spherocylinder, single vision, plano to plus or minus 4.00d sphere, over 6.00d cylinder, per lens	ASC
V2107	Spherocylinder, single vision, plus or minus 4.25 to plus or minus 7.00 sphere, 0.12 to 2.00d cylinder, per lens	ASC
V2108	Spherocylinder, single vision, plus or minus 4.25d to plus or minus 7.00d sphere, 2.12 to 4.00d cylinder, per lens	ASC
V2109	Spherocylinder, single vision, plus or minus 4.25 to plus or minus 7.00d sphere, 4.25 to 6.00d cylinder, per lens	ASC
V2110	Spherocylinder, single vision, plus or minus 4.25 to 7.00d sphere, over 6.00d cylinder, per lens	ASC
V2111	Spherocylinder, single vision, plus or minus 7.25 to plus or minus 12.00d sphere, 0.25 to 2.25d cylinder, per lens	ASC
V2112	Spherocylinder, single vision, plus or minus 7.25 to plus or minus 12.00d sphere, 2.25d to 4.00d cylinder, per lens	ASC
V2113	Spherocylinder, single vision, plus or minus 7.25 to plus or minus 12.00d sphere, 4.25 to 6.00d cylinder, per lens	ASC
V2114	Spherocylinder, single vision sphere over plus or minus 12.00d, per lens	ASC
V2115	Lenticular (myodisc), per lens, single vision	ASC
V2116	Lenticular lens, nonaspheric, per lens, single vision	ASC

V2117	Lenticular, aspheric, per lens, single vision	*ASC*
V2118	Aniseikonic lens, single vision	*ASC*
V2199	Not otherwise classified, single vision lens	*ASC*

Bifocal, Glass, or Plastic

V2200	Sphere, bifocal, plano to plus or minus 4.00d, per lens	*ASC*
V2201	Sphere, bifocal, plus or minus 4.12 to plus or minus 7.00d, per lens	*ASC*
V2202	Sphere, bifocal, plus or minus 7.12 to plus or minus 20.00d, per lens	*ASC*
V2203	Spherocylinder, bifocal, plano to plus or minus 4.00d sphere, 0.12 to 2.00d cylinder, per lens	*ASC*
V2204	Spherocylinder, bifocal, plano to plus or minus 4.00d sphere, 2.12 to 4.00d cylinder, per lens	*ASC*
V2205	Spherocylinder, bifocal, plano to plus or minus 4.00d sphere, 4.25 to 6.00d cylinder, per lens	*ASC*
V2206	Spherocylinder, bifocal, plano to plus or minus 4.00d sphere, over 6.00d cylinder, per lens	*ASC*
V2207	Spherocylinder, bifocal, plus or minus 4.25 to plus or minus 7.00d sphere, 0.12 to 2.00d cylinder, per lens	*ASC*
V2208	Spherocylinder, bifocal, plus or minus 4.25 to plus or minus 7.00d sphere, 2.12 to 4.00d cylinder, per lens	*ASC*
V2209	Spherocylinder, bifocal, plus or minus 4.25 to plus or minus 7.00d sphere, 4.25 to 6.00d cylinder, per lens	*ASC*
V2210	Spherocylinder, bifocal, plus or minus 4.25 to plus or minus 7.00d sphere, over 6.00d cylinder, per lens	*ASC*
V2211	Spherocylinder, bifocal, plus or minus 7.25 to plus or minus 12.00d sphere, 0.25 to 2.25d cylinder, per lens	*ASC*
V2212	Spherocylinder, bifocal, plus or minus 7.25 to plus or minus 12.00d sphere, 2.25 to 4.00d cylinder, per lens	*ASC*
V2213	Spherocylinder, bifocal, plus or minus 7.25 to plus or minus 12.00d sphere, 4.25 to 6.00d cylinder, per lens	*ASC*
V2214	Spherocylinder, bifocal, sphere over plus or minus 12.00d, per lens	*ASC*
V2215	Lenticular (myodisc), per lens, bifocal	*ASC*
V2216	Lenticular, nonaspheric, per lens, bifocal	*ASC*
V2217	Lenticular, aspheric lens, bifocal	*ASC*
V2218	Aniseikonic, per lens, bifocal	*ASC*
V2219	Bifocal seg width over 28mm	*ASC*
V2220	Bifocal add over 3.25d	*ASC*
V2299	Specialty bifocal (by report)	*ASC*

= Invalid Medicare Code (no grace period)

= Code may require certificate of medical necessity (CMN) or DMERC information form (DIF)

Trifocal, Glass, or Plastic

V2300	Sphere, trifocal, plano to plus or minus 4.00d, per lens	ASC
V2301	Sphere, trifocal, plus or minus 4.12 to plus or minus 7.00d per lens	ASC
V2302	Sphere, trifocal, plus or minus 7.12 to plus or minus 20.00, per lens	ASC
V2303	Spherocylinder, trifocal, plano to plus or minus 4.00d sphere, 0.12 to 2.00d cylinder, per lens	ASC
V2304	Spherocylinder, trifocal, plano to plus or minus 4.00d sphere, 2.25 to 4.00d cylinder, per lens	ASC
V2305	Spherocylinder, trifocal, plano to plus or minus 4.00d sphere, 4.25 to 6.00 cylinder, per lens	ASC
V2306	Spherocylinder, trifocal, plano to plus or minus 4.00d sphere, over 6.00d cylinder, per lens	ASC
V2307	Spherocylinder, trifocal, plus or minus 4.25 to plus or minus 7.00d sphere, 0.12 to 2.00d cylinder, per lens	ASC
V2308	Spherocylinder, trifocal, plus or minus 4.25 to plus or minus 7.00d sphere, 2.12 to 4.00d cylinder, per lens	ASC
V2309	Spherocylinder, trifocal, plus or minus 4.25 to plus or minus 7.00d sphere, 4.25 to 6.00d cylinder, per lens	ASC
V2310	Spherocylinder, trifocal, plus or minus 4.25 to plus or minus 7.00d sphere, over 6.00d cylinder, per lens	ASC
V2311	Spherocylinder, trifocal, plus or minus 7.25 to plus or minus 12.00d sphere, 0.25 to 2.25d cylinder, per lens	ASC
V2312	Spherocylinder, trifocal, plus or minus 7.25 to plus or minus 12.00d sphere, 2.25 to 4.00d cylinder, per lens	ASC
V2313	Spherocylinder, trifocal, plus or minus 7.25 to plus or minus 12.00d sphere, 4.25 to 6.00d cylinder, per lens	ASC
V2314	Spherocylinder, trifocal, sphere over plus or minus 12.00d, per lens	ASC
V2315	Lenticular (myodisc), per lens, trifocal	ASC
V2316	Lenticular nonaspheric, per lens, trifocal	ASC
V2317	Lenticular, aspheric lens, trifocal	ASC
V2318	Aniseikonic lens, trifocal	ASC
V2319	Trifocal seg width over 28 mm	ASC
V2320	Trifocal add over 3.25d	ASC
V2399	Specialty trifocal (by report)	ASC

Variable Asphericity Lens, Glass, or Plastic

V2410	Variable asphericity lens, single vision, full field, glass or plastic, per lens	ASC
V2430	Variable asphericity lens, bifocal, full field, glass or plastic, per lens	ASC
V2499	Variable sphericity lens, other type	ASC

V Codes

= Special Coverage Instructions Apply   = Carrier Discretion

= Noncovered by Medicare or Medicare Statute

Contact Lens

If procedure code 92391 or 92396 is reported, recode with specific lens type listed below (per lens).

V2500	Contact lens, PMMA, spherical, per lens	*ASC*
V2501	Contact lens, PMMA, toric or prism ballast, per lens	*ASC*
V2502	Contact lens, PMMA, bifocal, per lens	*ASC*
V2503	Contact lens, PMMA, color vision deficiency, per lens	*ASC*
V2510	Contact lens, gas permeable, spherical, per lens	*ASC*
V2511	Contact lens, gas permeable, toric, prism ballast, per lens	*ASC*
V2512	Contact lens, gas permeable, bifocal, per lens	*ASC*
V2513	Contact lens, gas permeable, extended wear, per lens	*ASC*
V2520	Contact lens, hydrophilic, spherical, per lens	*CIM 45-7, CIM 65-1, ASC*
V2521	Contact lens, hydrophilic, toric, or prism ballast, per lens	*CIM 45-7, CIM 65-1, ASC*
V2522	Contact lens, hydrophilic, bifocal, per lens	*CIM 45-7, CIM 65-1, ASC*
V2523	Contact lens, hydrophilic, extended wear, per lens	*CIM 45-7, CIM 65-1, ASC*
V2530	Contact lens, scleral, gas impermeable, per lens (for contact lens modification, see CPT Level I code 92325)	*CIM 45-7, CIM 65-1, ASC*
V2531	Contact lens, scleral, gas permeable, per lens (for contact lens modification, see CPT Level I code 92325)	*CIM 65-3, ASC*
V2599	Contact lens, other type	*ASC*

Vision Aids

If procedure code 92392 is reported, recode with specific systems below.

V2600	Hand held low vision aids and other nonspectacle mounted aids	*ASC*
V2610	Single lens spectacle mounted low vision aids	*ASC*
V2615	Telescopic and other compound lens system, including distance vision telescopic, near vision telescopes and compound microscopic lens system	*ASC*

Prosthetic Eye

V2623	Prosthetic eye, plastic, custom	*MCM 2133, ASC*
V2624	Polishing/resurfacing of ocular prosthesis	*ASC*
V2625	Enlargement of ocular prosthesis	*ASC*
V2626	Reduction of ocular prosthesis	*ASC*
V2627	Scleral cover shell	*CIM 65-3, ASC*
V2628	Fabrication and fitting of ocular conformer	*ASC*
V2629	Prosthetic eye, other type	*ASC*

= Invalid Medicare Code (no grace period)

= Code may require certificate of medical necessity (CMN) or DMERC information form (DIF)

Intraocular Lenses

V2630	Anterior chamber intraocular lens	*MCM 2130*
V2631	Iris supported intraocular lens	*MCM 2130*
V2632	Posterior chamber intraocular lens	*MCM 2130*

Miscellaneous

V2700	Balance lens, per lens	*ASC*
V2710	Slab off prism, glass or plastic, per lens	*ASC*
V2715	Prism, per lens	*ASC*
V2718	Press-on lens, Fresnell prism, per lens	*ASC*
V2730	Special base curve, glass or plastic, per lens	*ASC*
V2740	Tint, plastic, rose 1 or 2, per lens	*MCM 2130B, ASC*
V2741	Tint, plastic, other than rose 1 or 2, per lens	*MCM 2130B, ASC*
V2742	Tint, glass, rose 1 or 2, per lens	*MCM 2130B, ASC*
V2743	Tint, glass, other than rose 1 or 2, per lens	*MCM 2130B, ASC*
V2744	Tint, photochromatic, per lens	*MCM 2130B, ASC*
V2750	Antireflective coating, per lens	*MCM 2130B, ASC*
V2755	U-V lens, per lens	*MCM 2130B, ASC*
V2760	Scratch resistant coating, per lens	*ASC*
V2770	Occluder lens, per lens	*ASC*
V2780	Oversize lens, per lens	*ASC*
V2781	Progressive lens, per lens	*ASC*
V2785	Processing, preserving and transporting corneal tissue	
● **V2790**	Amniotic membrane for surgical reconstruction, per procedure	
V2799	Vision service, miscellaneous	*ASC*

Hearing Services V5000–V5999

Routine physical checkups for the purpose of prescribing, fitting or changing hearing aids and examinations for hearing aids are not covered by Medicare. These codes are for nonphysician services.

Hearing services fall under the jurisdiction of the local carrier unless incidental or otherwise noted.

V5008	Hearing screening	*MCM 2320*
V5010	Assessment for hearing aid	*Medicare Statute 1862.A7*
V5011	Fitting/orientation/checking of hearing aid	*Medicare Statute 1862.A7*
V5014	Repair/modification of a hearing aid	*Medicare Statute 1862.A7*
V5020	Conformity evaluation	*Medicare Statute 1862.A7*

V Codes

= Special Coverage Instructions Apply   = Carrier Discretion

= Noncovered by Medicare or Medicare Statute

V5030	Hearing aid, monaural, body worn, air conduction	
		Medicare Statute 1862.A7
V5040	Hearing aid, monaural, body worn, bone conduction	
		Medicare Statute 1862.A7
V5050	Hearing aid, monaural, in the ear	*Medicare Statute 1862.A7*
V5060	Hearing aid, monaural, behind the ear	*Medicare Statute 1862.A7*
V5070	Glasses, air conduction	*Medicare Statute 1862.A7*
V5080	Glasses, bone conduction	*Medicare Statute 1862.A7*
V5090	Dispensing fee, unspecified hearing aid	*Medicare Statute 1862.A7*
V5100	Hearing aid, bilateral, body worn	*Medicare Statute 1862.A7*
V5110	Dispensing fee, bilateral	*Medicare Statute 1862.A7*
V5120	Binaural, body	*Medicare Statute 1862.A7*
V5130	Binaural, in the ear	*Medicare Statute 1862.A7*
V5140	Binaural, behind the ear	*Medicare Statute 1862.A7*
V5150	Binaural, glasses	*Medicare Statute 1862.A7*
V5160	Dispensing fee, binaural	*Medicare Statute 1862.A7*
V5170	Hearing aid, CROS, in the ear	*Medicare Statute 1862.A7*
V5180	Hearing aid, CROS, behind the ear	*Medicare Statute 1862.A7*
V5190	Hearing aid, CROS, glasses	*Medicare Statute 1862.A7*
V5200	Dispensing fee, CROS	*Medicare Statute 1862.A7*
V5210	Hearing aid, BICROS, in the ear	*Medicare Statute 1862.A7*
V5220	Hearing aid, BICROS, behind the ear	*Medicare Statute 1862.A7*
V5230	Hearing aid, BICROS, glasses	*Medicare Statute 1862.A7*
V5240	Dispensing fee, BICROS	*Medicare Statute 1862.A7*
V5299	Hearing service, miscellaneous	*MCM 2320, ASC*

Speech-Language Pathology Services

V5336	Repair/modification of augmentative communicative system or device (excludes adaptive hearing aid)	*Medicare Statute 1862.A7*
V5362	Speech screening	*MCM 2320, ASC*
V5363	Language screening	*MCM 2320, ASC*
V5364	Dysphagia screening	*MCM 2320, ASC*

= Invalid Medicare Code (no grace period)

= Code may require certificate of medical necessity (CMN) or DMERC information form (DIF)

Appendix 1:

Modifiers

Under certain circumstances, the code chosen may require a modifier in order to report that the procedure has been altered by a specific circumstance.

Modifiers for Hospital Outpatient Services: Specific modifiers must be used when reporting outpatient services for accuracy in reimbursement, coding consistency, editing and to capture payment data. Modifiers indicated by a ◆ symbol are required by HCFA for reporting outpatient services provided to beneficiaries.

In HCPCS Level I, modifiers are two digits. Each modifier has an alternative code beginning with 099 that may be used instead. If the five-digit code is used, the modifier always begins with the first three numbers 099. For example:

30901*-50	Control nasal hemorrhage, anterior, simple (limited cautery and/or packing) any method, bilateral procedure
or	
30901*	Control nasal hemorrhage, anterior, simple (limited cautery and/or packing) any method
09950	Bilateral procedure

Level II of HCPCS also contains modifiers. These modifiers are either alphanumeric or two letters that include the range of letters from "-AA" to "-VP." For example:

E0260-NU	Hospital bed, semielectric (head and foot adjustment) with any type side rails, with mattress, new equipment

Keep in mind that CPT and national modifiers apply to both CPT and HCPCS Level II coding systems. When applicable, indicate the appropriate modifier on the claim. In some instances, a special report may be needed to clarify the use of the modifier to the third-party payer.

For ambulance services, there are separate one-letter codes that are used together to form a two-letter modifier. The first letter indicates the origin of the patient, and the second indicates the destination. For example:

A0302-SH	Ambulance service, BLS, emergency transport, all-inclusive (mileage and supplies) from the scene of an accident to a hospital

Modifiers -Q5 and -Q6 are used in conjunction with CPT codes to indicate whether the services rendered were provided through a reciprocal billing arrangement or by a locum tenens physician.

Below is a list of one-letter modifiers:

-D	Diagnostic or therapeutic site other than "P" or "H" when these are used as origin codes
-E	Residential, domiciliary, custodial facility (other than an 1819 facility)

-H	Hospital
-N	Skilled nursing facility (SNF) (1819 facility)
-P	Physician's office
-R	Residence
-S	Scene of accident or acute event
-X	(Destination code only). Intermediate stop at physician's office on the way to the hospital

Below is a list of two-letter modifiers:

-AA	Anesthesia services performed personally by anesthesiologist
-AD	Medical supervision by a physician: more than four concurrent anesthesia procedures
-AH	Clinical psychologist
-AJ	Clinical social worker
-AM	Physician, team member service
-AP	Determination of refractive state was not performed in the course of diagnostic ophthalmological examination
-AS	Physician assistant, nurse practitioner, or clinical nurse specialist services for assistant at surgery
-AT	Acute treatment (this modifier should be used when reporting service 98940, 98941, 98942)
-BP	The beneficiary has been informed of the purchase and rental options and has elected to purchase the item
-BR	The beneficiary has been informed of the purchase and rental options and has elected to rent the item
-BU	The beneficiary has been informed of the purchase and rental options and after 30 days has not informed the supplier of his/her decision
-CC	Procedure code change (use 'CC' when the procedure code submitted was changed either for administrative reasons or because an incorrect code was filed)
◆ -E1	Upper left, eyelid
◆ -E2	Lower left, eyelid
◆ -E3	Upper right, eyelid
◆ -E4	Lower right, eyelid
-EJ	Subsequent claims for a defined course of therapy, e.g., EPO, sodium hyaluronate, infliximab
-EM	Emergency reserve supply (for ESRD benefit only)

-EP	Service provided as part of medicaid early periodic screening diagnosis and treatment (EPSDT) program
-ET	Emergency treatment (dental procedures performed in emergency situations should show the modifier 'ET')
◆ -F1	Left hand, second digit
◆ -F2	Left hand, third digit
◆ -F3	Left hand, fourth digit
◆ -F4	Left hand, fifth digit
◆ -F5	Right hand, thumb
◆ -F6	Right hand, second digit
◆ -F7	Right hand, third digit
◆ -F8	Right hand, fourth digit
◆ -F9	Right hand, fifth digit
◆ -FA	Left hand, thumb
-FP	Service provided as part of medicaid family planning program
-G1	Most recent URR reading of less than 60
-G2	Most recent URR reading of 60 to 64.9
-G3	Most recent URR reading of 65 to 69.9
-G4	Most recent URR reading of 70 to 74.9
-G5	Most recent URR reading of 75 or greater
-G6	ESRD patient for whom less than six dialysis sessions have been provided in a month
-G7	Pregnancy resulted from rape or incest or pregnancy certified by physician as life threatening
-G8	Monitored anesthesia care (MAC) for deep complex, complicated, or markedly invasive surgical procedure
-G9	Monitored anesthesia care for patient who has history of severe cardio-pulmonary condition
-GA	Waiver of liability statement on file
-GC	This service has been performed in part by a resident under the direction of a teaching physician
-GE	This service has been performed by a resident without the presence of a teaching physician under the primary care exception
-GH	Diagnostic mammogram converted from screening mammogram on same day
-GJ	"OPT OUT" physician or practitioner emergency or urgent service

Appendix 1

-GN   Service delivered personally by a speech-language pathologist or under an outpatient speech-language pathology plan of care

-GO   Service delivered personally by an occupational therapist or under an outpatient occupational therapy plan of care

-GP   Service delivered personally by a physical therapist or under an outpatient physical therapy plan of care

-GT   Via interactive audio and video telecommunication systems

● -GU   Procedure performed in non fee schedule POS

-GX   Service not covered by Medicare

-K0   Lower extremity prosthesis functional level 0 — does not have the ability or potential to ambulate or transfer safely with or without assistance and a prosthesis does not enhance their quality of life or mobility

-K1   Lower extremity prosthesis functional level 1 — has the ability or potential to use a prosthesis for transfers or ambulation on level surfaces at fixed cadence. Typical of the limited and unlimited household ambulator

-K2   Lower extremity prosthesis functional level 2 — has the ability or potential for ambulation with the ability to traverse low level environmental barriers such as curbs, stairs or uneven surfaces. Typical of the limited community ambulator

-K3   Lower extremity prosthesis functional level 3 — has the ability or potential for ambulation with variable cadence. Typical of the community ambulator who has the ability to transverse most environmental barriers and may have vocational, therapeutic, or exercise activity that demands prosthetic utilization beyond simple locomotion

-K4   Lower extremity prosthesis functional level 4 — has the ability or potential for prosthetic ambulation that exceeds the basic ambulation skills, exhibiting high impact, stress, or energy levels, typical of the prosthetic demands of the child, active adult, or athlete

-KA   Add on option/accessory for wheelchair

-KH   DMEPOS item, initial claim, purchase or first month rental

-KI   DMEPOS item, second or third month rental

-KJ   DMEPOS item, parenteral enteral nutrition (PEN) pump or capped rental, months four to fifteen

-KM   Replacement of facial prosthesis including new impression/moulage

-KN   Replacement of facial prosthesis using previous master model

-KO   Single drug unit dose formulation

-KP   First drug of a multiple drug unit dose formulation

-KQ	Second or subsequent drug of a multiple drug unit dose formulation
-KS	Glucose monitor supply for diabetic beneficiary not treated with insulin
◆ -LC	Left circumflex coronary artery
◆ -LD	Left anterior descending coronary artery
-LL	Lease/rental (use the 'LL' modifier when DME equipment rental is to be applied against the purchase price)
-LR	Laboratory round trip
-LS	FDA-monitored intraocular lens implant
◆ -LT	Left side (used to identify procedures performed on the left side of the body)
-MS	Six month maintenance and servicing fee for reasonable and necessary parts and labor which are not covered under any manufacturer or supplier warranty
-NR	New when rented (use the 'NR' modifier when DME which was new at the time of rental is subsequently purchased)
-NU	New equipment
-PL	Progressive addition lenses
-Q2	HCFA/ORD demonstration project procedure/service
-Q3	Live kidney donor: services associated with postoperative medical complications directly related to the donation
-Q4	Service for ordering/referring physician qualifies as a service exemption
-Q5	Service furnished by a substitute physician under a reciprocal billing arrangement
-Q6	Service furnished by a locum tenens physician
-Q7	One Class A finding
-Q8	Two Class B findings
-Q9	One Class B and two Class C findings
-QA	FDA investigational device exemption
-QB	Physician providing service in a rural HPSA
-QC	Single channel monitoring
-QD	Recording and storage in solid state memory by a digital recorder
-QE	Prescribed amount of oxygen is less than 1 liter per minute (LPM)
-QF	Prescribed amount of oxygen exceeds 4 liters per minute (LPM) and portable oxygen is prescribed

-QG	Prescribed amount of oxygen is greater than 4 liters per minute (LPM)
-QH	Oxygen conserving device is being used with an oxygen delivery system
-QK	Medical direction of two, three, or four concurrent anesthesia procedures involving qualified individuals
-QL	Patient pronounced dead after ambulance called
◆ -QM	Ambulance service provided under arrangement by a provider of services
◆ -QN	Ambulance service furnished directly by a provider of services
-QP	Documentation is on file showing that the laboratory test(s) was ordered individually or ordered as a CPT-recognized panel other than automated profile codes 80002-80019, G0058, G0059, and G0060
● -QQ	Claim submitted with a written statement of intent
-QS	Monitored anesthesia care service
-QT	Recording and storage on tape by an analog tape recorder
-QU	Physician providing service in an urban HPSA
● -QV	Item or service provided as routine care in a Medicare qualifying trial
-QW	CLIA waived test
-QX	CRNA service: with medical direction by a physician
-QY	Medical direction of one certified registered nurse anesthetist (CRNA) by an anesthesiologist
-QZ	CRNA service: without medical direction by a physician
◆ -RC	Right coronary artery
-RP	Replacement and repair -RP may be used to indicate replacement of dme, orthotic and prosthetic devices which have been in use for sometime. The claim shows the code for the part, followed by the 'RP' modifier and the charge for the part
-RR	Rental (use the 'RR' modifier when DME is to be rented)
◆ -RT	Right side (used to identify procedures performed on the right side of the body)
-SF	Second opinion ordered by a professional review organization (PRO) per section 9401, p.l. 99-272 (100% reimbursement — no Medicare deductible or coinsurance)
-SG	Ambulatory surgical center (ASC) facility service
◆ -T1	Left foot, second digit
◆ -T2	Left foot, third digit
◆ -T3	Left foot, fourth digit
◆ -T4	Left foot, fifth digit

- ◆ -T5   Right foot, great toe

- ◆ -T6   Right foot, second digit

- ◆ -T7   Right foot, third digit

- ◆ -T8   Right foot, fourth digit

- ◆ -T9   Right foot, fifth digit

- ◆ -TA   Left foot, great toe

     -TC   Technical component. Under certain circumstances, a charge may be made for the technical component alone. Under those circumstances the technical component charge is identified by adding modifier 'TC' to the usual procedure number. Technical component charges are institutional charges and not billed separately by physicians. However, portable x-ray suppliers only bill for technical component and should utilize modifier TC. The charge data from portable x-ray suppliers will then be used to build customary and prevailing profiles.

     -UE   Used durable medical equipment

     -VP   Aphakic patient

Appendix 1

Appendix 2:

Summary of 2001 Additions, Deletions, and Revisions

A0030	Code deleted		**A0366**	Code deleted
A0040	Code deleted		**A0370**	Code deleted
A0050	Code deleted		**A0380**	Code deleted
A0300	Code deleted		**A0390**	Code deleted
A0302	Code deleted		**A0425**	Code added
A0304	Code deleted		**A0426**	Code added
A0306	Code deleted		**A0427**	Code added
A0308	Code deleted		**A0428**	Code added
A0310	Code deleted		**A0429**	Code added
A0320	Code deleted		**A0430**	Code added
A0322	Code deleted		**A0431**	Code added
A0324	Code deleted		**A0432**	Code added
A0326	Code deleted		**A0433**	Code added
A0328	Code deleted		**A0434**	Code added
A0330	Code deleted		**A0435**	Code added
A0340	Code deleted		**A0436**	Code added
A0342	Code deleted		**A4207**	Terminology revised
A0344	Code deleted		**A4290**	Code added
A0346	Code deleted		**A4319**	Code added
A0348	Code deleted		**A4324**	Code added
A0350	Code deleted		**A4325**	Code added
A0360	Code deleted		**A4331**	Code added
A0362	Code deleted		**A4332**	Code added
A0364	Code deleted		**A4333**	Code added

A4334	Code added		**A7506**	Code added
A4348	Code added		**A7507**	Code added
A4364	Terminology revised		**A7508**	Code added
A4365	Terminology revised		**A7509**	Code added
A4396	Code added		**A9508**	Code added
A4464	Code added		**A9510**	Code added
A4560	Code deleted		**A9700**	Code added
A4561	Code added		**A9900**	Terminology revised
A4562	Code added		**A9901**	Terminology revised
A4608	Code added		**B4150**	Terminology revised
A5065	Code deleted		**B4151**	Terminology revised
A5149	Code deleted		**B4152**	Terminology revised
A6020	Code deleted		**B4153**	Terminology revised
A6021	Code added		**B4154**	Terminology revised
A6022	Code added		**B4155**	Terminology revised
A6023	Code added		**B4156**	Terminology revised
A6024	Code added		**C1000**	Code added
A6222	Terminology revised		**C1001**	Code added
A6223	Terminology revised		**C1003**	Code added
A6224	Terminology revised		**C1004**	Code added
A6231	Code added		**C1005**	Code deleted
A6232	Code added		**C1006**	Code added
A6233	Code added		**C1007**	Code added
A7018	Code added		**C1008**	Code added
A7019	Code added		**C1009**	Code added
A7020	Code added		**C1010**	Code added
A7501	Code added		**C1011**	Code added
A7502	Code added		**C1012**	Code added
A7503	Code added		**C1013**	Code added
A7504	Code added		**C1014**	Code added
A7505	Code added			

C1016	Code added	**C1056**	Code added
C1017	Code added	**C1057**	Code added
C1018	Code added	**C1059**	Code added
C1019	Code added	**C1060**	Code added
C1024	Code added	**C1061**	Code added
C1025	Code added	**C1063**	Code added
C1026	Code added	**C1067**	Code added
C1027	Code added	**C1068**	Code added
C1028	Code added	**C1069**	Code added
C1029	Code added	**C1071**	Code added
C1030	Code added	**C1072**	Code added
C1031	Code added	**C1073**	Code added
C1033	Code added	**C1074**	Code added
C1034	Code added	**C1075**	Code added
C1035	Code added	**C1076**	Code added
C1036	Code added	**C1077**	Code added
C1037	Code added	**C1078**	Code added
C1038	Code added	**C1079**	Code added
C1039	Code added	**C1084**	Code added
C1040	Code added	**C1086**	Code added
C1042	Code added	**C1087**	Code added
C1043	Code added	**C1088**	Code added
C1045	Code added	**C1089**	Code added
C1047	Code added	**C1090**	Code added
C1048	Code added	**C1091**	Code added
C1050	Code added	**C1092**	Code added
C1051	Code added	**C1094**	Code added
C1053	Code added	**C1095**	Code added
C1054	Code added	**C1096**	Code added
C1055	Code added	**C1097**	Code added

Appendix 2

C1098	Code added	**C1129**	Code added
C1099	Code added	**C1130**	Code added
C1100	Code added	**C1131**	Code added
C1101	Code added	**C1132**	Code added
C1102	Code added	**C1133**	Code added
C1103	Code added	**C1134**	Code added
C1104	Code added	**C1135**	Code added
C1105	Code added	**C1136**	Code added
C1106	Code added	**C1137**	Code added
C1107	Code added	**C1143**	Code added
C1109	Code added	**C1144**	Code added
C1110	Code added	**C1145**	Code added
C1111	Code added	**C1146**	Code added
C1112	Code added	**C1147**	Code added
C1113	Code added	**C1148**	Code added
C1114	Code added	**C1149**	Code added
C1115	Code added	**C1151**	Code added
C1116	Code added	**C1152**	Code added
C1117	Code added	**C1153**	Code added
C1118	Code added	**C1154**	Code added
C1119	Code added	**C1155**	Code added
C1120	Code added	**C1156**	Code added
C1121	Code added	**C1157**	Code added
C1122	Code added	**C1158**	Code added
C1123	Code added	**C1159**	Code added
C1124	Code added	**C1160**	Code added
C1125	Code added	**C1161**	Code added
C1126	Code added	**C1162**	Code added
C1127	Code added	**C1163**	Code added
C1128	Code added	**C1164**	Code added

C1166	Code added		C1311	Code added
C1167	Code added		C1312	Code added
C1170	Code added		C1313	Code added
C1171	Code added		C1314	Code added
C1172	Code added		C1315	Code added
C1173	Code added		C1316	Code added
C1174	Code added		C1317	Code added
C1175	Code added		C1318	Code added
C1176	Code added		C1319	Code added
C1177	Code added		C1320	Code added
C1178	Code added		C1321	Code added
C1179	Code added		C1322	Code added
C1180	Code added		C1323	Code added
C1181	Code added		C1324	Code added
C1182	Code added		C1325	Code added
C1183	Code added		C1326	Code added
C1184	Code added		C1328	Code added
C1188	Code added		C1329	Code added
C1200	Code added		C1333	Code added
C1201	Code added		C1334	Code added
C1202	Code added		C1335	Code added
C1203	Code added		C1336	Code added
C1205	Code added		C1337	Code added
C1207	Code added		C1348	Code added
C1300	Code added		C1350	Code added
C1302	Code added		C1351	Code added
C1303	Code added		C1352	Code added
C1304	Code added		C1353	Code added
C1305	Code added		C1354	Code added
C1306	Code added		C1355	Code added

Appendix 2

C1356	Code added	C1702	Code added
C1357	Code added	C1703	Code added
C1358	Code added	C1704	Code added
C1359	Code added	C1705	Code added
C1360	Code added	C1706	Code added
C1361	Code added	C1707	Code added
C1362	Code added	C1708	Code added
C1363	Code added	C1709	Code added
C1364	Code added	C1710	Code added
C1365	Code added	C1711	Code added
C1366	Code added	C1712	Code added
C1367	Code added	C1790	Code added
C1368	Code added	C1791	Code added
C1369	Code added	C1792	Code added
C1370	Code added	C1793	Code added
C1371	Code added	C1794	Code added
C1372	Code added	C1795	Code added
C1375	Code added	C1796	Code added
C1376	Code added	C1797	Code added
C1377	Code added	C1798	Code added
C1378	Code added	C1799	Code added
C1379	Code added	C1800	Code added
C1420	Code added	C1801	Code added
C1421	Code added	C1802	Code added
C1450	Code added	C1803	Code added
C1451	Code added	C1804	Code added
C1500	Code added	C1805	Code added
C1531	Code deleted	C1806	Code added
C1700	Code added	C1810	Code added
C1701	Code added	C1811	Code added

C1812	Code added		C1935	Code added
C1850	Code added		C1936	Code added
C1851	Code added		C1937	Code added
C1852	Code added		C1938	Code added
C1853	Code added		C1939	Code added
C1854	Code added		C1940	Code added
C1855	Code added		C1941	Code added
C1856	Code added		C1942	Code added
C1857	Code added		C1943	Code added
C1858	Code added		C1944	Code added
C1859	Code added		C1945	Code added
C1860	Code added		C1946	Code added
C1861	Code added		C1947	Code added
C1862	Code added		C1948	Code added
C1863	Code added		C1949	Code added
C1864	Code added		C1979	Code added
C1865	Code added		C1980	Code added
C1866	Code added		C1981	Code added
C1867	Code added		C2000	Code added
C1868	Code added		C2001	Code added
C1869	Code added		C2002	Code added
C1870	Code added		C2003	Code added
C1871	Code added		C2004	Code added
C1872	Code added		C2005	Code added
C1873	Code added		C2006	Code added
C1929	Code added		C2007	Code added
C1930	Code added		C2008	Code added
C1931	Code added		C2009	Code added
C1932	Code added		C2010	Code added
C1933	Code added		C2011	Code added
C1934	Code added			

C2012	Code added		**C2605**	Code added
C2013	Code added		**C2606**	Code added
C2014	Code added		**C2607**	Code added
C2015	Code added		**C2608**	Code added
C2016	Code added		**C2609**	Code added
C2017	Code added		**C2610**	Code added
C2018	Code added		**C2611**	Code added
C2019	Code added		**C2612**	Code added
C2020	Code added		**C2676**	Code added
C2021	Code added		**C2700**	Code added
C2022	Code added		**C2701**	Code added
C2023	Code added		**C2702**	Code added
C2100	Code added		**C2703**	Code added
C2101	Code added		**C2704**	Code added
C2102	Code added		**C2801**	Code added
C2103	Code added		**C2802**	Code added
C2104	Code added		**C2803**	Code added
C2151	Code added		**C2804**	Code added
C2152	Code added		**C2805**	Code added
C2153	Code added		**C2806**	Code added
C2200	Code added		**C2807**	Code added
C2300	Code added		**C2808**	Code added
C2597	Code added		**C3001**	Code added
C2598	Code added		**C3002**	Code added
C2599	Code added		**C3003**	Code added
C2600	Code added		**C3004**	Code added
C2601	Code added		**C3400**	Code added
C2602	Code added		**C3401**	Code added
C2603	Code added		**C3500**	Code added
C2604	Code added		**C3510**	Code added

C3551	Code added		**C4310**	Code added
C3552	Code added		**C4311**	Code added
C3553	Code added		**C4312**	Code added
C3554	Code added		**C4313**	Code added
C3555	Code added		**C4314**	Code added
C3556	Code added		**C4315**	Code added
C3557	Code added		**C4316**	Code added
C3800	Code added		**C4317**	Code added
C3801	Code added		**C4600**	Code added
C3851	Code added		**C4601**	Code added
C4000	Code added		**C4602**	Code added
C4001	Code added		**C4603**	Code added
C4002	Code added		**C4604**	Code added
C4003	Code added		**C4605**	Code added
C4004	Code added		**C4606**	Code added
C4005	Code added		**C4607**	Code added
C4006	Code added		**C5000**	Code added
C4007	Code added		**C5001**	Code added
C4008	Code added		**C5002**	Code added
C4009	Code added		**C5003**	Code added
C4300	Code added		**C5004**	Code added
C4301	Code added		**C5005**	Code added
C4302	Code added		**C5006**	Code added
C4303	Code added		**C5007**	Code added
C4304	Code added		**C5008**	Code added
C4305	Code added		**C5009**	Code added
C4306	Code added		**C5010**	Code added
C4307	Code added		**C5011**	Code added
C4308	Code added		**C5012**	Code added
C4309	Code added		**C5013**	Code added

Appendix 2

C5014	Code added	**C5044**	Code added
C5015	Code added	**C5045**	Code added
C5016	Code added	**C5046**	Code added
C5017	Code added	**C5047**	Code added
C5018	Code added	**C5048**	Code added
C5019	Code added	**C5130**	Code added
C5020	Code added	**C5131**	Code added
C5021	Code added	**C5132**	Code added
C5022	Code added	**C5133**	Code added
C5023	Code added	**C5134**	Code added
C5024	Code added	**C5279**	Code added
C5025	Code added	**C5280**	Code added
C5026	Code added	**C5281**	Code added
C5027	Code added	**C5282**	Code added
C5028	Code added	**C5283**	Code added
C5029	Code added	**C5284**	Code added
C5030	Code added	**C5600**	Code added
C5031	Code added	**C5601**	Code added
C5032	Code added	**C6001**	Code added
C5033	Code added	**C6002**	Code added
C5034	Code added	**C6003**	Code added
C5035	Code added	**C6004**	Code added
C5036	Code added	**C6005**	Code added
C5037	Code added	**C6006**	Code added
C5038	Code added	**C6012**	Code added
C5039	Code added	**C6013**	Code added
C5040	Code added	**C6014**	Code added
C5041	Code added	**C6015**	Code added
C5042	Code added	**C6016**	Code added
C5043	Code added	**C6017**	Code added

C6018	Code added		C6056	Code added
C6019	Code added		C6057	Code added
C6020	Code added		C6058	Code added
C6021	Code added		C6080	Code added
C6022	Code added		C6200	Code added
C6023	Code added		C6201	Code added
C6024	Code added		C6202	Code added
C6025	Code added		C6203	Code added
C6026	Code added		C6204	Code added
C6027	Code added		C6205	Code added
C6028	Code added		C6206	Code added
C6029	Code added		C6207	Code added
C6030	Code added		C6208	Code added
C6031	Code added		C6209	Code added
C6032	Code added		C6210	Code added
C6033	Code added		C6300	Code added
C6034	Code added		C6500	Code added
C6035	Code added		C6501	Code added
C6036	Code added		C6525	Code added
C6037	Code added		C6600	Code added
C6038	Code added		C6650	Code added
C6039	Code added		C6651	Code added
C6040	Code added		C6652	Code added
C6041	Code added		C6700	Code added
C6050	Code added		C8099	Code added
C6051	Code added		C8100	Code added
C6052	Code added		C8102	Code added
C6053	Code added		C8103	Code added
C6054	Code added		C8500	Code added
C6055	Code added		C8501	Code added

Appendix 2

C8502	Code added		**C8533**	Code added
C8503	Code added		**C8534**	Code added
C8504	Code added		**C8535**	Code added
C8505	Code added		**C8536**	Code added
C8506	Code added		**C8539**	Code added
C8507	Code added		**C8540**	Code added
C8508	Code added		**C8541**	Code added
C8509	Code added		**C8542**	Code added
C8510	Code added		**C8543**	Code added
C8511	Code added		**C8550**	Code added
C8512	Code added		**C8551**	Code added
C8513	Code added		**C8552**	Code added
C8514	Code added		**C8597**	Code added
C8515	Code deleted		**C8598**	Code added
C8516	Code added		**C8599**	Code added
C8517	Code deleted		**C8600**	Code added
C8518	Code added		**C8650**	Code added
C8519	Code added		**C8724**	Code added
C8520	Code added		**C8725**	Code added
C8521	Code added		**C8748**	Code added
C8522	Code added		**C8749**	Code added
C8523	Code added		**C8750**	Code added
C8524	Code added		**C8775**	Code added
C8525	Code added		**C8776**	Code added
C8526	Code added		**C8777**	Code added
C8528	Code added		**C8800**	Code added
C8529	Code added		**C8801**	Code added
C8530	Code added		**C8802**	Code added
C8531	Code added		**C8830**	Code added
C8532	Code added		**C8890**	Code added

C8891	Code added	E0149	Code added
C9000	Code added	E0298	Code added
C9001	Code added	E0424	Terminology revised
C9002	Code added	E0431	Terminology revised
C9003	Code added	E0439	Terminology revised
C9004	Code added	E0441	Terminology revised
C9005	Code added	E0442	Terminology revised
C9006	Code added	E0443	Terminology revised
C9007	Code added	E0444	Terminology revised
C9008	Code added	E0571	Code added
C9009	Code added	E0572	Code added
C9010	Code added	E0574	Code added
C9011	Code added	E0575	Terminology revised
C9100	Code added	E0617	Code added
C9102	Code added	E0751	Code deleted
C9103	Code added	E0756	Code added
C9104	Code added	E0757	Code added
C9105	Code added	E0758	Code added
C9106	Code added	E0765	Code added
C9107	Code added	E0786	Code added
C9500	Code added	E0830	Code added
C9501	Code added	E1035	Code added
C9502	Code added	E1375	Code deleted
C9503	Code added	E1377	Code deleted
C9504	Code added	E1378	Code deleted
C9505	Code added	E1379	Code deleted
C9700	Code added	E1380	Code deleted
C9701	Code added	E1381	Code deleted
C9702	Code added	E1382	Code deleted
E0148	Code added	E1383	Code deleted

Appendix 2

E1384	Code deleted
E1385	Code deleted
E1800	Terminology revised
E1805	Terminology revised
E1810	Terminology revised
E1815	Terminology revised
E1825	Terminology revised
E1830	Terminology revised
G0108	Terminology revised
G0109	Terminology revised
G0159	Code deleted
G0160	Code deleted
G0161	Code deleted
G0169	Code deleted
G0170	Code deleted
G0171	Code deleted
G0172	Code deleted
G0173	Code added
G0174	Code added
G0175	Code added
G0176	Code added
G0177	Code added
G0178	Code added
G0179	Code added
G0180	Code added
G0181	Code added
G0182	Code added
G0183	Code deleted
G0184	Code added
G0185	Code added

G0186	Code added
G0187	Code added
G0188	Code added
G0190	Code added
G0191	Code added
G0192	Code added
G0193	Code added
G0194	Code added
G0195	Code added
G0196	Code added
G0197	Code added
G0198	Code added
G0199	Code added
G0200	Code added
G0201	Code added
G9001	Code added
G9002	Code added
G9003	Code added
G9004	Code added
G9005	Code added
G9006	Code added
G9007	Code added
G9008	Code added
G9016	Code added
H0001	Code added
H0002	Code added
H0003	Code added
H0004	Code added
H0005	Code added
H0006	Code added

H0007	Code added		J2543	Terminology revised
H0008	Code added		J2770	Code added
H0009	Code added		J2795	Code added
H0010	Code added		J2915	Code added
H0011	Code added		J2993	Code added
H0012	Code added		J2994	Code deleted
H0013	Code added		J2996	Code deleted
H0014	Code added		J2997	Code added
H0015	Code added		J3010	Terminology revised
H0016	Code added		J3485	Code added
H0017	Code added		J7330	Code added
H0018	Code added		J7505	Terminology revised
H0019	Code added		J7520	Code added
H0020	Code added		J7525	Code added
H0021	Code added		J7610	Code deleted
H0022	Code added		J7615	Code deleted
H0023	Code added		J7618	Terminology revised
H0024	Code added		J7619	Terminology revised
H0025	Code added		J7620	Code deleted
H0026	Code added		J7625	Code deleted
H0027	Code added		J7627	Code deleted
H0028	Code added		J7630	Code deleted
H0029	Code added		J7640	Code deleted
H0030	Code added		J7645	Code deleted
J0282	Code added		J7650	Code deleted
J0895	Terminology revised		J7651	Code deleted
J1100	Terminology revised		J7652	Code deleted
J1452	Code added		J7653	Code deleted
J1562	Code deleted		J7654	Code deleted
J1563	Code added		J7655	Code deleted

Appendix 2

J7660	Code deleted	**K0450**	Code deleted
J7665	Code deleted	**K0451**	Code deleted
J7670	Code deleted	**K0456**	Code deleted
J7672	Code deleted	**K0457**	Code deleted
J7675	Code deleted	**K0458**	Code deleted
J8700	Code added	**K0459**	Code deleted
J9160	Code added	**K0501**	Code deleted
J9180	Code added	**K0529**	Code deleted
J9219	Code added	**K0535**	Code deleted
K0182	Code deleted	**K0536**	Code deleted
K0269	Code deleted	**K0537**	Code deleted
K0270	Code deleted	**K0538**	Code added
K0280	Code deleted	**K0539**	Code added
K0281	Code deleted	**K0540**	Code added
K0283	Code deleted	**K0541**	Code added
K0407	Code deleted	**K0542**	Code added
K0408	Code deleted	**K0543**	Code added
K0409	Code deleted	**K0544**	Code added
K0410	Code deleted	**K0545**	Code added
K0411	Code deleted	**K0546**	Code added
K0440	Code deleted	**K0547**	Code added
K0441	Code deleted	**L1600**	Terminology revised
K0442	Code deleted	**L1610**	Terminology revised
K0443	Code deleted	**L1620**	Terminology revised
K0444	Code deleted	**L1630**	Terminology revised
K0445	Code deleted	**L1640**	Terminology revised
K0446	Code deleted	**L1650**	Terminology revised
K0447	Code deleted	**L1660**	Terminology revised
K0448	Code deleted	**L1680**	Terminology revised
K0449	Code deleted	**L1685**	Terminology revised

L1686	Terminology revised		**L1902**	Terminology revised
L1690	Terminology revised		**L1904**	Terminology revised
L1700	Terminology revised		**L1906**	Terminology revised
L1710	Terminology revised		**L1910**	Terminology revised
L1720	Terminology revised		**L1920**	Terminology revised
L1730	Terminology revised		**L1930**	Terminology revised
L1750	Terminology revised		**L1940**	Terminology revised
L1755	Terminology revised		**L1945**	Terminology revised
L1800	Terminology revised		**L1950**	Terminology revised
L1810	Terminology revised		**L1960**	Terminology revised
L1815	Terminology revised		**L1970**	Terminology revised
L1820	Terminology revised		**L1980**	Terminology revised
L1825	Terminology revised		**L1990**	Terminology revised
L1830	Terminology revised		**L2000**	Terminology revised
L1832	Terminology revised		**L2010**	Terminology revised
L1834	Terminology revised		**L2020**	Terminology revised
L1840	Terminology revised		**L2030**	Terminology revised
L1843	Terminology revised		**L2035**	Terminology revised
L1844	Terminology revised		**L2036**	Terminology revised
L1845	Terminology revised		**L2037**	Terminology revised
L1846	Terminology revised		**L2038**	Terminology revised
L1847	Terminology revised		**L2039**	Terminology revised
L1850	Terminology revised		**L2040**	Terminology revised
L1855	Terminology revised		**L2050**	Terminology revised
L1858	Terminology revised		**L2060**	Terminology revised
L1860	Terminology revised		**L2070**	Terminology revised
L1870	Terminology revised		**L2080**	Terminology revised
L1880	Terminology revised		**L2090**	Terminology revised
L1885	Terminology revised		**L2102**	Terminology revised
L1900	Terminology revised		**L2104**	Terminology revised

Appendix 2

L2106	Terminology revised	**L3908**	Terminology revised
L2108	Terminology revised	**L3910**	Terminology revised
L2114	Terminology revised	**L3912**	Terminology revised
L2116	Terminology revised	**L3914**	Terminology revised
L2122	Terminology revised	**L3916**	Terminology revised
L2124	Terminology revised	**L3918**	Terminology revised
L2126	Terminology revised	**L3920**	Terminology revised
L2128	Terminology revised	**L3922**	Terminology revised
L2132	Terminology revised	**L3923**	Code added
L2134	Terminology revised	**L3924**	Terminology revised
L2136	Terminology revised	**L3926**	Terminology revised
L3650	Terminology revised	**L3928**	Terminology revised
L3660	Terminology revised	**L3930**	Terminology revised
L3670	Terminology revised	**L3932**	Terminology revised
L3675	Terminology revised	**L3934**	Terminology revised
L3700	Terminology revised	**L3936**	Terminology revised
L3710	Terminology revised	**L3938**	Terminology revised
L3720	Terminology revised	**L3940**	Terminology revised
L3730	Terminology revised	**L3942**	Terminology revised
L3740	Terminology revised	**L3944**	Terminology revised
L3760	Code added	**L3946**	Terminology revised
L3800	Terminology revised	**L3948**	Terminology revised
L3805	Terminology revised	**L3950**	Terminology revised
L3807	Terminology revised	**L3952**	Terminology revised
L3900	Terminology revised	**L3954**	Terminology revised
L3901	Terminology revised	**L3960**	Terminology revised
L3902	Terminology revised	**L3962**	Terminology revised
L3904	Terminology revised	**L3963**	Terminology revised
L3906	Terminology revised	**L3964**	Terminology revised
L3907	Terminology revised	**L3965**	Terminology revised

L3966	Terminology revised		**P9017**	Terminology revised
L3968	Terminology revised		**P9018**	Code deleted
L3969	Terminology revised		**P9019**	Terminology revised
L3980	Terminology revised		**P9022**	Terminology revised
L3982	Terminology revised		**P9031**	Code added
L3984	Terminology revised		**P9032**	Code added
L3985	Terminology revised		**P9033**	Code added
L3986	Terminology revised		**P9034**	Code added
L4350	Terminology revised		**P9035**	Code added
L4360	Terminology revised		**P9036**	Code added
L4370	Terminology revised		**P9037**	Code added
L4380	Terminology revised		**P9038**	Code added
L4392	Terminology revised		**P9039**	Code added
L4396	Terminology revised		**P9040**	Code added
L4398	Terminology revised		**P9041**	Code added
L5674	Terminology revised		**P9042**	Code added
L5675	Terminology revised		**P9043**	Code added
L5979	Terminology revised		**P9044**	Code added
L8041	Code added		**Q0034**	Code deleted
L8042	Code added		**Q0082**	Code deleted
L8043	Code added		**Q0156**	Code deleted
L8044	Code added		**Q0157**	Code deleted
L8045	Code added		**Q0186**	Code deleted
L8046	Code added		**Q0188**	Code deleted
L8047	Code added		**Q1001**	Terminology revised
L8049	Code added		**Q2001**	Code added
L8603	Terminology revised		**Q2002**	Code added
L8606	Code added		**Q2003**	Code added
P9013	Code deleted		**Q2004**	Code added
P9016	Terminology revised		**Q2005**	Code added

Appendix 2

Q2006	Code added	**S0011**	Code deleted
Q2007	Code added	**S0085**	Code added
Q2008	Code added	**S0086**	Code added
Q2009	Code added	**S0097**	Code deleted
Q2010	Code added	**S0098**	Code deleted
Q2011	Code added	**S0156**	Code added
Q2012	Code added	**S0157**	Code added
Q2013	Code added	**S0220**	Code added
Q2014	Code added	**S0221**	Code added
Q2015	Code added	**S0630**	Code added
Q2016	Code added	**S0820**	Code added
Q2017	Code added	**S0830**	Code added
Q2018	Code added	**S1015**	Code added
Q2019	Code added	**S1016**	Code added
Q2020	Code added	**S2050**	Code deleted
Q2021	Code added	**S2060**	Code added
Q2022	Code added	**S2061**	Code added
Q3001	Code added	**S2102**	Code added
Q3002	Code added	**S2103**	Code added
Q3003	Code added	**S2109**	Code deleted
Q3004	Code added	**S2120**	Code added
Q3005	Code added	**S2140**	Code added
Q3006	Code added	**S2142**	Code added
Q3007	Code added	**S2180**	Code added
Q3008	Code added	**S2190**	Code deleted
Q3009	Code added	**S2202**	Code added
Q3010	Code added	**S2204**	Code deleted
Q3011	Code added	**S2220**	Code added
Q3012	Code added	**S2340**	Code added
S0010	Code deleted	**S2370**	Code added

S2371	Code added		S8105	Code added
S3620	Code added		S8210	Code added
S3700	Code added		S8300	Code deleted
S3708	Code added		S8400	Code added
S3902	Code added		S8402	Code added
S3904	Code added		S8405	Code added
S3906	Code added		S8999	Code added
S5000	Code added		S9007	Code added
S5001	Code added		S9015	Code added
S5002	Code added		S9025	Code added
S5003	Code added		S9033	Code deleted
S5010	Code added		S9035	Code added
S5011	Code added		S9061	Code added
S5012	Code added		S9088	Code added
S5013	Code added		S9200	Code added
S5014	Code added		S9210	Code added
S5016	Code added		S9220	Code added
S5017	Code added		S9225	Code added
S5018	Code added		S9230	Code added
S5019	Code added		S9300	Code added
S5020	Code added		S9308	Code added
S5021	Code added		S9310	Code added
S5022	Code added		S9395	Code added
S5025	Code added		S9420	Code added
S5503	Code added		S9423	Code added
S8001	Code added		S9425	Code added
S8048	Code deleted		S9435	Code added
S8060	Code deleted		S9526	Code added
S8080	Code added		S9533	Code added
S8085	Code added		S9535	Code added

S9539	Code added
S9545	Code added
S9550	Code added
S9555	Code added
V2790	Code added

Appendix 3:

HCPCS Table of Drugs
Introduction and Directions

The HCPCS 2000 Table of Drugs is designed to quickly and easily direct the user to drug names and their corresponding codes. Both generic and brand or trade names are alphabetically listed in the "Drug Name" column of the table. The associated J, K, or Q code is given only for the generic name of the drug. Brand or trade name drugs are cross-referenced to the appropriate generic drug name.

The "Amount" column lists the stated amount for the referenced generic drug as provided by the Health Care Financing Administration (HCFA). "Up to" listings are inclusive of all quantities up to and including the listed amount. All other listings are for the amount of the drug as listed. The editors recognize that the availability of some drugs in the quantities listed is dependent on many variables beyond the control of the clinical ordering clerk. The availability in your area of regularly used drugs in the most cost-effective quantities should be relayed to your third-party payers.

The "Route of Administration" column addresses the most common methods of delivering the referenced generic drug as described in current pharmaceutical literature. The official definitions for Level II drug codes generally describe administration other than by oral method. Therefore, with a handful of exceptions, oral-delivered options for most drugs are omitted from the Route of Administration column. The following abbreviations and listings are used in the Route of Administration column:

IA — Intra-arterial administration

IV — Intravenous administration

IM — Intramuscular administration

IT — Intrathecal

SC — Subcutaneous administration

INH — Administration by inhaled solution

INJ — Injection not otherwise specified

VAR — Various routes of administration

OTH — Other routes of administration

ORAL — Administered orally

Intravenous administration includes all methods, such as gravity infusion, injections, and timed pushes. When several routes of administration are listed, the first listing is simply the first, or most common, method as described in current reference literature. The "VAR" posting denotes various routes of administration and is used for drugs that are commonly administered into joints, cavities, tissues, or topical applications, in addition to other parenteral administrations. Listings posted with "OTH" alert the user to other administration methods, such as suppositories or catheter injections.

A dash (—) in a column signifies that no information is available to post for that particular listing.

Please be reminded that the Table of Drugs, as well as all HCPCS Level II National definitions and listings, constitutes a post-treatment medical reference for billing purposes only. Although the editors have exercised all normal precautions to ensure the accuracy of the table and related material, the use of any of this information to select medical treatment is entirely inappropriate.

A

	Amount	Route of Admin	Code
Abbokinase, *see* Urokinase			
Abbokinase, Open Cath, *see* Urokinase			
Abciximab	10 mg	IV	J0130
Abelcet, *see* Amphotericin B, any lipid formulation			
Acetazolamide sodium	up to 500 mg	IM, IV	J1120
Acetylcysteine	10%, per ml	INH	J7610
	20%, per ml	INH	J7615
Acetylcysteine, inhalation solution, unit dose form	per gram	INH	J7608
Achromycin, *see* Tetracycline			
ACTH, *see* Corticotropin			
Acthar, *see* Corticotropin			
Actimmune, *see* Interferon gamma 1-B			
Activase, *see* Alteplase recombinant			
Acyclovir sodium injection	50 mg	ORAL, IV	S0071
Adenocard, *see* Adenosine			
Adenosine	6 mg	IV	J0150
	90 mg	IV	J0151
Adrenalin Chloride, *see* Adrenalin, epinephrine			
Adrenalin, epinephrine	up to 1 ml ampule	SC, IM	J0170
Adriamycin PFS, *see* Doxorubicin HCl			
Adriamycin RDF, *see* Doxorubicin HCl			

	Amount	Route of Admin	Code
Adrucil, *see* Fluorouracil			
A-hydroCort, *see* Hydrocortisone sodium phosphate			
Akineton, *see* Biperiden			
Albumin Human, 5%	500 ml	IV	Q0156
Albumin Human, 25%	50 ml	IV	Q0157
Albumarc, *see* Albumin Human			
Albuterol, all formulations including separated isomers	per 1 mg	INH	J7618, J7619
Albuterol, sulfate	0.083%, per ml	INH	J7620
	0.5%, per ml	INH	J7625
Aldesleukin	per single use vial	IM, IV	J9015
Aldomet, *see* Methyldopate HCl			
Alferon N, *see* Interferon alfa-n3			
Alglucerase	per 10 units	IV	J0205
Alkaban-AQ, *see* Vinblastine sulfate			
Alkeran, *see* Melphalan, oral			
Alpha 1-proteinase inhibitor, human	per 10 mg	IV	J0256
Alprostadil	per 1.25 mcg	IV	J0270
Alprostadil, urethral suppository	—	OTH	J0275
Alteplase recombinant	per 10 mg	IV	J2996
Alupent, *see* Metaproterenol sulfate or Metaproterenol, compounded			
Amcort, *see* Triamcinolone diacetate			
A-methaPred, *see* Methylprednisolone sodium succinate			
Amicar, *see* Aminocaproic acid injection			
Amikacin Sulfate injection	100 mg	IV, IM	S0072
	500 mg	IV, IM	S0016
Amikin, *see* Amikacin sulfate injection			
Aminocaproic acid, injection	5 g	IV	S0017
Amifostine	500 mg	IV, INJ	J0207
Aminophylline/Aminophyllin	up to 250 mg	IV	J0280
Amitriptyline HCl	up to 20 mg	IM	J1320
Amobarbital	up to 125 mg	IM, IV	J0300
Amphotec, *see* Amphotericin B, any lipid formulation			

Appendix 3

	Amount	Route of Admin	Code
Amphotericin B	50 mg	IV	J0285
Amphotericin B, any lipid formulation	50 mg	IV	J0286
Ampicillin sodium	500 mg	IM, IV	J0290
Ampicillin sodium/sulbactam sodium	1.5 gm	IM, IV	J0295

Amygdalin, *see* Laetrile, Amygdalin, vitamin B-17

Amytal, *see* Amobarbital

Anabolin LA 100, *see* Nandrolone decanoate

Ancef, *see* Cefazolin sodium

Andrest 90-4, *see* Testosterone enanthate and estradiol valerate

Andro-Cyp, *see* Testosterone cypionate

Andro-Cyp 200, *see* Testosterone cypionate

Andro L.A. 200, *see* Testosterone enanthate

Andro-Estro 90-4, *see* Testosterone enanthate and estradiol valerate

Andro/Fem, *see* Testosterone cypionate and estradiol cypionate

Androgyn L.A., *see* Testosterone enanthate and estradiol valerate

Androlone-50, *see* Nandrolone phenpropionate

Androlone-D 100, *see* Nandrolone decanoate

Andronaq-50, *see* Testosterone suspension

Andronaq-LA, *see* Testosterone cypionate

Andronate-200, *see* Testosterone cypionate

Andronate-100, *see* Testosterone cypionate

Andropository 100, *see* Testosterone enanthate

Andryl 200, *see* Testosterone enanthate

Anectine, *see* Succinylcholine chloride

Anergan 25, *see* Promethazine HCl

Anergan 50, *see* Promethazine HCl

	Amount	Route of Admin	Code
Anistreplase	30 units	IV	J0350
Anti-inhibitor	per IU		J7198
Antispas, *see* Dicyclomine HCl			
Antithrombin III (human)	per IU	IV	J7197
A.P.L., *see* Chorionic gonadotropin			
Apresoline, *see* Hydralazine HCl			
AquaMEPHYTON, *see* Phytonadione			
Aralen, *see* Chloroquine HCl			
Aramine, *see* Metaraminol			
Arbutamine HCl	1 mg	IV	J0395
Aredia, *see* Pamidronate disodium			
Arfonad, *see* Trimethaphan camsylate			
Aristocort Forte, *see* Triamcinolone diacetate			
Aristocort Intralesional, *see* Triamcinolone diacetate			
Aristospan Intra-Articular, *see* Triamcinolone hexacetonide			
Aristospan Intralesional, *see* Triamcinolone hexacetonide			
Aromasin, *see* Exemestane			
Arrestin, *see* Trimethobenzamide HCl			
Asparaginase	10,000 units	IV, IM	J9020
Astramorph PF, *see* Morphine sulfate			
Astromorph, *see* Morphine sulfate			
Atgam, *see* Lymphocyte immune globulin			
Ativan, *see* Lorazepam			
Atropine sulfate	up to 0.3 mg	IV, IM, SC	J0460
Atropine, inhalation solution, concentrated form	per mg	INH	J7635
Atropine, inhalation solution, unit dose form	per mg	INH	J7636
Atrovent, *see* Ipratropium bromide			
Aurothioglucose	up to 50 mg	IM	J2910
Autoplex T, *see* Hemophilia clotting factors			
Azactam, *see* Aztreonam injection			
Azathioprine	50 mg	ORAL	J7500, K0119
Azathioprine, parenteral	100 mg	IV	J7501, K0120

	Amount	Route of Admin	Code
Azithromycin	500 mg	INJ	J0456
Azithromycin dihydrate, capsules/powder	1 g	ORAL	Q0144
Aztreonam, injection	500 mg	IV, IM	S0073

B

	Amount	Route of Admin	Code
Baclofen	10 mg	IT	J0475
	50 mcg	IT	J0476
Baclofen Intrathecal Refill Kit	per 500 mcg	IT	C9008
	per 2000 mcg	IT	C9009
	per 4000 mcg	IT	C9010
Baclofen Intrathecal Screening Kit	1 amp	IT	C9007
Bactocill, *see* Oxacillin sodium			
Bactrim IV, *see* Sulfamethoxazole and trimethoprim, injection			
BAL in oil, *see* Dimercaprol			
Banflex, *see* Orphenadrine citrate			
BCG (Bacillus Calmette and Guérin), live	per vial	IV	J9031
Becaplermin gel 0.01%	0.5 g	OTH	S0157
Bena-D 10, *see* Diphenhydramine HCl			
Bena-D 50, *see* Diphenhydramine HCl			
Benadryl, *see* Diphenhydramine HCl			
Benahist 10, *see* Diphenhydramine HCl			
Benahist 50, *see* Diphenhydramine HCl			
Ben-Allergin-50, *see* Diphenhydramine HCl			
Benoject-10, *see* Diphenhydramine HCl			
Benoject-50, *see* Diphenhydramine HCl			
Bentyl, *see* Dicyclomine			
Benzquinamide HCl	up to 50 mg	IM, IV	J0510
Benztropine mesylate	per 1 mg	IM, IV	J0515
Berubigen, *see* Vitamin B-12 cyanocobalamin			
Betalin 12, *see* Vitamin B-12 cyanocobalamin			
Betameth, *see* Betamethasone sodium phosphate			
Betamethasone acetate & betamethasone sodium phosphate	3 mg of each	IM	J0702

	Amount	Route of Admin	Code
Betamethasone sodium phosphate	4 mg	IM, IV	J0704
Betaseron, *see* Interferon beta-1b			
Bethanechol chloride	up to 5 mg	SC	J0520
Bicillin L-A, *see* Penicillin G benzathine			
Bicillin C-R 900/300, *see* Penicillin G procaine and penicillin G benzathine			
Bicillin C-R, *see* Penicillin G benzathine and penicillin G procaine			
BiCNU, *see* Carmustine			
Biperiden lactate	per 5 mg	IM, IV	J0190
Bitolterol mesylate 0.2%	per 10 ml	INH	J7627
Bitolterol mesylate, inhalation solution, concentrated form	per mg	INH	J7628
Bitolterol mesylate, inhalation solution, unit dose form	per mg	INH	J7629
Blenoxane, *see* Bleomycin sulfate			
Bleomycin sulfate	15 units	IM, IV, SC	J9040
Botulinum toxin type A	per unit	IM	J0585
Brethine, *see* Terbutaline sulfate or Terbutaline, compounded			
Bricanyl Subcutaneous, *see* Terbutaline sulfate			
Brompheniramine maleate	per 10 mg	IM, SC, IV	J0945
Bronkephrine, *see* Ethylnorepinephrine HCl			
Bronkosol, *see* Isoetharine HCl			
Bupivicaine HCl	30 ml	INJ	S0020
Bupivicaine hydrochloride, injection	30 mg	OTH	S0020
Busulfan (busulfex IV), injection	6 mg	IV	C1178
Butorphanol tartrate, injection	1 mg	IM, IV	S0009
Butorphanol tartrate, nasal spray	25 mg	Nasal spray	S0012

C

	Amount	Route of Admin	Code
Caffeine Citrate injection	per 1 mg	IM, IV	C9011
Caine-1, *see* Lidocaine HCl			
Caine-2, *see* Lidocaine HCl			

Appendix 3

	Amount	Route of Admin	Code
Calcijex, *see* Calcitriol			
Calcimar, *see* Calcitonin-salmon			
Calcitonin-salmon	up to 400 units	SC, IM	J0630
Calcitriol	1 mcg ampule	IM	J0635
Calcium Disodium Versenate, *see* Edetate calcium disodium			
Calcium EDTA, *see* Edetate calcium disodium			
Calcium gluconate	per 10 ml	IV	J0610
Calcium glycerophosphate and calcium lactate	per 10 ml	IM, SC	J0620
Capecitabine	150 mg	ORAL	J8520
	500 mg	ORAL	J8521
Calphosan, *see* Calcium glycerophosphate and calcium lactate			
Carbocaine, *see* Mepivacaine			
Carboplatin	50 mg	IV	J9045
Carmustine	100 mg	IV	J9050
Carnitor, *see* Levocarnitine			
Cefadyl, *see* Cephapirin Sodium			
Cefazolin sodium	500 mg	IV, IM	J0690
Cefizox, *see* Ceftizoxime soduim			
Cefobid, *see* Cefoperazone sodium injection			
Cefonicid sodium	1 g	IV	J0695
Cefoperazone sodium, injection	1 g	IV, IM	S0021
Cefotan, *see* Cefotetan disodium injection			
Cefotaxime sodium	per 1 g	IV, IM	J0698
Cefotetan disodium, injection	500 mg	IV, IM	S0074
Cefoxitin sodium	1 g	IV, IM	J0694
Ceftazidime	per 500 mg	IM, IV	J0713
Ceftizoxime soduim	per 500 mg	IV, IM	J0715
Ceftriaxone sodium	per 250 mg	IV, IM	J0696
Ceftoperazone sodium	1 g	INJ	S0021
Cefuroxime sodium, sterile	per 750 mg	IM, IV	J0697
Celestone Phosphate, *see* Betamethasone sodium phosphate			

	Amount	**Route of Admin**	**Code**
Celestone Soluspan, *see* Betamethasone acetate and betamethasone sodium phosphate			
CellCept, *see* Mycophenolate mofetil			
Cel-U-Jec, *see* Betamethasone sodium phosphate			
Cenacort Forte, *see* Triamcinolone diacetate			
Cenacort A-40, *see* Triamcinolone acetonide			
Cephalothin sodium	up to 1 g	IM, IV	J1890
Cephapirin sodium	up to 1 g	IV, IM	J0710
Cerebyx, *see* Fosphenytoin sodium injection			
Ceredase, *see* Alglucerase			
Cerezyme, *see* Imiglucerase			
Cerubidine, *see* Daunorubicin HCl			
Chlor-100, *see* Chlorpheniramine maleate			
Chloramphenicol sodium succinate	up to 1 g	IV	J0720
Chlordiazepoxide HCl	up to 100 mg	IM, IV	J1990
Chloromycetin Sodium Succinate, *see* Chloramphenicol sodium succinate			
Chlor-Pro, *see* Chlorpheniramine maleate			
Chlor-Pro 10, *see* Chlorpheniramine maleate			
Chloroprocaine HCl	per 30 ml	VAR	J2400
Chloroquine HCl	up to 250 mg	IM	J0390
Chlorothiazide sodium	per 500 mg	IV	J1205
Chlorpheniramine maleate	per 10 mg	IV, IM, SC	J0730
Chlorpromazine HCl	10 mg	ORAL	Q0171
	25 mg	ORAL	Q0172
	up to 50 mg	IM, IV	J3230
Chlorprothixene	up to 50 mg	IM	J3080
Chlortrimeton, *see* Chlorpheniramine maleate			
Chorex-5, *see* Chorionic gonadotropin			
Chorex-10, *see* Chorionic gonadotropin			

Appendix 3

	Amount	Route of Admin	Code
Chorignon, *see* Chorionic gonadotropin			
Chorionic gonadotropin	per 1000 USP units	IM	J0725
Choron 10, *see* Chorionic gonadotropin			
Cidofovir	375 mg	IV	J0740
Cimetidine HCl	300 mg	INJ	S0023
Cimetidine hydrochloride injection	300 mg	IV, IM	S0023
Cipro I.V., *see* Ciprofloxacin, injection			
Ciprofloxacin, injection	200 mg	IV	S0024
Cilastatin sodium, imipenem	per 250 mg	IV, IM	J0743
Cisplatin, powder or solution	per 10 mg	IV	J9060
Cisplatin	50 mg	IV	J9062
Cladribine	per mg	IV	J9065
Claforan, *see* Cefotaxime sodium			
Cleocin Phosphate, *see* clindamycin phosphate			
Clindamycin phosphate	300 mg	IV, IM	S0077
Clonidine HCl	1 mg	VAR, ORAL	J0735
Cobex, *see* Vitamin B-12 cyanocobalamin			
Codeine phosphate	per 30 mg	IM, IV, SC	J0745
Cogentin, *see* Benztropine mesylate			
Cognex, *see* Tacrine hydrochloride			
Colchicine	per 1 mg	IV	J0760
Colistimethate sodium	up to 150 mg	IM, IV	J0770
Coly-Mycin M, *see* Colistimethate sodium			
Compa-Z, *see* Prochlorperazine			
Compazine, *see* Prochlorperazine			
Cophene-B, *see* Brompheniramine maleate			
Copper contraceptive, intrauterine	—	OTH	J7300
Corgonject-5, *see* Chorionic gonadotropin			
Corticotropin	up to 40 units	IV, IM, SC	J0800
Cortisone acetate, *see* Cortisone			
Cortisone	up to 50 mg	IM	J0810
Cortrosyn, *see* Cosyntropin			

	Amount	Route of Admin	Code
Cosmegen, *see* Dactinomycin			
Cosyntropin	per 0.25 mg	IM, IV	J0835
Cotranzine, *see* Prochlorperazine			
Cromolyn sodium	per 20 mg	INH	J7630
Cromolyn sodium, inhalation solution	10 mg	INH	J7631
Crysticillin 300 A.S., *see* Penicillin G procaine			
Crysticillin 600 A.S., *see* Penicillin G procaine			
Cyclophosphamide	100 mg	IV	J9070
	200 mg	IV	J9080
	500 mg	IV	J9090
	1 g	IV	J9091
	2 g	IV	J9092
Cyclophosphamide, lyophilized	100 mg	IV	J9093
	200 mg	IV	J9094
	500 mg	IV	J9095
	1 g	IV	J9096
	2 g	IV	J9097
Cyclophosphamide, oral	25 mg	ORAL	J8530
Cyclosporine, oral	25 mg	ORAL	J7515
	100 mg	ORAL	J7502
	per 100 mg	ORAL	K0418
	25 mg	ORAL	K0121
Cyclosporine, parenteral	250 mg	IV	J7516
Cytarabine	100 mg	SC, IV	J9100
	500 mg	SC, IV	J9110
Cytarabine liposome, depocyt/liposomal cytarabine (ara-C cytosine arabinoside), Injection	10 mg	SC, IV	C1166
Cytomegalovirus immune globulin intravenous (human)	per vial	IV	J0850
Cytosar-U, *see* Ctarabine liposome			
Cytovene, *see* Ganciclovir sodium			
Cytoxan, *see* Cyclophosphamide; cyclophosphamide, lyophilized; and cyclophosphamide, oral			

Appendix 3

D

	Amount	Route of Admin	Code
D-5-W, infusion	1000 cc	IV	J7070
Dacarbazine	100 mg	IV	J9130
	200 mg	IV	J9140
Daclizumab	25 mg	OTH	J7513
Dactinomycin	0.5 mg	IV	J9120
Dalalone, *see* Dexamethasone sodium phosphate			
Dalalone L.A., *see* Dexamethasone acetate			
Dalteparin Sodium	per 2500 IU	SC	J1645
Daunorubicin citrate, liposomal formula	10 mg	IV	J9151
Daunorubicin HCl	10 mg	IV	J9150
Daunoxome, *see* Daunorubicin citrate			
DDAVP, *see* Desmopressin acetate			
Decadron Phosphate, *see* Dexamethasone sodium phosphate			
Decadron, *see* Dexamethasone sodium phosphate			
Decadron-LA, *see* Dexamethasone acetate			
Deca-Durabolin, *see* Nandrolone decanoate			
Decaject, *see* Dexamethasone sodium phosphate			
Decaject-L.A., *see* Dexamethasone acetate			
Decolone-50, *see* Nandrolone decanoate			
Decolone-100, *see* Nandrolone decanoate			
De-Comberol, *see* Testosterone cypionate and estradiol cypionate			
Deferoxamine mesylate	500 mg per 5 cc	IM, SC, IV	J0895
Dehist, *see* Brompheniramine maleate			
Deladumone OB, *see* Testosterone enanthate and estradiol valerate			
Deladumone, *see* Testosterone enanthate and estradiol valerate			
Delatest, *see* Testosterone enanthate			

	Amount	Route of Admin	Code
Delatestadiol, *see* Testosterone enanthate and estradiol valerate			
Delatestryl, *see* Testosterone enanthate			
Delta-Cortef, *see* Prednisolone, oral			
Delestrogen, *see* Estradiol valerate			
Delta-Cortef, *see* Prednisone			
Deltasone, *see* Prednisone			
Demadex, *see* Torsemide			
Demerol HCl, *see* Meperidine HCl			
Denileukin diftitox	300 mcg	IV	**C1084**
DepAndro 100, *see* Testosterone cypionate			
DepAndro 200, *see* Testosterone cypionate			
DepAndrogyn, *see* Testosterone cypionate and estradiol cypionate			
DepGynogen, *see* Depo-estradiol cypionate			
DepMedalone 40, *see* Methylprednisolone acetate			
DepMedalone 80, *see* Methylprednisolone acetate			
Depo-estradiol cypionate	up to 5 mg	IM	**J1000**
Depogen, *see* Depo-estradiol cypionate			
Depoject, *see* Methyprednisolone acetate			
Depo-Medrol, *see* Methylprednisolone acetate			
Depopred-40, *see* Methylprednisolone acetate			
Depopred-80, *see* Methylprednisolone acetate			
Depo-Provera, *see* Medroxyprogesterone acetate			
Depotest, *see* Testosterone cypionate			
Depo-Testadiol, *see* Testosterone cypionate and estradiol cypionate			
Depotestogen, *see* Testosterone cypionate and estradiol cypionate			
Depo-Testosterone, *see* Testosterone cypionate			

Appendix 3

	Amount	Route of Admin	Code
Desferal Mesylate, *see* Deferoxamine mesylate			
Desmopressin acetate	1 mcg	IV, SC	J2597
Dexacen-4, *see* Dexamethasone sodium phosphate			
Dexamethasone acetate	8 mg per ml	VAR	J1095
Dexamethosone sodium phosphate	1 mg	ORAL	J1100
Dexasone, *see* Dexamethasone sodium phosphate			
Dexasone L.A., *see* Dexamethasone acetate			
Dexone, *see* Dexamethasone sodium phosphate			
Dexone LA, *see* Dexamethasone acetate			
Dexamethasone, inhalation solution, concentrated form	per mg	INH	J7637
Dexamethasone, inhalation solution, unit dose form	per mg	INH	J7638
Dexamethasone sodium phosphate	1 mg	IM, IV, ORAL	J1100
Dexrazoxane HCl	per 250 mg	IV	J1190
Dextran 40	500 ml	IV	J7100
Dextran 75	500 ml	IV	J7110
Dextrose/normal saline solution 5%)	500 ml = 1 unit	IV	J7042
Dextrose/water (5%)	500 ml = 1 unit	IV	J7060
Dextrose 5% and normal saline 45%	1000 ml	IV	S5010
Dextrose 5% in lactated ringer's	1000 ml	IV	S5011
Dextrose 5% with potassium chloride	1000 ml	IV	S5012
Dextrose 5%/45% NS w/ potassium chloride & magnesium sulfate	1000 ml	IV	S5013, S5014
D.H.E. 45, *see* Dihydroergotamine			
Diamox, *see* Acetazolamide sodium			
Diazepam	up to 5 mg	IM, IV	J3360
Diazoxide	up to 300 mg	IV	J1730
Dibent, *see* Dicyclomine HCl			
Dicyclomine HCl	up to 20 mg	IM	J0500
Didronel, *see* Etidronate disodium			

	Amount	Route of Admin	Code
Diethylstilbestrol diphosphate	250 mg	IV	J9165
Diflucan, *see* Fluconazole			
Digoxin	up to 0.5 mg	IM, IV	J1160
Dihydrex, *see* Diphenhydramine HCl			
Dihydroergotamine mesylate	per 1 mg	IM, IV	J1110
Dilantin, *see* Phenytoin sodium			
Dilaudid, *see* Hydromorphone HCl			
Dilocaine, *see* Lidocaine HCl			
Dilomine, *see* Dicyclomine HCl			
Dilor, *see* Dyphylline			
Dimenhydrinate	up to 50 mg	IM, IV	J1240
Dimercaprol	per 100 mg	IM	J0470
Dimethyl sulfoxide, *see* DMSO, Dimethylsulfoxide			
Dinate, *see* Dimenhydrinate			
Dioval, *see* Estradiol valerate			
Dioval 40, *see* Estradiol valerate			
Dioval XX, *see* Estradiol valerate			
Diphenacen-50, *see* Diphenhydramine HCl			
Diphenhydramine HCl	up to 50 mg	IV, IM	J1200
	50 mg	ORAL	Q0163
Dipyridamole	per 10 mg	IV	J1245
Disotate, *see* Endrate ethylenediamine-tetra-acetic acid			
Di-Spaz, *see* Dicyclomine HCl			
Ditate-DS, *see* Testosterone enanthate and estradiol valerate			
Diuril Sodium, *see* Chlorothiazide sodium			
D-Med 80, *see* Methylprednisolone acetate			
DMSO, Dimethyl sulfoxide	50%, 50 ml	OTH	J1212
Dobutamine HCl	per 250 mg	IV	J1250
Dobutrex, *see* Dobutamine HCl			
Docetaxel	20 mg		J9170
Dolasetron mesylate	100 mg	ORAL	Q0180
	10 mg	INJ	J1260
Dolophine HCl, *see* Methadone HCl			

	Amount	Route of Admin	Code
Dommanate, *see* Dimenhydrinate			
Dornase alpha, inhalation solution, unit dose form	per mg	INH	J7639
Doxorubicin HCl	10 mg	IV	J9000
Doxorubicin HCl, all lipid formulations	10 mg		J9001
Dramamine, *see* Dimenhydrinate			
Dramanate, *see* Dimenhydrinate			
Dramilin, *see* Dimenhydrinate			
Dramocen, *see* Dimenhydrinate			
Dramoject, *see* Dimenhydrinate			
Dronabinol	2.5 mg	ORAL	Q0167
	5 mg	ORAL	Q0168
Droperidol	up to 5 mg	IM, IV	J1790
Drug administered through a metered dose inhaler	—	INH	J3535
Droperidol and fentanyl citrate	up to 2 ml ampule	IM, IV	J1810
DTIC-Dome, *see* Dacarbazine			
Dua-Gen L.A., *see* Testosterone enanthate and estradiol valerate cypionate			
Duoval P.A., *see* Testosterone enanthate and estradiol valerate			
Durabolin, *see* Nandrolone phenpropionate			
Dura-Estrin, *see* Depo-estradiol cypionate			
Duracillin A.S., *see* Penicillin G procaine			
Duragen-10, *see* Estradiol valerate			
Duragen-20, *see* Estradiol valerate			
Duragen-40, *see* Estradiol valerate			
Duralone-40, *see* Methylprednisolone acetate			
Duralone-80, *see* Methylprednisolone acetate			
Duralutin, *see* Hydroxyprogesterone Caproate			
Duramorph, *see* Morphine sulfate			
Duratest-100, *see* Testosterone cypionate			
Duratest-200, *see* Testosterone cypionate			

	Amount	Route of Admin	Code
Duratestrin, *see* Testosterone cypionate and estradiol cypionate			
Durathate-200, *see* Testosterone enanthate			
Dymenate, *see* Dimenhydrinate			
Dyphylline	up to 500 mg	IM	J1180

E

	Amount	Route of Admin	Code
Edetate calcium disodium	up to 1000 mg	IV, SC, IM	J0600
Edetate Disodium		IV	
Elavil, *see* Amitriptyline HCl			
Ellence, *see* Epirubicin hydrochloride			
Elspar, *see* Asparaginase			
Eminase, *see* Anistreplase			
Emete-Con, *see* Benzquinamide			
Endrate ethylenediamine-tetra-acetic acid EDTA	—	IV	J3520
Enovil, *see* Amitriptyline HCl			
Enoxaparin sodium,	10 mg	SC	J1650
Epinephrine, adrenalin	up to 1 ml amp	SC, IM	J0170
Epinephrine, via DME	2.25%, per ml	INH	J7640
Epirubicin hydrochloride injection	2 mg	IV	C1167
Epoetin alpha, for non-ESRD use	per 1000 units	IV, SC	Q0136
Epoetin alpha, EPO for chronic renal failure, based on HCT, injection	Per 1000 units	IV, SC	Q9920–Q9940
Epoetin Alpha (Non-ESRD use) injection	Per 1000 units	IV, SC	Q0136
Epogen, *see* Epoetin alpha			
Epoprostenol	0.5 mg	IV	J1325
Eptifibatide	5 mg	INJ	J1327
Ergonovine maleate	up to 0.2 mg	IM, IV	J1330
Erythromycin gluceptate	250 mg	IV	J1362
Erythromycin lactobionate	500 mg	IV	J1364
Estra-D, *see* Depo-estradiol cypionate			
Estra-L 20, *see* Estradiol valerate			
Estra-L 40, *see* Estradiol valerate			

Appendix 3

	Amount	Route of Admin	Code
Estra-Testrin, *see* Testosterone enanthate and estradiol valerate			
Estradiol Cypionate, *see* Depo-estradiol cypionate			
Estradiol L.A., *see* Estradiol valerate			
Estradiol L.A. 20, *see* Estradiol valerate			
Estradiol L.A. 40, *see* Estradiol valerate			
Estradiol valerate	up to 10 mg	IM	J1380
	up to 20 mg	IM	J1390
	up to 40 mg	IM	J0970
Estro-Cyp, *see* Depo-estradiol cypionate			
Estrogen, conjugated	per 25 mg	IV, IM	J1410
Estroject L.A., *see* Depo-estradiol cypionate			
Estrone	per 1 mg	IM	J1435
Estrone 5, *see* Estrone			
Estrone Aqueous, *see* Estrone			
Estronol, *see* Estrone			
Estronol-L.A., *see* Depo-estradiol cypionate			
Etanercept	25 mg	INJ	J1438
Ethylnorepinephrine HCl	1 ml	SC, IM	J0590
Etidronate disodium	per 300 mg	IV	J1436
Etoposide	10 mg	IV	J9181
	100 mg	IV	J9182
Etoposide, oral	50 mg	ORAL	J8560
Everone, *see* Testosterone Enanthate			
Exemestane	25 mg	ORAL	S0156

F

	Amount	Route of Admin	Code
Factor, hemophilia clotting, not otherwise specified		INJ	J7199
Factor VIIIa (coagulation-factor, recombinant)	per 1.2 mg	IV	Q0187
Factor VIII	per IU	IV	J7190
Factor VIII (anti-hemophilic factor (porcine))	per IU	IV	J7191
Factor VIII, recombinant	per IU	IV	J7192

	Amount	Route of Admin	Code
Factor IX, complex	per IU	IV	J7194
Factor IX, non-recombinant	per IU		Q0160
Factor IX, recombinant	per IU		Q0161
Factrel, *see* Gonadorelin HCl			
Famotidine, injection	20 mg	IV	S0028
Fat emulsion 10%, with administration set	250 ml	IV	S5002
Fat emulsion 20%, with administration set	250 ml	IV	S5003
Feiba VH Immuno, *see* Factors, other hemophilia clotting			
Fentanyl citrate	up to 2 ml	IM, IV	J3010
Feostat, *see* Iron dextran			
Feronim, *see* Iron dextran			
Filgrastim (G-CSF)	300 mcg	SC, IV	J1440
	480 mcg	SC, IV	J1441
Flagyl IV RTU, *see* Metronidazole injection			
Flexoject, *see* Orphenadrine citrate			
Flexon, *see* Orphenadrine citrate			
Floxin IV, *See* Ofloxacin			
Fluconazole	200 mg	IV	J1450
	400 mg	IV	S0029
Floxuridine	500 mg	IV	J9200
Fludara, *see* Fludarabine phosphate			
Fludarabine phosphate	50 mg	IV	J9185
Fluorouracil	500 mg	IV	J9190
Fluphenazine decanoate	up to 25 mg	IM, SC	J2680
Folex, *see* Methotrexate sodium			
Folex PFS, *see* Methotrexate sodium			
Follutein, *see* Chorionic gonadotropin			
Fortaz, *see* Ceftazidime			
Foscarnet sodium	per 1000 mg	IV	J1455
Foscavir, *see* Foscarnet sodium			
Fosphenytoin sodium	750 mg	IV, IM	S0078
Fragmin, *see* Dalteparin			
FUDR, *see* Floxuridine			
Furomide M.D., *see* Furosemide			
Furosemide	up to 20 mg	IM, IV	J1940

Appendix 3

G

	Amount	Route of Admin	Code
Gamma globulin	1 cc	IM	J1460
	2 cc	IM	J1470
	3 cc	IM	J1480
	4 cc	IM	J1490
	5 cc	IM	J1500
	6 cc	IM	J1510
	7 cc	IM	J1520
	8 cc	IM	J1530
	9 cc	IM	J1540
	10 cc	IM	J1550
	over 10 cc	IM	J1560
Gamulin RH, see Rho(D) immune globulin			
Ganciclovir	4.5 mg	OTH	J7310
Ganciclovir sodium	500 mg	IV	J1570
Ganisetron HCl	1 mg	ORAL	Q0166
Garamycin, gentamicin	up to 80 mg	IM, IV	J1580
Gatifloxacin, injection	200 mg	IV	S0085
Gemcitabine HCl	200 mg		J9201
Gemtuzumab ozogramicin, injection	5 mg	IV	C9004
Gemzar, See Gemtuzumab ozogramicin injection			
GenESA, see Arbutumine HCL			
Gentamicin Sulfate, see Garamycin, gentamicin			
Gentran, see Dextran 40			
Gentran 75, see Dextran 75			
Gesterol 50, see Progesterone			
Gesterol L.A. 250, see Hydroxyprogesterone Caproate			
Glucagon HCl	per 1 mg	SC, IM, IV	J1610
Glukor, see Chorionic gonadotropin			
Glycopyrrolate, inhalation solution, concentrated form	per mg	INH	J7642
Glycopyrrolate, inhalation solution, unit dose form	per mg	INH	J7643
Gold sodium thiomalate	up to 50 mg	IM	J1600
Gonadorelin HCl	per 100 mcg	SC, IV	J1620

	Amount	Route of Admin	Code
Gonic, *see* Chorionic gonadotropin			
Goserelin acetate implant	per 3.6 mg	SC	J9202
Granisetron HCl	1 mg	ORAL	Q0166
	100 mcg	IV	J1626
Growth Hormone therapy (e.g., protropin, humatrope)	5 mg to 10 mg vial	IM, SQ	S5022
Gynogen L.A. "10," *see* Estradiol valerate			
Gynogen L.A. "20," *see* Estradiol valerate			
Gynogen L.A. "40," *see* Estradiol valerate			

H

	Amount	Route of Admin	Code
H-BIG, *see* Hepatitis B immune globulin	per 1 mg	IM	C9105
Haldol, *see* Haloperidol			
Haloperidol	up to 5 mg	IM, IV	J1630
Haloperidol decanoate	per 50 mg	IM	J1631
Hematran, *see* Iron dextran			
Hemofil M, *see* Factor VIII			
Hemophilia clotting factors (e.g., anti-inhibitors), other	per IU	IV	J7196
Hep-Lock, *see* Heparin sodium (heparin lock flush)			
Hep-Lock U/P, *see* Heparin sodium (heparin lock flush)			
Heparin sodium	1000 units	IV, SC	J1644
Heparin sodium (heparin lock flush)	10 units	IV	J1642
Hepatitis B immune globulin injection	per 1 mg	IM, SQ	S5022
Hexadrol Phosphate, *see* Dexamethasone sodium phosphate			
Histaject, *see* Brompheniramine maleate			
Histerone 50, *see* Testosterone suspension			
Histerone 100, *see* Testosterone suspension			
Humatrope, *see* Somatropin			
Hyaluronidase	up to 150 units	SC, IV	J3470

Appendix 3

	Amount	Route of Admin	Code
Hybolin Improved, *see* Nandrolone phenpropionate			
Hybolin Decanoate, *see* Nandrolone decanoate			
Hydeltra-T.B.A., *see* Prednisolone tebutate			
Hydeltrasol, *see* Prednisolone sodium phosphate			
Hydextran, *see* Iron dextran			
Hydralazine HCl	up to 20 mg	IV, IM	J0360
Hydrate, *see* Dimenhydrinate			
Hydrochlorides of opium alkaloids	up to 20 mg	IM, SC	J2480
Hydrocortisone acetate	up to 25 mg	IV, IM, SC	J1700
Hydrocortisone sodium phosphate	up to 50 mg	IV, IM, SC	J1710
Hydrocortisone succinate sodium	up to 100 mg	IV, IM, SC	J1720
Hydrocortone Acetate, *see* Hydrocortisone acetate			
Hydrocortone Phosphate, *see* Hydrocortisone sodium phosphate			
Hydromorphone HCl	up to 4 mg	SC, IM, IV	J1170
Hydroxyprogesterone caproate	25 mg/ml	IM	J1739
	250 mg/ml	IM	J1741
Hydroxyzine HCl	up to 25 mg	IM	J3410
Hydroxyzine pamoate	25 mg	ORAL	Q0177
	50 mg	ORAL	Q0178
Hylan G-F 20	16 mg	OTH	J7320
Hylutin, *see* Hydroxyprogesterone Caproate			
Hyoscyamine sulfate	up to 0.25 mg	SC, IM, IV	J1980
Hyper-Hep, *see* Hepatitis B immune globulin			
Hyperstat IV, *see* Diazoxide			
Hyprogest 250, *see* Hydroxyprogesterone caproate			
Hyrexin-50, *see* Diphenhydramine HCl			
Hyzine-50, *see* Hydroxyzine HCl			

	Amount	Route of Admin	Code
I			
Ibutilide fumarate	1 mg	INJ	S0097
Idamycin, *see* Idarubicin HCl			
Idarubicin HCl	5 mg	IV	J9211
Ibutilide fumarate	1 mg		J1742
Ifex, *see* Ifosfamide			
Ifosfamide	per 1 g	IV	J9208
IL-2, *see* Aldesleukin			
Ilotycin, *see* Erythromycin gluceptate			
Imfergen, *see* Iron dextran			
Imferon, *see* Iron dextran			
Imiglucerase	per unit	IV	J1785
Imipramine HCl	up to 25 mg	IM	J3270
Imitrex, *see* Sumatriptan succinate			
Immune globulin	per 500 mg	IV	J1561
Immune globulin intravenous (human) 10%	5 g	IV	J1562
Immunosuppressive drug, not otherwise classified			J7599
Imuran, *see* Azathioprine			
Inapsine, *see* Droperidol			
Infed			
Infliximab	10 mg	INJ	J1745
Inderal, *see* Propranolol HCl			
Innohep, *see* Tinzaparin sodium injection			
Innovar, *see* Droperidol with fentanyl citrate			
Insulin	up to 100 units	SC	J1820
Intal, *see* Cromolyn sodium or Cromolyn sodium, compounded			
Interferon alfa-2a, recombinant	3 million units	SC, IM	J9213
Interferon alfa-2b, recombinant	1 million units	SC, IM	J9214
Interferon alfa-n3 (human leukocyte derived)	250,000 IU	IM	J9215
Interferon alfacon-1, recombinant	1 mcg	IM	J9212
Interferon beta 1a	33 mcg	IM	J1825
Interferon beta-1b	0.25 mg	SC	J1830
Interferon gamma-1b	3 million units	SC	J9216

Appendix 3

	Amount	Route of Admin	Code
Intrauterine copper contraceptive, *see* Copper contraceptive, intrauterine			
Ipratropium bromide 0.2%	per ml	INH	J7645
Ipratropium bromide, inhalation solution, unit dose form	per mg	INH	J0518
Irinotecan	20 mg		J9206
Irodex, *see* Iron dextran			
Iron dextran	50 mg	INJ	J1750
Isocaine HCl, *see* Mepivacaine			
Isoetharine HCl	0.1% per ml	INH	J7650
	0.125% per ml	INH	J7651
	0.167% per ml	INH	J7652
	0.2% per ml	INH	J7653
	0.25% per ml	INH	J7654
	1.0% per ml	INH	J7655
Isoetharine HCl, inhalation solution, concentrated form	per mg	INH	J7648
Isoetharine HCl, inhalation solution, unit dose form	per mg	INH	J7649
Isoproterenol HCl	0.5% per ml	INH	J7660
	1.0%, per ml	INH	J7665
Isoproterenol HCl, inhalation solution, concentrated form	per mg	INH	J7658
Isoproterenol HCl, inhalation solution, unit dose form	per mg	INH	J7659
Isuprel, *see* Isoproterenol HCl			
Itraconazole injection	200 mg	ORAL	**S0096**

J

Jenamicin, *see* Garamycin, gentamicin

K

Kabikinase, *see* Streptokinase

	Amount	Route of Admin	Code
Kanamycin sulfate	up to 75 mg	IM, IV	**J1850**
Kanamycin sulfate	up to 500 mg	IM, IV	**J1840**
Kantrex, *see* Kanamycin sulfate			

	Amount	Route of Admin	Code
Keflin, *see* Cephalothin sodium			
Kefurox, *see* Cufuroxime sodium			
Kefzol, *see* Cefazolin sodium			
Kenaject-40, *see* Triamcinolone acetonide			
Kenalog-10, *see* Triamcinolone acetonide			
Kenalog-40, *see* Triamcinolone acetonide			
Kestrone 5, *see* Estrone			
Ketorolac tromethamine	per 15 mg	IM, IV	J1885
Key-Pred 25, *see* Prednisolone acetate			
Key-Pred 50, *see* Prednisolone acetate			
Key-Pred-SP, *see* Prednisolone sodium phosphate			
K-Feron, *see* Iron dextran			
K-Flex, *see* Orphenadrine citrate			
Klebcil, *see* Kanamycin sulfate			
Koate-HP, *see* Factor VIII			
Kogenate, *see* Factor VIII			
Konakion, *see* Phytonadione			
Konyne-80, *see* Factor IX, complex			
Kutapressin	up to 2 ml	SC, IM	J1910

L

	Amount	Route of Admin	Code
L.A.E. 20, *see* Estradiol valerate			
Laetrile, Amygdalin, vitamin B-17	—	—	J3570
Lanoxin, *see* Digoxin			
Largon, *see* Propiomazine HCl			
Lasix, *see* Furosemide			
L-Caine, *see* Lidocaine HCl			
Leucovorin calcium	per 50 mg	IM, IV	J0640
Leukine, *see* Sargramostim (GM-CSF)			
Leuprolide acetate (for depot suspension)	3.75 mg	IM	J1950
	7.5 mg	IM	J9217
Leuprolide acetate	per 1 mg	IM	J9218
Leustatin, *see* Cladribine			

	Amount	Route of Admin	Code
Levaquin, *see* Levofloxacin			
Levocarnitine	per 1 gm	IV	**J1955**
Levo-Dromoran, *see* Levorphanol tartrate			
Levofloxacin	250 mg	IV	**J1956**
Levoprome, *see* Methotrimeprazine			
Levorphanol tartrate	up to 2 mg	SC, IV	**J1960**
Levsin, *see* Hyoscyamine sulfate			
Librium, *see* Chlordiazepoxide HCl			
Lidocaine HCl	50 cc	VAR	**J2000**
Lidoject-1, *see* Lidocaine HCl			
Lidoject-2, *see* Lidocaine HCl			
Lincocin, *see* Lincomycin HCl			
Lincomycin HCl	up to 300 mg	IV	**J2010**
Linezolid, injection	per 200 mg	IV	**C9001**
Liquaemin Sodium, *see* Heparin sodium			
Lioresal, *see* Baclofen			
Lioresal Intrathecal, *see* Baclofen intrathecal			
LMD (10%), *see* Dextran 40			
Lovenox, *see* Enoxaparin sodium			
Lorazepam	2 mg	IM, IV	**J2060**
Lufyllin, *see* Dyphylline			
Luminal Sodium	up to 120 mg	IM, IV	**J2560**
Lupron, *see* Leuprolide acetate			
Lymphocyte immune globulin, anti-thymocyte globulin	50 mg/ml, 5 ml ea	IV	**J7504**
	250 mg	IV	**K0123**
Lymphocyte immune globulin anti-thymocyte globulin (equine) ATG, LIG	per 25 mg	IV	**C9104**
Lyophilized, *see* Cyclophosphamide lyophilized			

M

	Amount	Route of Admin	Code
Magnesium sulfate	500 mg	IM, IV	**J3475**
Mannitol	25% in 50 ml	IV	**J2150**

	Amount	Route of Admin	Code
Marcaine, *see* Bupivicaine hydrochloride injection			
Marmine, *see* Dimenhydrinate			
Mechlorethamine HCl (nitrogen mustard), HN2	10 mg	IV	J9230
Medralone 40, *see* Methylprednisolone acetate			
Medralone 80, *see* Methylprednisolone acetate			
Medrol, *see* Methylprednisolone			
Medroxyprogesterone acetate	100 mg	IM	J1050
	150 mg	IM	J1055
Mefoxin, *see* Cefoxitin sodium			
Melphalan HCl	50 mg	IV	J9245
Melphalan, oral	2 mg	ORAL	J8600
Menoject LA, *see* Testosterone cypionate and estradiol cypionate			
Mepergan Injection, *see* Meperdine and promethazine HCl			
Meperidine HCl	per 100 mg	IM, IV, SC	J2175
Meperidine and promethazine HCl	up to 50 mg	IM, IV	J2180
Mephentermine sulfate	up to 30 mg	IM, IV	J3450
Mepivacaine	per 10 ml	VAR	J0670`
Mesna	200 mg	IV	J9209
Mesnex, *see* Mesna			
Metaprel, *see* Metaproterenol sulfate			
Metaproterenol, inhalation solution, concentrated form	per 10 mg	INH	J7668
Metaproterenol, inhalation solution, unit dose form	per 10 mg	INH	J7669
Metaproterenol sulfate	0.4%, per 2.5 ml	INH	J7670
	0.6%, per 2.5 ml	INH	J7672
	5.0%, per ml	INH	J7675
Metaraminol bitartrate	per 10 mg	IV, IM, SC	J0380
Methadone HCl	up to 10 mg	IM, SC	J1230
Methergine, *see* Methylergonovine maleate			
Methicillin sodium	up to 1 g	IM, IV	J2970
Methocarbamol	up to 10 ml	IV, IM	J2800
Methotrexate, oral	2.5 mg	ORAL	J8610

	Amount	Route of Admin	Code
Methotrexate sodium	5 mg	IV, IM, IT, IA	J9250
	50 mg	IV, IM, IT, IA	J9260
Methotrexate LPF, *see* Methotrexate sodium			
Methotrimeprazine	up to 20 mg	IM	J1970
Methoxamine HCl	up to 20 mg	IM, IV	J3390
Methyldopate HCl	up to 250 mg	IV	J0210
Methylergonovine maleate	up to 0.2 mg		J2210
Methylprednisolone, oral	per 4 mg	ORAL	J7509
Methylprednisolone acetate	20 mg	IM	J1020
	40 mg	IM	J1030
	80 mg	IM	J1040
Methylprednisolone sodium succinate	up to 40 mg	IM, IV	J2920
	up to 125 mg	IM, IV	J2930
Metoclopramide HCl	up to 10 mg	IV	J2765
Metronidazole injection	500 mg	IV	S0030
Metocurine iodide	up to 2 mg	IV	J2240
Metubine iodine, *see* Metocurine iodide			
Miacalcin, *see* Calcitonin-salmon			
Midazolam HCl	per 1 mg	IM, IV	J2250
Milrinone lactate	5 mg	IV	J2260
Mithracin, *see* Plicamycin			
Mitomycin	5 mg	IV	J9280
	20 mg	IV	J9290
	40 mg	IV	J9291
Mitoxantrone HCl	per 5 mg	IV	J9293
Monarc-M, *see* Factor VIII			
Monocid, *see* Cefonicic sodium			
Monoclate-P, *see* Factor VIII			
Monoclonal antibodies, parenteral	amp, 5 mg/5 ml, 5 ml ea	IV	J7505
Morphine sulfate	up to 10 mg	IM, IV, SC	J2270
	100 mg	IT, IV, SC	J2271
Morphine sulfate, preservative-free	per 10 mg	SC, IM, IV	J2275
M-Prednisol-40, *see* Methylprednisolone acetate			
M-Prednisol-80, *see* Methylprednisolone acetate			

	Amount	Route of Admin	Code
Mucomyst, *see* Acetylcysteine or Acetylcysteine, compounded			
Mucosol, *see* Acetylcysteine			
Mustargen, *see* Mechlorethamine HCl			
Mutamycin, *see* Mitomycin			
Mycophenolate mofetil	250 mg	ORAL	J7517
Myleran, *see* Busulfan (busulfex IV) injection			
Myochrysine, *see* Gold sodium thiomalate			
Myolin, *see* Orphenadrine citrate			

N

	Amount	Route of Admin	Code
Nafcillin sodium, injection	2 g	IV, IM	S0032
Nalbuphine HCl	per 10 mg	IM, IV, SC	J2300
Nallpen, Unipen , *see* Nafcillin sodium injection			
Naloxone HCl	per 1 mg	IM, IV, SC	J2310
Nandrobolic, *see* Nandrolone phenpropionate			
Nandrobolic L.A., *see* Nandrolone decanoate			
Nandrolone decanoate	up to 50 mg	IM	J2320
	up to 100 mg	IM	J2321
	up to 200 mg	IM	J2322
Nandrolone phenpropionate	up to 50 mg	IM	J0340
Narcan, *see* Naloxone HCl			
Nasahist B, *see* Brompheniramine maleate			
Nasal vaccine inhalation	—	INH	J3530
Navane, *see* Thiothixene			
Navelbine, *see* Vinorelbine tartrate			
ND Stat, *see* Brompheniramine maleate			
Nebcin, *see* Tobramycin sulfate			
NebuPent, *see* Pentamidine isethionate			
Nembutal Sodium Solution, *see* Pentobarbital sodium			
Neocyten, *see* Orphenadrine citrate			

Appendix 3

	Amount	Route of Admin	Code
Neo-Durabolic, *see* Nandrolone decanoate			
Neoquess, *see* Dicyclomine HCl			
Neoral, *see* Cyclosporine, for microemulsion			
Neosar, *see* Cyclophosphamide			
Neostigmine methylsulfate	up to 0.5 mg	IM, IV, SC	J2710
Neo-Synephrine, *see* Phenylephrine HCl			
Neupogen, *see* Filgrastim (G-CSF)			
Neutrexin, *see* Trimetrexate glucuronate			
Nervocaine 1%, *see* Lidocaine HCl			
Nervocaine 2%, *see* Lidocaine HCl			
Nesacaine, *see* Chloroprocaine HCl			
Nesacaine-MPF, *see* Chloroprocaine HCl			
Niacinamide, niacin	up to 100 mg	IV, SC, IM	J2350
Nicotinic Acid, *see* Niacinamide, niacin			
Nicotinamide, *see* Niacinamide, niacin			
Nipent, *see* Pentostatin			
Norditropin, *see* Somatropin			
Nordryl, *see* Diphenhydramine HCl			
Nor-Feran, *see* Iron dextran			
Norflex, *see* Orphenadrine citrate			
Norzine, *see* Thiethylperazine maleate			
Not otherwise classified drugs	—	—	J3490
	—	other than INH	J7799
	—	INH	J7699
Not otherwise classified drugs, anti-emetic	—	ORAL	Q0181
Not otherwise classified drugs, anti-neoplastic	—	—	J9999
Not otherwise classified drugs, chemotherapeutic	—	ORAL	J8999
Not otherwise classified drugs, immunosuppressive	—	—	J7599

	Amount	Route of Admin	Code
Not otherwise classified drugs, nonchemotherapeutic	—	ORAL	J8499

Novantrone, *see* Mitoxantrone HCl

NPH, *see* Insulin

Nubain, *see* Nalbuphine HCl

Nulicaine, *see* Lidocaine HCl

Numorphan, *see* Oxymorphone HCl

Numorphan H.P., *see* Oxymorphone HCl

Nutropin, *see* Somatropin

Nutropin AQ, *see* Somatropin

O

	Amount	Route of Admin	Code
Octreotide acetate	1 mg	SC	C1207, J2352
Oculinum, *see* Botulinum toxin type A			
Odansetron HCl	1 mg	IV	J2405
Ofloxacin, injection	400 mg	IV	S0034
O-Flex, *see* Orphenadrine citrate			
Omnipen-N, *see* Ampicillin			
Oncaspar, *see* Pegaspargase			
Oncovin, *see* Vincristine sulfate			
Ondansetron HCl	8 mg	ORAL	Q0179
Ontak, IV, *see* Denileukin diftitox			
Oprelvekin	5mg	INJ	J2355
Oraminic II, *see* Brompheniramine maleate			
Ormazine, *see* Chlorpromazine HCl			
Orphenadrine citrate	up to 60 mg	IV, IM	J2360
Orphenate, *see* Orphenadrine citrate			
Or-Tyl, *see* Dicyclomine			
Oxacillin sodium	up to 250 mg	IM, IV	J2700
Oxymorphone HCl	up to 1 mg	IV, SC, IM	J2410
Oxytetracycline HCl	up to 50 mg	IM	J2460
Oxytocin	up to 10 units	IV, IM	J2590

© 2000 Ingenix Publishing Group

P

	Amount	Route of Admin	Code
Paclitaxel	30 mg	IV	J9265
Palivizumab-RSV-IGM	50 mg	IM	C9003
Pamidronate disodium	per 30 mg	IV	J2430
Panglobulin, *see* Immune globulin intravenous			
Pantopon, *see* Hydrochlorides of opium alkaloids			
Papaverine HCl	up to 60 mg	IV, IM	J2440
Paricalcitrol	5 mcg	INJ	J2500
Paragard T 380 A, *see* Copper contraceptive, intrauterine			
Paraplatin, *see* Carboplatin			
Pegaspargase	per single dose vial	IM, IV	J9266
Peg-L-asparaginase, *see* Pegaspargase			
Penicillin G benzathine	up to 600,000 units	IM	J0560
	up to 1,200,000 units	IM	J0570
	up to 2,400,000 units	IM	J0580
Penicillin G benzathine and penicillin G procaine	up to 600,000 units	IM	J0530
	up to 1,200,000 units	IM	J0540
	up to 2,400,000 units	IM	J0550
Penicillin G potassium	up to 600,000 units	IM, IV	J2540
Penicillin G procaine, aqueous	up to 600,000 units	IM	J2510
Pentacarinat, *see* Pentamidine isethionate			
Pentagastrin	per 2 ml	SC	J2512
Pentam 300, *see* Pentamidine isethionate			
Pentamidine isethionate	per 300 mg	INH	J2545
	per 300 mg	IV, IM	S0080, S0081
Pentazocine HCl	up to 30 mg	IM, SC, IV	J3070
Pentobarbital sodium	per 50 mg	IM, IV	J2515
Pentostatin	per 10 mg	IV	J9268
Pepcid, *see* Famotidine injection			
Peptavlon, *see* Pentagastrin			

	Amount	Route of Admin	Code
Perfluoron	per 2 ml	INJ	C8890
	per 5 ml or 7 ml vial	INJ	C8891
Permapen, *see* Penicillin G benzathine			
Perphenazine	up to 5 mg	IM, IV	J3310
	4 mg	ORAL	Q0175
	8 mg	ORAL	Q0176
Persantine IV, *see* Dipyridamole			
Pfizerpen, *see* Penicillin G potassium			
Pfizerpen A.S., *see* Penicillin G procaine			
PGE₁, *see* Alprostadil			
Phenazine 25, *see* Promethazine HCl			
Phenazine 50, *see* Promethazine HCl			
Phenergan, *see* Promethazine HCl			
Phenobarbital sodium	up to 120 mg	IM, IV	J2560
Phentolamine mesylate	up to 5 mg	IM, IV	J2760
Phenylephrine HCl	up to 1 ml	SC, IM, IV	J2370
Phenytoin sodium	per 50 mg	IM, IV	J1165
Phytonadione	per 1mg	IM, SC, IV	J3430
Piperacillin sodium	500 mg	INJ	S0081
Piperacillin sodium/tazobactam sodium	1.125 g	INJ	J2543
Pitocin, *see* Oxytocin			
Plantinol AQ, *see* Cisplatin			
Platinol, *see* Cisplatin			
Plicamycin	2,500 mcg	IV	J9270
Polocaine, *see* Mepivacaine			
Polycillin-N, *see* Ampicillin			
Porfimer sodium	75 mg		J9600
Potassium chloride	per 2 mEq	IV	J3480
Pralidoxime chloride	up to 1 g	IV, IM, SC	J2730
Predalone T.B.A., *see* Prednisolone tebutate			
Predalone-50, *see* Prednisolone acetate			
Predcor-25, *see* Prednisolone acetate			
Predcor-50, *see* Prednisolone acetate			
Predicort-50, *see* Prednisolone acetate			

Appendix 3

	Amount	Route of Admin	Code
Prednisone	any dose, 100 tabl	ORAL	J7506
	tab, 5 mg	ORAL	K0125
Prednisol TBA, *see* Prednisolone tebutate			
Prednisolone, oral	5 mg	ORAL	J7510
Prednisolone acetate	up to 1 ml	IM	J2650
Prednisolone sodium phosphate	up to 20 mg	IV, IM	J2640
Prednisolone tebutate	up to 20 mg	VAR	J1690
Predoject-50, *see* Prednisolone acetate			
Pregnyl, *see* Chorionic gonadotropin			
Premarin Intravenous, *see* Estrogen, conjugated			
Prescription, anti-emetic, for use in conjunction with oral anti-cancer drug NOS		ORAL, OTH	K0415
Prescription, chemotherapeutic, not otherwise specified	—	ORAL	J8999
Prescription drug, brand name			S5001
Prescription drug, generic			S5000
Prescription, nonchemotherapeutic, not otherwise specified	—	ORAL	J8999
Primacor, *see* Milrinone lactate			
Primaxin I.M., *see* Cilastatin sodium, imipenem			
Primaxin I.V., *see* Cilastatin sodium,z imipenem			
Priscoline HCl, *see* Tolazoline HCl			
Pro-Depo, *see* Hydroxyprogesterone Caproate			
Procainamide HCl	up to 1 g	IM, IV	J2690
Prochlorperazine	up to 10 mg	IM, IV	J0780
Prochlorperazine maleate	10 mg	ORAL	Q0165
	5 mg	ORAL	Q0164
Procrit, *see* Epoetin alpha			
Profasi HP, *see* Chorionic gonadotropin			
Proferdex, *see* Iron dextran			
Profilnine Heat-Treated, *see* Factor IX			
Progestaject, *see* Progesterone			
Progesterone	per 50 mg	IM	J2675
Prograf, *see* tacrolimus, injection			

	Amount	Route of Admin	Code
Prograf, *see* Tacrolimus, oral and parenteral			
Prokine, *see* Sargramostim (GM-CSF)			
Prolastin, *see* Alpha 1-proteinase inhibitor, human			
Proleukin, *see* Aldesleukin			
Prolixin Decanoate, *see* Fluphenazine decanoate			
Promazine HCl	up to 25 mg	IM	J2950
Promethazine HCl	12.5 mg	ORAL	Q0169
	25 mg	ORAL	Q0170
	up to 50 mg	IM, IV	J2550
Pronestyl, *see* Procainamide HCl			
Propiomazine HCl	up to 20 mg	IV, IM	J1930
Proplex T, *see* Factor IX			
Proplex SX-T, *see* Factor IX			
Propranolol HCl	up to 1 mg	IV	J1800
Prorex-25, *see* Promethazine HCl			
Prorex-50, *see* Promethazine HCl			
Prostaglandin E$_1$, *see* Alprostadil			
Prostaphlin, *see* Procainamide HCl			
Prostigmin, *see* Neostigmine methylsulfate			
Prostin VR Pediatric, *see* Alprostadil			
Protamine sulfate	per 10 mg	IV	J2720
Protirelin	per 250 mcg	IV	J2725
Prothazine, *see* Promethazine HCl			
Protopam Chloride, *see* Pralidoxime chloride			
Protropin, *See* Somatrem			
Proventil, *see* Albuterol sulfate, compounded			
Prozine-50, *see* Promazine HCl			

Q

Quelicin, *see* Succinylcholine chloride

Appendix 3

R

	Amount	Route of Admin	Code
Rantidine HCl	25 mg	INJ	J2780
Rapamune, *see* Sirolimus			
Recombinate, *see* Factor VIII			
Redisol, *see* Vitamin B-12 cyanocobalamin			
Regitine, *see* Phentolamine mesylate			
Reglan, *see* Metoclopramide HCl			
Regranex Gel, *see* Becaplermin gel			
Regular, *see* Insulin			
Relefact TRH, *see* Protirelin			
Rep-Pred 40, *see* Methylprednisolone acetate			
Rep-Pred 80, *see* Methylprednisolone acetate			
Respiratory syncytial virus immune globulin	50 mg	IV	J1565
Retavase, *see* Retaplase			
Reteplase	37.6 mg	IV	J2994
Reteplase, injection	18.8 mg	IV	C9005
Retravase, *see* Reteplase, injection			
Rheomacrodex, *see* Dextran 40			
Rhesonativ, *see* Rho(D) immune globulin, human			
Rheumatrex Dose Pack, *see* Methotrexate, oral			
Rho(D) immune globulin	100 IU	IV	J2792
Rho(D) immune globulin, human	1 dose package	IM	J2790
RhoGAM, *see* Rho(D) immune globulin, human			
Ringer's lactate infusion	up to 1000 cc	IV	J7120
Rituximab	100 mg		J9310
Robaxin, *see* Methocarbamol			
Rocephin, *see* Ceftriaxone sodium			
Roferon-A, *see* Interferon alfa-2A, recombinant			
Rubex, *see* Doxorubicin HCl			
Rubramin PC, *see* Vitamin B-12 cyanocobalamin			

S

	Amount	Route of Admin	Code
Saizen, *see* Somatropin			
Saline hypertonic solution	50 or 100 meq, 20 cc vial	IV, IM	J7130
Saline solution	5% dextrose, 500 ml	IV	J7042
	infusion, 250 cc	IV	J7050
	infusion, 1000 cc	IV	J7030
Saline solution, sterile	500 ml = 1 unit	IV, OTH	J7040
	up to 5 cc	IV, OTH	J7051
Sandimmune, *see* Cyclosporine			
Sandostatin, *see* Octreotide acetate			
Sargramostim (GM-CSF)	50 mcg	IV	J2820
Secobarbital sodium	up to 250 mg	IM, IV	J2860
Seconal, *see* Secobarbital sodium			
Sensorcaine, *see* Bupivicaine hydrochloride injection			
Septra IV, *see* Sulfamethoxazole and trimethoprim, injection			
Serostim, *see* Somatropin			
Sildenafil citrate	25 mg	ORAL	S0090
Selestoject, *see* Betamethasone sodium phosphate			
Sinusol-B, *see* Brompheniramine maleate			
Sirolimus	per 1 mg/ml	ORAL	C9106
SMZ-TMP, *see* Sulfamethoxazole and trimethoprim, injection			
Sodium chloride, 0.9%	per 2 ml	IV	J2912
Sodium ferric gluconate complex in sucrose	62.5 mg	INJ	S0098
Sodium hyaluronate	20 mg	OTH	J7315
Solganal, *see* Aurothioglucose			
Solu-Cortef, *see* Hydrocortisone sodium phosphate			
Solu-Medrol, *see* Methylprednisolone sodium succinate			
Solurex, *see* Dexamethasone sodium phosphate			
Solurex LA, *see* Dexamethasone acetate			

Appendix 3

	Amount	Route of Admin	Code
Somatrem	5 mg	INJ	S0010
Somatrem, *see* Growth hormone therapy (e.g., protropin humatrope)			
Somatrem injection	5 mg	IM	Q2015
Somatropin	1 mg	SC, IM	Q2016
	5 mg	INJ	S0011
Sparine, *see* Promazine HCl			
Spasmoject, *see* Dicyclomine HCl			
Spectinomycin HCl	up to 2 g	IM	J3320
Sporanox, *see* Itraconazole injection			
Stadol, *see* Butorphanol tartrate injection			
Stadol NS, *see* Butorphanol tartrate nasal spray			
Staphcillin, *see* Methicillin sodium			
Stilphostrol, *see* Diethylstilbestrol diphosphate			
Streptase, *see* Streptokinase			
Streptokinase	per 250,000 IU	IV	J2995
Streptomycin Sulfate, *see* Streptomycin			
Streptomycin	up to 1 g	IM	J3000
Streptozocin	1 gm	IV	J9320
Sublimaze, *see* Fentanyl citrate			
Succinylcholine chloride	up to 20 mg	IV, IM	J0330
Sucostrin, *see* Succinycholine chloride			
Sulfamethoxazole and trimethoprim	10 ml	INJ, IV	S0039
Sulfatrim, *see* Sulfamethoxazole and trimethoprim injection			
Sumatriptan succinate	6 mg	SC	J3030
Sus-Phrine, *see* Adrenalin, epinephrine			
Synagis, *see* Palivizumab RSV IGM			
Syntocionon, *see* Oxytocin			
Sytobex, *see* Vitamin B-12 cyanocobalamin			

	Amount	Route of Admin	Code

T

	Amount	Route of Admin	Code
Tacrine hydrochloride	10mg	ORAL	S0014
Tacrolimus, injection	per 5 mg (1 amp)	IV	C9006
Tacrolimus, oral	per 1 mg	ORAL	J7507
	per 5 mg	ORAL	J7508
Tacrolimus, parenteral	5 mg	IV	J7525

Tagamet HCl, *see* Cimetidine hydrochloride injection

Talwin, *see* Pentazocine HCl

Taractan, *see* Chlorprothixene

Taxol, *see* Paclitaxel

TEEV, *see* Testosterone enanthate and estradiol valerate

Temodar, *see* Temozolmide

Temozolmide	5 mg	ORAL	C1086
Tenecteplase	per 50 mg vial	IV	C9002

Tequin injection, *see* Gatifloxacin injection

Terbutaline sulface, inhalation solution, concentrated form	per mg	INH	J7680
Terbutaline sulface, inhalation solution, unit dose form	per mg	INH	J7681
Terbutaline sulfate	up to 1 mg	SC	J3105

Terramycin IM, *see* Oxytetracycline HCl

Testa-C, *see* Testosterone cypionate

Testadiate, *see* Testosterone enanthate and estradiol valerate

Testadiate-Depo, *see* Testosterone cypionate

Testaject-LA, *see* Testosterone cypionate

Testaqua, *see* Testosterone suspension

Test-Estro Cypionates, *see* Testosterone cypionate and estradiol cypionate

Test-Estro-C, *see* Testosterone cypionate and estradiol cypionate

Testex, *see* Testosterone propionate

	Amount	Route of Admin	Code
Testoject-50, *see* Testosterone suspension			
Testoject-LA, *see* Testosterone cypionate			
Testone LA 200, *see* Testosterone enanthate			
Testone LA 100, *see* Testosterone enanthate			
Testosterone Aqueous, *see* Testosterone suspension			
Testosterone enanthate and estradiol valerate	up to 1 cc	IM	J0900
Testosterone enanthate	up to 100 mg	IM	J3120
	up to 200 mg	IM	J3130
Testosterone cypionate			
	1 cc, 50 mg	IM	J1090
	up to 100 mg	IM	J1070
	1 cc, 200 mg	IM	J1080
Testosterone cypionate and estradiol cypionate	up to 1 ml	IM	J1060
Testosterone propionate	up to 100 mg	IM	J3150
Testosterone suspension	up to 50 mg	IM	J3140
Testradiol 90/4, *see* Testosterone enanthate and estradiol valerate			
Testrin PA, *see* Testosterone enanthate			
Tetanus immune globulin, human	up to 250 units	IM	J1670
Tetracycline	up to 250 mg	IM, IV	J0120
Theelin Aqueous, *see* Estrone			
Theophylline	per 40 mg	IV	J2810
TheraCys, *see* BCG live			
Thiethylperazine	10 mg	ORAL	Q0174
Thiethylperazine maleate	up to 10 mg	IM	J3280
Thiotepa	15 mg	IV	J9340
Thiothixene	up to 4 mg	IM	J2330
Thorazine, *see* Chlorpromazine HCl			
Thypinone, *see* Protirelin			
Thyrotropin alpha injection	0.9 mg	IM, SC	J3240
Thytropar, *see* Thyrotropin			
Ticarcillin disodium and clavulanate potassium, injection	3.1 g	IV, IM	S0040

	Amount	Route of Admin	Code
Tice BCG, *see* BCG live			
Ticon, *see* Trimethobenzamide HCl			
Tigan, *see* Trimethobenzamide HCl			
Tiject-20, *see* Trimethobenzamide HCl			
Timentin , *See* Ticarcillin disodium and clavulanate potassium injection			
Tinzaparin sodium injection	per 2 mg vial	SC	C9107
Tirofiban HCl	12.5 mg	INJ	J3245
TNKase, *see* Tenecteplase			
Tobramycin	300 mg	INH	J7681
Tobramycin sulfate	up to 80 mg	IM, IV	J3260
Tofranil, *see* Imipramine HCl			
Tolazoline HCl	up to 25 mg	IV	J2670
Topotecan	4 mg		J9350
Toradol, *see* Ketorolac tromethamine			
Torecan, *see* Thiethylperazine maleate			
Tornalate, *see* Bitolterol mesylate			
Torsemide	10 mg/ml	IV	J3265
Totacillin-N, *see* Ampicillin			
Trastuzumab	10 mg		J9355
Tri-Kort, *see* Triamcinolone acetonide			
Triam-A, *see* Triamcinolone acetonide			
Triamcinolone acetonide	per 10 mg	IM	J3301
Triamcinolone diacetate	per 5 mg	IM	J3302
Triamcinolone hexacetonide	per 5 mg	VAR	J3303
Triamcinolone, inhalation solution, concetrated form	per mg	INH	J7683
Triamcinolone, inhalation solution, unit dose form	per mg	INH	J7684
Triflupromazine HCl	up to 20 mg	IM, IV	J3400
Trilafon, *see* Perphenazine			
Trilog, *see* Triamcinolone acetonide			
Trilone, *see* Triamcinolone diacetate			
Trimethaphan camsylate	up to 500 mg	IV	J0400
Trimethobenzamide HCl	up to 200 mg	IM	J3250
	250 mg	ORAL	Q0173
Trimetrexate glucuronate	per 25 mg	IV	J3305
Trobicin, *see* Spectinomycin HCl			

Appendix 3

	Amount	Route of Admin	Code

U

Ultrazine-10, *see* Prochlorperazine

Unasyn, *see* Ampicillin sodium/ sulbactam sodium

Unclassified drugs (*see also* Not elsewhere classified)	—	—	J3490
Urea	up to 40 g	IV	J3350

Ureaphil, *see* Urea

Urecholine, *see* Bethanechol chloride

Urokinase	5,000 IU vial	IV	J3364
	250,000 IU vial	IV	J3365

V

V-Gan 25, *see* Promethazine HCl

V-Gan 50, *see* Promethazine HCl

Valergen 10, *see* Estradiol valerate

Valergen 20, *see* Estradiol valerate

Valergen 40, *see* Estradiol valerate

Valertest No. 1, *see* Testosterone enanthate and estradiol valerate

Valertest No. 2, *see* Testosterone enanthate and estradiol valerate

Valium, *see* Diazepam

Valrubicin	200 mg	Intravesical	J9357

Vancocin, *see* Vancomycin HCl

Vancoled, *see* Vancomycin HCl

Vancomycin HCl	500 mg	IV, IM	J3370

Vasoxyl, *see* Methoxamine HCl

Velban, *see* Vinblastine sulfate

Velsar, *see* Vinblastine sulfate

Ventolin, *see* Albuterol sulfate

VePesid, *see* Etoposide and Etoposide, oral

Versed, *see* Midazolam HCl

Verteporfin	15mg	IV	C1203, S0086

Vesprin, *see* Triflupromazine HCl

Viagra, *see* Sildenafil citrate

	Amount	Route of Admin	Code
Vinblastine sulfate	1 mg	IV	J9360
Vincasar PFS, *see* Vincristine sulfate			
Vincristine sulfate	1 mg	IV	J9370
	2 mg	IV	J9375
	5 mg	IV	J9380
Vinorelbine tartrate	per 10 mg	IV	J9390
Vistaject-25, *see* Hydroxyzine HCl			
Vistaril, *see* Hydroxyzine HCl			
Visudyne, *see* Verteporfin			
Vitamin K, *see* Phytonadione			
Vitamin B-12 cyanocobalamin	up to 1000 mcg	IM, SC	J3420
Vitrasert, *see* Ganciclovir			

W

Wehamine, *see* Dimenhydrinate

Wehdryl, *see* Diphenhydramine HCl

Wellcovorin, *see* Leucovorin calcium

Wyamine Sulfate, *see* Mephentermine sulfate

Wycillin, *see* Penicillin G procaine

Wydase, *see* Hyaluronidase

X

Xylocaine HCl, *see* Lidocaine HCl

Z

Zanosar, *see* Streptozocin

Zetran, *see* Diazepam

Zinacef, *see* Cefuroxime sodium

Zinecard, *see* Dexrazoxane

Zithromax, *see* Azithromycin, Azithromycin-dihydrate

Zofran, *see* Ondansetron HCl

Zoladex, *see* Goserelin acetate implant

Zolicef, *see* Cefazolin sodium

Zovirax, *see* Acyclovir sodium injection

Zyvox, *see* Linezolid

Appendix 4:

CIM, MCM References

CIM References

35-5   Cellular therapy

This therapy is not covered under Medicare.

35-10   Hyperbaric oxygen therapy

Hyperbaric oxygen therapy (HBO) is a modality in which the entire body is exposed to oxygen under increased atmospheric pressure. This modality is covered by Medicare when administered in a chamber (including the one man unit.)

The list of conditions for which the above modality is covered includes: acute carbon monoxide intoxication, decompression illness, gas embolism, gas gangrene, acute traumatic peripheral ischemia, crush injuries and suturing of severed limbs, progressive necrotizing infections (necrotizing fasciitis), acute peripheral arterial insufficiency, preparation and preservation of compromised skin grafts, chronic refractory osteomyelitis that is unresponsive to conventional medical and surgical management, osteoradionecrosis as an adjunct to conventional treatment, soft tissue radionecrosis as an adjunct to conventional treatment, cyanide poisoning and actinomycosis (only as an adjunct to conventional therapy when the disease process is refractory to antibiotics and surgical treatment).

Coverage of HBO therapy specifically excludes cutaneous, decubitus, and stasis ulcers; chronic peripheral vascular insufficiency; anaerobic septicemia and infection other than clostridial; skin burns (thermal); senility; myocardial infarction; cardiogenic shock; sickle cell anemia; acute thermal and chemical pulmonary damage, i.e., smoke inhalation with pulmonary insufficiency; acute or chronic cerebral vascular insufficiency; hepatic necrosis; aerobic septicemia; nonvascular causes of chronic brain syndrome (Pick's disease, Alzheimer's disease, Korsakoff's disease); tetanus; systemic aerobic infection; organ transplantation and storage; pulmonary emphysema; exceptional blood loss anemia; Multiple Sclerosis; and acute cerebral edema.

HBO therapy is not covered for any conditions other than those listed above.

HBO therapy must be clinically practical and should not replace standard therapeutic measures. Treatment may range from less than one week to several months in duration. The average duration of treatment is from two to four weeks. If treatment continues for more than two months, medical necessity should be documented and will be evaluated before payment is made for the services.

The topical application of oxygen is not covered by Medicare because its clinical efficacy has not been established.

For HBO therapy to be covered under the Medicare program the physician must be in constant attendance during the entire treatment. This requirement applies in all settings.

Cardiopulmonary resuscitation team coverage must be immediately available during the hours of the hyperbaric chamber operations.

35-13 Prolotherapy, joint sclerotherapy and ligamentous injections with sclerosing agents

These therapies are not covered under Medicare because the medical effectiveness for their use has not been verified.

35-20 Treatment of motor function disorders with electric nerve stimulation

Although electric nerve stimulation has been employed to control chronic intractable pain for some time, its use in the treatment of motor function disorders, such as multiple sclerosis, is a recent innovation, and the medical effectiveness of such therapy has not been verified by scientifically controlled studies. Therefore, electric nerve stimulation use to treat motor function disorders cannot be considered reasonable and necessary. The stimulator and the services related to its implantation are not covered by Medicare.

Medicare coverage of deep brain stimulation by implantation of a stimulator device is not prohibited. Therefore, coverage of deep brain stimulation provided by an implanted deep brain stimulator is at the carrier's discretion.

35-27 Biofeedback therapy

Biofeedback therapy is covered by Medicare only when it is reasonable and necessary for re-education of specific muscle groups or for treating pathological muscle abnormalities of spasticity, incapacitating muscle spasm or weakness and when more conventional treatments such as heat, cold, massage, exercise and support have not been successful.

Biofeedback therapy for treating ordinary muscle tension or psychosomatic conditions is not covered.

35-34 Fabric wrapping of abdominal aneurysms

Fabric wrapping is not covered under Medicare.

35-46 Assessing patient's suitability for electrical nerve stimulation therapy

Electrical nerve stimulation is used to assess a patient's suitability for ongoing treatment with a transcutaneous or an implanted nerve stimulator. If transcutaneous nerve stimulation (TENS) significantly alleviates pain, it may be considered as primary treatment. If no relief or greater discomfort than the original pain is produced, then electrical nerve stimulation therapy is ruled out. In cases where TENS produces incomplete relief, further evaluation with percutaneous electrical nerve stimulation (PENS) may be considered to determine whether an implanted peripheral nerve stimulator would provide significant relief from pain.

The patient's suitability for electrical nerve stimulation therapy is assessed during a one-month trial period. If the trial period is longer, medical necessity must be documented.

Usually, the physician or physical therapist furnishes the assessment equipment. If the patient rents the equipment, Medicare may pay for the rental and for the services of the physician or physical therapist who is evaluating its use. The combined payment should not exceed the amount paid for the total service, which would include the stimulator furnished by the physician or therapist.

Since electrical nerve stimulators do not prevent pain but only alleviate pain, a patient can be taught how to employ the stimulator safely and effectively without direct physician supervision. Therefore, it is inappropriate for a patient to visit his or her physician, physical therapist, or an outpatient clinic on a continuous basis for treatment.

35-47 Breast reconstruction following mastectomy

Medicare program payment may be made for breast reconstruction surgery of the affected and the contralateral unaffected breast following the removal of a breast for any medical reason. A mastectomy may be simple, modified, radical, subtotal, total, unilateral or bilateral, and must be coded to reflect the appropriate procedure. It is considered a safe and effective noncosmetic procedure.

Breast reconstruction solely for cosmetic reasons is not covered.

35-48 Osteogenic stimulation

Electrical stimulation to augment bone repair can be performed invasively or noninvasively. Medicare covers the noninvasive stimulator for nonunion of long bone fractures, failed fusion (where a minimum of nine months has elapsed since the last surgery), congenital pseudarthrosis and as an adjunct to spinal fusion surgery for patients at high risk of pseudarthrosis due to previously failed spinal fusion at the same site or for those undergoing multiple level fusion. A multiple level fusion involves three or more vertebrae (e.g., L3-L5, L4-S1, etc.). The invasive device is covered for nonunion of long bone fractures and as an adjunct to spinal fusion for patients at high risk of pseudarthrosis due to previously failed spinal fusion at the same site or for those undergoing multiple level fusion. A multiple level fusion involves three or more vertebrae (e.g., L3-L5, L4-S1, etc.). Nonunion is considered to exist only after six or more months without healing of the fracture.

Nonunion of long bone fractures, for both noninvasive and invasive devices, is considered to exist only when serial radiographs have confirmed that fracture healing has ceased for three or more months prior to starting treatment with the electrical osteogenic stimulator. Serial radiographs must include a minimum of two sets of radiographs, each including multiple views of the fracture site, separated by a minimum of 90 days.

There is insufficient evidence to support the medical necessity of using an ultrasonic osteogenic stimulator. Therefore, the device is not covered, because it is not considered reasonable and necessary.

35-61 Transsexual surgery

Transsexual surgery, also known as sex reassignment surgery or intersex surgery, is the culmination of a series of procedures designed to change the anatomy of transsexuals to conform to their gender identity. Transsexual surgery for sex reassignment of transsexuals is controversial.

Because of the lack of well controlled, long term studies of the safety and effectiveness of the surgical procedures and attendant therapies for transsexualism, the treatment is considered experimental. Moreover, there is a high rate of serious complications for these surgical procedures. For these reasons, transsexual surgery is not covered.

35-64 Chelation therapy for treatment of atherosclerosis

Chelation therapy is not covered under Medicare.

This therapy may also be referred to as chemoendarterectomy and may show a diagnosis other than atherosclerosis, such as arteriosclerosis or calcinosis. Claims employing such variant terms will also be denied coverage.

35-65 Gastric freezing

Gastric freezing is not covered under Medicare.

35-74 Enhanced external counterpulsation (EECP) for severe angina-Covered (Effective for services performed on or after July 1, 1999)

Enhanced external counterpulsation (EECP) is a non-invasive outpatient treatment for coronary artery disease refractory to medical and/or surgical therapy. Although these and similar devices are cleared by the FDA for use in treating a variety of conditions, including stable or unstable angina pectoris, acute myocardial infarction and cardiogenic shock, Medicare coverage is limited to its use in patients with stable angina pectoris, since only that use has developed sufficient evidence to demonstrate its medical effectiveness. Other uses of this device and similar devices remain non-covered. In addition, the non-coverage of hydraulic versions of these types of devices remains in force.

Coverage is further limited to those enhanced external counterpulsation systems that heve sufficiently demonstrated their medical effectiveness in treating patients with severe angina in well designed clinical trials. Note that a 501(k) clearance by the FDA does not, by itself, satisfy this requirement.

Coverage is provided for the use of EECP for patients who have been diagnosed with disabling angina (Class III or Class IV, Canadian Cardiovascular Society Classification or equivalent classification)who, in the opinion of a cardiologist or cardiothoracic surgeon, are not readily amenable to surgical intervention, such as PTCA or cardiac bypass because: (1)their condition is inoperable, or at a high risk of operative complications or post-operative failure; (2) their coronary anatomy is not readily amenable to such procedures; or (3)they have co-morbid states which create excessive risk.

A full course of therapy usually consists of 35 one-hour treatments, which may be offered once or twice daily (usually 5 days per week). This service must be rendered under the direct supervision of a physician.

Appendix 4

35-77 Neuromuscular electrical stimulation (NMES) in the treatment of disuse atrophy

Coverage for NMES is limited to:

- treatment of disuse atrophy when nerve supply to the muscle is intact, including brain, spinal cord and peripheral nerves; and,

- other nonneurological reasons for atrophy caused by disuse, which can result from casting or splinting of a limb, contracture due to scarring of soft tissue as in burn lesions and hip replacement surgery (until orthotic training begins). (See also Coverage Issues Manual 45-25.)

35-90 Extracorporeal immunoadsorption (ECI) using protein A columns for the treatment of patients with idiopathic thrombocytopenia purpura (ITP) failing other treatments

Extracorporeal immunoadsorption (ECI), using protein A columns, is used to selectively remove circulating immune complexes (CIC) and immunoglobulins (IgG) from patients with diseases related to these substances.

Medicare covers the use of Protein A columns for the treatment of ITP. In addition, Medicare will cover Protein A columns for the treatment of rheumatoid arthritis (RA) for patients with severe RA (e.g., patient disease is active, having > 5 swollen joints, > 20 tender joints, and morning stiffness > 60 minutes) and for patients who have a course of a minimum of three Disease Modifying Anti-Rheumatic Drugs (DMARDs). Failure does not include intolerance.

Other uses of these columns are currently considered to be investigational and, therefore, not reasonable and necessary under the Medicare law. (See §1862(a)(1)(A) of the Act.)

35-93 Lung volume reduction surgery (reduction pneumoplasty, also called lung shaving or lung contouring)

Lung volume reduction surgery (LVRS) is performed on patients with emphysema and chronic obstructive pulmonary disease (COPD) to allow the underlying compressed lung to expand and establish improved respiratory function. It may also be offered as a "bridge to transplant" for patients who may not have been considered candidates for a lung transplant.

Unilateral or bilateral lung volume reduction surgery by open or thoracoscopic approach is not covered in most cases.

However, the Health Care Financing Administration (HCFA) and the National Heart, Lung and Blood Institute (NHLBI) has approved a multicenter, randomized clinical trial regarding the safety and effectiveness of LVRS. Medicare will cover LVRS under those limited circumstances when it is provided to a Medicare beneficiary under the protocols established for the clinical trials and where the care is furnished in facilities that are approved as meeting the criteria established by HCFA and NHLBI for this study.

Coverage to those beneficiaries who participate in the HCFA/NHLBI trial consists of services integral to the study and for which the Medicare statute does not prohibit. This includes tests performed to determine whether a beneficiary qualifies for randomization, LVRS and follow-up tests that are necessary during participation in the study (e.g., pulmonary rehabilitation and pulmonary function testing). Medicare will not cover those services that are prohibited (e.g., oral steroids provided as part of a physician's service because they are self-administrable).

35-96 Cryosurgery of prostate (Effective for services performed on or after July 1, 1999)

Cryosurgery of the prostate gland, also known as cryosurgical ablation of the prostate (CSAP), destroys prostate tissue by applying extremely cold temperatures in order to reduce the size of the prostate gland. It is safe and effective, as well as medically necessary and appropriate, as primary treatment for patients with clinically localized prostate cancer, Stages T1–T3.

35-99 Abortion

Abortions are not covered Medicare procedures except if the pregnancy is the result of an act of rape or incest; or where a woman suffers from a physical disorder, physical injury, or physical illness, including a life-endangering physical condition caused by or arising from the pregnancy that would, as certified by a physician, place the woman in danger of death unless an abortion is performed.

This restricted coverage applies to CPT codes 59840, 59841, 59850, 59851, 59852, 59855, 59856, 59857, and 59866.

45-4 Vitamin B-12 injections to strengthen tendons, ligaments, etc., of the foot

Vitamin B-12 injections to strengthen tendons, ligaments, etc., of the foot are not covered under Medicare.

45-7 Hydrophilic contact lens for corneal bandage

Some hydrophilic contact lenses are used as moist corneal bandages for the treatment of acute or chronic corneal pathology (e.g., bullous keratopathy, dry eyes, corneal ulcers and erosion, keratitis, corneal edema, descemetocele, corneal ectasis, Mooren's ulcer, anterior corneal dystrophy, neurotrophic keratoconjunctivitis) and for other therapeutic reasons.

FDA-approved hydrophilic contact lenses that are used as a supply incident to a physician's service are covered by Medicare. Payment for the lens is included in the payment for the physician's service to which the lens is incident. (See also Coverage Issues Manual 65-1.)

45-10 Laetrile and related substances

Laetrile and other drugs characterized as "nitrilosides" are not covered under Medicare.

45-16 Certain drugs distributed by the National Cancer Institute (effective for services furnished on or after 10/1/80)

The Division of Cancer Treatment of the National Cancer Institute (NCI), with the Food and Drug Administration, approves and distributes certain drugs for use in treating terminally ill cancer patients. One group of these drugs, designated as Group C drugs are not limited to use in clinical trials for the purpose of testing their efficacy. Drugs are classified as Group C if evidence demonstrates their efficacy within a tumor type and that they can be safely administered.

Physicians can receive Group C drugs if they are registered as an investigator with the NCI, submit a written request for the drug and indicate the disease to be treated. NCI guidelines are followed when use of the drug and adverse reactions are reported to the Division of Cancer Treatment. Under Medicare, Group C drugs and the related hospital stay are covered services if all other applicable coverage requirements are met.

45-20 Ethylenediamine-tetra-acetic (EDTA) chelation therapy for treatment of atherosclerosis

The use of EDTA as a chelating agent to treat atherosclerosis, arteriosclerosis, calcinosis or a similar generalized condition not listed by the FDA as an approved use is considered experimental and is not covered by Medicare.

45-24 Antiinhibitor coagulant complex (AICC)

AICC is a drug used to treat hemophilia in patients with factor VIII inhibitor antibodies. It is safe and effective when furnished to patients with hemophilia A and inhibitor antibodies to factor VIII with major bleeding episodes and who fail to respond to other less expensive therapies.

45-25 Supplies used in the delivery of transcutaneous electrical nerve stimulation (TENS) and neuromuscular electrical stimulation (NMES)

TENS and/or NMES can be delivered using conventional electrodes, adhesive tapes and lead wires. It might be medically necessary, however, for certain patients to use a form-fitting conductive garment with conductive fibers separated from the patient's skin by layers of fabric. These FDA-approved garments may be covered if prescribed by a physician, and one of the following medical conditions is met:

- The patient has such a large area to stimulate that conventional electrodes, adhesive tape and lead wires are not feasible.

- The patient needs the garment to treat chronic intractable pain because the areas to be stimulated are inaccessible.

- A documented medical condition, such as a skin problem, precludes the application of conventional electrodes.

- The patient requires stimulation beneath a cast either to treat disuse atrophy where the nerve supply to the muscle is intact, or to treat chronic intractable pain.

- There is a medical need for rehabilitation strengthening based on a written plan of rehabilitation following an injury where the nerve supply to the muscle is intact.

A conductive garment is not covered for use with TENS during the trial period (one month) unless the patient has documented skin problems prior to the start of the trial period and it is medically necessary. (See also Coverage Issues Manual 35-77.)

50-1 Cardiac pacemaker evaluation services

Medicare covers a variety of services for the postimplant follow-up and evaluation of implanted cardiac pacemakers. The guidelines apply to lithium battery-powered pacemakers.

The physician determines how often a patient's pacemaker is to be monitored. If a commercial monitoring service or hospital outpatient department is used, the physician should issue a prescription that is renewed at least annually to ensure proper monitoring frequency.

The definition of transtelephonic monitoring of cardiac pacemakers stipulates:

- a minimum 30-second readable strip of the pacemaker in the free running mode;

- unless contraindicated, a minimum 30-second readable strip of the pacemaker in the magnetic mode; and

- a minimum 30 seconds of readable ECG strip.

The following guidelines describe the maximum monitoring frequency for various kinds of pacemakers that is allowable by Medicare without claim review. More frequent monitoring may be covered if it is documented as medically necessary.

Guideline I: Maximum monitoring frequency guideline that applies to the majority of pacemakers in use.

Single-chamber pacemakers:

- First month: every two weeks

- Second through 36th month: every eight weeks

- 37th month to failure: every four weeks.

Dual-chamber pacemakers:

- First month: every two weeks

- Second through sixth month: every four weeks

- Seventh through 36th month: every eight weeks

- 37th month to failure: every four weeks.

Guideline II: Maximum monitoring frequency that applies to pacemaker systems that meet the standards of the Inter-Society Commission for Heart Disease Resources.

Single-chamber pacemakers:

- First month: every two weeks

- Second through 48th month: every twelve weeks

- 49th month through 72nd month: every eight weeks

- Thereafter: every four weeks.

Dual-chamber pacemakers:

- First month: every two weeks

- Second through 30th month: every twelve weeks

- 31st through 48th month: every eight weeks

- Thereafter: every four weeks.

Pacemaker clinic services are covered as separate services or in conjunction with transtelephonic monitoring. The services include the physical examination of patients and pacemaker reprogramming. The type of monitoring, whether

transtelephonic or through clinic visits, does not preclude concurrent use of the other. The frequency of clinic visits depends on the patient's physician and the medical condition of the patient.

Monitoring guidelines that are useful for screening lithium-battery pacemakers

Single-chamber pacemakers: twice in the first six months following implant, then once every 12 months.

Dual-chamber pacemakers: twice in the first six months, then once every six months.

50-4   Gravlee jet washer

The use of this diagnostic device is appropriate if the patient shows clinical symptoms or signs suggesting endometrial disease (e.g., irregular or heavy vaginal bleeding).

Medicare does not cover the washer or related diagnostic services furnished with an examination of an asymptomatic patient. Medicare precludes payment for routine physical checkups.

50-15   Electrocardiographic services

Electrocardiographic services rendered by a physician or incidental to his or her services, or by an approved laboratory or supplier of portable x-ray services, may be covered under Medicare. EKG services are covered for the signs, symptoms or other reasons necessitating services.

EKG services are not covered on a screening basis or as part of a routine exam.

EKG services furnished by a laboratory or a portable x-ray supplier must identify the physician ordering the service. If the charge includes the tracing and its interpretation, the identity of the interpreting physician must be provided. No separate services rendered by a physician are allowed unless the physician is the patient's attending or consulting physician.

EKGs taken in an emergency in which the patient is or may be experiencing a heart attack would be covered as a laboratory or diagnostic service by a portable x-ray supplier as long as a physician was in attendance at the time or immediately thereafter.

When the EKG is performed in the home and the supplier's charge is higher than that for the same services performed in a laboratory or portable x-ray supplier's office, the medical need for home services must be documented.

Long-term EKG monitoring-This diagnostic procedure provides a continuous record of the electrocardiographic activity while the patient is engaged in daily activities. It also is known as long-term EKG recording, Holter recording or dynamic electrocardiography. Recording up to 24 hours is usually adequate to detect transient arrhythmias and to provide diagnostic information-longer periods require documentation. Monitoring is valid for inpatient and outpatient diagnoses and therapy and reduces the length of stay for postcoronary infarct patients in intensive care and may result in an earlier discharge from the hospital.

Documentation must include a diagnostic impression statement by the referring physician, with an indication of the patient's relevant signs and symptoms.

This diagnostic procedure is warranted for:

- detecting transient episodes of cardiac dysrhythmia and permitting the correlation of the episodes with cardiovascular symptomatology;

- patients with symptoms of obscure etiology suggestive of cardiac arrhythmia, including palpitations, chest pain, dizziness, light-headedness, near syncope, syncope, transient ischemic episodes, dyspnea and shortness of breath;

- instituting arrhythmic drug therapy to evaluate response during administration or to evaluate a response to a change of dosage before or after the discontinuation of antiarrhythmic medication;

- assessing patients with coronary artery disease by making it possible to document the etiology of such symptoms as chest pain and shortness of breath;

- patients recovering from an acute myocardial infarction or coronary insufficiency before and after discharge from the hospital;

Appendix 4

- identifying patients at a higher risk of dying suddenly following an acute myocardial infarction;

- the high-risk patient with known cardiovascular disease who advances to a substantially higher level of activity that might trigger increased or new types of arrhythmias necessitating treatment, especially when there is documentation that acute phase arrhythmias have not totally disappeared during convalescence; and,

- patients with an internal pacemaker only if they have symptoms suggestive of arrhythmia that are not revealed by the standard EKG or rhythm strip.

Patient-activated EKG recorders-These devices permit the patient to record an EKG upon manifestation of symptoms or in response to a physician's order. Most permit voice recording to describe the symptom, activity and transtelephonic transmission to a physician's office, clinic, hospital, etc.

Services connected with patient-activated EKG recorders are covered as an alternative to long-term EKG monitoring for detecting and characterizing symptomatic arrhythmias, regulation of antiarrhythmic drug therapy, etc. Use of this device for evaluating symptoms such as obscure etiology suggestive of cardiac arrhythmia is covered. Recorders are useful for inpatient and outpatient diagnoses and therapy. They are not covered for outpatient monitoring of a recently discharged postinfarct patient.

Computer analyzed electrocardiograms-Computer interpretation of EKGs improves the quality and availability of cardiology services. The services are reimbursable when furnished under the coverage guidelines of other electrocardiographic services.

When the laboratory or portable x-ray supplier's charge includes the physician review and certification of the printout, the certifying physician must be identified before reimbursement can be made. When the reviewing physician is not identified, no professional component is involved. When there is a charge for the physician component, it should be substantially less than the physician interpretation of the conventional EKG tracing.

Transtelephonic electrocardiographic transmissions-Coverage includes transtelephonic electrocardiographic (EKG) transmissions as a diagnostic service. Coverage is limited to the physician's interpretation of the transmission, including charges for equipment rental. Devices must be capable of transmitting EKG leads I, II and III, and must be sufficiently comparable to readings obtained by a conventional EKG to permit proper interpretation of abnormal cardiac rhythms.

Covered uses of transtelephonic EKGs include the following:

- To detect, characterize and document symptomatic transient arrhythmias

- To overcome problems in regulating antiarrhythmic drug dosage

- To carry out early posthospital monitoring of patients discharged after myocardial infarction (only if 24-hour coverage is provided)

- Other uses, subject to medical review.

Written justification for use in excess of 30 consecutive days for the detection of transient arrhythmias is required.

Payment is not made for posthospital monitoring of myocardial infarction patients unless there is 24-hour coverage at the monitoring site and an experienced EKG technician. Tape recording devices do not meet this criteria. The technicians must have immediate access to a physician and know when and how to contact available facilities in an emergency.

50-16   Hemorheograph

The hemorheograph is a diagnostic instrument that is safe and effective for determining the adequacy of skin perfusion prior to the performance of minor surgical procedures on the extremities, including minor podiatric procedures, and as an adjunct to the evaluation of patients suspected of having peripheral vascular disease. Program payment may be made only for those services employing the hemorheograph performed for preoperative and postoperative diagnostic evaluation of suspected peripheral artery disease.

50-20   Diagnostic Pap smears (effective for services performed on or after May 15, 1978)

Diagnostic Pap smears and related services are covered under Medicare Part B when ordered by a physician for one of the following conditions:

- Previous cancer of the cervix, uterus or vagina that has been or is presently being treated

- Previous abnormal Pap smear

- Abnormal findings of the vagina, cervix, uterus, ovaries or adnexa

- Significant complaint pertaining to the female reproductive system

- Any signs or symptoms that the physician judges to be reasonably related to a gynecologic disorder. The carrier's medical staff determines whether a previous malignancy at another site is an indication for a diagnostic Pap smear or whether the test must be considered a screening Pap smear.

50-24   Hair analysis

Hair analysis is not covered under Medicare.

50-34   Obsolete or unreliable diagnostic tests

The following diagnostic tests have been replaced by more advanced procedures. Only with documented medical necessity will the following procedures be covered by Medicare:

- Amylase, blood isoenzymes, electrophoretic

Appendix 4

- Bendien's test for cancer and tuberculosis
- Bolen's test for cancer
- Calcium saturation clotting time
- Calcium, feces, 24-hour quantitative
- Capillary fragility test (Rumpel-Leede)
- Cephalin flocculation
- Chromium, blood
- Chymotrypsin, duodenal contents
- Circulation time, one test
- Colloidal gold
- Congo red, blood
- Gastrianalysis, pepsin
- Gastrianalysis, tubeless
- Guanase, blood
- Hormones, adrenocorticotropin quantitative animal tests
- Hormones, adrenocorticotropin quantitative bioassay
- Phonocardiography diagnostic tests
- Rehfuss test for gastric acidity
- Serum seromucoid assay for cancer and other diseases
- Skin test, actinomycosis
- Skin test, brucellosis
- Skin test, cat scratch fever
- Skin test, lymphopathic a venereum
- Skin test, psittacosis
- Skin test, trichinosis
- Starch, feces, screening
- Thymol turbidity, blood
- Vectorcardiography diagnostic tests
- Zinc sulfate turbidity, blood

50-36 Positron emission tomography (PET or PETT) scans (effective for services performed on or after March 14, 1995)

Positron emission tomography (PET) or positron emission transverse tomography (PETT) is used to produce cross-sectional tomographic images by detecting radioactivity from a radioactive tracer substance (radiopharmaceutical) that is injected into the patient.

Medicare used to consider PET scans experimental, however, one use of the PET scans, imaging of the perfusion of the heart using Rubidium 82 (Rb 82), may be covered as dictated by two factors.

- A PET scan is no longer considered experimental for this single use, but it duplicates other forms of diagnostic testing that are covered also. It is not clear when PET scans may be substituted as a primary form of diagnostic testing rather than as a confirming or medically necessary additional test.

- The FDA has approved only Rubidium 82 for general PET scan use. Some uses of PET will not be covered due to the lack of approval of the radiopharmaceuticals involved in those uses.

The FDA has approved another radiopharmaceutical (deoxy-2-Flouro-D-glucose (FDG)) on a restricted basis and Medicare will not consider coverage at this time due to the restrictions.

The coverage requirements that must be met to assure PET scans are medically necessary, do not unnecessarily duplicate other covered diagnostic tests and do not involve investigational drugs or procedures using investigational drugs are:

- approved sites-PET scans may be covered only at PET imaging centers using PET scanners that are FDA approved.

- coverage is limited to rest alone or rest with pharmacologic stress PET scans used for noninvasive imaging of the perfusion of the heart for the diagnosis and management of patients with known or suspected coronary artery disease using FDA-approved Rubidium 82.

- the PET scan, whether rest alone or rest with stress, is used in place of but not in addition to a single photon emission computed tomography (SPECT) or is used following a SPECT that was found to be inconclusive.

PET scans using Rb 82 are not covered for routine screening of an asymptomatic patient, regardless of the level of risk factors applicable to the patient.

Claims must be submitted with the proper codes and modifiers to indicate the results of the PET scan. The detailed information required for appropriate billing is found in the G codes used for PET billing. PET scan claims must be backed up with medical records indicating the patient's age, sex and height, and body size and type, which indicated a need for the PET scan.

Appendix 4

50-42 Ambulatory blood pressure monitoring with fully and semiautomatic (patient-activated) portable monitors

The clinical usefulness of ambulatory blood pressure monitoring data has not been clearly established, although it is a safe and accurate means of measuring blood pressure. Program payment may not be made for fully and semiautomatic (patient-activated) portable monitors at this time.

50-44 Bone (mineral) density studies (effective for services rendered on or after March 4, 1983)

Bone (mineral) density studies are used to evaluate diseases of bone and/or the responses of bone diseases to treatment. The studies assess bone mass or density associated with such diseases as osteoporosis, osteomalacia and renal osteodystrophy. Various single or combined methods of measurement may be required to: (a) diagnose bone disease, (b) monitor the course of bone changes with disease progression, or (c) monitor the course of bone changes with therapy. Bone density is usually studied by using photodensitometry, single or dual photon absorptiometry, or bone biopsy.

A. Single Photon Absorptiometry-A noninvasive radiological technique that measures absorption of a monochromatic photon beam by bone material. The device is placed directly on the patient, uses a low dose of radionuclide and measures the mass absorption efficiency of the energy used. It provides a quantitative measurement of the bone mineral of cortical and trabecular bone, and is used in assessing an individual's treatment response at appropriate intervals. Single photon absorptiometry is covered under Medicare when used to assess changes in the bone density of patients with osteodystrophy or osteoporosis when performed on the same individual at intervals of six to 12 months.

B. Bone Biopsy-A physiologic test, which is a surgical, invasive procedure. A small sample of bone (usually from the ilium) is removed, generally by a biopsy needle. The biopsy sample is then examined histologically, and provides a qualitative measurement of the bone mineral of trabecular bone. This procedure is used to ascertain a differential diagnosis of bone disorders and to differentiate osteomalacia from osteoporosis. Bone biopsy is covered under Medicare no more than four times per patient, unless there is special justification given. When used more than four times on a patient, bone biopsy leaves a defect in the pelvis and may produce some patient discomfort.

C. Photodensitometry-(radiographic absorptiometry)-A noninvasive radiological procedure that attempts to assess bone mass by measuring the optical density of extremity radiographs with a photodensitometer, usually with a reference to a standard density wedge placed on the film at the time of exposure. This procedure provides a quantitative measurement of the bone mineral of cortical bone, and is used to monitor gross bone change.

Dual Photon Absorptiometry — A noninvasive radiological technique that measures absorption of a dichromatic beam by bone material. This procedure is not covered under Medicare because it is still considered to be in the investigational stage.

50-50 Displacement cardiography

Displacement cardiography, including cardiokymography and photokymography, is a noninvasive diagnostic test used to evaluate coronary artery disease.

A. Cardiokymography-(Effective for services rendered on or after 10/12/88) is a covered service only when used as an adjunct to electrocardiographic stress testing in evaluating coronary artery disease when the following clinical indications are present:

■ Male patients-atypical angina pectoris or nonischemic chest pain

■ Female patients-angina, either typical or atypical

B. Photokymography-This test is not covered under the Medicare program.

50-54 Cardiac output monitoring by electrical bioimpedance

This diagnostic method is still investigational and is not covered under Medicare.

50-55 Prostate cancer screening tests-Covered (Effective for services furnished on or after January 1, 2000).

A. General-Section 4103 of the Balanced Budget Act of 1997 provides for coverage of certain prostate cancer screening tests subject to certain coverage, frequency, and payment limitations. Effective for services furnished on or after January 1, 2000. Medicare will cover prostate cancer screening test/procedures for early detection of prostate cancer. Coverage of prostate cancer screening tests includes the following procedures furnished to an individual for the early detection of prostate cancer:

■ Screening digital rectal examination; and

■ Screening prostate specific antigen blood test.

B. Screening digital rectal examinations- Screening digital rectal examinations (HCPCS code G0102) are covered at a frequency of once every twelve months for men who have attained age 50 (at least 11 months have passed following the month in which the last Medicare-covered screening digital rectal examination was performed). Screening digital rectal examination means a clinical examination of an individual's prostate for nodules or other abnormalities of the prostate. This screening must be performed by a doctor of medicine or osteopathy, or by a physician assistant, nurse practitioner, clinical nurse specialist, or certified nurse midwife who is authorized under state law to perform the examination, fully knowledgeable about the beneficiary's medical condition, and would be responsible for using the results of any examination performed in the overall management of the beneficiary's specific medical problem.

C. Screening prostate specific antigen tests- Screening prostate specific antigen tests (code G0103) are covered at a frequency of once every

Appendix 4

twelve months for men who have attained age 50 (at least 11 months have passed following the month in which the last Medicare-covered screening prostate specific antigen test was performed). Screening prostate specific antigen tests (PSA) means a test to detect the marker for adenocarcinoma of prostate. PSA is a reliable immunocytochemical marker for primary and metastatic adenocarcinoma of prostate. This screening must be ordered by the beneficiary's physician or by the beneficiary's physician assistant, nurse practitioner, clinical nurse specialist, or certified nurse midwife, who is fully knowledgeable about the beneficiary's medical condition, and would be responsible for using the results of any examination (test) performed in the overall management of the beneficiary's specific medical problem.

55-1 Water purification and softening systems used in conjunction with home dialysis

Water purification systems-Water used for home dialysis does not need to be sterile but should be chemically free of heavy trace metals and/or organic contaminants and free of bacteria. Water purification systems that are used in conjunction with home dialysis, either peritoneal or hemodialysis, are covered under Medicare. Two types of systems meet the requirements:

- Deionization- removes organic substances, mineral salts of magnesium and calcium, compounds of fluoride and chloride from tap water, using filtration and ion exchange.

- Reverse osmosis- removes impurities from tap water using pressure to force water through a porous membrane.

Use of these systems together is medically unnecessary, and spare deionization tanks are not covered because they are a precautionary supply rather than a requirement for treatment.

Activated carbon filters used as a component of water purification to remove unsafe concentrations of chlorine and chloramines are covered when prescribed by a physician.

Water-softening system- The water-softening system used with home dialysis is excluded from Medicare coverage because it is not reasonable and necessary. The system does not adequately remove heavy metal contaminants, such as arsenic, that may be present in trace amounts.

A water-softening system used to pretreat water that will be purified by a reverse osmosis (RO) unit for home dialysis may be covered under Medicare. The manufacturer of the RO must have standards for the quality of water entering the system (e.g., the water must be of a certain quality for the unit to perform as intended). The water-softening system may also be covered if the patient's water is of a lesser quality than required and the softener is used only to soften water entering the RO unit.

Developing need when a water-softening system is replaced with a water purification unit in an existing home dialysis system- In some cases, the installation of a water purification system is not medically necessary. The physician must provide the reason for the changes, with supporting documentation, such as the supplier's recommendations or a water analysis. A purification system may be ordered if medical community standards for water quality are raised or the water quality itself deteriorates.

60-3   White cane for use by a blind person

The white cane is not covered by Medicare.

60-4   Home use of oxygen

Home oxygen use is covered under the durable medical equipment (DME) benefit and is considered reasonable and necessary only for patients with significant hypoxemia who meet specified medical documentation, laboratory evidence and health condition requirements.

Medical documentation -Initial claims must include the completed certification form HCFA-484 (Attending Physician's Certification of Medical Necessity for Home Oxygen Therapy) so that HCFA may determine whether coverage criteria have been met and that the service provided reflects what the physician prescribed and other medical documentation. The certification must include the results of specific testing before Medicare coverage can be determined.

The medical prescription and HCFA-484 must be completed by the attending physician, or by an employee of the physician using information in the patient's medical record for the physician's review and signature. Hospital discharge coordinators, nurses and medical social workers have no authority to prescribe the services or to enter medical or prescription information in items 1 through 6 on the HCFA-484. Suppliers may not enter this information either.

Initial claims also must be supported by medical documentation (written prescription from the attending physician) unless it is an electronic claim. In the case of electronic claims, separate documentation is required.

The attending physician's prescription or other medical documentation also must indicate that other treatments (e.g., medical and physical therapy directed at secretions, bronchospasm and infection) were tried unsuccessfully and that oxygen therapy is still required. The patient must be examined within a month of the start of therapy. The prescription must specify a disease requiring home use of oxygen, the oxygen flow rate and an estimate of the frequency, duration of use (two liters per minute, 10 minutes per hour, 12 hours a day) and the duration of need (six months, lifetime).

A prescription for "oxygen PRN" or "oxygen as needed" does not satisfy Medicare requirements for documenting reasonable and necessary services.

Medical review will occur when flow rates are greater than two liters per minute. If the physician specifies a type of system to be used (e.g., gas, liquid or concentrator), the medical reasons for selecting the system must be specified. A change in the oxygen requirements must be supported by new documentation written by the patient's attending physician. Periodic and continuing medical necessity reviews are conducted on patients with indefinite or extended periods of necessity.

Appendix 4

Also, earlier recertification and testing are required for patients who initially tested with an arterial blood gas at or above a partial pressure of 55 or an arterial oxygen saturation percent at or above 89.

Laboratory evidence -Initial oxygen therapy claims must include a blood gas study ordered and evaluated by the attending physician. This is usually a measurement of the partial pressure of oxygen (PO2) in arterial blood. A measurement of arterial oxygen saturation obtained by ear or pulse oximetry is acceptable when ordered and evaluated by the attending physician and performed under his supervision or by a qualified provider or supplier of laboratory services. A DME supplier is not considered qualified. The conditions under which the laboratory tests are performed (e.g., resting, sleeping, while exercising, on room air or oxygen, the amount and the body position during testing), must be in writing and submitted with the initial claim.

If both arterial blood gas and oximetry studies are used to document medical necessity and results of these tests conflict, the arterial blood gas pressure is preferred.

Preferred sources of laboratory evidence are existing physician and/or hospital records reflecting the patient's medical condition. Subsequent blood gas tests that appear to duplicate the hospital test will be denied as not medically reasonable and necessary.

Covered blood gas values -Medical documentation will be reviewed to determine if coverage is available under one of three groups.

Group I covers patients with significant hypoxemia evidenced by:

- arterial PO2 at or below 55 millimeters of mercury (mm Hg), arterial oxygen saturation at or below 88 percent, taken at rest, breathing room air;

- arterial PO2 at or below 55 mm Hg, or an arterial oxygen saturation at or below 88 percent, taken during sleep for a patient demonstrating arterial PO2 at or above 56 mm Hg or an arterial oxygen saturation at or above 89 percent, while awake; or a greater than normal fall in oxygen level during sleep associated with symptoms such as impairment of cognitive processes, nocturnal restlessness or insomnia. Coverage is provided only for nocturnal use; or,

- arterial PO2 at or below 55 mm Hg, arterial oxygen saturation at or below 88 percent, taken during exercise for a patient who demonstrates an arterial PO2 at or above 56 mm Hg or an arterial oxygen saturation at or above 89 percent during the day while at rest.

Group II covers patients with arterial PO2 at 56-59 mm Hg or whose arterial blood oxygen saturation is 89 percent, if there is evidence of:

- dependent edema suggesting congestive heart failure;

- "P" pulmonale on EKG (P wave greater than 3 mm in standard leads II, III or AVF); or,

- erythrocythemia with a hematocrit greater than 56 percent.

Group III indicates that a home program of oxygen use is not medically necessary for patients with arterial PO2 levels at or above 60 mm Hg or arterial blood saturation at or above 90 percent. For claims in this category to be reimbursed, medical documentation must rebut the above presumptions, and each case will be medically reviewed.

Health conditions -Coverage is available to patients with significant hypoxemia in the chronic stable state if the attending physician has determined that the patient has one of the following health conditions:

- The patient meets the blood gas evidence as previously specified.

- The patient has tried alternative treatments without complete success.

- The patient has a health condition for which oxygen therapy may be covered (see section Conditions for which oxygen therapy may be covered).

Conditions for which oxygen therapy may be covered-Oxygen therapy may be covered for severe lung disease, such as chronic obstructive pulmonary disease and diffuse interstitial lung disease, whether of known or unknown etiology; cystic fibrosis; bronchiectasis; widespread pulmonary neoplasm; or hypoxia-related symptoms or findings that may improve with oxygen therapy. Examples include pulmonary hypertension, recurring congestive heart failure due to chronic cor pulmonale, erythrocytosis, impairment of the cognitive process, nocturnal restlessness and morning headache.

Conditions for which oxygen therapy is not covered-No coverage is offered for angina pectoris in the absence of hypoxemia, breathlessness without cor pulmonale or evidence of hypoxemia, severe peripheral vascular disease from desaturation in one or more extremities and terminal illnesses that do not affect the lungs.

Portable oxygen systems-Patients may qualify for a portable oxygen system alone or to complement a stationary system. The medical documentation must describe the patient's activities or exercise routine and the medical necessity for a portable, rather than a stationary system.

Respiratory therapists are not covered under the provisions for oxygen services.

60-5   Power-operated vehicles that may be used as wheelchairs

A wheelchair may be covered if it is medically necessary, and the patient is unable to operate one manually. A specialist in physical medicine, orthopaedic surgery, neurology or rheumatology must evaluate the patient's medical and physical condition and prescribe the vehicle to ensure it is required and that the patient is capable of using it safely. A prescription from the beneficiary's physician is acceptable if a specialist is more than one day's round trip from the patient's home or the patient's condition precludes travel. All claims for power-operated wheelchairs require a medical review by Medicare.

Appendix 4

60-6 Specially sized wheelchairs

Specially sized wheelchairs may be covered by Medicare. For example, a narrow wheelchair may be necessary due to narrow doorways or a patient's slender build. A physician's certification or prescription is not required when a specially sized wheelchair is needed to accommodate the place of use or physical size of the patient.

60-7 Self-contained pacemaker monitors

Medicare will pay for the rental or purchase of the following pacemaker monitors when prescribed by a physician:

- digital electronic pacemaker monitor

- audible/visible signal pacemaker monitor

Regular visits to an outpatient department should be minimal for patients who monitor their pacemakers. Therefore, medical necessity of these visits must be documented.

60-8 Seat lift

The rental or purchase of a medically necessary seat lift is covered by Medicare when prescribed by a physician for patients with severe arthritis of the hip or knee, muscular dystrophy or other neuromuscular diseases. Units that also feature a recliner are paid up to the amount of the seat lift.

On or after Jan. 1, 1991, Medicare durable medical equipment (DME) does not include seat lift chairs (Medicare program memorandum B-91-3 [Feb. 1991]). The lift mechanism is covered as DME. Some lift mechanisms are equipped with a seat that should be considered an integral part of the lift mechanism. The E codes available for seat lift mechanisms are:

- E0628 Separate lift mechanism for use with patient-owned furniture-electric.

- E0629 Separate seat lift mechanism for use with patient-owned furniture-nonelectric.

- E0627 Seat lift mechanism incorporated into a combination lift chair.

Devices with a spring release mechanism are not covered.

60-9 Durable medical equipment (DME) reference list

Appendix 8 defines Medicare coverage for each DME item and the conditions of payment coverage for the rental and purchase of the DME. Coverage for items that do not fall into the generic categories is left to carrier discretion.

60-11 Home blood glucose monitors

Coverage for home monitors varies depending on the type of device and the medical condition of the patient. The following describes the conditions of coverage:

- Reflectance colorimeter devices are used for measuring blood glucose levels in clinical settings and are not covered for home use.

- Blood glucose monitors that use a reflectance meter designed for diabetic patients at home may be covered as durable medical equipment subject to conditions and limitations.

- Lancets, reagent strips and other supplies used for the proper functioning of the monitoring device are covered.

- Patients must be insulin-dependent diabetics, and there must be physician documentation of poor diabetic control. The physician must state that the patient (or responsible family member) is capable of being trained to use the device. The device is designed for home use rather than clinical use.

- Special blood glucose monitoring systems designed for those patients with visual impairments are covered if the patient meets the above conditions. The physician must certify that the visual impairment is severe enough to require a special monitoring system. These systems feature voice synthesizers, automatic timers and specially designed equipment to enable easy access.

Identify claims for special blood glucose monitoring systems with HCPCS Level II code E0609.

60-14   Infusion pumps

External infusion pumps are covered for:

- iron poisoning-to administer deferoxamine to treat acute iron poisoning and iron overload;

- thromboembolic disease-to administer heparin to treat thromboembolic disease and/or pulmonary embolism;

- chemotherapy for liver cancer-to treat primary hepatocellular carcinoma or colorectal cancer if the disease is unresectable or the patient refuses surgical excision of the tumor; and

- morphine-to treat intractable pain caused by cancer in either an inpatient or an outpatient setting, including a hospice.

- Continuous subcutaneous insulin infusion pumps (CSII)

Medicare covers the treatment of Type I diabetes in the home setting, which includes the infusion pump, drugs and related supplies. However, patients must meet criterion A or B:

A. The patient has completed a diabetes education program and been on a program of multiple daily injections of insulin (i.e., at least three injections per day), with frequent self-adjustments of insulin dose, for at least six months prior to the insulin pump. The patient must have documented frequency of glucose self-testing on an average of at least four times per day during the two months prior to initiation of

Appendix 4

the insulin pump, and meets one or more of the following criteria while on the multiple daily injection regimen:

- Glycosylated hemoglobin level(HbAlc) > 7.0%

- History of recurring hypoglycemia

- Wide fluctuations in blood glucose before mealtime

- Dawn phenomenon with fasting blood sugars frequently exceeding 200 mg/dl

- History of severe glycemic excursions

- The patient with Type I diabetes has been on a pump prior to enrollment in Medicare and has documented frequency of glucose self-testing an average of at least 4 times per day during the month prior to Medicare enrollment.

B.
- Type I diabetes needs to be documented by a C-peptide level < 0.5

- Continued coverage of the insulin pump would require that the patient has been seen and evaluated by the treating physician at least every 3 months

- The pump must be ordered by and follow-up care of the patient must be managed by a physician who manages multiple patients with CSII and who works closely with a team including nurses, diabetes educators, and dietitians knowledgeable in the use of CSII.

Subcutaneous insulin infusion pumps will continue to be denied as not medically necessary and reasonable for all Type II diabetics including insulin-requiring Type II diabetics.

Payment may also be made for drugs necessary for the effective use of an external infusion pump as long as the drug being used with the pump is itself reasonable and necessary for the patient's treatment. Other uses of external infusion pumps are covered if the contractor's medical staff verifies the appropriateness of the therapy and of the prescribed pump for the individual patient.

Implantable infusion pumps are covered:

- for intraarterial infusion of 5-FUdR to treat liver cancer in patients with primary hepatocellular carcinoma or Duke's Class D colorectal cancer; when the metastasis is limited to the liver; and when the disease is unresectable or the patient refuses surgical excision of the tumor.

- to administer antispasmodic drugs intrathecally (e.g., baclofen) to treat chronic intractable spasticity if the patient is unresponsive to less invasive therapy. Examples of less invasive therapies include a six-week trial whereby oral antispasmodic drugs fail to control the spasticity adequately or produce intolerable side effects; the patient responded favorably to a trial intrathecal dose of the antispasmodic drug.

- to administer opioid drugs (e.g., morphine) intrathecally or epidurally to treat severe chronic intractable pain of malignant or nonmalignant origin, when the patient is expected to live at least three months but is unresponsive to less invasive therapy. The patient's history must show an unresponsiveness to noninvasive methods of pain control such as systemic opioids and the elimination of physical and behavioral problems that may cause exaggerated reactions to pain.

The patient must undergo a preliminary trial of intraspinal opioid drug administration with a temporary intrathecal/epidural catheter to substantiate pain relief, and degree of side effects including effects on daily living and the patient's acceptance of the drugs.

- for other uses when the contractor's medical staff can validate that the drug is reasonable and necessary to treat the patient, administration of the drug by implantable infusion pump is medically necessary and the FDA has approved the pump for use with the drug being administered.

It is not appropriate to implant an infusion pump for patients who are allergic or hypersensitive to the drug (e.g., oral baclofen, morphine, etc.), have an infection, cannot support the weight and bulk of the device and have other implanted programmable devices, since crosstalk between devices may change the prescription.

Drugs necessary for the effective use of the pump are covered if they are reasonable and necessary for the patient's treatment.

Medicare does not cover:

- the subcutaneous infusion of insulin using an external infusion pump in the treatment of diabetes or the administration of vancomycin; or

- the heparin implantable infusion pump in the treatment of recurrent thromboembolic disease.

60-15   Safety roller

Safety rollers are covered by Medicare for some patients who are obese, have severe neurological disorders or restricted use of one hand, making it impossible to use a wheeled walker that does not have the sophisticated braking system found on the safety rollers. Documentation must support medical necessity.

Safety rollers come under medical review for determining whether the features are necessary, covered and reimbursable. If a patient can use a standard wheeled walker, the charge for the safety roller is reduced to that of a standard wheeled walker.

In the case of patients with medical documentation indicating severe neurological disorders, which make it impossible for them to use a standard wheeled walker, a reasonable charge for the safety roller may be determined without relating it to the reasonable charge for the standard wheeled walker.

Appendix 4

60-16 Pneumatic compression devices (used for lymphedema)

In the home setting, the segmental and nonsegmental compression devices are covered only for the treatment of generalized, refractory lymphedema.

Pneumatic compression devices are covered only as a treatment of last resort (i.e., other less intensive treatments such as leg or arm elevation, and custom fabricated gradient pressure stockings or sleeves must have been tried first and found inadequate). These devices must be prescribed by a physician and be used with appropriate physician oversight. This must include physician evaluation of the patient's condition to determine medical necessity, suitable instruction in the operation of the machine, a treatment plan defining the pressure to be used, frequency and duration of use and ongoing monitoring and response to treatment.

The medical necessity determination must include the patient's diagnosis and prognosis; symptoms and objective findings (i.e., measurements that establish the severity of the condition; the reason the device is required; treatments that have been tried and failed; and the clinical response to initial treatment with the device).

Payment is made for the least expensive medically appropriate device. The nonsegmented (HCPCS E0650) or segmented (HCPCS E0651) compression device without manual control of pressure is the least costly alternative that meets the clinical needs of the individual. The segmented device with manual control (HCPCS E0652) is covered only when there are unique characteristics that prevent the individual from receiving satisfactory pneumatic treatment using a less costly device (e.g., significant sensitive skin scars, the presence of contracture, pain caused by a clinical condition requiring the more costly manual control device).

Pneumatic compression devices may be medically appropriate for patients with generalized, refractory edema from venous insufficiency with lymphatic obstruction, (i.e., recurrent cellulitis with secondary scarring of the lymphatic system) with significant ulceration of the lower extremities, who have received repeated, standard treatment from a physician using a compression bandage system, but failed to heal after six months of continuous treatment. The medical problem must be evident from the medical information submitted.

60-17 Continuous positive airway pressure (CPAP)

CPAP is covered under Medicare when used on adult patients. Initial claims must be supported by medical documentation such as a prescription from the patient's physician that specifies that the patient's diagnosis is moderate or severe obstructive sleep apnea (OSA) and surgery is the likely alternative. The medical documentation must support a diagnosis of OSA-at least 30 episodes of apnea, each lasting a minimum of 10 seconds during 6-7 hours of recorded sleep.

60-18 Hospital beds

A physician's prescription and other documentation in the medical record as required by the contractor's medical staff must establish the medical necessity of a hospital bed. Medical necessity is established if the patient's condition requires positioning of the body or requires special attachments that cannot be fixed and used on a regular bed. The physician's prescription must accompany the initial claim and include the medical condition, severity and frequency of the symptoms that necessitate a hospital bed for positioning. The prescription must describe the patient's condition and specify the attachments that require a hospital bed.

A variable height feature on a hospital bed may be approved for severe arthritis and other injuries to the lower extremities to assist the patient to ambulate; severe cardiac conditions to avoid strain of jumping up or down from bed; spinal cord injuries, quadriplegic and paraplegic patients, multiple limb amputee and stroke patients to assist transfer from bed to a wheelchair; and other severely debilitating diseases and conditions to assist the patient to ambulate.

Electric-powered hospital-bed adjustments may be required to lower or raise the head and feet and may be covered if the patient requires a frequent change in body position and/or there is an immediate need for a change in position, and the patient can operate the adjustment controls. Exceptions regarding the requirement that the patient operate the controls may be made for patients with spinal cord injuries or brain damage.

If the patient's condition requires bedside rails, they can be covered as an integral part of the hospital bed.

60-19 Air-fluidized bed (effective for services rendered on or after July 30, 1990)

Medicare payment for home use of the air-fluidized bed for treatment of pressure sores can be made if use of the bed is reasonable and necessary for the individual patient. The attending physician must submit a written order to the supplier prior to the delivery of the equipment in order for it to be covered. Reasonable and necessary use of an air-fluidized bed requires that:

- the patient has a stage 3 (full-thickness tissue loss) or stage 4 (deep tissue destruction) pressure sore;

- the patient is bedridden or chair-bound due to severely limited mobility;

- the patient would require institutionalization without the air-fluidized bed;

- the physician has provided a written order for the air-fluidized bed based on a comprehensive assessment and evaluation of the patient after conservative treatment has been tried without success;

- a trained adult care giver is available to assist the patient with activities of daily living, fluid balance, dry skin care, repositioning, recognition and management of altered mental status, dietary needs, prescribed treatments and management and support of the air-fluidized bed system and its problems, such as leakage;

Appendix 4

- a physician directs the home treatment regimen, reevaluates and recertifies the need for the air-fluidized bed on a monthly basis; and all other alternative equipment has been considered and ruled out.

Coverage is not provided if:

- the patient has coexisting pulmonary disease (the lack of firm back support makes coughing ineffective and dry air inhalation thickens pulmonary secretions);

- the patient requires treatment with wet soaks or moist wound dressings that are not protected with an impervious covering such as plastic wrap;

- the care giver is unwilling or unable to provide the required care on an air-fluidized bed;

- structural support is inadequate to support the weight of the air-fluidized bed system (it generally weighs 1,600 pounds or more);

- the electrical system is insufficient for the increase in energy consumption; or

- other known contraindications exist.

65-1 Hydrophilic contact lenses

Hydrophilic contact lenses are eyeglasses and are not covered under Medicare when used in treating nondiseased eyes with spherical ametrophia, refractive and/or corneal astigmatism.

Payment may be made under the prosthetic device benefit when an FDA-approved device is prescribed for an aphakic patient. An FDA letter of approval or other FDA-published material will be accepted as evidence of FDA approval.

65-3 Scleral shell

The scleral shell or shield is a term for different types of hard scleral contact lenses. A scleral shell fits over the entire exposed surface of the eye. The shell may forestall the need for surgical enucleation and prosthetic implant and act to support the surrounding orbital tissue. The device essentially serves as an artificial eye and may be covered by Medicare.

Scleral shells are occasionally used with artificial tears to treat "dry eye" of diverse etiology. Tears dry at a rapid rate and are continually replaced by the lacrimal gland. When the gland fails, the half-life of artificial tears may be prolonged by using the scleral contact lens as a protective barrier against the drying action of the atmosphere. The frequent installation of artificial tears can be avoided. The lens acts as a substitute for the diseased lacrimal gland and is covered as a prosthetic device when used to treat "dry eye."

65-5   Electronic speech aids

Electronic speech aids (oral tube model or the throat contact device) are covered under Part B as prosthetic devices when the patient has had a laryngectomy or his or her larynx is permanently inoperative.

65-7   Intraocular Lenses (IOLs)

An intraocular lens, or pseudophakos, is an artificial lens which may be implanted to replace the natural lens after cataract surgery. Intraocular lens implantation services, as well as the lens itself, may be covered if reasonable and necessary for the individual. Implantation services may include hospital, surgical, and other medical services, including pre-implantation ultrasound (A-scan) eye measurement of one or both eyes.

65-8   Electrical nerve stimulators

Two classifications of nerve stimulators are used to treat chronic intractable pain: implanted peripheral nerve stimulators and central nervous system stimulators.

Payment is made for implanted peripheral nerve stimulators under the prosthetic device benefit. Use of this stimulator involves implantation of electrodes around a selected peripheral nerve. Implantation requires surgery and usually necessitates an operating room. When peripheral nerve stimulators are used to assess the patient's suitability for continued treatment with an electric nerve stimulator, such use of the stimulator is covered as part of the total diagnostic service rather than as a prosthesis (see also Medicare Coverage Issues Manual 35-46).

Central nervous system stimulators (dorsal column and deep brain stimulators) are covered for therapies that relieve chronic intractable pain.

No payment is made for either implantation unless all of the conditions below are present:

- The implantation is used as a last resort for patients with chronic intractable pain.

- Other treatment modalities have been tried and did not prove satisfactory or are contraindicated for the patient.

- The patient underwent psychological and physical screening, evaluation and diagnosis by a multidisciplinary team prior to implantation.

- All facilities, equipment and professional and support personnel required for the proper diagnosis, treatment, training and follow-up of the patient must be available.

- Demonstration of pain relief with a temporary implanted electrode preceded permanent implantation.

65-9   Incontinence control devices

Mechanical/hydraulic incontinence control devices-This class of device achieves control of urination by compression of the urethra. It safely and effectively manages urinary incontinence in patients with permanent anatomic and neurological dysfunctions of the bladder. The device is covered when its use is reasonable and necessary for the individual patient.

Collagen implant-The collagen implant is a prosthetic device used to treat stress urinary incontinence resulting from intrinsic sphincter deficiency (ISD), whereby the urethral sphincter is unable to contract and generate sufficient resistance in the bladder. The implant is injected into the submucosal tissues of the urethra and/or the bladder neck and into tissues adjacent to the urethra. Prior to collagen implant therapy, a skin test for collagen sensitivity must be administered and evaluated over a four-week period. Physicians must have urology training in the use of a cystoscope and complete a collagen implant training program.

Evaluation requirements for the establishment of a diagnosis of ISD-For male patients, the evaluation must include a complete history and physical examination and a simple cystometrogram to determine that the bladder fills and stores properly. The patient then is asked to stand upright with a full bladder and to cough or otherwise exert abdominal pressure on his bladder. A diagnosis of ISD is established if the patient leaks. For female patients, the evaluation must include a complete history and physical examination (including a pelvic exam) and a simple cystometrogram to rule out abnormalities of bladder compliance and abnormalities of urethral support. Also, an abdominal leak point pressure (ALLP) test is performed. If the patient has an ALLP of less than 100 cm H2O, the diagnosis of ISD is established.

Coverage of the implant and the procedure to inject it is limited to the following patients with stress urinary incontinence due to ISD:

- male or female patients with congenital sphincter weakness secondary to conditions such as myelomeningocele or epispadias

- male or female patients with acquired sphincter weakness secondary to spinal cord lesions

- male patients following trauma, including prostatectomy and/or radiation

- female patients without urethral hypermobility and with abdominal leak point pressures of 100 cm H2O or less.

Patients whose incontinence does not improve with five injection procedures are considered treatment failures and no further treatment of urinary incontinence by collagen implant is covered. Patients who have a reoccurrence of incontinence following successful treatment with collagen 6-12 months previously may benefit from additional treatment sessions. Coverage of additional sessions may be allowed but must be supported by medical justification.

Electronic stimulators-Pelvic floor electrical stimulators are not covered as a treatment (as a bladder pacer or a retraining mechanism) for urinary incontinence.

65-10 Enteral and parenteral nutritional therapy covered as a prosthetic device

Medicare coverage for nutritional therapy is provided under the prosthetic device benefit provision. The patient must have a permanently inoperative internal body organ or function.

Enteral and parenteral nutritional therapy is not covered for temporary impairments. The test of permanence will be considered met, however, if the medical record and the attending physician indicate that the impairment will be of indefinite duration.

Supplies, equipment and nutrients related to enteral and parenteral nutrition therapy are covered under the following conditions:

Parenteral nutrition therapy -Daily therapy is reasonable and necessary for patients with a severe pathology of the alimentary tract that does not allow absorption of sufficient nutrients to maintain weight and strength equal to the patient's general condition. Parenteral nutrition can be provided in the patient's home by specially trained nonprofessional persons.

Services provided by nonphysician professionals are not covered, except as services furnished incident to a physician's services.

A physician's written order or prescription is required for coverage. Documentation must support the medical necessity for the prosthetic device. Coverage is approved on a case-by-case basis and at periodic intervals of no more than three months. If the claim involves an infusion pump, sufficient evidence of medical necessity must be provided.

Nutrient solutions for parenteral therapy are covered. Medicare pays for one month's supply at a time. Medicare pays the reasonable charge for the solution components unless a signed statement from the attending physician establishes that the beneficiary cannot mix the solution safely or effectively, and there is no responsible person who can do so. In that case, premixed solutions may be covered.

Enteral nutrition therapy-Enteral nutrition is considered reasonable and necessary for a patient with a functioning gastrointestinal tract that, due to pathology or to nonfunction of the structures that normally permit food to reach the digestive tract, does not allow the patient to maintain weight and strength. Therapy can be given by nasogastric, jejunostomy or gastrostomy tubes and can be provided safely in the home by nonprofessionals who have undergone training. Reimbursement is not available for any nonphysician professionals, except as services furnished incidental to a physician's services.

Coverage, which requires a physician's written order or prescription, is approved on a case-by-case basis. Documentation must support the medical necessity of the prosthetic device. Claims are reviewed every three months.

Nutrient solutions for enteral therapy are covered. Medicare pays for one month's supply at a time. If the claim involves a pump, sufficient evidence of medical necessity must be provided.

Appendix 4

Nutritional supplements of daily protein and caloric intake between meals are not covered under Medicare Part B.

65-11 Bladder stimulators (pacemakers)-Not covered

There are a number of devices available to induce emptying of the bladder by using electrical current which forces the muscles of the bladder to contract.

The use of spinal cord electrical stimulators, rectal electrical stimulators, and bladder wall stimulators is not considered reasonable and necessary. Therefore, no program payment may be made for these devices or their implantation.

65-14 Cochlear implantation

Medicare coverage is provided for cochlear implantation for patients meeting all of the following criteria:

- diagnosis of severe to profound sensorineural/hearing impairment with limited benefit from appropriate hearing aid

- cognitive ability to use auditory clues and a willingness to undergo an extended program of rehabilitation

- freedom from middle ear infection, an accessible cochlear lumen that is structurally suited to implantation and freedom from lesions in the auditory nerve and acoustic areas of the central nervous system

- no contraindications to surgery

Adults-Cochlear implants may be covered for adults (over age 18) for prelinguistically, perilinguistically and postlinguistically deafened adults. Postlinguistically deafened adults must demonstrate test scores of 30 percent or less on sentence recognition from tape recorded tests in the patient's best listening condition.

Children-Cochlear implants may be covered for children aged 2-17, prelinguistically and postlinguistically deafened. Bilateral profound sensorineural deafness must be demonstrated by the inability to improve on age appropriate closed-set word identification tasks with amplification.

65-16 Tracheostomy speaking valve

A tracheostomy speaking valve is covered under Medicare as an "add on" element that enhances the function and effectiveness of a trachea tube as a prosthetic device.

70-1 Corset used as a hernia support

A hernia support (e.g., corset or truss), which meets the definition of a brace, is covered under the Medicare Part B benefit.

70-2 Sykes Hernia Control

The Sykes Hernia Control (a spring type, "u"-shaped, strapless truss) is not functionally better than a conventional truss and is covered and paid for based on the reimbursement for a conventional truss.

70-3   Prosthetic Shoe

A prosthetic shoe (a device used when all or a substantial portion of the front part of the foot is missing) can be covered as a terminal device; i.e., a structural supplement replacing a totally or substantially absent hand or foot. The coverage of artificial arms and legs includes payment for terminal devices such as hands or hooks even though the patient may not require an artificial limb. The function of the prosthetic shoe is quite distinct from that of excluded orthopedic shoe and supportive foot devices which are used by individuals whose feet, although impaired, are essentially intact.

Appendix 4

MCM References

2005.1 When Part B expenses are incurred, physicians' expense for surgery, childbirth, and treatment for infertility

Medicare covers all expenses for surgical and obstetrical care, including preoperative/prenatal examinations and tests and postoperative/postnatal services are considered incurred on the date of surgery or delivery, as appropriate. This policy applies whether the physician bills on a package charge basis, or itemizes the bill separately.

Infertility is a condition sufficiently at variance with the usual state of health to make it appropriate for a person who normally is expected to be fertile to seek medical consultation and treatment. Reasonable and necessary services associated with treatment for infertility are covered under Medicare.

2005.2 When Part B expenses are incurred; physicians' expense for allergy treatment

Allergists typically bill separately for the initial diagnostic work-up and for the treatment. When it is necessary for the physician to provide treatment over an extended period, the allergist may bill a lump sum for all treatments. It also is common for the entire physician's charge to be divided over the period of treatment and billed periodically. Expenses for allergists are incurred when the services are rendered. When the allergist bills periodically for a course of treatment, it is assumed that the physician's periodic bill relates to services rendered prior to the billing date. No payment is made for that portion of the fee or charge relating to services that were not rendered, as in the case of a patient who dies while undergoing treatment. The physician may need to provide documentation for the dates of service and charges for each.

2049 Services and supplies; drugs and biologicals (formerly MCM 2050.5)

Drugs and biologicals, except those that are necessary to the effective use of an item of DME or prosthetic device, or are specifically covered (e.g., EPO and drugs used as immunosuppressive therapy), are covered only if they meet all of the following requirements:

- They are defined as a drug or biologicals as defined by statute.

- The drug cannot be self-administered based on how the drug or biological is usually administered. For example, if the physician gives the patient a pill or oral medication that the patient usually self-administers, or if the physician gives the patient an injection that is usually self-administered, the medication or injection is excluded from coverage. However, if the injection is administered in an emergency situation (e.g., diabetic oma), the drug is covered.

Whole blood cannot be self-administered and is covered incident to a physician service.

- Blood clotting factors for hemophilia patients who are able to self-administer the factors to control bleeding without supervision are covered as an exception. Hemophilia encompasses Factor VIII deficiency (classic hemophilia), Factor IX deficiency (also called plasma thromboplastin component (PTC) or Christmas factor deficiency) and Von Willebrand's disease.

- Antigens that have been prepared for a particular patient may be covered if the antigen is prepared by a physician and the antigen is administered according to a treatment plan following examination of the patient. A reasonable supply of antigens is considered to cover a period of not more than 12 weeks.

- The drug or biological is not excluded as an immunization.

Vaccinations or inoculations are considered immunizations unless they are directly related to the treatment of an injury or direct exposure to a disease or condition. In the absence of injury or direct exposure, preventive immunizations (vaccination or inoculation) against such diseases as smallpox, polio, diphtheria, etc., are not covered. However, pneumococcal, hepatitis B and influenza virus vaccines are exceptions to this rule.

Pneumococcal vaccine and its administration are covered if it is ordered by a physician who is a doctor of medicine or osteopathy. The physician does not have to be present to meet this requirement if a standing order exists specifying:

- the person's age, health and vaccination status;

- a signed consent must be obtained;

- the vaccine may be administered only to persons at high risk* of pneumococcal disease who have been previously vaccinated; and

- a record of vaccination must be provided.

*High-risk individuals are people age 65 and older, immunocompetent adults who are at increased risk of pneumococcal disease or complications because of a chronic illness and individuals with compromised immune systems.

Hepatitis B vaccine and its administration furnished to a Medicare beneficiary at *high or **intermediate risk of contracting hepatitis B are covered.

*High-risk individuals are end stage renal disease (ESRD) patients, hemophiliacs who receive Factor VIII or IX concentrates, clients of institutions for the mentally retarded, persons who live in the same household as a Hepatitis B Virus (HBV) carrier, homosexual men and illicit injectable drug abusers.

**Intermediate-risk individuals are staff in institutions for the mentally retarded and workers in health care professions who have frequent contact with blood or blood-derived body fluids during routine work.

EXCEPTION: Individuals identified above would not be considered at high or intermediate risk of contracting hepatitis B, however, if there is laboratory evidence positive for antibodies to hepatitis B.

The vaccine may be administered upon the order of a doctor of medicine or osteopathy by home health agencies, skilled nursing facilities, ESRD facilities, hospital outpatient departments, persons recognized under the incident to physicians' services provision of law, and doctors of medicine and osteopathy

Influenza virus vaccine and its administration are covered when furnished in compliance with applicable State law by any provider or any entity or individual with a Medicare supplier number. These vaccines are administered once a year . The beneficiary may receive the vaccine upon request without a physician's order or supervision.

■ It must be safe, effective, reasonable and necessary for the diagnosis or treatment of the illness or injury for which it is administered. Determinations as to whether an injection is reasonable and necessary are made with the advice of medical consultants and with reference to accepted standards of medical practice and the medical circumstances of the individual case.

　• Medications given for a purpose other than to treat the specific condition (except for certain immunizations), illness or injury are not covered.

　• Medication administered by injection is not covered if oral administration is the accepted or preferred method of administration and is standard medical practice.

　• Injections are not covered if the frequency or duration of the injections exceed accepted standards of medical practice.

■ It must meet the requirements for coverage of items furnished by a physician and administered by him or incident to a physician's services, by personnel employed by him under his personal supervision. The charge for the drug or biological must be included in the physician's bill, and the cost of the drug or biological must represent an expense to the physician. Drugs and biologicals furnished by other health professionals may also meet these requirements.

■ It has not been determined by the FDA to be less than effective for the indications on the label.

■ Immunosuppressive drugs are covered for one year following discharge from a hospital for a Medicare-covered organ transplant in addition to prescription drugs that are used in conjunction with immunosuppressive drugs as approved by the FDA.

■ Epoetin (EPO) is covered to treat anemia induced by AZT, anemia associated with chronic renal failure, anemia caused by chemotherapy in patients with nonmyeloid malignancies when furnished incident to a physician's service. All ESRD patients initiating EPO treatment with anemia associated with chronic renal failure and having a hematocrit less than 30 percent or hemoglobin less than 10 are considered for EPO therapy. For a patient who has been receiving EPO from the facility or the physician, a hematocrit of between 30 and 36 percent is considered. Also, patients with severe angina, severe pulmonary distress, or severe hypotension may require EPO to prevent adverse symptoms even if they have higher hematocrit or hemoglobin levels.

EPO is covered also for the treatment of anemia for patients with chronic renal failure who are on dialysis if it is administered in the renal dialysis facility, self-administered in the home by the patient or administered by a patient caregiver competent to administer the drug. A dialysis patient using EPO in the home must have a current care plan that monitors diet, fluid intake and adequate provision of supplemental iron, evaluates hematocrit and iron stores, reevaluates the dialysis prescription, provides a method for physician and facility follow-up on blood tests and for informing the physician, provides training to the patient to identify signs of hypotension and hypertension and discontinues EPO if the hypertension is uncontrollable.

- Coverage is extended to oral anti-cancer drugs that are prescribed as anti-neoplastic chemotherapeutic agents. Self-administered antiemetics are covered when they are necessary for the administration and absorption of the anti-neoplastic agent. The oral anti-cancer drug must be approved by the FDA.

To be covered under Part B, an oral anti-cancer drug must be prescribed by a physician or other practitioner licensed under State law to prescribe such drugs as anti-cancer chemotherapeutic agents, be a drug or biological that has been approved by the FDA, have the same active ingredients as a non-self-administrable anti-cancer chemotherapeutic drug or biological that is covered when furnished incident to a physician's service, be used for the same indications as the non-self-administrable version of the drug and be reasonable and necessary for the individual patient.

- Anti-cancer chemotherapeutic regimen for a medically accepted indication is a combination of anti-cancer agents, which has been clinically recognized for the treatment of a specific type of cancer. A cancer treatment regimen includes drugs used to treat toxicities or side effects of the cancer treatment regimen when the drug is administered incident to a chemotherapy treatment. Anti-cancer chemotherapeutic regimen is covered under the following conditions. The drugs and biologicals must have approved labeling for use by the FDA, the American Hospital Formulary Service Drug Information or the American Medical Association Drug Evaluations United States Pharmacopoeia Drug Information. Use may also be supported by clinical research that appears in peer reviewed medical literature.

If a use is identified as "not indicated" by HCFA, FDA, one or more of the three compendia mentioned above or based on peer reviewed medical literature, the off-label usage is not supported and the drug is not covered. Also, a drug that has been determined by the Food and Drug Administration (FDA) to lack substantial evidence of safety and effectiveness for all labeled indications is not covered.

The Balanced Budget Act of 1997 extends coverage of oral anti-emetic drugs approved by FDA for use as anti-emetics. The oral anti-emetic must either be administered by the treating physician or in accordance with a written order from the physician as part of a cancer chemotherapy

Appendix 4

regimen. Oral anti-emetic drug administered with a particular chemotherapy treatment must be initiated within two hours of the administration of the chemotherapeutic agent and may be continued for a period not to exceed 48 hours from that time. The oral anti-emetic drug provided must be used as a full therapeutic replacement for the intravenous anti-emetic drugs that would have otherwise been administered at the time of the chemotherapy treatment.

Only drugs pursuant to a physician's order at the time of the chemotherapy treatment qualify for this benefit. The dispensed number of dosage units may not exceed a loading dose administered within two hours of that treatment, plus a supply of additional dosage units not to exceed 48 hours of therapy. However, more than one oral anti-emetic drug may be prescribed and will be covered for concurrent usage within these parameters if more than one oral drug is needed to fully replace the intravenous drugs that would otherwise have been given.

Prescription and nonprescription drugs and biologicals purchased by or dispensed to a patient are not covered.

The Food and Drug Administration (FDA) determined that some companies operating as retail pharmacies were mass producing compounded drugs beyond the normal scope of pharmaceutical practice in violation of FFDCA. The FDA found companies operating as unsanctioned drug manufacturers and producing unapproved drugs. The manufacturing and processing procedures have not been approved by the FDA and there is no assurance that the drugs are safe and effective.

Medicare limits coverage of drugs to those that are reasonable and necessary and that have received final marketing approval by the FDA, unless instructed otherwise by HCFA.

Also, services related to the use of noncovered drugs are not covered by Medicare. If DME or a prosthetic device is used to administer a noncovered drug, coverage is denied for both the nonapproved drug and the DME or prosthetic device.

The Medicare Carriers Manual provides a list of companies the FDA has identified as producing unapproved compounded drugs in violation of the FFDCA.

2051B Services incident to a physician's service to homebound patients under general physician supervision; covered services

In medically underserved areas, some physicians direct nurses and other paramedical personnel to provide services under general supervision. The physician need not be physically present when the service is performed; however, it must be performed under his overall supervision and control. These services are covered if paramedical personnel meet state requirements, the patient is homebound and the services performed are an integral part of the physician's service to the patient.

The following services are covered:

- Injections

- Venipuncture

- EKGs

- Therapeutic exercises

- Insertion and sterile irrigation of a catheter

- Changing of catheters and collection of catheterized specimen for urinalysis and culture

- Dressing changes, the most chronic conditions being decubitus care and gangrene

- Replacement and/or insertion of nasogastric tubes

- Removal of fecal impaction, including enemas

- Sputum collection for gram stain and culture and possible acid-fast and/or fungal stain and culture

- Paraffin bath therapy for hands and/or feet in rheumatoid arthritis or osteoarthritis

- Teaching and training of the patient about the care of colostomy and ileostomy, permanent tracheostomy, testing urine and care of the feet (diabetic patients only), blood pressure monitoring. Teaching and training services can be covered only when providing knowledge essential for chronically ill patients to participate in their own treatment.

2070.1G Independent Laboratory Service to a Patient in His Home or an Institution

A visit by an independent laboratory technician to obtain a specimen or to perform a venipuncture or take an EKG tracing is considered medically necessary only if:

- the patient was confined to the facility (other than a hospital) or to his or her home or other place of residence; and

- the facility did not have on-duty personnel qualified to perform this service and the service is of the type that requires the skills of a laboratory technician.

Messenger services for the purpose of pick-up only of the specimen (e.g., urine or sputum), do not require the skills of a laboratory technician and would not be covered. (This policy is intended for independent laboratories only.)

2070.4 Coverage of portable x-ray services not under the direct supervision of a physician

Diagnostix-ray services furnished by a portable x-ray supplier are covered under Medicare Part B when furnished in the patient's home, in a nonparticipating institution, in participating SNFs and hospitals when the

Appendix 4

services are not covered under Part A hospital insurance (i.e., when the services are not furnished by the participating institution either directly or under arrangements that provide for the institution to bill for the services).

The services must be performed under the general supervision of a physician and conditions of health and safety must be met.

Coverage for portable x-ray includes: skeletal films involving arms and legs, pelvis, vertebral column and skull; chest films not involving the use of contrast media (except routine screening procedures and tests in connection with routine physical examinations); and abdominal films which do not involve the use of contrast media.

Procedures and examinations which are not covered under the portable x-ray provision include procedures involving: fluoroscopy, the use of contrast media, requiring the administration of a substance to the patient or injection of a substance into the patient and/or special manipulation of the patient, requiring special medical skill or knowledge possessed by a doctor of medicine or doctor of osteopathy or requiring medical judgement to be exercised, requiring special technical competency and/or special equipment or materials, routine screening procedures and procedures which are not of a diagnostic nature.

Portable x-ray tests must be provided on the written order of a physician. Claims for services must contain the name of the physician who ordered the service, and claims for services involving the chest must also contain the reason the x-ray test was required.

An electrocardiogram tracing by an approved supplier of portable x-ray services may be covered as an other diagnostic test.

2079 Surgical dressings, and splints, casts and other devices used for reductions of fractures and dislocations

Surgical dressings are limited to primary and secondary dressings required to treat a wound caused by or treated by a surgical procedure performed by a physician or other health care professional as allowed under state law. Primary dressings are therapeutic and protective coverings applied directly to skin lesions or openings. Secondary dressings are materials that have a therapeutic or protective function to secure a primary dressing. These items include adhesive tape, roll gauze, bandages and disposable compression materials. Items such as transparent film may be used as a primary or a secondary dressing.

Surgical dressings required after debridement of a wound are covered, as long as the debridement was reasonable and necessary. Surgical dressings are covered for as long as they are medically necessary.

Surgical dressings applied first by the physician, certified nurse midwife, physician assistant, nurse practitioner or clinical nurse specialist are considered incident to the professional service rendered. If the patient obtains a surgical dressing from a supplier (pharmacy) based on a physician's order, the dressing is covered under the Part B benefit.

Splints and casts include dental splints.

Elastic stockings, support hose, foot coverings, leotards, knee supports, surgical leggings, gauntlets and pressure garments for the arms and hands are used as secondary dressings and are not covered as surgical dressings.

2100.1 Durable medical equipment (DME)-general; definition of durable medical equipment

Durable medical equipment (DME) can withstand repeated use (i.e., the type of item which could normally be rented) and is used primarily to serve a medical purpose. It generally is not useful in the absence of an illness or injury, and is appropriate for use in the home. All requirements must be met before an item can be considered to be DME.

Expendable medical supplies, such as incontinent pads, lamb's wool pads, catheters, ace bandages, elastic stockings, surgical face masks, irrigating kits, sheets and bags, are not considered to be DME.

Equipment that is presumptively medical are items such as hospital beds, wheelchairs, hemodialysis equipment, iron lungs, respirators, intermittent positive pressure breathing machines, medical regulators, oxygen tents, crutches, canes, trapeze bars, walkers, inhalators, nebulizers, commodes, suction machines and traction equipment.

Hemodialysis is classified as a prosthetic device but it meets the definition of DME also. The reimbursement for the rental or purchase of hemodialysis equipment for home use is made under the DME benefit provisions.

Equipment used for nonmedical purposes is not covered under Medicare. Such equipment includes items used to control or enhance the environment, such as air conditioners, heaters, humidifiers, dehumidifiers and electric air cleaners. Equipment used for convenience (elevators, stairway elevators, posture chairs), physical fitness (exercycle), first aid, precautionary equipment (preset portable oxygen units, self-help devices such as safety grab bars), training equipment (speech teaching machines, Braille training texts) are nonmedical in nature and are not covered.

Specified items of equipment may be covered under certain conditions even though they do not meet the definition of DME. Therapeutic benefit must be clearly established in the medical documentation and a physician must be supervising its use for the equipment to be considered. These items include gel pads and pressure and water mattresses for patients who have bed sores or are highly likely to develop such ulcerations, and heat lamps where the medical need for heat therapy has been established.

2100.4 Durable medical equipment; repairs, maintenance, replacement and delivery

Payment may be made for repairs, maintenance, replacement and delivery of medically required DME that the beneficiary owns or is buying, including equipment that was used before the patient enrolled in the Part B program.

Separately itemized charges for repair, maintenance and replacement of rented equipment are not covered except for conditions related to leased renal dialysis equipment.

Appendix 4

Payment is not made for repair, maintenance and replacement of purchased equipment requiring frequent and substantial servicing, capped rental equipment, or oxygen equipment.

Repairs to equipment being purchased or already owned are covered to make the equipment serviceable. If the repair expense exceeds the purchase or rental price of a replacement item for the remaining period of medical need, no payment will be made for the excess amount.

Maintenance-Routine servicing such as testing, cleaning, regulating and checking, is not covered. Extensive maintenance performed by authorized technicians based on the manufacturer's recommendations is covered as a repair. Examples include breaking down sealed components and performing tests using specialized equipment.

Replacement-Replacement equipment owned or being purchased by the beneficiary is covered in case of loss, irreparable damage or wear or a change in the patient's condition. Replacement equipment due to loss or irreparable damage does not require a physician's order if it is appropriate. Replacing equipment due to wear or a change in the patient's condition must have a current physician's order.

Delivery-Reasonable charges for delivering DME are covered if the supplier customarily charges separately for delivery and if it is common practice among local suppliers.

Leased renal dialysis equipment-Reimbursement may be made for repairing and maintaining home dialysis equipment leased from the manufacturer if the rental charge does not include a margin to recover these costs. The patient also must be free to secure economical repairs locally. Separately itemized repair costs are excluded from reimbursement for medical equipment, retail, supply and rental companies. The patient looks to the DME supplier for repairs, maintenance and replacement of home dialysis equipment.

Medicare payment is made only after the initial warranty period has expired. Routine periodic servicing, testing and cleaning of leased dialysis equipment is not covered. Extensive maintenance and necessary repairs of leased equipment is covered under the Medicare program.

Travel related to the repair of leased dialysis equipment is covered if the repairman customarily charges for travel and if it is common practice in the area. The location of other qualified repairmen will be considered in determining the allowance for travel.

2100.5 Durable medical equipment; coverage of supplies and accessories

Reimbursement may be made for supplies that are necessary for the effective use of DME and are reasonable for the treatment of the illness or injury or to improve the functioning of a malformed body part. Supplies include oxygen, drugs and biologicals directly entered into the equipment to achieve the therapeutic benefit or proper functioning of the DME (e.g., tumor chemotherapy agents used with an infusion pump or heparin used in home dialysis). The drug or biological must be reasonable and necessary.

Replacement of essential accessories, such as hoses, tubes, mouthpieces, etc., may be reimbursed if the patient owns or is purchasing the equipment.

2120.1 Ambulance service; vehicle and crew requirements

Vehicle-The ambulance must be designed and equipped for transporting the sick or injured and include patient care equipment, such as a stretcher, clean linens, first-aid supplies, oxygen equipment and other safety and lifesaving equipment required by state or local authorities.

Crew-The ambulance crew must have at least two members, one of which has medical training equivalent to the standard and advanced Red Cross training. This includes ambulance service training, experience acquired in military service, completion of a recognized first-aid course or on-the-job training sufficient to ensure proficiency in handling a wide range of patient care services.

Compliance-The vehicle and personnel supplier must provide a statement that describes the first-aid, safety and other patient-care items in the vehicle, the extent of first-aid training of the personnel and the supplier's agreement to notify Medicare of any changes that could affect coverage. Documentation must show that the ambulance is equipped according to state and local guidelines. This documentation includes a copy of the letter, license, permit and certificates issued by the authorities.

Equipment and supplies-Reusable devices, such as backboards, neck boards and inflatable leg and arm splints, are considered part of general ambulance services and included in the charge for the trip. A separate reasonable charge may be recognized for nonreusable items and disposable supplies, such as oxygen, gauze and dressings, that are required in patient care during the trip.

2120.4 Ambulance service; air ambulance service

Air ambulance services are covered when:

- the point of pickup is inaccessible by land vehicle;

- distances or other obstacles are involved in getting the patient to the nearest hospital with appropriate facilities (e.g., for cases in which transportation by land ambulance is contraindicated); and

- all other conditions of coverage are met.

An air ambulance can be covered for cases in which the patient's condition and other circumstances necessitated the use of this transportation. When a land ambulance could have sufficed, air ambulance reimbursement is based on the amount payable for land ambulance.

Medical appropriateness-Appropriateness is established when the time needed to transport a patient by land, or the instability of transportation by land, poses a threat to the patient's condition/survival. The following is an advisory list of cases where air ambulance could be justified:

- Intracranial bleeding, requiring neurosurgical intervention

Appendix 4

- Cardiogenic shock

- Burns requiring treatment in a burn center

- Conditions requiring treatment in an hyperbaric oxygen unit

- Multiple severe injuries or life-threatening trauma

Time-When it would take a land ambulance 30 to 60 minutes or more to transport an emergency patient, consider an air ambulance appropriate.

Appropriate facility-The patient must be transported for treatment to the nearest appropriate facility that is capable of providing the required level of care for the patient's illness and that has available the type of physician or physician specialist needed to treat the patient's condition.

Hospital to hospital transport-Transfer from one hospital to another is warranted if the medical appropriateness criteria are met (e.g., ground transportation would endanger the patient, or the transferring hospital does not have the appropriate facilities to provide the medical services the patient needs, such as trauma units, burn units or cardiac care units). Services are covered only if the hospital to which the patient is being transferred is the nearest available with appropriate facilities.

Special coverage rule-An air ambulance is not covered for transport to a facility that is not an acute care hospital, such as a physician's office, nursing facility or the patient's home.

Special payment limitations-Payment for an air ambulance when a land ambulance would have sufficed is based on the amount payable for the land ambulance, if less costly. If the air ambulance was appropriate but the patient could have been treated at a nearer hospital than the one to which the patient was transported, the payment is limited to the distance to the nearest hospital.

Documentation-Adequate documentation is necessary to support air ambulance services. All air ambulance claims are reviewed for medical appropriateness.

2125   Coverage guidelines for ambulance service claims

Ambulance services may be reimbursed by Medicare when the following criteria have been met:

- The patient was transported by an approved ambulance services supplier.

- The patient was suffering from an illness or injury which did not permit transportation by any other means.

- The patient was transported from his or her residence, or other place where need arose, to a hospital or skilled nursing home; a skilled nursing home to a hospital or hospital to a skilled nursing home; a hospital to a hospital or a skilled nursing home to a skilled nursing home; a hospital or skilled nursing home to the patient's residence;

round trip for hospital or skilled nursing facility inpatient to the nearest hospital or nonhospital treatment facility.

In any case, medical documentation must establish that the above conditions for coverage are met. Specifically, the ambulance supplier must be listed in the Medicare carrier's table of approved ambulance companies. Medical documentation must establish medical need, and the claim should show points of pickup and destination.

Ambulance service to a physician's office or physician-directed clinic is not covered by Medicare.

2125.1 Coverage guidelines for ambulance service claims; patient was transported by an approved ambulance service provider

Condition-The patient was transported by an approved supplier of ambulance services.

Documentation-The ambulance supplier is listed in the Medicare carrier's table of approved ambulance companies.

2130 Prosthetic devices

General-Prosthetic devices (other than dental) which replace all or part of an internal body organ (including contiguous tissue), or replace all or part of the function of a permanently inoperative or malfunctioning internal body organ, are covered when furnished on a physician's order. This does not require a determination that there is no possibility that the patient's condition may improve in the future. If the medical record and the judgement of the attending physician indicate that the condition is of long and indefinite duration, the test of permanence is met. The device may also be covered as a supply item when furnished incident to a physician's service.

These devices include cardiac pacemakers, prosthetic lenses, breast prostheses (including surgical brassiere) for post-mastectomy patients, maxillofacial devices and devices that replace all or part of the ear or nose. A urinary collection and retention system, with or without a tube, is a prosthetic device replacing bladder function in the case of permanent urinary incontinence. A Foley catheter is also a prosthetic device for a patient with permanent urinary incontinence.

Chucks, diapers, or rubber sheets are supplies and are not covered under this rule.

Medicare does not cover a prosthetic device dispensed to a patient prior to the time at which the patient undergoes the procedure that makes it necessary to use the device.

Colostomy bags-These and other ostomy bags-and necessary accoutrements required for attachment, including irrigation and flushing equipment and other items and supplies directly related to ostomy care-are covered as prosthetic devices.

Accessories and/or supplies used directly with an enteral or parenteral device to achieve the therapeutic benefit of the prosthesis or assure the

Appendix 4

proper functioning of the device are covered subject to the guidelines provided in CIM section 65-10 through 65-10.3. Covered items include catheters, filters, extension tubing, infusion bottles, pumps (either food or infusion), intravenous (IV) pole, needles, syringes, dressings, tape, heparin sodium (parenteral only), volumetric monitors (parenteral only) and parenteral and enteral nutrient solutions.

Baby food and other regular grocery products that can be blenderized and used with the enteral system are not covered.

Some items qualify as durable medical equipment (e.g., food pump, IV pole).

Coverage of prosthetic devices includes replacement of and repairs to the devices.

Prosthetic lenses-The lens of an eye is considered an internal body organ. Prostheses replacing the lens of an eye include postsurgical lenses used during convalescence from eye surgery in which the lens of an eye was removed. Permanent lenses are also covered by individuals lacking the organic lens of the eye because of surgical removal or congenital absence. Prosthetic lenses obtained on or after the beneficiary's date of entitlement to Part B benefits can be covered even if the surgical removal of the crystalline lens occurred before entitlement.

The following combinations of prosthetic lenses are covered when determined to be medically necessary by a physician to restore the vision provided by the crystalline lens of the eye:

■ Prosthetic bifocal lenses in frames

■ Prosthetic lenses in frames for far vision, and prosthetic lenses in frames for near vision

■ Prosthetic contact lens for far vision. When this is prescribed, payment will be made for the contact lenses and 1) prosthetic lenses in frames for near vision to be worn at the same time as the contact lenses, 2) prosthetic lenses in frames for far vision to be worn when the contacts have been removed.

Payment will be made for prosthetic lenses which have ultraviolet absorbing or reflecting properties instead of untinted prosthetic lenses if it has been determined that such lenses are medically reasonable and necessary for the patient.

Cataract sunglasses are not covered in addition to the regular untinted prosthetic lenses since the sunglasses duplicate the restoration of vision function performed by the regular prosthetic lens.

For services provided on or after March 12, 1990, payment for intraocular lenses (IOLs) inserted during or subsequent to cataract surgery is included with the payment for facility services furnished in connection with the covered surgery. Payment is allowed for no more than one pair of conventional eyeglasses or contact lenses following each cataract surgery with IOL insertion.

Dentures-Dentures are covered only when a denture or a portion thereof is an integral, built-in part of a covered prosthesis (e.g., an obturator to fill an opening in the palate).

Supplies, repairs, adjustments and replacements-Supplies that are necessary for the effective use of the prosthetic device are covered (e.g., batteries needed to operate an artificial larynx). Adjustment to a prosthetic device required by wear or by a change in the patient's condition are covered when ordered by a physician. The same conditions that apply to the repair and replacement of durable medical equipment apply to the prosthetic device.

Supplies, adjustments, repairs and replacements are covered as long as the device continues to be medically necessary.

2130A   Prosthetic devices; general

Prosthetic devices that replace all or part of an internal body organ or the function of a permanently inoperative or malfunctioning internal body organ are covered when furnished on a physician's order. If the medical record and attending physician indicate the condition will be indefinite, the test of permanence is met.

Medicare does not cover a prosthetic device dispensed to a patient prior to the time at which the patient undergoes the procedure that makes the use of the device necessary. For example, no separate payment may be made for an IOL or pacemaker a physician dispenses during an office visit prior to surgery.

Medicare-covered prosthetic devices include: cardiac pacemakers; prosthetic lenses; breast prostheses for postmastectomy patients; maxillofacial devices and devices that replace all or part of the ear or nose; urinary collection and retention systems with or without a tube and colostomy bags and necessary accoutrements required for attachment, including irrigation and flushing equipment and other items and supplies directly related to ostomy care whether or not the attachment bag is required.

Accessories and/or supplies used directly with an enteral or parenteral device to achieve the therapeutic benefit of the device or ensure proper functioning are covered according to guidelines established in CIM section 65-10 through 65-10.3. These items include catheters, filters, extension tubing, infusion bottles, pumps (food or infusion), intravenous pole, needles, syringes, dressings, tape, heparin sodium (parenteral only), volumetric monitors (parenteral only) and parenteral and enteral nutrient solutions.

The coverage of prosthetic devices includes replacement of and repairs to such devices.

2130B   Prosthetic devices; prosthetic lenses

The term "internal body organ" includes the lens of an eye. Prostheses replacing the lens of an eye include postsurgical lenses customarily used during convalescence from eye surgery in which the lens of the eye was removed. Permanent lenses are covered when required for individuals lacking the organic lens of the eye due to surgical removal or congenital absence.

To restore the vision provided by the crystalline lens of the eye, one of the following prosthetic lenses or combinations is covered when medically necessary: prosthetic bifocal lenses in frames; prosthetic lenses in frames for far vision and in frames for near vision; or when prosthetic contact lenses for far vision are prescribed, contact lenses and prosthetic lenses in frames for near vision to be worn at the same time as the contact lenses and prosthetic lenses in frames to be worn when the contacts have been removed. Lenses with ultraviolet absorbing or reflecting properties are covered in lieu of regular untinted lenses if they are medically reasonable and necessary. Cataract sunglasses obtained in addition to regular prosthetic lenses are not covered.

No more than one pair of conventional eyeglasses or conventional contact lenses furnished after each cataract surgery with insertion of an intraocular lens is covered.

2130D   Prosthetic devices; supplies, repairs, adjustments and replacement

Payment may be made for supplies necessary for the effective use of a prosthetic device (e.g., batteries needed to operate an artificial larynx).

Adjustment to a prosthetic device required by wear or a change in the patient's condition is covered when ordered by a physician.

The guidelines for repairing and replacing prosthetic devices are, to the extent possible, covered under the provisions related to DME. Payment is not allowed, however, for more than one pair of conventional eyeglasses or contact lenses following each cataract surgery with IOL insertion.

Necessary supplies, adjustments, repairs and replacements are covered even when the device had been in use prior to the patient's enrollment in Part B, as long as the device continues to be medically required.

2133   Leg, arm, back and neck braces, trusses and artificial legs, arms and eyes

Appliances are covered when furnished incidental to physician's services or on a physician's order.

Braces include rigid and semirigid devices used for supporting a weak or deformed body part or restricting or eliminating motion in a diseased or injured part of the body. Back braces include, but are not limited to, special corsets, sacroiliac, sacrolumbar and dorsolumbar corsets and belts. A terminal device (e.g., hand or hook) is covered whether or not an artificial limb is required.

Elastic stockings, garter belts and similar devices are not considered braces.

Stump stockings and harnesses, including replacements, are covered when they are essential to the effective use of the artificial limb.

Adjustments made to an artificial limb or other appliance that are required by wear or a change in the patient's condition are covered when ordered by a physician.

The guidelines for the repair and replacement of artificial limbs, braces, etc., are, to the extent possible, covered under the provisions relating to DME. Adjustments, repairs and replacements are covered even when the item had been in use prior to the patient's enrollment in Part B, as long as the item continues to be medically required.

2134   Therapeutic shoes for individuals with diabetes

Therapeutic shoes-either depth or custom-molded-with inserts are covered by Medicare for individuals with diabetes as long as certification and prescription requirements are met. Coverage includes a pair of shoes even if only one foot is affected by diabetic foot disease. Each shoe is equipped to provide protection for the affected limb, as well as the remaining limb.

Submit claims for therapeutic shoes for diabetics to the Durable Medical Equipment Regional Carrier (DMERC) for processing.

The following items are covered:

- custom-molded shoes-constructed over a positive model of the patient's foot; shoes made from leather or other suitable material; shoes with removable inserts that can be altered or replaced as the patient's condition requires; shoes that have some form of closure.

- depth shoes-full-length, heel-to-toe filler that, when removed, provides at least 3/16 inch of additional depth; used to accommodate custom-molded or customized inserts; shoes made from leather or other suitable material; have some form of closure; are available in full and half sizes with at least three widths, and the sole is graded to the size and width of the upper portion of the shoe according to the American last sizing schedule (the numerical shoe sizing system used for shoes sold in the United States) or the equivalent.

- inserts-total contact, multiple density, removable inlays that are molded to the patient's foot or a model of the patient's foot; are constructed of suitable material. Inserts may be covered and dispensed independently of diabetic shoes as long as the supplier verifies in writing that the patient has either custom-molded or depth shoes for the insert.

Limitations-Within one calendar year, coverage includes no more than one pair of custom-molded shoes, including inserts, and two additional pairs of inserts; or no more than one pair of depth shoes and three pairs of inserts, not including the noncustomized removable inserts that are provided with the shoe.

Coverage of diabetic shoes and brace-Orthopedic shoes are covered only if they are an integral part of a leg brace. When an individual qualifies for both diabetic shoes and a leg brace, these items are covered separately, as long as his or her respective coverage requirements is met.

Appendix 4

Substitution of modifications for inserts-Modifications of custom-molded or depth shoes may be substituted for inserts in any combination. The payment for the modification will not exceed that of the inserts. The following are the most common shoe modifications available:

- rigid rocker bottoms-exterior elevations with apex positions for 51 percent to 75 percent distance measured from the back end of the heel. Apex height helps eliminate pressure at the metatarsal heads. The heel is tapered off in the back to cause the heel to strike in the middle.

- roller bottoms (sole or bar)-the heel is tapered from the apex to the front tip of the sole.

- metatarsal bars-an exterior bar placed behind the metatarsal heads to remove pressure from the heads. The bars come in various shapes, heights and construction.

- wedges-hind foot, forefoot, or both and in the middle or side. Wedges transfer weight while standing or during ambulation to the opposite side of the foot for added support, stabilization, equalized weight distribution or balance.

- offset heels-a heel flanged at its base in the middle, side or a combination that is extended upward to the shoe to stabilize extreme positions of the hind foot.

- other modifications-flared heels, velcro closures, inserts for missing toes.

Separate inserts-Inserts may be covered and dispensed independently of diabetic shoes if the footwear meets the definition for depth shoes and custom-molded shoes. The supplier must verify in writing that the patient has appropriate footwear into which the insert is to be placed.

Certification-A physician or doctor of medicine or osteopathy responsible for diagnosing and treating the diabetic condition must certify in a plan of care the need for the diabetic shoes. Documentation must include the patient's medical record indicating diabetes; certification that the patient is being treated under a comprehensive plan of care and that diabetic shoes are necessary; the patient has one or more of the following conditions:

- peripheral neuropathy with evidence of callus formation

- history of preulcerative calluses

- history of previous ulceration

- foot deformity

- previous amputation of the foot or part of the foot

- poor circulation

The specific footwear and inserts must be prescribed by a podiatrist or other qualified physician who is knowledgeable about fitting diabetic shoes based on the physician's certification statement.

Payment for the certification of diabetic shoes and for the prescription of the shoes is considered to be included in the payment for the visit or consultation during which these services are provided. If the sole purpose of an encounter with the beneficiary is to dispense or fit the shoes, then no payment may be made for a visit or consultation provided on the same day by the same physician. Thus, a separate payment is not made for certification of the need for diabetic shoes, the prescribing of diabetic shoes or the fitting of diabetic shoes unless the physician documents that these services were not the sole purpose of the visit or consultation.

2136 Dental services

Items and services related to the care, treatment, filling, removal or replacement of teeth or structures directly supporting the teeth are not covered, including periodontium, gingivae, dentogingival junction, periodontal membrane, cementum of the teeth and alveolar process. For an otherwise noncovered procedure or service performed by a dentist incident to and as an integral part of a covered procedure or service performed by him/her, the total service performed by the dentist is covered.

The extraction of teeth to prepare for radiation treatment of neoplastic disease is covered. In this case, the dentist extracts the patient's teeth and a radiologist administers the radiation treatments.

When an excluded service is the primary procedure, it is not covered by Medicare regardless of complexity or difficulty (e.g., the extraction of a tooth). An alveoplasty and a frenectomy are excluded from coverage when either is performed in connection with a noncovered service. The removal of a torus palatinus may be a covered service on rare occasions, but this service is usually performed in connection with an excluded service and is noncovered as such.

Coverage for anesthesia, diagnostic-rays and other related procedures depends on whether the primary procedure is covered. The hospitalization or nonhospitalization of a patient has no bearing on the coverage or exclusion of a dental procedure.

2150 Clinical Psychologist Services

Medicare makes direct payment to the hospital for services furnished to hospital patients. However, services furnished incident to the professional services to hospital patients are paid to the hospital as "incident to" services.

To qualify as a CP, a practitioner must meet the following requirements:

- hold a doctoral degree in psychology

- be licensed or certified, on the basis of the doctoral degree in psychology, by the state of practice, at the independent practice level of psychology to furnish diagnostic, assessment, preventive, and therapeutic services directly to individuals

CPs may provide diagnostic and therapeutic services that the CP is legally authorized to perform in accordance with state laws and regulations. CPs are paid based on the fee schedule for diagnostic and therapeutic services.

Services and supplies furnished incident to a CP's services include:

- mental health services that are commonly furnished in CPs' offices

- an integral, although incidental, part of professional services performed by the CP

- performed under the direct personal supervision of the CP

- furnished without charge or included in the CP's bill

CP services are not covered unless "reasonable and necessary for the diagnosis or treatment of an illness or injury or to improve the functioning of a malformed body member."

A CP must attempt to consult with the patient's physician within a reasonable time after receiving the consent. If the CP's attempts to consult directly with the physician are not successful, the CP must notify the physician within a reasonable time that services are being furnished to the patient. Additionally, the CP must document, in the patient's medical record, the date the patient consented or declined consent to consultations, the date of consultation, or, if attempts to consult did not succeed, that date and manner of notification to the physician.

The only exception to the consultation requirement for CPs is in cases where the patient's primary care or attending physician refers the patient to the CP. Also, neither a CP nor a primary care or attending physician may bill Medicare or the patient for this required consultation.

2152   Clinical Social Worker Services

Medicare covers services provided by a clinical social worker (CSW) only under assignment. The amount payable cannot exceed 80 percent of the lesser of the actual charge for the services or 75 percent of the amount paid to a psychologist for the same service.

According to Medicare guidelines, a clinical social worker must:

- possesses a master's or doctor's degree in social work

- performed at least two years of supervised clinical social work

and either be:

- licensed or certified as a clinical social worker by the state where services are performed; or

- in a state that does not provide for licensure or certification, completed at least two years or 3,000 hours of post master's degree supervised clinical social work practice under the supervision of a master's level social worker in an appropriate setting such as a hospital, SNF, or clinic.

A clinical social worker may provide services for the diagnosis and treatment of mental illnesses. Services furnished to an inpatient of a hospital or an inpatient of a SNF. Services covered by Part B include:

■ services that are otherwise covered if furnished by a physician, or as incident to a physician's service

■ performed by a person who meets the definition of a CSW

■ not otherwise excluded from coverage.

Services of a CSW are not covered when furnished to inpatients of a hospital or to inpatients of a SNF if the services furnished in the SNF are those that the SNF is required to furnish as a condition of participation in Medicare.

2210   Reimbursable physical therapy

To be covered, physical therapy services must relate directly to an active written treatment plan established by the physician after consultation with a qualified physical therapist and must be reasonable and necessary for the treatment of the patient's illness or injury.

The plan of treatment for outpatient services may be established by the physician or qualified physical therapist providing the services.

Services related to activities for the general good and welfare of patients (e.g., general exercises to promote overall fitness and flexibility, and activities to provide diversion or general motivation) are not considered physical therapy under Medicare.

The following conditions of coverage constitute reasonable and necessary physical therapy services:

■ The services must be specific and effective treatment for the patient's conditions based on accepted medical practices.

■ The services and patient's condition must warrant the use of a qualified physical therapist or someone under his or her supervision. Services that do not require qualified physical therapists or their supervision are not considered reasonable or necessary.

■ The development, implementation, management and evaluation of a patient care plan because the beneficiary's condition requires the skills of a physical therapist to meet the beneficiary's needs, promote recovery and ensure medical safety. Where the skills of a physical therapist are needed to manage and periodically reevaluate the appropriateness of a maintenance program because of an identified danger to the patient, those reasonable and necessary management and evaluation services could be covered, even if the skills of a therapist are not needed to carry out the activities performed as part of the maintenance program.

Appendix 4

- The skills of a physical therapist are needed to treat the illness or injury. A beneficiary's diagnosis or prognosis should never be the sole factor in deciding that a service is or is not skilled.

- A service that ordinarily would be performed by nonskilled personnel could be considered a skilled physical therapy service in cases in which there is clear documentation that, because of special medical complications, a skilled physical therapist is required to perform or supervise the service. The importance of a particular service to a beneficiary or the frequency with which it must be performed is not a key factor in determining whether the service is to be considered skilled or nonskilled.

- It is expected that the condition will improve significantly within reasonable time frames based on the physician's assessment and consultation with the qualified physical therapist, or the services must be necessary to establish a safe and effective maintenance program for an individual with a specific disease.

- The amount, frequency and duration of the services are reasonable.

2210.3 Reimbursable physical therapy; application of guidelines

Heat treatments, such as hot packs, hydrocollator, infrared treatments, paraffin and whirlpool baths, do not normally require the skills of a qualified physical therapist. However, if the patient's condition is complicated by circulatory deficiency, areas of desensitization, open wounds or other complications, heat treatments would be considered part of the therapy service.

Gait evaluation and training for a patient whose ability to walk is impaired by neurological, muscular or skeletal abnormality are covered if the skills of a physical therapist are required and the training can be expected to significantly improve a patient's ability to walk.

Ultrasound, shortwave and microwave diathermy treatments must always be performed by qualified physical therapists.

Range of motion tests may be performed only by a qualified physical therapist and, therefore, such tests would constitute physical therapy.

Therapeutic exercises must be performed by or under the supervision of a physical therapist. Range of motion exercises requiring the skills of a qualified physical therapist are covered when they are part of the active treatment of a specific disease that has resulted in lost or restricted mobility.

2217 Covered occupational therapy

Occupational therapy is medically prescribed treatment concerned with improving or restoring functions impaired by illness or injury, or functions that have been permanently lost or reduced by illness or injury. The goal of the therapy is to improve the patient's ability to perform the tasks required for independent functioning. Covered occupational therapy services must relate directly to a written plan of treatment established by a physician.

Therapy may involve:

- evaluating and reevaluating a patient's level of function by administering diagnostic and prognostic tests;

- selecting and teaching task-oriented therapeutic activities to restore physical function;

- planning, implementation and supervision of individual therapeutic activity programs as a part of an overall active treatment program for a patient with diagnosed psychiatric illness;

- planning and implementation of therapeutic tasks and activities to restore sensory-integrative function;

- teaching of compensatory techniques to improve the level of independence in the activities of independent living; design, fabrication and fitting of orthotic and self-help devices; and

- vocational and prevocational assessment and training.

The qualified occupational therapist evaluates and reevaluates a patient's level of function, determines whether an occupational therapy program can reasonably be expected to improve, restore or compensate for lost function and recommends a plan of treatment to the physician.

2251   Coverage of chiropractic services

Coverage of chiropractic services is limited to treatment (also referred to as correction) by means of manual manipulation (i.e., by hands only-also referred to as spine or spinal adjustment by manual means, spine or spinal manipulation, manual adjustment or vertebral manipulation or adjustment). No other diagnostic or therapeutic service is covered.

Manual manipulation must be directed to the spine to correct subluxation demonstrated by an x-ray. Medicare defines subluxation as incomplete dislocation, off-centering, misalignment, fixation or abnormal spacing of the vertebrae anatomically demonstrated on x-ray.

Manual devices (i.e., those that are hand-held with the thrust of the force of the device being controlled manually) may be used by chiropractors in performing manual manipulation of the spine. However, no additional payment for the use of the device or extra charge for the device itself is covered by Medicare.

The x-ray is considered reasonably proximate if taken no more than 12 months prior to, or three months following, the initial course of treatment. In cases of chronic subluxation, such as scoliosis, an older x-ray may be acceptable if there are reasonable grounds to conclude that the condition is permanent.

The patient must have a neuromusculoskeletal condition that requires treatment, and the services rendered must have a direct therapeutic relationship to the condition. The primary diagnosis must be subluxation with the precise level of the subluxation and description of the pertinent

Appendix 4

symptoms specified by the chiropractor to substantiate a claim for manipulation of the spine.

Treatment parameters-There should be improvement, arrest or retarded deterioration in the condition within a reasonable and predictable time period. Acute subluxation problems may require as many as three months of treatment. A chronic spinal joint condition implies a longer treatment time but not with higher frequency.

Carriers have developed treatment parameters under which coverage will be terminated for lack of reasonable expectations that continued treatment will be beneficial. Reimbursement under Medicare is limited to no more than one treatment per day unless documentation of reasonable and necessary additional treatment is submitted.

2300 General exclusions

Medicare does not pay for items and services that are: not reasonable and necessary, under no legal obligation to be paid for or provided, furnished or paid for by government instrumentalities, not provided within the United States, resulting from war, for personal comfort, routing services and appliances, supportive devices for feet, custodial care, cosmetic surgery, charges by immediate relatives or members of the household, dental services, paid or expected to be paid under workers' compensation, nonphysician services provided to a hospital inpatient that were not provided directly or arranged for by the hospital.

2303 Services not reasonable and necessary

Items and services that are not reasonable and necessary for the diagnosis and treatment of illness or injury, or to improve the functioning of a malformed body part are not covered by Medicare. For example, payment cannot be made for the rental of a special hospital bed to be used by the patient in the home unless it is reasonable and necessary for the patient's treatment. Medical devices that have not been approved by the FDA are considered investigational and are not covered. Medical procedures or services performed using such devices are not covered.

2320 Routine services and appliances

Routine physical checkups; eyeglasses, contact lenses and eye examinations for the purpose of prescribing, fitting or changing eyeglasses; eye refractions; hearing aids; and examinations for hearing aids and immunizations are not covered under Medicare.

The routine physical checkup exclusion applies to examinations performed without relationship to treatment or diagnosis for a specific illness, symptom, complaint or injury and examinations required by other third-party payers.

Exclusions apply to eyeglasses or contact lenses, and eye examinations for prescribing, fitting or changing eyeglasses or contact lenses for refractive errors. The exclusions do not apply to physicians' services performed due to an eye disease, to postsurgical prosthetic lenses used to convalesce from eye surgery in which the lens was removed, or to permanent prosthetic lenses required by an individual lacking the organic lens of the eye.

Coverage of services rendered by an ophthalmologist is dependent on the purpose of the exam rather than the diagnosis of the patient's condition.

Vaccinations or inoculations are not covered with the exception of pneumococcal pneumonia, hepatitis B and influenza. Antirabies treatment, tetanus antitoxin or booster vaccine, botulin vaccine, antivenin and immune globulin are covered when they are directly related to injury or direct exposure.

2323 **Foot care and supportive devices for the feet**

Foot care services are not covered for the following services under Medicare:

Treatment of flat foot-The term "flat foot" is a condition where one or more arches have flattened out. The care or correction of flat feet is not covered.

Treatment of subluxations of the foot-Subluxations of the foot are partial dislocations or displacements of joint surfaces, tendons, ligaments or muscles of the foot. Surgical and nonsurgical treatments for the purpose of correcting a subluxated structure in the foot are not covered under Medicare. This exclusion does not apply to medical or surgical treatment of subluxation of the ankle joint (talo-crural joint).

Routine foot care-This includes the cutting or removal of corns or calluses, nail trimming, cutting, clipping or debriding and other hygenic and preventive maintenance, cleansing, soaking and other services performed in the absence of localized illness, injury or symptoms involving the foot. Treatment of fungal infection of the toenail is considered routine and not covered in the absence of clinical evidence of mycosis of the toenail and compelling medical evidence documenting that the patient has a marked limitation of ambulation requiring active treatment of the foot or a nonambulatory patient has a condition that is likely to result in medical complications in the absence of treatment.

Supportive devices for the feet-Orthopedic shoes and other supportive devices for the feet are not covered except if they are an integral part of a leg brace.

The following foot care services are covered under Medicare:

Reasonable and necessary medical or surgical services, diagnosis and treatment of symptomatic conditions such as osteoarthritis, bursitis (including bunion), tendonitis, etc., associated with the partial displacement of foot structures are covered. Surgical correction of a subluxated foot structure that is an integral part of the treatment of a foot injury or that is undertaken to improve the function of the foot or to alleviate an induced or associated symptomatic condition is covered.

Certain foot care procedures considered routine (cutting or removal of corns, calluses or nails) may be hazardous when performed by a nonprofessional person on patients with a systemic condition such as metabolic, neurologic or peripheral vascular disease that resulted in severe circulating embarrassment or areas of desensitization in the legs or feet.

Appendix 4

Services ordinarily considered routine are also covered if performed as a necessary and integral part of an otherwise covered service, such as the diagnosis and treatment of diabetic ulcers, wounds and infections.

The treatment of warts is covered, including plantar warts.

Treatment of mycotic nails may be covered in the absence of a systemic condition. For ambulatory patients, the physician must document clinical evidence of mycosis of the toenail, and that the patient has a clearly defined limit in ambulating, pain or secondary infection caused by the thickening and dystrophy of the infected toenail plate. For nonambulatory patients, the physician must document clinical evidence of mycosis of the toenail and pain or secondary infection caused by the thickening and dystrophy of the infected toenail plate.

2323C Systemic conditions; routine foot care

The following are examples of the types of systemic conditions (i.e., metabolic, neurologic and peripheral vascular diseases) that may justify Medicare coverage for routine foot care. Routine foot procedures performed for conditions noted with an asterisk (*) are reimbursable if the patient is under the active care of a doctor of medicine or osteopathy:

- *Diabetes mellitus

- Arteriosclerosis obliterans

- Buerger's disease

- *Chronic thrombophlebitis

- Peripheral neuropathies involving the feet, with associated:

    - *malnutrition and vitamin deficiency (general malnutrition, alcoholism, malabsorption, pernicious anemia);

    - *carcinoma;

    - *diabetes mellitus;

    - *drugs and toxins;

    - *multiple sclerosis;

    - *uremia;

    - traumatic injury;

    - leprosy or neurosyphilis; and

    - hereditary disorders (hereditary sensory radicular neuropathy, angiokeratoma corporis diffusum [Fabry's], amyloid neuropathy).

Services normally considered routine, such as diagnosis and treatment of diabetic ulcers, wounds and infections, also are covered if performed as necessary and integral parts of otherwise covered services.

2323D   Supportive devices for feet

Orthopedic shoes and other supportive devices for the feet are covered if the shoe is an integral part of a leg brace and its expense is included with the brace. Also, coverage applies to therapeutic shoes furnished to diabetics.

2329   Cosmetic surgery

Cosmetic surgery or expenses incurred in connection with such surgery are not covered. Cosmetic surgery includes any surgical procedure directed at improving appearance, except when required for the prompt (i.e., as soon as medically feasible) repair of accidental injury or for the improvement of the functioning of a malformed body member. For example, this exclusion does not apply to surgery in connection with treatment of severe burns, to repair of the face following a serious automobile accident, or to surgery for therapeutic purposes that coincidentally serves some cosmetic purpose.

2336   Dental services and exclusions

Items and services in connection with the care, treatment, filling, removal or replacement of teeth, or structures directly supporting the teeth are not covered under Medicare. However, payment may be made for other services of a dentist.

2455A   Medical insurance blood deductible; general

Program payment is not made for the first three units (pints) of whole blood or packed red cells received by a beneficiary in a calendar year. After the three-unit deductible has been met, payment may be made for all blood charges subject to normal coverage and reasonable charge criteria. Blood can be covered under Part B only when furnished incident to a physician's services.

2455B   Medical insurance blood deductible; application of the blood deductible

The blood deductible applies only to whole blood and packed red cells. Other components, such a platelets, fibrinogen, plasma, gamma globulin and serum albumin, are not subject to the blood deductible and are covered biologicals.

There is also a Part A blood deductible applicable to the first three pints of whole blood or equivalent units of packed red cells received by a beneficiary in a benefit period. The Part A and Part B blood deductibles are applied separately.

The blood deductible applies to only the charges for blood and not the administration of the blood or packed cells. Payment for the administration charges for all covered units of blood includes the first three furnished in a calendar year. In order for a pint of blood to be counted toward the deductible, it must be medically necessary and furnished incident to a physician's services.

Appendix 4

2470 Outpatient mental health treatment limitation

The amount of expenses that may be recognized for Part B deductible and payment purposes is limited to 62.5 percent of the Medicare-allowed amount for those services, regardless of the actual expenses a beneficiary incurs for treatment of mental, psychoneurotic and personality disorders while the beneficiary is not an inpatient of a hospital at the time such expenses are incurred. This limitation is called the outpatient mental health treatment limitation. Expenses for diagnostic services (e.g., psychiatric testing and evaluation to diagnose the patient's illness) are not subject to this limitation. This limitation applies only to therapeutic services and to services performed to evaluate the progress of a course of treatment for a diagnosed condition, as described in the Medicare Carriers Manual section 2472.3.

3045.4 Effect of assignment upon purchase of cataract glasses from participating physician or supplier

A participating physician or supplier (ophthalmologist, optometrist or optician) who accepts assignment on cataract glasses with deluxe frames may charge the Medicare patient the difference between his or her usual charge for glasses with standard frames and the usual charge for deluxe frames, in addition to the applicable deductible and coinsurance on glasses with standard frames. The patient must be informed in advance of the price difference and sign a statement agreeing to pay the extra charge.

3045.7 Mandatory Assignment and Other Requirements for Home Dialysis Supplies and Equipment Paid Under Method II

Deny payment for supplies and equipment if any of the following conditions are met:

- supplier has not accepted assignment (use EOMB message no. 4.9)

- supplies were furnished by a second supplier

- monthly limit has been paid

- claim is marked as non-assigned and evidence clearly shows that the supplier intends not to accept assignment

3060.6 Payment Under Reciprocal Billing Arrangements

The patient's regular physician may submit the claim, and (if assignment is accepted) receive the Part B payment, for covered visit services (including emergency visits and related services) which the regular physician arranges to be provided by a substitute physician on an occasional reciprocal basis, if:

- the regular physician is unavailable to provide the visit services

- the Medicare patient has arranged or seeks to receive the visit services from the regular physician

- the substitute physician does not provide the visit services to Medicare patients over a continuous period of longer than 60 days

- the regular physician identifies the services as substitute physician services meeting the requirements of this section by entering in item 24d of Form HCFA 1500 HCPCS Q5 modifier (service furnished by a substitute physician under a reciprocal billing arrangement) after the procedure code.

3060.7 Payment Under Locum Tenens Arrangements.--

Medicare allows a regular physician to bill for the services of "locum tenens" physicians. A regular physician is the physician that is normally scheduled to see a patient and includes physician specialists (such as, a cardiologist, oncologist, urologist, etc.).

A patient's regular physician may submit the claim, and (if assignment is accepted) receive the Part B payment for covered visit services (including emergency visits and related services) of a locum tenens, if:

- the regular physician is unavailable to provide the visit services

- the Medicare beneficiary has arranged or seeks to receive the visit services from the regular physician

- the regular physician pays the locum tenens for his/her services on a per diem or similar fee-for-time basis

- The substitute physician does not provide the visit services to Medicare patients over a continuous period of longer than 60 days; and

- The regular physician identifies the services as substitute physician services meeting the requirements of this section by entering HCPCS Q6 modifier (service furnished by a locum tenens physician) after the procedure code.

If the only substitution services a physician performs in connection with an operation are post- operative services furnished during the period covered by the global fee, these services need not be identified on the claim as substitution services.

3312 Evidence of medical necessity for durable medical equipment

For certain items or services billed to the DME Regional Carrier (DMERC), the supplier must receive a signed Certificate of Medical Necessity (CMN) from the treating physician.

The following is a list of the items or services currently requiring a CMN:

- Home oxygen therapy

- Hospital beds

- Support surfaces

- Motorized wheelchairs

- Manual wheelchairs

- Continuous positive airway pressure (CPAP) devices

- Lymphedema pumps (pneumaticompression devices)

- Osteogenesis stimulators

- Transcutaneous electrical nerve stimulators (TENS)

- Seat lift mechanisms

- Power operated vehicles

- Infusion pumps

- Parenteral nutrition

- Enteral nutrition

- Manual and motorized wheelchairs

The physician must supply the following information: estimated length of need (in months) the physician expects the patient to require use of the ordered item, the diagnosis codes that represents the primary reason for ordering this item and additional diagnosis codes that would further describe the medical necessity for the item.

3350.3 Claims Coding Requirements

Physicians must indicate that their services were provided in an incentive-eligible rural or urban HPSA by using one of the following modifiers:

- QB — physician providing a service in a rural HPSA; or

- QU — physician providing a service in an urban HPSA.

The incentive payment is 10 percent of the amount actually paid, not the approved amount. Pay the incentive payment for services identified on either assigned or unassigned claims. Do not include the incentive payment with each claim payment. Establish a quarterly schedule for issuing incentive payments. These payments are taxable and must be reported to the IRS. Prepare a list to accompany each payment. Include a line item for each assigned claim represented in the incentive check and a "summary" item showing the number of unassigned claims represented. The sum of the line items and the "summary" item should equal the amount of the check.

4107 Durable medical equipment-billing and payment considerations under the fee schedule

Reimbursement for DME, prosthetics and orthotics is made under a fee schedule. The equipment is grouped into one of six classes:

- Inexpensive or other routinely purchased DME

- Items requiring frequent and substantial servicing

- Customized items

- Prosthetic and orthotic devices

- Capped rental items

- Oxygen and oxygen equipment

4107.6 Durable medical equipment-written order prior to delivery

The equipment listed for the following E codes is covered when the supplier has a written order in hand prior to delivery.

E0180	E0189	E0181	E0192
E0182	E0720	E0184	E0730
E0185	E1230	E0188	

4107.8 Durable medical equipment-EOMB messages

Explanation of Medicare benefits (EOMB) messages explain the payment amount allowed on a DME claim. The messages are for general DME items when payment is reduced for a line item, inexpensive or frequently purchased equipment, items requiring frequent and substantial servicing, customized items and other prosthetic and orthotic devices, capped rental items, oxygen and oxygen equipment, and items requiring a written order prior to delivery.

4107.9 Durable medical equipment-oxygen HCPCS codes effective Jan. 1, 1989

Old Codes	New Codes	Definition
Q0036	E1377-E1385,E1397	Oxygen concentrator, See notes (1) High humidity
Q0038	E0400, E0405	Oxygen contents, gaseous, per unit (for use with owned gaseous stationary systems or when both a stationary and portable gaseous system are owned; 1 unit = 50 cubic ft.)
Q0039	E0410, E0415O	Oxygen contents, liquid, per unit, (for use with owned stationary liquid systems or when both a stationary and portable liquid system are owned; 1 unit = 10 lbs.)
Q0040	E0416	Portable oxygen contents, per unit (for use only with portable gaseous systems when no stationary gas system is used; 1 unit = 5 cubic ft.)

Appendix 4

Old Codes	New Codes	Definition
Q0041	None	Portable oxygen contents, liquid, per unit (for use only with portable liquid systems when no stationary liquid system is used; 1 unit = 1 lb.)
Q0042	E0425	Stationary compressed See note (3)gas system rental, includes contents (per unit), regulator with flow gauge, humidifier, nebulizer, cannula or mask & tubing; 1 unit = 50 cubic ft.
E0425	Same	No change
E0430	Same	No change
E0435	Same	No change in terminology, but and (8)see note (7).
Q0043	E0440	Stationary liquid (see note (3) oxygen system rental), includes contents (per unit), use of reservoir, contents indicator, flowmeter, humidifier, nebulizer, cannula or mask and tubing; 1 unit of contents = 10 lbs.
Q0440	Same	No change
E0455	Same	No change See note (6)
E0555	Same	No change
E0580	Same	No change See note (6)
E1351	Same	No change See note (6)
E1352	Same	No change
E1353	Same	No change
E1354	Same	No change
E1371	Same	No change
E1374	Same	No change
E1400	E1388-E1396	Same as Q0014
E1401	E1388-E1396	Same as Q0015
E1402	Same	No change
E1403	Same	No change
E1404	Same	No change

Old Codes	New Codes	Definition
E1405	Q0037	Combine the fee See note (10)schedule amounts for the stationary oxygen system and the nebulizer with a compressor and heater (code E0585) to determine the fee schedule amount to apply to oxygen enrichers with a heater (code E1405)
E1406	Q0037	Combine the fee schedule amounts for the stationary oxygen system and the nebulizer with only a compressor (i.e., without a heater, code E0570) to determine the fee schedule amount to apply to oxygen enrichers without a heater (code E1406)

4120   **Foot Care**

The exclusion of foot care is determined by the nature of the service. When an itemized bill shows both covered and noncovered services not integrally related to the covered service, the portion of noncovered charges will be denied. For example, if a bill shows surgery for an ingrown toe and also removal of calluses, the additional charge for the removal of calluses will be denied. The following are exceptional situations, which may warrant payment:

■   incidental noncovered services performed as a necessary and integral part of, and secondary to, a covered procedure,

■   initial diagnostic services performed in connection with a specific symptom or complaint

■   routine type foot care when the patient has a systemic disease of sufficient severity, Medicare Carriers Manual section 2323C

■   evidence available discloses certain physical and/or clinical findings consistent with the diagnosis of severe peripheral involvement. The following findings are pertinent:

Class A findings:

•   Nontraumatic amputation of foot or integral skeletal portion thereof

Class B findings:

•   Absent posterior tibial pulse

•   Advanced trophic changes

Appendix 4

- Absent doralis pedis pulse

Class C findings:

- Claudication
- Temperature changes
- Edema
- Paresthesia
- Burning

The claim may be paid if the physician identifies a Class A finding, two Class B findings, or one Class B and two CLass C findings.

4173   Positron emission tomography (PET) scans

For dates of service on or after March 14, 1995, PET scans were covered for only one use, imaging of the perfusion of the heart using Rubidium 82 (Rb82).

For dates of service on or after January 1, 1998 coverage is available for PET scans for the characterization of solitary pulmonary nodules and for the initial staging of lung cancer.

All other uses of PET scans remain not covered.

4174   Cryosurgery of the Prostate Gland

Cryosurgery of the prostate gland, also known as cryosurgical ablation of the prostate (CSAP), destroys prostate tissue by applying extremely cold temperatures in order to reduce the size of the prostate gland. Medicare covers cryosurgery of the prostate gland only as primary treatment for patients with clinically localized prostate cancer, stages T1-T3.

Providers must submit claims for cryosurgery of the prostate gland and for the accompanying ultrasonic guidance on Health Insurance Claim Form HCFA-1500 or electronic equivalent.

Pay for cryosurgery of the prostate gland and for the accompanying ultrasonic guidance only for the codes and services noted and only as required below.

HCPCS Code TOS* Description	Requirements	Payment ICD-9-CM Code Description	Methodology/ Fee Schedule
G0160; TOS=2 Cryosurgical ablation of localized prostate cancer, primary treatment only (postoperative irrigations and aspiration of sloughing tissue included)	Pay 1. For this service only as a primary treatment for patients with clinically localized prostate cancer, stages T1-T3. 2. For only one claim for this service per beneficiary per date of service.	185 Malignant neoplasm of prostate	Refer to the Medicare physician fee schedule including applicable quarterly database updates. This code has a 90-day global indicator.
G0161**; G0161-26;Pay for this service G0161-TC; TOS=6 Ultrasonic guidance for interstitial cryosurgical probes	185 1. Only when you have already paid for a claim for G0160 for the same patient on the same day.*** 2. Only once per corresponding claim for G0160.	Malignant neoplasm of prostate	Refer to the Medicare physician fee schedule including applicable quarterly database updates.

**Providers must report component services with the -26 (professional component) or -TC (technical component) modifier when appropriate. Physicians or qualified nonphysician practitioners performing both the professional and the technical components for such services must bill without the modifier, unless the service is provided in a health professional shortage area.

***Note: Advise providers of this payment requirement and recommend that they coordinate the billing of their claims to avoid delays resulting from a claim for G0161 preceding the corresponding claim for G0160.

4182   Prostate Cancer Screening Tests and Procedures

Medicare covers prostate cancer screening tests and procedures for the early detection of prostate cancer. Coverage currently consists of the following tests and procedures furnished to an individual for the early detection of prostate cancer:

A.   Screening Digital Rectal Examination is a clinical examination of an individual's prostate for nodules or other abnormalities of the prostate

B.   Screening Prostate Specific Antigen (PSA) blood test to detect the marker for adenocarcinoma of the prostate

For more information regarding coverage of prostate cancer screening tests and procedures, refer to §50-55 of the Coverage Issues Manual.

Appendix 4

The following table lists coverable codes and services for prostate cancer screening tests and procedures. Pay for these services according to the appropriate fee schedule when all of the requirements noted are met.

HCPCS Code TOS* Description	Requirements	Methodology/ Fee Schedule
1. G0102; TOS=1	Prostate cancer screening; digital rectal examination Performed on a male Medicare beneficiary over 50 years of age (i.e., for services starting at least one day after the beneficiary attained age 50).	Refer to the Medicare physician fee schedule
		Apply deductible and coinsurance
	Performed by one of the following , who is authorized under State law to perform the examination, is fully knowledgeable about the beneficiary, and is responsible for explaining the results of the examination to the beneficiary:	Claims from Physicians for these examinations where assignment was not taken are subject to Medicare Limiting Charge
	a. Doctor of medicine or osteopathy	
	b. Qualified physician assistant	
	c. Qualified nurse practitioner	
	d. Qualified clinical nurse specialist	
	e. Qualified certified nurse midwife	

HCPCS Code TOS* Description	Requirements	Methodology/ Fee Schedule
G0103;TOS=5 Prostate cancer screening; PSA test	Performed at a frequency no greater than once every 12 months. Performed on a male Medicare beneficiary over 50 years of age (i.e., for services starting at least one day after the beneficiary attained age 50)	Refer to the clinical laboratory fee schedule; payment for this test is the same as for code "84153, PSA; total." Do not apply deductible and coinsurance.

Ordered by one of the following, who is authorized under State law to perform the examination, is fully knowledgeable about the beneficiary, and is responsible for explaining the results of the examination to the beneficiary:

a. Physician (doctor of medicine or osteopathy)

b. Qualified physicianassistant

c. Qualified nurse practitioner

d. Qualified clinical nursespecialist

e. Qualified certified nursemidwife

Performed at a frequency no greater than once every 12 months.

Once a beneficiary has received any (or all) of the covered prostate cancer screening test/procedures, he may receive another (or all) of such test/procedures after 11 full months have passed. To determine the 11-month period, start your count beginning with the month after the month in which any (or all) of the previous covered screening test/procedures was performed.

EXAMPLE: The beneficiary received a screening PSA test on February 25, 2000. Start your count beginning March 2000. The beneficiary is eligible

Appendix 4

to receive another screening PSA test on February 1, 2001 (the month after 11 months have passed.)

4273.1 Epoetin alfa (EPO)

The drug EPO is covered under Part B if administered incident to a physician's services, effective June 1, 1989. EPO is used to treat anemia associated with chronic renal failure, including patients who are, and are not, on dialysis.

Completion of initial claim for EPO-The following information is required with initial claims:

- ICD-9-CM diagnosis (must also correlate with the procedure).

- Hematocrit (HCT)

Use the following Q codes to provide simultaneous reporting of the patient's latest hematocrit or Hgb reading before administration of EPO.

Q9920-Injection of EPO, per 1,000 units at patient HCT of 20 or less.

Q9921-Q9939-Injection of EPO per 1,000 units at patient HCT of 21 to 39.

For HCT levels of 21 or more, up to 39, a Q code that includes the actual HCT levels is used. To convert Hgb to the corresponding HCT value for Q-code reporting, multiply the Hgb value by 3 and round to the nearest whole number. Use the whole number to determine the Q-code assignment.

For example, if the patient's Hgb is 8.2-8.4, multiply the Hgb value by a factor of 3 and round to the nearest whole number. Code Q9925 should be used since the HCT value is calculated to be 25.

Q9940-Injection of EPO, per 1,000 units at patient HCT of 40 or above.

- Units administered-A standard unit of EPO is 1,000. Use a unit entry on the claim to reflect each unit of 1,000. If the dosage does not round to an even multiple of 1,000, round down dosages of 0 to 499 and round up dosages of 500 to 999.

- Date of the patient's most recent HCT or Hgb.

- Most recent HCT or Hgb level prior to initiation of EPO therapy.

- Date of most recent HCT or Hgb level prior to initiation of EPO therapy.

- Patient's most recent serum creatine within the last month, prior to initiation of EPO therapy.

- Date of most recent serum creatine prior to initiation of EPO therapy.

- Patient's weight in kilograms.

- Patient's starting dose per kilogram, usually 50 to 100 units per kilogram.

4450   Parenteral and enteral nutrition (PEN)

A completed certification of medical necessity must accompany and support claims for PEN to establish coverage criteria and that the PEN provided is consistent with the attending physician's prescription. The initial certification is valid for three months. The diagnosis must show a functional impairment that precludes the enteral patient from swallowing and the parenteral patient from absorbing nutrients.

Medical information should include the patient's general condition, estimated duration of therapy and other treatments or therapies; the patient's clinical assessment relating to the need for PEN therapy; and nutritional support therapy.

Revised certifications are necessary when there is a change in the attending physician's orders in the category of nutrients and/or calories prescribed; a change in the daily volume of parenteral solutions; a change in home-mix to pre-mix to home-mix parenteral solutions; a change from enteral to parenteral or parenteral to enteral therapy; or a change in the method of infusion.

Nutrients-Category IB of enteral nutrients contains products that are natural intact protein/protein isolates commonly known as blenderized nutrients. Additional documentation is required to justify the necessity of category IB nutrients.

Pumps-Enteral nutrition may be administered by syringe, gravity or pump. Use of pumps must be medically justified.

Supplies-Enteral care kits contain all the necessary supplies for the enteral patient using the syringe, gravity or pump method of nutrient administraton. Parenteral care kits and their components are considered all-inclusive items necessary to administer therapy during a monthly period.

4603   Screening Pap Smear and Pelvic Examinations

Medicare provides coverage every three years for a screening Pap smear or more frequent coverage for women (1) at high risk for cervical or vaginal cancer, or (2) of childbearing age who have had a Pap smear during any of the preceding three years indicating the presence of cervical or vaginal cancer or other abnormality.

Screening Pap smears are covered when ordered and collected by a doctor of medicine or osteopathy, or other authorized practitioner (e.g., a certified nurse midwife, physician assistant, nurse practitioner, or clinical nurse specialist, who is authorized under state law to perform the examination) under one of the following conditions:

- beneficiary has not had a screening Pap smear test during the preceding 3 years

- evidence (on the basis of her medical history or other findings) that she is of childbearing age and has had an examination that indicated the presence of cervical or vaginal cancer or other abnormalities during any of the preceding three years; or that she is at high risk of developing cervical or vaginal cancer. The high risk factors for cervical and vaginal cancer are:

Cervical cancer high risk factors are:

- early onset of sexual activity (under 16 years of age)

- multiple sexual partners (five or more in a lifetime)

- history of a sexually transmitted disease (including HIV infection)

- fewer than three negative Pap smears within the previous 7 years

Vaginal cancer high risk factors are:

- DES (diethylstilbestrol)-exposed daughters of women who took DES during pregnancy

Payment is not made for a screening Pap smear for women at high risk or who qualify for coverage under the childbearing provision more frequently than once every 11 months after the month that the last screening Pap smear covered by Medicare was performed.

The following HCPCS codes can be used for screening Pap smear:

Q0091--Screening Pap smear, obtaining, preparing and conveyance of cervical or vaginal smear to laboratory

This service is paid under physician fee schedule and the Part B deductible is waived

P3000--Screening Papanicolaou smear, cervical or vaginal, up to three smears, by a technician under the physician supervision

P3001--Screening Papanicolaou smear, cervical or vaginal, up to three smears requiring interpretation by a physician

P3000 and P3001 are paid under the clinical diagnostic laboratory fee schedule

G0123--Screening cytopathology, cervical or vaginal collected in preservation fluid, automated thin layer preparation, screening by cytotechnologist under physician supervision

G0124--Screening cytopathology, cervical or vaginal, collected n preservation fluid, automated thin layer preparation, requiring interpretation by physician

G0141--Screening cytopathology smears, cervical or vaginal, performed by automated system, with manual rescreening, requiring interpretation by physician

G0143--Screening cytopathology, cervical or vaginal, collected in preservative fluid, automated thin layer preparation, with manual evaluate and reevaluation by cytotechnologist under physician supervision

G0144--Screening cytopathology, cervical or vaginal, collected in preservative fluid, automated thin layer preparation, with manual evaluation and computer-assisted reevaluation by cytotechnologist under physician supervision

G0145--Screening cytopathology, cervical or vaginal, collected in preservative fluid, automated thin layer preparation, with manual evaluation and computer-assisted reevaluation using cell selection and review under physician supervision

G0147--Screening cytopathology smears, cervical or vaginal; performed by automated system under physician supervision

G0148--Screening cytopathology smears, cervical or vaginal, performed by automated system with manual reevaluation.

Medicare provides coverage of a screening pelvic examination for all female beneficiaries. A screening pelvic examination should include at least seven of the following eleven elements:

■ inspection and palpation of breasts for masses or lumps, tenderness, symmetry, or nipple discharge

■ digital rectal examination including sphincter tone, presence of hemorrhoids, and rectal masses

■ pelvic examination (with or without specimen collection for smears and cultures) including:

■ external genitalia (for example, general appearance, hair distribution, or lesions)

■ urethral meatus (for example, size, location, lesions, or prolapse)

■ urethra (for example, masses, tenderness, or scarring)

■ bladder (for example, fullness, masses, or tenderness)

■ vagina (for example, general appearance, estrogen effect, discharge, lesions, pelvic support, cystocele, or rectocele)

■ cervix (for example, general appearance, lesions or discharge

■ uterus (for example, size, contour, position, mobility, tenderness, consistency, descent, or support)

■ adnexa/parametria (for example, masses, tenderness, organomegaly, or nodularity)

■ anus and perineum.

Medicare Part B pays for a screening pelvic examination if it is performed by a doctor of medicine or osteopathy, or by a certified nurse midwife, or a physician assistant, nurse practitioner, or clinical nurse specialist authorized under state law to perform the examination. This examination does not have to be ordered by a physician or other authorized practitioner.

Payment may be made for a screening pelvic examination performed on an asymptomatic woman only if the individual has not had a screening pelvic examination paid for by Medicare during the preceding 35 months following the month in which the last Medicare-covered screening pelvic examination was performed.

Payment may be made for a screening pelvic examination performed more frequently than once every 36 months if the test is performed by a physician or other practitioner and there is evidence that the woman is at high risk (on the basis of her medical history or other findings) of developing cervical cancer, or vaginal cancer. The high risk factors for cervical and vaginal cancer are:

Cervical cancer high risk factors:

■ early onset of sexual activity (under 16 years of age)

■ multiple sexual partners (five or more in a lifetime)

■ history of a sexually transmitted disease (including HIV infection)

■ fewer than three negative Pap smears within the previous 7 years

Vaginal cancer high risk factors:

■ DES (diethylstilbestrol)-exposed daughters of women who took DES during pregnancy.

Payment may also be made for a screening pelvic examination performed more frequently than once every 36 months if the examination is performed by a physician or other practitioner, for a woman of childbearing age, who has had such an examination that indicated the presence of cervical or vaginal cancer or other abnormality during any of the preceding three years. Payment is not made for a screening pelvic examination for women at high risk or who qualify for coverage under the childbearing provision more frequently than once every 11 months after the month that the last screening pelvic examination covered by Medicare was performed.

Pelvic examinations will be paid under the physician fee schedule.

Use code G0101 for cervical or vaginal cancer screening, pelvic and clinical breast examination). This service is paid under the physician fee schedule.

A separately identifiable Evaluation and Management service and Q0091 or G0101 can be billed by the same physician on the same date of service. Modifier 25 must be used in these . When this happens both procedure codes should be shown as separate line items on the claim. These services can also be performed separately on separate office visits.

■ A covered evaluation and management visit and code Q0091 may be reported by the same physician for the same date of service if the evaluation and management visit is for a separately identifiable service. In this case, the 25 modifier must be reported with the evaluation and management service and the medical records must clearly document the evaluation and management service reported.

- A covered evaluation and management visit and code G0101 may be reported by the same physician for the same date of service if the evaluation and management visit is for a separately identifiable service. In this case, the 25 modifier must be reported with the evaluation and management service and the medical records must clearly document the evaluation and management service reported.

4900   **National Emphysema Treatment Trial (NETT)**

The National Heart, Lung, and Blood Institute (NHLBI), part of the National Institutes of Health (NIH) are conducting a study to examine the role of lung volume reduction surgery (LVRS) and evaluate the long-term outcome of the procedure on function, morbidity, and mortality, as well as to define appropriate patient selection criteria. The Health Care Financing Administration (HCFA) entered into an interagency agreement with NHLBI to cosponsor the study by providing payment for the clinical procedures provided in the trial to Medicare beneficiaries. NETT physicians screen patients to determine eligibility for participation in the study. NHLBI will evaluate the effectiveness of treatment for qualified patients randomized into two treatment groups:

A. Those receiving maximal medical therapy, including pulmonary rehabilitation services

B. Those receiving maximal medical therapy, including pulmonary rehabilitation services, and LVRS

In general, Medicare covers NETT services:

ÿ performed on Medicare beneficiaries

ÿ integral to the NETT study

ÿ not prohibited from coverage by Medicare statute.

The evaluation and surgery portions of this study must be performed at one of the 17 participating centers. Pulmonary rehabilitation may be performed at one of these centers or at a satellite location closer to the patient's residence, as identified by the participating center and reported to HCFA.

Claims for NETT services and procedures are to be submitted on Health Insurance Claim Form HCFA-1500 or electronic equivalent. Providers must submit all NETT claims with a demonstration number of 30.

For claims with the demonstration ID number of 30, Medicare pays as appropriate for CPT and HCPCS codes for services integral to the study and not precluded from Medicare coverage. For those codes for which professional and technical modifiers apply, providers must report component services with the -26 (professional component) or -TC (technical component) modifier when appropriate depending on the setting and the diagnostic service furnished. Physicians performing both the professional and the technical components for such services must bill using the appropriate code without the modifier.

Appendix 4

Report one of the following codes and services for lung volume reduction surgery. Payment for these surgical services includes payment for patient visits associated with postoperative management and completing forms such as the Interim History (HI), Surgical Summary Report (XS) and the Postoperative Summary Report (XP). Do not pay separately for these visits.

32491 Removal of lung, other than total pneumonectomy; excision- Lung volume plication of emphysematous lung(s) (bullous or non-bullous) reduction for lung volume reduction, sternal split or transthoracic approach, with or without any pleural procedure

32655 Thoracoscopy, surgical; with excision-plication of bullae, Thoracoscopy, including any pleural procedure surgical

32663 Thoracoscopy, surgical; with lobectomy, total or segmental Thoracoscopy, surgical

Pay for claims for the following services and codes only as appropriate for the NETT study:

G0110 training, individual

G0111 NETT PulmRehab; education/skills NETT pulm-rehab educ; group training, group

G0112 NETT PulmRehab; nutritional NETT; nutrition guid, initial guidance - initial

G0113 NETT PulmRehab; nutritional NETT; nutrition guid, subseqnt guidance - subsequent

G0114 NETT PulmRehab; psychosocial NETT; psychosocial consult consultation

G0115 NETT PulmRehab; psychological NETT; psychological testing testing

G0116 NETT PulmRehab; psychosocial NETT; psychosocial counsel counseling, individual

32491 Removal of lung, other than total Lung volume reduction pneumonectomy; excision- plication of emphysematous lung(s) (bullous or non-bullous) for lung volume reduction, sternal split or transthoracic approach, with or without any pleural procedure

Medicare does not pay separately for patient visits included in the payment for lung volume reduction surgery, i.e., patient visits associated with postoperative management and completing forms such as Interim History (HI), Surgical Summary Report (XS) and the Postoperative Summary Report (XP).

5114.1D Payment for diagnostic laboratory services; specimen collection fee

Separate charges made by physicians, independent laboratories or hospital laboratories for drawing or collecting specimens are allowed up to $3 whether the specimens are referred to physicians or other laboratories for testing. Only one collection fee is allowed for each patient encounter.

Series are treated as a single encounter. Specimen collection fees are allowed in drawing blood through venipuncture or collecting a urine sample through catheterization.

A specimen collection fee for physicians is allowed only where it is accepted practice among physicians in the locality to make separate charges for drawing or collecting a specimen, and it is the customary practice of the physician performing such services.

A specimen collection fee is not allowed where the cost of collecting the specimen is minimal, such as in the case of a throat culture or a routine capillary puncture for clotting or bleeding time. A fee for stool specimen collection for an occult blood test is not allowed. When a stool specimen is collected during a rectal examination, the collection is an incidental by-product of the examination. Costs for items such as gloves are accounted for in the visit payment.

Payment for routine handling charges where a specimen is referred by one laboratory to another is not allowed. Preparatory services are considered an integral part of the testing process and the costs are included in the total testing service charge.

A specimen collection fee is allowed when it is medically necessary for a laboratory technician to draw a specimen from a nursing home or homebound patient. The technician must personally draw the specimen. If the patient is not confined to the facility or the facility has on-duty personnel qualified to perform the collection, a specimen collection fee is not permitted.

Special rules and reimbursement factors apply to dialysis patients. ESRDs are paid by the fiscal intermediaries. Carriers never pay specimen collection fees to an ESRD.

5114.1K Payment for diagnostic laboratory services; travel allowance

A travel allowance can be made to cover the costs of collecting a specimen from a nursing home or homebound patient. The allowance is permitted only where the specimen collection fee is also payable. That is, no travel allowance is permitted if a technician merely picks up the specimen. The trip to the home or nursing home must be solely for the purpose of drawing a specimen, otherwise the travel costs are associated with the other purposes of the trip.

The allowance reflects the technician's salary and travel costs. The following HCPCS Level II codes are used:

- P9603 Travel allowance-one way, in connection with medically necessary laboratory specimen collection drawn from homebound or nursing home-bound patients, prorated miles actually travelled (carrier allowance on per mile basis); or

- P9604 Travel allowance-one way, in connection with medically necessary laboratory specimen collection drawn from homebound or nursing home-bound patient; prorated trip charge (carrier allowance on flat fee basis).

Appendix 4

Round trips are identified using the modifier "-LR." Carrier payment allowances for additional travel (e.g., to a distant nursing home) can be extended to all circumstances in which travel is required. Otherwise, establish an appropriate allowance based on:

- the current federal mileage allowance for operating personal automobiles, plus

- a personnel allowance per mile to cover personnel costs based on an estimate of average hourly wages and average driving speed.

Travel allowance amounts claimed by suppliers are prorated by the total number of patients (Medicare and non-Medicare) from whom specimens are drawn or picked up in a given trip.

15022 Payment conditions for radiology services

F: Low osmolar contrast media (LOCM):

Payment Criteria-Make separate payments for LOCM (HCPCS Level II codes A4644, A4645 and A4646) in the case of all medically necessary intrathecal radiologic procedures furnished to nonhospital patients. In the case of intra-arterial and intravenous radiologic procedures, pay separately for LOCM only when it is used for nonhospital patients with one or more of the following characteristics:

- A history of previous adverse reaction to contrast material, with the exception of a sensation of heat, flushing, or a single episode of nausea or vomiting;

- A history of asthma or allergy;

- Significant cardiac dysfunction including recent or imminent cardiac decompensation, severe arrhythmia, unstable angina hypertension;

- Generalized severe debilitation; or

- Sickle cell disease.

A LOCM pharmaceutical is considered to be a supply that is an integral part of the diagnostic test. Determine payment in the same manner as for a drug furnished incident to a physician's service, with the following additional requirement: Reduce the lower of the estimated actual acquisition cost or the national average wholesale price by 8 percent to take into account the fact that the TRVUs (technical component relative value units) of the procedure codes reflect less expensive contrast media.

If the beneficiary does not meet any of these criteria, the payment for contrast media is considered to be bundled into the TC of the procedure, and the beneficiary may not be billed for LOCM.

G: Portable X-ray services:

Services furnished by portable X-ray suppliers may have as many as four components.

■ Professional Component of radiologic services furnished by portable x-ray suppliers is paid for on the same basis as other physician fee schedule services.

■ Technical Component of radiology services furnished by portable x-ray suppliers under the fee schedule on the same basis as TC services.

■ Transportation Component (HCPCS Level II Codes R0070-R0076) represents the transportation of the equipment to the patient. Establish local RVUs for the transportation R codes based on your knowledge of the nature of the service furnished. Allow only a single transportation payment for each trip the portable x-ray supplier makes to a particular location, and prorate the single fee schedule transportation payment among all patients receiving the services. Further, for services furnished on or after Jan. 1, 1997, no separate payment is made under HCPCS Level II code R0076 for the transportation of EKG equipment by portable x-ray suppliers or any other entity.

■ Set-Up Component (HCPCS Level II Code Q0092) is paid for each radiologic procedure (other than retakes of the same procedure) during both single patient and multiple patient trips under HCPCS Level II code Q0092. No payment is made for the set-up payment for EKG services furnished by the portable x-ray supplier.

15030   Supplies

Make a separate payment for supplies furnished in connection with a procedure only under the following conditions:

■ the supply (A4550, A4200 and A4263) is separately billed for in conjunction with the appropriate procedure under the Medicare Physician Fee Schedule, or

■ the supply is a pharmaceutical or radiopharmaceutical diagnostic imaging agent (including codes A4641 through A4647); pharmacologistressing agent (code J1245); or therapeutic radionuclide used in diagnostic radiologic procedures (including diagnostic nuclear medicine), other diagnostic tests, clinical brachytherapy procedures, or therapeutic nuclear medicine procedures.

Appendix 5:

HCPCS Level II Codes Deleted Prior to 2000

Code	Narrative
A0010	See codes A0302, A0322, A0342 or A0362
A0020	See code A0380
A0060	See code A0420
A0070	See code A0422
A0150	No reference
A0215	No reference
A0220	See code A0308 or A0310
A0221	See code A0390
A0222	No reference
A0223	See codes A0348, A0350, A0368 or A0370
A4190	See codes A6257-A6259
A4200	See codes A6216-A6230, A6266-A6404
A4201	See code 99070
A4202	See codes A6263, A6405
A4203	See codes A6264, A6406
A4204	See codes A6234-A6241, A6251-A6256
A4205	See codes A6242-A6248
A4216	See code 99070
A4252	See codes A4649, 99070
A4341	See code A4338

Code	Narrative
A4342	See code A4338
A4343	See code A4338
A4345	See code A4338
A4348	See code A4357
A4349	See code A4358
A4350	See codes A4649, 99090
A4360	See codes A4421, 99070
A4363	No reference
A4366	See codes A4421, 99070
A4369	See codes A4421, 99070
A4370	See code A4455
A4380	See codes A4421, 99070
A4390	See codes A4421, 99070
A4430	See codes A4421, 99070
A4440	See code A4421
A4450	See code A4454
A4453	See code A4454
A4555	See codes A6234-A6256
A4581	No reference
A4610	See codes A4221-A4222, J7699, J7799, Q0132 See also Drugs
A4648	See codes A4644-A4646
A9180	No reference

Appendix 5

Code	Narrative	Code	Narrative
A9250	No reference	D3940	See codes D3351, D3352, D3353
A9260	No reference	D4250	No reference
A9280	No reference	D4261	See code D4263
A9290	No reference	D4262	See codes D4263-D4264
B4099	See code B9998	D4268	See codes D4266 and D4267
B4157	See code B9998		
B4188	See code B9999	D4272	See code D4240
B4192	See code B9999	D4340	See code D4341
B4196	See code B9999	D4345	See code D4341
B4198	See code B9999	D5215	See code D5213
B4514	See code B9999	D5216	See code D5214
D0110	See codes D0140-D0160	D5280	See code D5281
D0130	See codes D0140-D0160	D5917	See code D5919
D0275	See code D0270	D5918	See codes D5926, D5927, D5928, D5929
D0410	See code D0415		
D0420	See code D0425	D5920	See code D5923
D0471	No reference	D5921	See code L8611
D1202	See code D1205	D5956	See codes D5931, D5932, D5933, D5936
D2210	No reference		
D2540	See code D2543 or D2544	D5957	See codes D5952, D5953
D2640	See codes D2642-D2644	D5971	See codes D6010-D6199
D2660	See codes D2622-D2664	D5972	See codes D6010-D6199
D2810	No reference	D5973	See code D6040
D2953	See code D2952	D5974	See codes 21248, 21249
D3340	See code D3330	D5976	See code D6050
D3350	See code D3351	D6030	See codes 21248, 21249
D3411	See code D3426	D6540	See codes D6543, D6544
D3440	See code D3999	D7271	No reference
		D7470	No reference

Code	Narrative	Code	Narrative
D7942	No reference	E0405	See code E0441
D7992	See code D7999	E0410	See code E0442
D7993	See code 21208	E0415	See code E0442
D7994	See CPT	E0416	See code E0443
D8110	See code D8210	E0451	See code E0450
D8120	See code D8220	E0452	No reference
D8360	See codes D8050, D8060	E0453	No reference
D8370	See codes D8050, D8060	E0456	See code E0457
D8460	See code D8070	E0458	See code E0460
D8470	See code D8070	E0461	See code E0460
D8480	See code D8070	E0505	See code E0500
D8560	See code D8090	E0510	See code E0500
D8570	See code D8090	E0515	See code E0500
D8580	See code D8090	E0620	See codes E0627, E0628, E0629
D8650	No reference	E0670	No reference
D8750	No reference	E0674	See code E0460
D9240	No reference	E0750	See code E0751 or E0753
D9960	See code 99080	E0777	See code B9000
E0150	See code A4635	E0778	See code B9002
E0151	See code A4636	E0779	See code B9004
E0152	See code A4637	E0780	See code B9006
E0183	See codes E0176-E0178	E0790	See code E0791
E0190	See codes E0186, E0187, E0196	E1005	See code A4631
E0195	See code A4640	E1030	See code E1031
E0237	See codes E0217 and E0218	E1035	See code E1031
E0252	See codes E0250, E0290	E1036	See code E1031
E0330	See codes A5149, E1399	E1040	See code E1031
E0400	See code E0441	E1067	See code E1399

Code	Narrative	Code	Narrative
E1080	See code E1211	G0021	See code 21077
E1081	See code E1212	G0054	See CPT
E1082	See code E1213	G0055	See CPT
E1299	See code E1298	G0056	See CPT
E1350	See code E1340	G0057	See CPT
E1351	See code A4615	G0061	See code 32491
E1352	See code A4616	G0133	No reference
E1354	See code A4617	H5000	No reference
E1356	See code A4618	H5010	See codes 90806, 90807, 90818, 90819
E1371	See code A4619		
E1373	See code A4621	H5020	See code 90853
E1374	See code A4620	H5025	See code 90853
E1388	No reference	H5030	See code 90899
E1389	No reference	H5040	No reference
E1390	No reference	H5050	No reference
E1391	No reference	H5060	No reference
E1392	No reference	H5090	No reference
E1393	No reference	H5100	No reference
E1394	No reference	H5110	No reference
E1395	No reference	H5120	No reference
E1396	No reference	H5130	No reference
E1400	No reference	H5160	No reference
E1401	No reference	H5170	No reference
E1402	No reference	H5180	No reference
E1403	No reference	H5190	No reference
E1404	No reference	H5200	No reference
G0003	See codes G0004-G0007 and G0015-G0016	H5220	See code 99241
		H5230	See code 99242
G0020	See code 21076	H5240	See code 99243

Code	Narrative	Code	Narrative
H5299	See code 97799	J0830	See code J3490
J0110	See codes 90782-90788	J0840	See code J3490
J0130	See code J0800	J0860	See code J3490
J0140	See code J0800	J0870	See code J3490
J0160	See code J3490	J0880	See code J3490
J0180	See code J3490	J0890	See code J1100
J0200	See code J3490	J0950	See code J3490
J0220	See code 95180	J0960	See code J3130
J0230	See code 95180	J0980	See code J3490
J0240	See code 95180	J0990	See code J2175
J0250	See code J3490	J0995	See code J3420
J0255	See code J3420	J1010	See code J3490
J0260	See code J3490	J1130	See code J3490
J0310	See code J3490	J1140	See code J3490
J0320	See code J3490	J1150	See code J3490
J0410	See code J3490	J1155	See code J3490
J0420	See codes J3301-J3303	J1210	See codes J0530, J0580, J2510, J2540
J0430	See codes J3301-J3303	J1220	See code J3490
J0440	See code J3490	J1260	See code J0900
J0450	See code J3490	J1270	See code J0900
J0480	See code J3490	J1280	See code J0340
J0490	See code J1200	J1290	See code J2510
J0650	See code J3490	J1300	See code J3490
J0660	See code J3490	J1310	See code J1000
J0680	See code J3490	J1340	See code J3490
J0700	See code J0702 or J0704	J1350	See code J3490
J0750	See code J0515	J1360	See codes J1362 and J1364
J0790	See code J3490	J1370	See code J3490
J0820	See code J3490		

Appendix 5

Code	Narrative	Code	Narrative
J1400	See code J3490	J2130	See code J3490
J1405	See code J9999	J2140	See code J3490
J1420	See code J1435	J2160	See code J3490
J1430	See code J3490	J2170	See code J3490
J1450	See code J1435	J2190	See code J3490
J1590	See code J0725	J2200	See code J3490
J1640	See code J1644	J2220	No reference
J1660	See code J3490	J2230	See code J3490
J1680	See code J2640	J2280	See code J0720
J1740	See code J3490	J2290	See code J1600
J1750	See code J3490	J2340	See code J3490
J1760	No reference	J2380	See code J3490
J1770	No reference	J2390	See code J1180
J1780	No reference	J2420	See code J3490
J1860	See code J3430	J2450	See code J3490
J1870	See codes J3301-J3303	J2470	See code J1644
J1880	See codes J3301-J3303	J2490	See code J3490
J1900	See code J3430	J2495	See code J3490
J1920	See code J1160	J2500	See code J0290
J2020	See code J1644	J2520	See code J3490
J2030	See code J3490	J2530	See code J0560
J2040	See code J1644	J2570	See code J3490
J2050	See code J3490	J2580	See code J3490
J2070	See code J3490	J2595	See code J3490
J2080	See code J3490	J2600	See code J3490
J2090	See code J1180	J2610	See code P9018
J2100	See code J2560	J2620	See code J0290
J2110	See code J3490	J2630	See code J2650
J2120	See code J3490	J2655	See code J1410

Code	Narrative	Code	Narrative
J2660	See code J0290	J3180	See code 90703
J2672	See code J3490	J3190	See code J0120
J2740	See code J3490	J3200	See code J1435
J2750	See code 90726	J3210	See code J3490
J2770	See code J3490	J3220	See code J3490
J2780	See code J3490	J3290	See code J0290
J2825	See code J3490	J3300	See codes J3301-J3303
J2830	See code J3490	J3330	See code J3490
J2840	See code J3490	J3340	See code J3490
J2850	See code J3490	J3355	See code J3490
J2870	See code J3490	J3380	See code J3490
J2880	See code J3490	J3440	See code J3490
J2890	See code J3490	J3460	See code J2510
J2900	See code J3490	J3500	No reference
J2914	See code J3490	J3510	See code M0075
J2940	See code J3490	J3540	See codes 90782, 90784
J2960	See code J3490	J3550	See code 90783
J2975	See code J3490	J3560	See code J3490
J2980	See code J3400	J6015	See code 90749
J2990	See codes J2640, J2650	J6025	See code 90725
J3020	See code J0330	J6045	See code 90749
J3040	See code J3490	J7000	See codes 95120, 95125
J3050	See code J3490	J7010	See code 95120
J3060	See code J3430	J7020	See code 95125
J3090	See code J3490	J7080	See codes 90780, 90781
J3100	See code J2460	J7090	See codes 90780, 90781
J3110	See code J3490	J7140	See code J8499
J3160	See code J3490	J7150	See code J8999
J3170	See code J3490	J7160	See code J3490

Code	Narrative	Code	Narrative
J7170	See code J3490	K0118	See code A4595
J7180	See code J3490	K0119	No reference
J7195	See code J3490	K0120	No reference
J7196	No reference	K0121	No reference
J7320	See code 95130	K0122	No reference
J7330	See code 95130	K0123	No reference
J7340	See codes 95130-95134	K0124	See code J7505
J7350	See code 95130	K0125	See code J7506
J7502	See code K0418	K0126	See code L4390
J7503	No reference	K0127	See code L4392
J9010	See code J9000	K0128	See code L4394
J9030	See code 90728	K0129	See code L4396
J9160	See code J9999	K0130	See code L4398
J9162	See code J1050	K0131	See code A4258
J9180	See code J9295	K0132	See codes K0410, K0411
J9210	See code J9999	K0133	See code A4351
J9212	No reference	K0134	See code A4352
J9219	See code J9999	K0135	See code A4351
J9220	See code J9999	K0136	See code A4352
J9240	See code J0150	K0137	No reference
J9295	See code J9999	K0138	No reference
J9300	No reference	K0139	No reference
J9310	See code J9165	K0147	See code B4085
J9330	See code J9999	K0148	See codes K0242-K0249
J9381	See code J0696	K0149	See codes K0234-K0241
K0109	No reference	K0150	See codes K0196-K0199
K0110	See code A4221	K0151	See codes K0209-K0215
K0111	See code A4222	K0152	See codes A6196-A6406
K0117	No reference	K0153	See codes K0203-K0205

Code	Narrative	Code	Narrative
K0154	See code A6154	K0199	See code A6199
K0162	See code V2781	K0203	See code A6203
K0163	See code L7900	K0204	See code A6204
K0164	See code A4628	K0205	See code A6205
K0165	See code A4629	K0206	See code A6206
K0166	See code J7509	K0207	See code A6207
K0167	See code J7510	K0208	See code A6208
K0168	No reference	K0209	See code A6209
K0169	No reference	K0210	See code A6210
K0170	No reference	K0211	See code A6211
K0171	No reference	K0212	See code A6212
K0172	No reference	K0213	See code A6213
K0173	No reference	K0214	See code A6214
K0174	No reference	K0215	See code A6215
K0175	No reference	K0216	See code A6216
K0176	No reference	K0217	See code A6217
K0177	No reference	K0218	See code A6218
K0178	No reference	K0219	See code A6219
K0179	No reference	K0220	See code A6220
K0180	No reference	K0221	See code A6221
K0181	No reference	K0222	See code A6222
K0190	No reference	K0223	See code A6223
K0191	No reference	K0224	See code A6224
K0192	No reference	K0228	See code A6228
K0193	No reference	K0229	See code A6229
K0194	No reference	K0230	See code A6230
K0196	See code A6196	K0234	See code A6234
K0197	See code A6197	K0235	See code A6235
K0198	See code A6198	K0236	See code A6236

Appendix 5

Code	Narrative	Code	Narrative
K0237	See code A6237	K0266	See code A6266
K0238	See code A6238	K0267	See code A4254
K0239	See code A6239	K0271	See codes A5064, K0419, K0420
K0240	See code A6240		
K0241	See code A6241	K0272	See codes A5062, K0421, K0422
K0242	See code A6242	K0273	See codes A5074, K0423, K0424
K0243	See code A6243		
K0244	See code A6244	K0274	See codes A5072, K0425, K0426, K0427
K0245	See code A6245	K0275	See codes A5093, K0428
K0246	See code A6246	K0276	See codes A5093, K0428
K0247	See code A6247	K0277	No reference
K0248	See code A6248	K0278	No reference
K0249	See code A6262	K0279	No reference
K0250	See code A6250	K0282	See code K0182
K0251	See code A6251	K0284	No reference
K0252	See code A6252	K0285	See code L7520
K0253	See code A6253	K0400	No reference
K0254	See code A6254	K0401	No reference
K0255	See code A6255	K0402	See code A6402
K0256	See code A6256	K0403	See code A6403
K0257	See code A6257	K0404	See code A6404
K0258	See code A6258	K0405	See code A6405
K0259	See code A6259	K0406	See code A6406
K0260	See code A6260	K0412	No reference
K0261	See code A6261	K0417	No reference
K0262	See code A6262	K0418	No reference
K0263	See code A6263	K0419	No reference
K0264	See code A6264	K0420	No reference
K0265	See code A6265		

Code	Narrative	Code	Narrative
K0421	No reference	K0513	No reference
K0422	No reference	K0514	No reference
K0423	No reference	K0515	No reference
K0424	No reference	K0516	No reference
K0425	No reference	K0518	No reference
K0426	No reference	K0519	No reference
K0427	No reference	K0520	No reference
K0428	No reference	K0521	No reference
K0429	No reference	K0522	No reference
K0430	No reference	K0523	No reference
K0431	No reference	K0524	No reference
K0432	No reference	K0525	No reference
K0433	No reference	K0526	No reference
K0434	No reference	K0527	No reference
K0435	No reference	K0528	No reference
K0436	No reference	K0530	No reference
K0437	No reference	L0800	See code L1499
K0438	No reference	L1670	See code L2999
K0439	No reference	L1740	See code L1685
K0453	No reference	L2100	See codes L2102, L2104
K0503	No reference	L2110	See codes L2102, L2180
K0504	No reference	L2120	See codes L2106, L2114, L2116
K0505	No reference		
K0506	No reference	L2130	See code L2999
K0507	No reference	L2140	See codes L2122, L2124
K0508	No reference	L2150	See code L2134
K0509	No reference	L2160	See code L2999
K0511	No reference	L2400	See code L2999
K0512	No reference	L2410	See code L2999

Code	Narrative		Code	Narrative
L2420	See code L2999		L7150	See codes L6890, L6945, L7025
L2440	See code L2385		L7160	See codes L7170, L7185, L7186
L2450	See codes L2390, L2395			
L2460	See code L2999		L7165	See codes L7180, L7190, L7191
L2470	See code L2999			
L2475	See code L2415		L7200	See codes L6890, L6950, L7010
L2480	See code L2395		L7250	See codes L6890, L6955, L7025
L2490	See codes L2390, L2492			
L2495	See codes L2795, L2800, L2810		L7300	See codes L6890, L6960, L7010
L2560	See code L2999		L7350	See codes L6890, L6965, L7025
L2626	See codes L2627, L2628			
L4200	See code L4205		L9999	No reference
L4310	No reference		M0009	See code 99499
L4320	No reference		M0019	See code 99499
L4390	No reference		M0021	See code 99231
L5110	See code L5639		M0022	See code 99233
L5612	See code L5999		M0023	See code 99431
L5703	See code L5976		M0024	See codes 99231-99233
L5708	See codes L5982, L5984		M0029	See code 99499
L5709	See code L5986		M0039	See code 99499
L6760	See code L7499		M0049	See code 99499
L6785	See code L7499		M0050	See code 99499
L6869	See code L6868		M0051	See code 99499
L7000	See codes L6890, L6930, L7010		M0052	See code 99499
			M0053	See code 99499
L7050	See codes L6890, L6935, L7025		M0054	See code 99499
			M0059	See code 99499
L7100	See codes L6890, L6940, L7010		M0070	See code 99199
			M0071	See code 99199

Code	Narrative	Code	Narrative
M0072	See code 99199	M0728	See code 98928
M0080	See code 77605	M0730	See code 98929
M0101	No reference	M0799	See code 97799
M0260	See codes 42820-42826, 69420-69421	M0900	See codes 36800-36861
		M0910	See code 36489
M0261	See codes 42820-42826, 69420-69421	M0916	See code 90999
M0299	See code 92599	M0920	See code 90999
M0399	See code 93799	M0928	See code 90999
M0520	See code 93734	M0931	See code 90999
M0525	See code 93040	M0932	See code 90999
M0526	See code 93000	M0936	See code 90999
M0530	See code 93268	M0937	See code 90999
M0535	See code 93268	M0945	See codes 90918-90921
M0540	See code 93278	M0974	See code 90989
M0560	See codes 93965-93971	M0978	See code 90993
M0575	See code 95819	M0982	See code 90989
M0580	See code 95999	M0994	See codes 90945, 90947
M0585	See code 95999	M9999	See code 99199
M0590	See code 95829	P0999	See code 89399
M0592	See code 94760	P2032	See code 84999
M0601	See code 90830	P7020	See code 87999
M0702	See code 98925	P9005	No reference
M0704	See code 98926	P9006	See codes 88000-88399
M0706	See code 98927	P9007	See codes 99000, 99001
M0708	See code 98928	P9014	No reference
M0710	See code 98929	P9015	No reference
M0722	See code 98925	P9023	See code J7190
M0724	See code 98926	P9024	No reference
M0726	See code 98927	P9605	See code G0001

Appendix 5

Code	Narrative	Code	Narrative
P9610	No reference	**Q0032**	See code 93237
Q0004	See code J7500	**Q0036**	See codes E1377-E1385
Q0005	See code J7501	**Q0037**	See codes E1405-E1406
Q0006	See code J7502	**Q0038**	See code E0441
Q0007	See code J7503	**Q0039**	See code E0442
Q0008	See code J7504	**Q0040**	See code E0443
Q0009	See code J7505	**Q0041**	See code E0444
Q0010	See code E0651	**Q0042**	See code E0424
Q0011	See code E0652	**Q0043**	See code E0439
Q0012	See code E0667	**Q0044**	See code M0064
Q0013	See code E0668	**Q0045**	See code 00147
Q0014	See code E1400	**Q0046**	See code E0434
Q0015	See code E1401	**Q0047**	See code 00103
Q0016	See code E1402	**Q0048**	See code J7196
Q0017	See code E1403	**Q0049**	See code E0194
Q0018	See code E1404	**Q0050**	See code B4189
Q0019	See code 93224	**Q0051**	See code B4193
Q0020	See code 93225	**Q0052**	See code B4197
Q0021	See code 93226	**Q0053**	See code B4199
Q0022	See code 93227	**Q0054**	See code B5200
Q0023	See code 93230	**Q0055**	See code B5100
Q0024	See code 93231	**Q0056**	See code B5000
Q0025	See code 93232	**Q0057**	See code J9217
Q0026	See code 93233	**Q0059**	See code 56340
Q0027	See code 93235	**Q0060**	See code P3000
Q0028	See code 93236	**Q0061**	See code P3001
Q0029	See code 93237	**Q0062**	See code 56341
Q0030	See code 93235	**Q0063**	See code Q0091
Q0031	See code 93236	**Q0064**	See code 77781

Code	Narrative	Code	Narrative
Q0065	See code 77782	Q0120	See code A5503
Q0066	See code M0302	Q0121	See code A5504
Q0067	See code 77784	Q0122	See code A5505
Q0068	No reference	Q0123	See code A5506
Q0069	See code 70553	Q0124	See codes G0008, G0009 or G0010
Q0070	See code 72156	Q0125	See code J9265
Q0071	See code 72157	Q0126	See codes 87449, 87450
Q0072	See code 72158	Q0127	See code J8530
Q0073	See code L8642	Q0128	See code J8560
Q0074	See code L8612	Q0129	See code J8610
Q0076	See code 77783	Q0130	See code J8600
Q0077	See code J2545	Q0132	No reference
Q0078	See code E0628	Q0133	See code A5507
Q0079	See code E0629	Q0134	See code L8603
Q0080	See code E0627	Q0135	See code A4643
Q0087	See code J0895	Q0137	See code J1095
Q0088	See code J0635	Q0138	See code J1095
Q0089	See code J3365	Q0139	See code J2597
Q0090	See code J0694	Q0140	See code J3480
Q0093	See codes J1440, J1441	Q0141	See code J3475
Q0094	See code J2820	Q0142	See code A9505
Q0105	See code A4644	Q0143	See code A9500
Q0106	See code A4645	Q0159	No reference
Q0107	See code A4646	Q0162	No reference
Q0108	See code 99360	Q0182	No reference
Q0116	See CPT	R0009	See code 76499
Q0117	See code A5500	R0059	See code 76499
Q0118	See code A5501	R0065	See code 78999
Q0119	See code A5502		

Appendix 5

Code	Narrative		Code	Narrative
R0085	See code 76499		V5001	See code 92557
R0109	See code 76499		V5002	See code 92584
R0129	See code 76499		V5003	See code 92599
R0159	See code 76499		V5012	See code 69930
R0209	See code 76499		V5016	See code 92599
R0259	See code 76499		V5301	See code 92506
R0309	See code 76499		V5310	See code 92506
R0359	See code 76499		V5321	See code 92506
R0599	See code 76499		V5322	See code 92506
V2620	See code V2629		V5330	See code 92507
V2621	See code V2629		V5335	See code 92507
V2622	See code V2629		V5360	See code 92599
V5000	See code 92553			

Appendix 6:

National Average Payment

The following table represents commercial and/or Medicare national average payment (NAP) for services, supplies (DME, orthotics, prosthetics, etc.), drugs and non—physician procedures reported using HCPCS Level II codes. Not all HCPCS Level II codes are included in this listing since data concerning the commercial and Medicare national average payments were not available. Please remember these are average payments and do not represent actual payment applicable to specific carriers, localities or third party payers. The NAP should be used as a broad benchmark tool only.

For the commercial NAP, the average 60th percentile value for the code was calculated by taking the summation of the fees for each code at the 60th percentile across all of geographical areas and dividing by the number of areas.

The Medicare data shown is the average of the floor and ceiling limits of those procedures fee amounts (Medicare Physician Fee Schedule Data Base FY1997 without the geographical practice cost index factor), or the national amount from the Clinical Lab Fee Schedule. The average 60th percentile value for the HCPCS code was calculated by taking the summation of the fees for each code at the 60th percentile across all geographical areas and dividing by the number of areas.

Code	Commercial	Medicare	Code	Commercial	Medicare
A0021	9.28	0.00	A0200	0.00	0.00
A0030	0.00	0.00	A0210	0.00	0.00
A0040	0.00	0.00	A0225	309.20	0.00
A0050	0.00	0.00	A0300	222.24	0.00
A0080	0.00	0.00	A0302	229.19	0.00
A0090	0.00	0.00	A0304	259.73	0.00
A0100	0.00	0.00	A0306	273.26	0.00
A0110	0.00	0.00	A0308	267.84	0.00
A0120	0.00	0.00	A0310	290.65	0.00
A0130	0.00	0.00	A0320	190.54	0.00
A0140	0.00	0.00	A0322	198.66	0.00
A0160	0.31	0.00	A0324	193.25	0.00
A0170	0.00	0.00	A0326	211.80	0.00
A0180	0.00	0.00	A0328	203.30	0.00
A0190	0.00	0.00	A0330	225.33	0.00

Code	Commercial	Medicare	Code	Commercial	Medicare
A0340	206.78	0.00	A4214	2.98	1.54
A0342	211.03	0.00	A4215	0.00	0.00
A0344	227.65	0.00	A4220	0.00	0.00
A0346	244.65	0.00	A4221	0.00	19.97
A0348	237.31	0.00	A4222	0.00	41.23
A0350	254.70	0.00	A4230	0.00	0.00
A0360	161.17	0.00	A4231	0.00	0.00
A0362	167.74	0.00	A4232	0.00	2.34
A0364	164.65	0.00	A4244	1.49	0.00
A0366	186.29	0.00	A4245	4.58	0.00
A0368	175.08	0.00	A4246	5.06	0.00
A0370	198.27	0.00	A4247	7.71	0.00
A0380	7.73	0.00	A4250	28.52	0.00
A0382	7.73	0.00	A4253	48.70	0.00
A0384	38.65	0.00	A4254	9.12	0.00
A0390	7.73	0.00	A4255	2.80	3.63
A0392	38.65	0.00	A4256	15.47	10.10
A0394	18.55	0.00	A4258	25.67	15.92
A0396	30.92	0.00	A4259	10.78	11.24
A0398	7.73	0.00	A4260	605.17	0.00
A0420	0.00	0.00	A4261	0.00	0.00
A0422	28.60	0.00	A4262	0.83	0.00
A0424	0.00	0.00	A4263	65.21	19.04
A0888	0.00	0.00	A4265	3.73	2.99
A0999	0.00	0.00	A4270	0.00	0.00
A4206	0.30	0.00	A4280	8.29	4.91
A4207	0.00	0.00	A4300	0.00	19.04
A4208	0.27	0.00	A4301	0.00	0.00
A4209	0.43	0.00	A4305	21.47	0.00
A4210	1409.30	0.00	A4306	29.45	0.00
A4211	0.00	0.00	A4310	6.68	6.82
A4212	13.70	0.00	A4311	22.45	13.10
A4213	1.46	0.00	A4312	27.41	15.91

Code	Commercial	Medicare	Code	Commercial	Medicare
A4313	35.28	16.35	A4367	9.78	6.49
A4314	23.74	22.31	A4368	0.78	0.23
A4315	31.02	23.28	A4369	5.01	2.13
A4316	43.11	25.06	A4370	7.23	3.02
A4320	4.82	4.70	A4371	4.97	3.22
A4321	0.00	0.00	A4372	5.49	3.68
A4322	2.35	2.69	A4373	9.67	5.54
A4323	13.18	7.74	A4374	0.00	7.45
A4326	0.00	9.52	A4375	0.00	15.15
A4327	0.00	39.37	A4376	0.00	41.98
A4328	14.92	9.22	A4377	0.00	3.79
A4329	35.61	22.48	A4378	0.00	27.13
A4330	9.95	6.31	A4379	0.00	13.26
A4335	0.00	0.00	A4380	0.00	32.93
A4338	9.57	10.82	A4381	0.00	4.07
A4340	18.82	28.01	A4382	0.00	21.72
A4344	16.20	14.13	A4383	0.00	24.88
A4346	28.19	17.29	A4384	0.00	8.49
A4347	21.27	17.95	A4385	5.72	4.50
A4351	2.74	1.60	A4386	8.02	5.93
A4352	11.61	5.66	A4387	0.00	3.54
A4353	6.62	6.17	A4388	4.15	3.85
A4354	12.73	10.41	A4389	3.93	5.48
A4355	9.12	7.87	A4390	0.00	8.48
A4356	53.93	40.26	A4391	0.00	6.23
A4357	7.91	8.56	A4392	0.00	5.87
A4358	6.43	5.86	A4393	0.00	8.10
A4359	46.42	27.03	A4394	4.34	2.27
A4361	23.21	16.21	A4395	0.08	0.04
A4362	4.97	3.05	A4397	6.07	4.23
A4363	5.01	3.47	A4398	6.67	12.18
A4364	1.69	2.59	A4399	18.24	10.82
A4365	12.72	9.99	A4400	49.34	43.13

Code	Commercial	Medicare	Code	Commercial	Medicare
A4402	0.58	1.40	A4613-RR	21.55	12.73
A4404	2.79	1.49	A4613-UE	155.85	92.02
A4421	0.00	0.00	A4613-NU	215.54	127.24
A4454	3.32	2.30	A4614	0.00	20.98
A4455	1.41	1.26	A4615	2.49	0.00
A4460	5.84	1.06	A4616	1.03	0.00
A4462	19.70	2.90	A4617	13.26	0.00
A4465	15.07	0.00	A4618	12.85	0.00
A4470	10.28	0.00	A4619	2.90	1.12
A4480	8.22	0.00	A4620	4.61	0.00
A4481	0.00	0.34	A4621	0.00	1.28
A4483-UE	0.00	0.00	A4622	86.22	50.53
A4483-RR	0.00	0.00	A4623	9.95	5.78
A4483-NU	0.00	0.00	A4624	4.11	0.00
A4490	11.01	0.00	A4625	9.95	6.12
A4495	11.01	0.00	A4626	4.97	2.82
A4500	8.21	0.00	A4627	27.41	0.00
A4510	19.90	0.00	A4628	1.13	0.00
A4550	48.08	19.04	A4629	6.63	4.09
A4554	4.97	0.00	A4630	6.85	0.00
A4556	12.44	10.71	A4631	150.88	0.00
A4557	12.85	18.62	A4635	6.13	0.00
A4558	5.52	4.81	A4636	5.31	0.00
A4560	27.75	21.55	A4637	3.15	0.00
A4565	11.61	0.00	A4640	77.93	0.00
A4570	28.19	0.00	A4641	0.00	0.00
A4572	18.24	0.00	A4642	0.00	0.00
A4575	0.00	0.00	A4643	0.00	0.00
A4580	0.00	0.00	A4644	0.00	0.00
A4590	63.42	0.00	A4645	0.00	0.00
A4595	17.41	25.42	A4646	0.00	0.00
A4611	286.83	0.00	A4647	149.22	0.00
A4612	119.38	0.00	A4649	0.00	0.00

Code	Commercial	Medicare	Code	Commercial	Medicare
A4650	0.00	0.00	A4901	0.00	0.00
A4655	0.00	0.00	A4905	0.00	0.00
A4660	21.64	0.00	A4910	0.00	0.00
A4663	41.45	0.00	A4912	13.70	0.00
A4670	106.11	0.00	A4913	0.00	0.00
A4680	107.77	0.00	A4914	26.03	0.00
A4690	1068.63	0.00	A4918	0.00	0.00
A4700	0.00	0.00	A4919	0.00	0.00
A4705	16.58	0.00	A4920	0.00	0.00
A4712	16.85	0.00	A4921	0.00	0.00
A4714	66.32	0.00	A4927	6.63	0.00
A4730	0.00	0.00	A5051	2.75	2.05
A4735	0.00	0.00	A5052	3.68	1.47
A4740	0.00	0.00	A5053	4.11	1.53
A4750	20.56	0.00	A5054	1.38	1.49
A4755	0.00	0.00	A5055	2.44	1.26
A4760	0.00	0.00	A5061	4.06	2.38
A4765	0.00	0.00	A5062	4.78	1.96
A4770	0.00	0.00	A5063	2.74	1.97
A4771	0.00	0.00	A5064	56.37	0.00
A4772	43.11	0.00	A5065	8.90	0.00
A4773	27.34	0.00	A5071	8.22	3.84
A4774	0.00	0.00	A5072	4.97	3.11
A4780	0.00	0.00	A5073	5.34	2.81
A4790	0.00	0.00	A5074	8.29	0.00
A4800	11.94	0.00	A5075	6.63	0.00
A4820	0.00	0.00	A5081	2.74	2.91
A4850	74.00	0.00	A5082	18.24	10.49
A4860	0.00	0.00	A5093	10.64	1.72
A4870	0.00	0.00	A5102	9.04	19.91
A4880	382.30	0.00	A5105	58.93	35.97
A4890	0.00	0.00	A5112	9.88	30.55
A4900	0.00	0.00	A5113	8.26	4.14

Code	Commercial	Medicare	Code	Commercial	Medicare
A5114	6.63	7.88	A6208	0.00	0.00
A5119	16.58	9.58	A6209	11.61	6.61
A5121	9.88	6.59	A6210	29.84	17.57
A5122	19.90	11.34	A6211	43.11	25.91
A5123	8.29	5.00	A6212	14.92	8.56
A5126	1.34	1.17	A6213	34.82	0.00
A5131	16.45	13.99	A6214	14.92	9.09
A5149	0.00	0.00	A6215	0.00	0.00
A5200	0.00	9.97	A6216	0.41	0.04
A5500	0.00	0.00	A6217	0.56	0.00
A5501	0.00	0.00	A6218	0.66	0.00
A5502	0.00	0.00	A6219	1.66	0.84
A5503	0.00	0.00	A6220	3.32	2.27
A5504	0.00	0.00	A6221	0.00	0.00
A5505	0.00	0.00	A6222	0.85	1.88
A5506	0.00	0.00	A6223	3.32	2.13
A5507	0.00	0.00	A6224	4.97	3.18
A5508	0.00	0.00	A6228	3.12	0.00
A6020	0.00	0.00	A6229	3.73	3.18
A6025	39.79	0.00	A6230	5.14	0.00
A6154	10.51	12.68	A6234	7.76	5.77
A6196	11.61	6.49	A6235	17.24	14.84
A6197	24.87	14.51	A6236	28.45	24.04
A6198	0.00	0.00	A6237	9.32	6.97
A6199	8.29	4.66	A6238	23.01	20.11
A6200	1.66	8.38	A6239	0.00	0.00
A6201	3.32	18.35	A6240	18.24	10.81
A6202	0.00	30.78	A6241	2.60	2.26
A6203	4.97	2.95	A6242	8.29	5.36
A6204	6.63	5.50	A6243	18.24	10.87
A6205	0.00	0.00	A6244	58.03	34.65
A6206	7.26	0.00	A6245	8.85	6.41
A6207	11.61	6.47	A6246	14.92	8.75

Code	Commercial	Medicare	Code	Commercial	Medicare
A6247	34.82	20.98	A7009	64.66	0.00
A6248	24.87	14.33	A7010	36.48	0.00
A6250	0.00	0.00	A7011	33.13	0.00
A6251	3.32	1.76	A7012	5.80	0.00
A6252	3.83	2.87	A7013	1.24	0.00
A6253	5.70	5.60	A7014	7.05	0.00
A6254	4.79	1.07	A7015	2.90	0.00
A6255	0.00	2.68	A7016	11.19	0.00
A6256	0.00	0.00	A7017	0.00	0.00
A6257	3.56	1.35	A9150	0.00	0.00
A6258	6.63	3.79	A9160	0.00	0.00
A6259	16.58	9.65	A9170	0.00	0.00
A6260	1.74	0.00	A9190	0.00	0.00
A6261	6.60	0.00	A9270	0.00	0.00
A6262	1.66	0.00	A9300	0.00	0.00
A6263	0.45	0.26	A9500	0.00	0.00
A6264	0.75	0.42	A9502	0.00	0.00
A6265	0.00	0.11	A9503	0.00	0.00
A6266	2.93	1.69	A9504	0.00	0.00
A6402	0.56	0.11	A9505	0.00	0.00
A6403	0.66	0.38	A9507	0.00	0.00
A6404	0.86	0.00	A9600	965.45	0.00
A6405	0.91	0.30	A9605	0.00	0.00
A6406	0.99	0.70	A9900	0.00	0.00
A7000	14.92	0.00	A9901	0.00	0.00
A7001	50.57	0.00	B4034	0.00	0.00
A7002	5.80	0.00	B4035	0.00	0.00
A7003	4.15	0.00	B4036	0.00	0.00
A7004	2.90	0.00	B4081	33.86	0.00
A7005	47.67	0.00	B4082	17.92	0.00
A7006	14.51	0.00	B4083	4.51	0.00
A7007	7.05	0.00	B4084	27.41	0.00
A7008	16.99	0.00	B4085	41.62	0.00

Appendix 6

Code	Commercial	Medicare	Code	Commercial	Medicare
B4150	3.65	0.00	B9004-RR	28.42	0.00
B4151	3.65	0.00	B9006-NU	0.00	0.00
B4152	3.43	0.00	B9006-UE	0.00	0.00
B4153	12.65	0.00	B9006-RR	16.58	0.00
B4154	17.13	0.00	B9998	0.00	0.00
B4155	32.40	0.00	B9999	0.00	0.00
B4156	12.37	0.00	E0100-UE	16.65	14.83
B4164	36.81	0.00	E0100-NU	20.90	18.60
B4168	70.48	0.00	E0100-RR	8.16	5.25
B4172	105.65	0.00	E0105-UE	29.96	33.40
B4176	120.59	0.00	E0105-NU	33.29	43.33
B4178	152.95	0.00	E0105-RR	11.10	7.81
B4180	50.42	0.00	E0110-RR	21.88	14.12
B4184	111.32	0.00	E0110-NU	57.18	68.46
B4186	146.22	0.00	E0110-UE	51.46	51.34
B4189	175.80	0.00	E0111-RR	14.37	7.43
B4193	189.97	0.00	E0111-NU	62.69	46.99
B4197	196.94	0.00	E0111-UE	48.32	36.26
B4199	208.13	0.00	E0112-UE	13.94	24.90
B4216	0.00	0.00	E0112-NU	15.48	32.65
B4220	0.00	0.00	E0112-RR	13.71	8.76
B4222	0.00	0.00	E0113-RR	6.53	4.54
B4224	32.38	0.00	E0113-NU	29.06	18.64
B5000	113.90	0.00	E0113-UE	18.28	13.99
B5100	141.11	0.00	E0114-RR	14.37	7.57
B5200	0.00	0.00	E0114-NU	32.15	41.63
B9000-RR	124.35	0.00	E0114-UE	28.94	31.47
B9000-UE	824.03	0.00	E0116-NU	39.18	24.47
B9000-NU	1284.95	0.00	E0116-UE	28.73	18.41
B9002-RR	169.95	0.00	E0116-RR	10.45	4.77
B9002-NU	1382.77	0.00	E0130-NU	85.54	61.96
B9004-UE	0.00	0.00	E0130-RR	22.20	14.84
B9004-NU	0.00	0.00	E0130-UE	68.57	48.28

Code	Commercial	Medicare	Code	Commercial	Medicare
E0135-UE	46.81	56.75	E0156-UE	26.12	17.51
E0135-RR	23.51	15.22	E0157-RR	10.45	7.92
E0135-NU	59.87	73.97	E0157-NU	97.95	72.28
E0141-UE	25.95	76.30	E0157-UE	78.36	54.22
E0141-RR	26.77	19.73	E0158-UE	26.45	21.43
E0141-NU	39.01	101.72	E0158-RR	3.59	3.13
E0142-RR	31.34	23.32	E0158-NU	35.26	28.39
E0142-UE	133.87	115.56	E0159	31.30	0.00
E0142-NU	167.49	151.73	E0160-RR	5.22	3.82
E0143-RR	29.71	19.06	E0160-UE	32.00	21.86
E0143-UE	115.91	79.38	E0160-NU	39.83	29.16
E0143-NU	144.97	106.08	E0161-UE	25.14	17.34
E0144	0.00	0.00	E0161-NU	31.34	23.14
E0145-NU	195.90	0.00	E0161-RR	3.92	3.15
E0145-UE	156.72	0.00	E0162-UE	146.27	99.69
E0145-RR	28.41	18.31	E0162-RR	18.28	13.49
E0146-NU	186.11	0.00	E0162-NU	182.84	128.55
E0146-RR	19.59	16.80	E0163-NU	143.66	97.31
E0146-UE	148.88	0.00	E0163-RR	33.63	21.55
E0147-NU	470.16	507.15	E0163-UE	104.48	75.03
E0147-UE	376.13	380.38	E0164-UE	186.43	120.04
E0147-RR	51.59	50.71	E0164-NU	248.47	160.06
E0153-UE	58.77	45.90	E0164-RR	36.24	23.32
E0153-NU	84.89	61.22	E0165-NU	220.71	0.00
E0153-RR	9.14	6.91	E0165-RR	25.47	16.39
E0154-UE	68.57	47.27	E0165-UE	176.31	0.00
E0154-NU	85.54	62.20	E0166-RR	36.57	27.48
E0154-RR	10.45	7.56	E0166-UE	241.61	0.00
E0155-RR	5.22	3.39	E0166-NU	302.99	0.00
E0155-NU	43.42	27.85	E0167-NU	16.33	10.59
E0155-UE	32.98	21.22	E0167-UE	12.41	7.97
E0156-RR	5.88	2.98	E0167-RR	2.61	1.12
E0156-NU	32.65	23.32	E0175-NU	90.77	58.43

Code	Commercial	Medicare	Code	Commercial	Medicare
E0175-UE	66.93	43.01	E0187-NU	261.20	0.00
E0175-RR	9.14	5.85	E0187-RR	26.12	20.48
E0176-NU	130.60	94.50	E0188	53.55	0.00
E0176-RR	19.59	12.49	E0189	0.00	0.00
E0176-UE	104.48	70.25	E0191-RR	1.96	0.90
E0177-NU	127.99	93.65	E0191-NU	6.86	8.82
E0177-UE	97.95	70.25	E0192-UE	359.15	256.09
E0177-RR	19.59	10.72	E0192-NU	457.10	341.46
E0178-UE	111.01	80.29	E0192-RR	60.08	34.39
E0178-RR	20.90	13.24	E0193-RR	1484.39	797.12
E0178-NU	163.25	107.06	E0194-UE	0.00	0.00
E0179-NU	19.59	10.55	E0194-NU	0.00	0.00
E0179-UE	13.06	8.30	E0194-RR	3918.00	2871.28
E0179-RR	1.96	1.10	E0196-UE	293.85	0.00
E0180-UE	287.32	0.00	E0196-RR	39.18	28.66
E0180-NU	457.10	0.00	E0196-NU	391.80	0.00
E0180-RR	50.61	19.16	E0197-NU	261.20	195.50
E0181-RR	31.34	21.24	E0197-UE	228.55	171.72
E0181-UE	272.95	0.00	E0197-RR	36.57	26.98
E0181-NU	342.17	0.00	E0198-NU	287.32	195.50
E0182-NU	326.50	0.00	E0198-UE	202.43	148.35
E0182-UE	269.04	0.00	E0198-RR	31.34	20.25
E0182-RR	31.34	23.10	E0199-NU	45.71	28.27
E0184-RR	33.96	21.68	E0199-RR	5.22	2.82
E0184-UE	195.90	131.75	E0199-UE	32.65	21.21
E0184-NU	261.20	171.78	E0200-NU	127.66	69.95
E0185-NU	424.45	282.21	E0200-RR	17.30	9.49
E0185-UE	300.38	216.59	E0200-UE	95.99	52.49
E0185-RR	54.85	39.65	E0202-RR	124.72	55.24
E0186-NU	228.55	0.00	E0205-RR	28.73	18.84
E0186-UE	113.62	0.00	E0205-UE	182.84	128.41
E0186-RR	19.59	17.91	E0205-NU	235.08	171.22
E0187-UE	222.02	0.00	E0210-NU	37.87	28.79

Code	Commercial	Medicare	Code	Commercial	Medicare
E0210-RR	4.90	2.71	E0242	69.54	0.00
E0210-UE	28.73	21.60	E0243	55.18	0.00
E0215-RR	10.45	6.54	E0244	41.79	0.00
E0215-UE	71.18	46.88	E0245	68.89	0.00
E0215-NU	86.20	62.50	E0246	94.03	0.00
E0217-RR	50.93	48.77	E0249-NU	117.54	87.88
E0217-UE	330.42	328.49	E0249-RR	15.02	9.65
E0217-NU	440.78	438.03	E0249-UE	87.50	65.91
E0218-UE	330.42	0.00	E0250-RR	117.54	86.26
E0218-RR	50.93	0.00	E0250-NU	1567.20	0.00
E0218-NU	440.78	0.00	E0250-UE	1015.09	0.00
E0220-RR	1.31	0.79	E0251-RR	87.50	65.36
E0220-UE	8.82	5.59	E0251-UE	700.02	0.00
E0220-NU	11.75	7.47	E0251-NU	875.02	0.00
E0225-NU	458.41	342.90	E0255-NU	1632.50	0.00
E0225-RR	45.84	33.80	E0255-UE	1222.42	0.00
E0225-UE	343.48	257.17	E0255-RR	142.35	103.65
E0230-NU	11.75	7.49	E0256-UE	783.60	0.00
E0230-UE	9.80	5.60	E0256-RR	97.95	73.54
E0230-RR	2.29	0.84	E0256-NU	979.50	0.00
E0235-UE	208.63	0.00	E0260-UE	1311.22	0.00
E0235-NU	278.18	0.00	E0260-NU	1697.80	0.00
E0235-RR	27.75	15.22	E0260-RR	208.96	148.15
E0236-RR	71.18	39.05	E0261-NU	1567.20	0.00
E0236-UE	293.85	0.00	E0261-RR	163.25	120.82
E0236-NU	366.99	0.00	E0261-UE	1044.80	0.00
E0238-RR	6.86	2.39	E0265-UE	1306.00	0.00
E0238-UE	28.47	17.54	E0265-NU	2017.77	0.00
E0238-NU	35.59	23.86	E0265-RR	242.92	176.36
E0239-UE	397.02	297.68	E0266-NU	2089.60	0.00
E0239-NU	528.93	396.88	E0266-UE	1436.60	0.00
E0239-RR	53.55	39.69	E0266-RR	208.96	156.68
E0241	30.69	0.00	E0270-RR	0.00	0.00

Code	Commercial	Medicare	Code	Commercial	Medicare
E0270-NU	0.00	0.00	E0292-UE	794.05	0.00
E0270-UE	0.00	0.00	E0292-NU	992.56	0.00
E0271-RR	27.43	20.35	E0293-NU	848.90	0.00
E0271-UE	203.74	153.04	E0293-UE	620.35	0.00
E0271-NU	261.20	195.89	E0293-RR	84.89	63.09
E0272-UE	177.62	133.28	E0294-UE	1044.80	0.00
E0272-NU	237.69	178.56	E0294-RR	156.72	115.28
E0272-RR	24.81	18.64	E0294-NU	1520.18	0.00
E0273-UE	26.12	0.00	E0295-NU	1409.17	0.00
E0273-RR	13.06	0.00	E0295-RR	154.11	112.36
E0273-NU	33.30	0.00	E0295-UE	914.20	0.00
E0274-RR	23.51	0.00	E0296-UE	1546.30	0.00
E0274-NU	53.55	0.00	E0296-RR	193.29	144.88
E0274-UE	43.10	0.00	E0296-NU	1932.88	0.00
E0275-UE	11.10	10.13	E0297-RR	165.86	124.11
E0275-NU	14.37	13.51	E0297-NU	1658.62	0.00
E0275-RR	2.61	1.40	E0297-UE	1110.10	0.00
E0276-RR	2.61	1.38	E0305-RR	20.90	15.69
E0276-UE	13.06	9.28	E0305-NU	208.96	0.00
E0276-NU	13.71	11.74	E0305-UE	150.19	0.00
E0277-NU	0.00	0.00	E0310-RR	27.43	20.08
E0277-RR	966.44	669.98	E0310-UE	180.23	129.62
E0277-UE	0.00	0.00	E0310-NU	235.08	171.29
E0280-RR	5.22	3.63	E0315	0.00	0.00
E0280-UE	36.57	25.28	E0325-UE	6.53	5.90
E0280-NU	47.02	33.70	E0325-RR	3.92	1.33
E0290-RR	88.81	65.94	E0325-NU	9.80	8.91
E0290-UE	731.36	0.00	E0326-UE	7.84	6.94
E0290-NU	914.20	0.00	E0326-NU	13.06	9.27
E0291-NU	653.00	0.00	E0326-RR	3.92	1.06
E0291-UE	483.22	0.00	E0350-RR	0.00	0.00
E0291-RR	65.30	47.91	E0350-NU	0.00	0.00
E0292-RR	99.26	74.15	E0350-UE	0.00	0.00

Code	Commercial	Medicare	Code	Commercial	Medicare
E0352	0.00	0.00	E0457-NU	940.97	542.17
E0370	0.00	0.00	E0457-UE	705.89	406.61
E0371	0.00	0.00	E0457-RR	94.03	54.22
E0372	0.00	0.00	E0459-UE	522.73	0.00
E0373	0.00	0.00	E0459-NU	697.08	0.00
E0424-RR	331.72	211.64	E0459-RR	69.87	44.90
E0425-UE	3134.40	0.00	E0460-RR	0.00	647.23
E0425-NU	4153.08	0.00	E0460-UE	0.00	0.00
E0430-UE	1410.48	0.00	E0460-NU	0.00	0.00
E0430-NU	1880.64	0.00	E0462-NU	3992.44	0.00
E0431-RR	54.20	33.27	E0462-UE	2994.33	0.00
E0434-RR	54.20	33.27	E0462-RR	399.31	257.11
E0435-NU	1292.94	0.00	E0480-RR	58.77	38.76
E0435-UE	969.71	0.00	E0480-NU	565.50	0.00
E0439-RR	331.72	211.64	E0480-UE	496.28	0.00
E0440-UE	1968.80	0.00	E0500-NU	1436.60	0.00
E0440-NU	2625.06	0.00	E0500-RR	130.60	96.85
E0441	32.65	150.75	E0500-UE	946.85	0.00
E0442	2.38	150.75	E0550-NU	365.68	0.00
E0443	18.28	19.81	E0550-RR	60.08	44.23
E0444	2.38	19.81	E0550-UE	292.54	0.00
E0450-NU	0.00	0.00	E0555-UE	7.84	0.00
E0450-RR	0.00	842.15	E0555-NU	9.14	0.00
E0450-UE	0.00	0.00	E0555-RR	6.53	0.00
E0452-RR	380.05	226.39	E0560-NU	202.43	151.33
E0452-NU	3526.20	0.00	E0560-UE	178.92	113.50
E0452-UE	2807.90	0.00	E0560-RR	28.41	17.73
E0453-RR	0.00	566.58	E0565-NU	705.24	0.00
E0453-UE	0.00	0.00	E0565-UE	496.28	0.00
E0453-NU	0.00	0.00	E0565-RR	70.52	53.84
E0455-RR	0.00	0.00	E0570-UE	85.54	0.00
E0455-NU	0.00	0.00	E0570-NU	213.53	0.00
E0455-UE	0.00	0.00	E0570-RR	23.51	17.41

Code	Commercial	Medicare	Code	Commercial	Medicare
E0575-NU	561.58	0.00	E0615-UE	424.45	316.85
E0575-UE	365.68	0.00	E0615-RR	71.83	51.61
E0575-RR	56.16	90.68	E0615-NU	566.80	422.46
E0580-UE	24.81	88.69	E0616	0.00	0.00
E0580-NU	26.12	118.26	E0621-NU	114.93	84.69
E0580-RR	23.51	11.82	E0621-RR	11.75	8.16
E0585-RR	40.49	30.94	E0621-UE	87.50	63.84
E0585-UE	261.20	0.00	E0625-NU	0.00	0.00
E0585-NU	404.86	0.00	E0625-RR	0.00	0.00
E0590	0.00	0.00	E0625-UE	0.00	0.00
E0600-UE	297.77	0.00	E0627-NU	532.20	297.62
E0600-RR	54.85	40.39	E0627-RR	53.22	29.77
E0600-NU	496.28	0.00	E0627-UE	399.31	223.22
E0601-RR	154.11	98.56	E0628-UE	399.31	223.22
E0601-UE	848.90	0.00	E0628-RR	53.22	29.77
E0601-NU	1418.32	0.00	E0628-NU	532.20	297.62
E0602	0.00	0.00	E0629-UE	399.31	218.82
E0605-RR	4.24	2.71	E0629-RR	53.22	29.18
E0605-NU	38.20	23.32	E0629-NU	532.20	291.78
E0605-UE	29.71	19.20	E0630-NU	1332.12	0.00
E0606-UE	235.73	0.00	E0630-UE	946.85	0.00
E0606-NU	314.09	0.00	E0630-RR	124.07	89.89
E0606-RR	31.34	20.24	E0635-UE	1319.06	0.00
E0607-RR	6.27	0.00	E0635-NU	1932.88	0.00
E0607-NU	62.69	0.00	E0635-RR	193.29	107.95
E0607-UE	56.42	0.00	E0650-RR	112.97	78.41
E0608-RR	356.54	247.36	E0650-UE	639.94	476.58
E0609-RR	0.00	56.75	E0650-NU	980.81	635.44
E0609-NU	0.00	567.48	E0651-RR	117.54	82.78
E0609-UE	0.00	425.62	E0651-UE	829.31	607.74
E0610-UE	215.49	157.41	E0651-NU	1090.51	810.32
E0610-RR	31.34	22.14	E0652-UE	4571.00	3504.93
E0610-NU	313.44	209.87	E0652-RR	653.00	462.28

Code	Commercial	Medicare	Code	Commercial	Medicare
E0652-NU	6787.28	4677.42	E0730-NU	296.46	326.94
E0655-UE	101.87	71.51	E0730-UE	163.25	0.00
E0655-RR	15.67	11.18	E0730-RR	100.89	0.00
E0655-NU	133.21	95.22	E0731-RR	0.00	0.00
E0660-RR	23.51	14.67	E0731-UE	0.00	0.00
E0660-NU	191.98	140.94	E0731-NU	0.00	314.71
E0660-UE	146.27	105.70	E0740	0.00	0.00
E0665-NU	163.25	120.87	E0744-UE	633.41	0.00
E0665-UE	124.07	90.77	E0744-NU	698.71	0.00
E0665-RR	18.28	12.41	E0744-RR	104.48	80.79
E0666-NU	169.78	121.83	E0745-UE	351.31	0.00
E0666-RR	19.59	12.56	E0745-NU	439.47	0.00
E0666-UE	127.99	91.39	E0745-RR	147.58	78.97
E0667-UE	370.90	214.25	E0746-RR	0.00	0.00
E0667-NU	585.09	285.66	E0746-NU	0.00	0.00
E0667-RR	47.02	32.25	E0746-UE	0.00	0.00
E0668-RR	56.16	38.48	E0747-RR	564.85	309.25
E0668-NU	528.93	389.87	E0747-UE	4223.93	2312.17
E0668-UE	402.25	292.40	E0747-NU	5685.34	3112.03
E0669-RR	26.12	16.18	E0748	0.00	0.00
E0669-NU	222.02	161.74	E0749	4128.59	0.00
E0669-UE	167.17	121.33	E0751	0.00	5590.81
E0671	0.00	0.00	E0753	0.00	1264.16
E0672	0.00	0.00	E0755	0.00	0.00
E0673	0.00	0.00	E0760	0.00	0.00
E0690-RR	169.78	124.17	E0776-NU	172.39	126.31
E0690-NU	1612.91	1202.36	E0776-RR	26.12	16.46
E0690-UE	1208.05	899.65	E0776-UE	127.99	92.92
E0700	0.00	0.00	E0779	0.00	0.00
E0710	0.00	0.00	E0780	0.00	0.00
E0720-RR	82.93	0.00	E0781-RR	280.79	233.69
E0720-UE	158.03	0.00	E0782	5560.30	0.00
E0720-NU	287.97	324.31	E0783	0.00	0.00

Appendix 6

Code	Commercial	Medicare	Code	Commercial	Medicare
E0784	3656.80	0.00	E0920-RR	57.46	40.71
E0785	0.00	375.49	E0920-NU	574.64	0.00
E0791-UE	0.00	0.00	E0930-UE	403.55	0.00
E0791-NU	0.00	0.00	E0930-RR	54.85	40.31
E0791-RR	0.00	278.98	E0930-NU	548.52	0.00
E0840-RR	22.20	14.39	E0935-RR	0.00	20.06
E0840-NU	94.03	64.65	E0940-UE	302.99	0.00
E0840-UE	67.91	48.46	E0940-NU	428.37	0.00
E0850-RR	20.90	12.73	E0940-RR	45.71	30.68
E0850-NU	143.99	92.69	E0941-UE	404.86	0.00
E0850-UE	108.07	69.53	E0941-NU	535.46	0.00
E0855-RR	52.24	44.34	E0941-RR	53.55	38.31
E0855-NU	522.40	443.47	E0942-UE	20.24	13.13
E0855-UE	391.80	332.60	E0942-NU	27.10	17.51
E0860-UE	32.45	26.04	E0942-RR	3.27	2.06
E0860-RR	11.75	5.75	E0943-RR	4.57	2.86
E0860-NU	36.06	33.99	E0943-NU	41.79	24.41
E0870-RR	20.90	11.82	E0943-UE	35.26	18.30
E0870-NU	141.05	102.62	E0944-RR	6.20	4.06
E0870-UE	109.70	77.31	E0944-UE	24.76	30.36
E0880-NU	154.11	110.76	E0944-NU	27.52	40.48
E0880-RR	28.73	17.39	E0945-NU	60.73	39.11
E0880-UE	117.54	83.84	E0945-UE	47.02	30.27
E0890-RR	52.89	28.96	E0945-RR	6.20	3.91
E0890-UE	126.68	85.57	E0946-NU	810.37	0.00
E0890-NU	154.11	106.24	E0946-UE	607.94	0.00
E0900-RR	44.40	24.38	E0946-RR	80.97	52.20
E0900-NU	82.76	113.04	E0947-NU	783.60	535.08
E0900-UE	73.31	84.81	E0947-RR	78.36	55.49
E0910-NU	302.67	0.00	E0947-UE	587.70	401.30
E0910-RR	30.36	17.64	E0948-UE	515.87	365.01
E0910-UE	226.92	0.00	E0948-NU	744.42	517.54
E0920-UE	476.69	0.00	E0948-RR	74.44	51.74

Code	Commercial	Medicare	Code	Commercial	Medicare
E0950-RR	15.67	9.18	E0965-UE	82.28	56.10
E0950-UE	106.77	68.79	E0965-NU	114.93	74.77
E0950-NU	142.35	91.72	E0965-RR	13.71	7.49
E0951-NU	25.79	16.62	E0966-NU	91.42	62.97
E0951-RR	2.61	1.72	E0966-UE	62.69	47.22
E0951-UE	19.26	12.47	E0966-RR	9.14	6.20
E0952-NU	30.36	16.62	E0967-UE	127.99	87.46
E0952-RR	3.27	1.73	E0967-RR	18.94	11.96
E0952-UE	22.86	12.47	E0967-NU	185.45	116.58
E0953-RR	5.88	3.54	E0968-RR	24.49	15.82
E0953-UE	43.42	25.86	E0968-UE	156.72	0.00
E0953-NU	58.12	36.09	E0968-NU	245.85	0.00
E0954-RR	7.51	4.16	E0969-UE	160.96	103.65
E0954-UE	33.96	27.70	E0969-NU	214.51	138.19
E0954-NU	58.77	36.91	E0969-RR	21.22	13.68
E0958-UE	527.62	0.00	E0970-UE	49.63	31.88
E0958-NU	703.28	0.00	E0970-NU	65.95	42.49
E0958-RR	70.20	38.50	E0970-RR	5.88	3.79
E0959-NU	117.54	78.01	E0971-NU	88.81	58.00
E0959-RR	14.37	7.84	E0971-RR	12.08	6.59
E0959-UE	91.42	59.05	E0971-UE	58.77	43.50
E0961-NU	48.00	26.24	E0972-NU	70.52	48.63
E0961-UE	35.92	19.70	E0972-RR	9.14	4.95
E0961-RR	5.22	2.74	E0972-UE	52.24	35.61
E0962-RR	9.47	5.25	E0973-RR	13.39	9.65
E0962-NU	84.24	52.49	E0973-UE	101.87	76.08
E0962-UE	62.69	39.36	E0973-NU	141.05	101.44
E0963-RR	11.75	6.38	E0974-UE	81.30	52.28
E0963-NU	99.91	62.69	E0974-NU	108.40	69.71
E0963-UE	75.10	47.13	E0974-RR	11.43	7.33
E0964-NU	97.95	69.95	E0975-RR	6.86	4.37
E0964-RR	12.73	7.05	E0975-NU	69.54	43.89
E0964-UE	75.75	52.49	E0975-UE	52.24	32.93

Code	Commercial	Medicare	Code	Commercial	Medicare
E0976-UE	52.24	33.22	E0996-RR	4.57	2.42
E0976-NU	59.42	44.31	E0996-UE	30.04	19.24
E0976-RR	6.86	4.37	E0996-NU	39.18	25.16
E0977-UE	65.30	43.31	E0997-NU	91.42	58.68
E0977-NU	84.89	57.71	E0997-RR	9.14	6.29
E0977-RR	10.12	5.56	E0997-UE	65.30	44.02
E0978-UE	47.67	29.62	E0998-NU	47.02	33.77
E0978-NU	63.67	39.48	E0998-UE	36.57	25.35
E0978-RR	6.53	3.93	E0998-RR	5.55	3.50
E0979-NU	46.36	29.81	E0999-NU	143.66	101.44
E0979-RR	4.57	2.99	E0999-UE	111.01	76.08
E0979-UE	34.61	22.36	E0999-RR	15.67	10.14
E0980-RR	4.57	2.91	E1000-RR	6.53	3.50
E0980-UE	33.63	21.76	E1000-UE	37.22	23.82
E0980-NU	45.38	29.16	E1000-NU	49.63	31.77
E0990-UE	124.07	80.94	E1001-NU	127.99	86.51
E0990-NU	156.72	103.61	E1001-RR	14.04	9.09
E0990-RR	18.28	11.66	E1001-UE	102.85	64.89
E0991-NU	62.69	40.48	E1031-UE	519.14	0.00
E0991-RR	7.18	3.88	E1031-NU	691.85	0.00
E0991-UE	47.02	30.52	E1031-RR	69.22	44.57
E0992-UE	83.58	62.97	E1050-RR	146.27	89.85
E0992-RR	13.06	8.16	E1050-NU	1641.32	0.00
E0992-NU	130.60	83.94	E1050-UE	1231.23	0.00
E0993-NU	58.77	41.02	E1060-RR	148.88	111.23
E0993-UE	44.40	30.90	E1060-NU	1765.39	0.00
E0993-RR	6.53	4.09	E1060-UE	1323.96	0.00
E0994-UE	19.92	11.67	E1065-RR	362.09	233.19
E0994-RR	2.61	1.58	E1065-UE	2987.15	1923.79
E0994-NU	26.77	15.56	E1065-NU	3982.97	2565.05
E0995-UE	36.57	20.10	E1066-UE	254.67	174.44
E0995-RR	4.90	2.69	E1066-NU	365.68	232.59
E0995-NU	41.79	26.82	E1066-RR	36.57	23.32

Code	Commercial	Medicare	Code	Commercial	Medicare
E1069-UE	117.54	74.34	E1092-RR	154.11	113.38
E1069-RR	18.28	9.96	E1093-NU	1403.95	0.00
E1069-NU	134.19	99.13	E1093-UE	1044.80	0.00
E1070-NU	1765.39	0.00	E1093-RR	143.66	97.51
E1070-RR	143.66	96.64	E1100-RR	151.17	91.59
E1070-UE	1323.96	0.00	E1100-NU	1510.39	0.00
E1083-UE	829.31	0.00	E1100-UE	1132.96	0.00
E1083-RR	113.62	69.47	E1110-RR	129.29	89.69
E1083-NU	1136.22	0.00	E1110-UE	940.32	0.00
E1084-RR	112.32	86.55	E1110-NU	1292.94	0.00
E1084-NU	1371.30	0.00	E1130-RR	65.30	41.20
E1084-UE	979.50	0.00	E1130-NU	653.00	0.00
E1085-RR	101.87	61.06	E1130-UE	496.28	0.00
E1085-UE	731.36	0.00	E1140-UE	666.06	0.00
E1085-NU	1018.68	0.00	E1140-NU	940.32	0.00
E1086-RR	112.97	74.15	E1140-RR	94.03	63.38
E1086-NU	1240.70	0.00	E1150-UE	653.00	0.00
E1086-UE	901.14	0.00	E1150-NU	986.03	0.00
E1087-NU	1567.20	0.00	E1150-RR	95.34	71.97
E1087-RR	156.72	111.62	E1160-UE	574.64	0.00
E1087-UE	1142.75	0.00	E1160-RR	75.10	55.14
E1088-NU	1808.81	0.00	E1160-NU	822.78	0.00
E1088-RR	180.23	133.02	E1170-UE	917.79	0.00
E1088-UE	1240.70	0.00	E1170-RR	122.44	78.80
E1089-UE	1235.15	0.00	E1170-NU	1223.72	0.00
E1089-NU	1646.87	0.00	E1171-NU	1291.96	0.00
E1089-RR	164.56	106.05	E1171-UE	969.05	0.00
E1090-NU	1697.80	0.00	E1171-RR	129.29	70.72
E1090-RR	164.56	120.14	E1172-UE	1183.89	0.00
E1090-UE	1240.70	0.00	E1172-NU	1578.63	0.00
E1091	0.00	0.00	E1172-RR	158.03	86.42
E1092-UE	1240.70	0.00	E1180-RR	138.76	89.41
E1092-NU	1697.80	0.00	E1180-NU	1388.28	0.00

Code	Commercial	Medicare	Code	Commercial	Medicare
E1180-UE	1041.21	0.00	E1224-NU	1070.92	0.00
E1190-RR	150.19	103.29	E1224-UE	718.30	0.00
E1190-UE	1097.04	0.00	E1225-NU	655.94	0.00
E1190-NU	1501.90	0.00	E1225-UE	492.04	0.00
E1195-RR	186.43	110.85	E1225-RR	65.63	39.88
E1195-NU	1864.32	0.00	E1226-UE	509.34	361.04
E1195-UE	1398.40	0.00	E1226-RR	71.83	49.55
E1200-RR	134.84	76.76	E1226-NU	718.30	481.42
E1200-UE	1010.19	0.00	E1227-NU	380.05	244.84
E1200-NU	1347.14	0.00	E1227-RR	37.87	24.48
E1210-UE	4221.97	0.00	E1227-UE	285.03	183.65
E1210-NU	5629.19	0.00	E1228-RR	41.47	24.72
E1210-RR	562.89	362.50	E1228-UE	311.81	0.00
E1211-NU	5733.67	0.00	E1228-NU	415.63	0.00
E1211-RR	573.33	369.25	E1230-NU	3236.92	1995.56
E1211-UE	4300.33	0.00	E1230-RR	323.56	196.26
E1212-NU	5557.36	0.00	E1230-UE	2883.32	1578.26
E1212-RR	555.70	357.88	E1240-RR	124.07	90.89
E1212-UE	4167.77	0.00	E1240-NU	1240.70	0.00
E1213-RR	597.50	384.88	E1240-UE	888.08	0.00
E1213-NU	5976.58	0.00	E1250-NU	1005.62	0.00
E1213-UE	4482.19	0.00	E1250-RR	91.42	67.05
E1220	0.00	0.00	E1250-UE	796.66	0.00
E1221-RR	64.97	41.91	E1260-NU	1175.40	0.00
E1221-NU	651.04	0.00	E1260-UE	927.26	0.00
E1221-UE	488.44	0.00	E1260-RR	117.54	82.24
E1222-NU	875.02	0.00	E1270-RR	103.17	69.65
E1222-RR	87.50	59.81	E1270-UE	757.48	0.00
E1222-UE	629.49	0.00	E1270-NU	1031.74	0.00
E1223-NU	940.32	0.00	E1280-RR	156.72	115.81
E1223-RR	94.03	65.30	E1280-NU	1567.20	0.00
E1223-UE	672.59	0.00	E1280-UE	1123.16	0.00
E1224-RR	101.87	71.61	E1285-UE	1110.10	0.00

Code	Commercial	Medicare	Code	Commercial	Medicare
E1285-NU	1514.96	0.00	E1375-RR	53.55	36.82
E1285-RR	151.50	106.40	E1375-NU	267.73	201.26
E1290-UE	1142.75	0.00	E1375-UE	239.65	153.02
E1290-RR	156.72	110.42	E1377-UE	0.00	0.00
E1290-NU	1567.20	0.00	E1377-NU	2350.80	0.00
E1295-NU	1528.02	0.00	E1377-RR	287.32	0.00
E1295-UE	1110.10	0.00	E1378-RR	287.32	0.00
E1295-RR	152.80	107.17	E1378-NU	0.00	0.00
E1296-NU	653.00	433.79	E1378-UE	0.00	0.00
E1296-UE	457.10	325.35	E1379-NU	0.00	0.00
E1296-RR	65.30	44.07	E1379-UE	0.00	0.00
E1297-UE	104.48	69.22	E1379-RR	287.32	0.00
E1297-NU	133.21	92.29	E1380-RR	287.32	0.00
E1297-RR	15.67	10.25	E1380-NU	0.00	0.00
E1298-RR	57.46	38.25	E1380-UE	0.00	0.00
E1298-UE	391.80	280.33	E1381-NU	0.00	0.00
E1298-NU	522.40	373.79	E1381-RR	287.32	0.00
E1300-RR	0.00	0.00	E1381-UE	0.00	0.00
E1300-UE	0.00	0.00	E1382-UE	0.00	0.00
E1300-NU	0.00	0.00	E1382-NU	0.00	0.00
E1310-UE	2285.50	1420.97	E1382-RR	287.32	0.00
E1310-NU	3069.10	1894.63	E1383-RR	287.32	0.00
E1310-RR	228.55	162.05	E1383-UE	0.00	0.00
E1340	0.00	0.00	E1383-NU	0.00	0.00
E1353-NU	97.95	0.00	E1384-UE	0.00	0.00
E1353-UE	78.36	0.00	E1384-RR	287.32	0.00
E1353-RR	5.22	0.00	E1384-NU	0.00	0.00
E1355-RR	7.84	0.00	E1385-NU	0.00	0.00
E1355-NU	66.61	0.00	E1385-RR	287.32	0.00
E1355-UE	53.55	0.00	E1385-UE	0.00	0.00
E1372-RR	33.96	20.90	E1390-RR	316.05	211.64
E1372-NU	215.49	143.84	E1390-NU	2403.04	0.00
E1372-UE	160.64	106.47	E1399	0.00	0.00

Code	Commercial	Medicare	Code	Commercial	Medicare
E1400-NU	2403.04	0.00	E1550-NU	0.00	0.00
E1400-UE	0.00	0.00	E1550-RR	0.00	0.00
E1400-RR	316.05	211.64	E1550-UE	0.00	0.00
E1401-RR	316.05	211.64	E1560-RR	0.00	0.00
E1401-NU	2403.04	0.00	E1560-NU	0.00	0.00
E1401-UE	0.00	0.00	E1560-UE	0.00	0.00
E1402-NU	2403.04	0.00	E1570-UE	0.00	0.00
E1402-UE	0.00	0.00	E1570-NU	0.00	0.00
E1402-RR	316.05	211.64	E1570-RR	0.00	0.00
E1403-NU	2403.04	0.00	E1575-UE	0.00	0.00
E1403-UE	0.00	0.00	E1575-NU	0.00	0.00
E1403-RR	316.05	211.64	E1575-RR	0.00	0.00
E1404-NU	2403.04	0.00	E1580-NU	0.00	0.00
E1404-RR	316.05	211.64	E1580-UE	0.00	0.00
E1404-UE	0.00	0.00	E1580-RR	0.00	0.00
E1405-NU	0.00	0.00	E1590-RR	0.00	0.00
E1405-UE	0.00	0.00	E1590-UE	0.00	0.00
E1405-RR	313.44	0.00	E1590-NU	0.00	0.00
E1406-UE	0.00	0.00	E1592-UE	0.00	0.00
E1406-NU	0.00	0.00	E1592-NU	0.00	0.00
E1406-RR	130.60	0.00	E1592-RR	0.00	0.00
E1510-NU	0.00	0.00	E1594-NU	0.00	0.00
E1510-UE	0.00	0.00	E1594-RR	0.00	0.00
E1510-RR	0.00	0.00	E1594-UE	0.00	0.00
E1520-RR	0.00	0.00	E1600-UE	0.00	0.00
E1520-NU	0.00	0.00	E1600-NU	0.00	0.00
E1520-UE	0.00	0.00	E1600-RR	0.00	0.00
E1530-NU	0.00	0.00	E1610-UE	0.00	0.00
E1530-UE	0.00	0.00	E1610-NU	0.00	0.00
E1530-RR	0.00	0.00	E1610-RR	0.00	0.00
E1540-RR	0.00	0.00	E1615-NU	0.00	0.00
E1540-UE	0.00	0.00	E1615-RR	0.00	0.00
E1540-NU	0.00	0.00	E1615-UE	0.00	0.00

Code	Commercial	Medicare	Code	Commercial	Medicare
E1620-NU	0.00	0.00	E1830	0.00	0.00
E1620-RR	0.00	0.00	E1900	0.00	0.00
E1620-UE	0.00	0.00	G0001	7.41	0.00
E1625-UE	0.00	0.00	G0002	40.41	89.34
E1625-RR	0.00	0.00	G0004	251.89	318.17
E1625-NU	0.00	0.00	G0005	49.84	48.70
E1630-NU	0.00	0.00	G0006	101.03	237.99
E1630-UE	0.00	0.00	G0007	101.03	31.49
E1630-RR	0.00	0.00	G0008	10.78	0.00
E1632-UE	0.00	0.00	G0009	10.78	0.00
E1632-NU	0.00	0.00	G0010	10.78	0.00
E1632-RR	0.00	0.00	G0015	83.51	237.99
E1635-NU	0.00	0.00	G0016	64.66	32.59
E1635-UE	0.00	0.00	G0025	44.45	19.04
E1635-RR	0.00	0.00	G0026	13.24	5.90
E1636-NU	0.00	0.00	G0027	24.25	8.99
E1636-RR	0.00	0.00	G0030	0.00	0.00
E1636-UE	0.00	0.00	G0031	0.00	0.00
E1640-NU	0.00	0.00	G0032	0.00	0.00
E1640-UE	0.00	0.00	G0033	0.00	0.00
E1640-RR	0.00	0.00	G0034	0.00	0.00
E1699	0.00	0.00	G0035	0.00	0.00
E1700-UE	354.25	228.19	G0036	0.00	0.00
E1700-RR	46.36	29.84	G0037	0.00	0.00
E1700-NU	472.45	304.25	G0038	0.00	0.00
E1701	16.98	9.36	G0039	0.00	0.00
E1702	31.02	19.91	G0040	0.00	0.00
E1800	0.00	0.00	G0041	0.00	0.00
E1805	0.00	0.00	G0042	0.00	0.00
E1810	0.00	0.00	G0043	0.00	0.00
E1815	0.00	0.00	G0044	0.00	0.00
E1820	0.00	0.00	G0045	0.00	0.00
E1825	0.00	0.00	G0046	0.00	0.00

Code	Commercial	Medicare	Code	Commercial	Medicare
G0047	0.00	0.00	G0144	22.90	0.00
G0050	0.00	33.32	G0145	24.92	0.00
G0101	57.92	33.32	G0147	22.90	0.00
G0102	0.00	9.52	G0148	23.91	0.00
G0103	67.35	25.42	G0151	0.00	0.00
G0104	191.27	95.56	G0152	0.00	0.00
G0105	696.40	331.72	G0153	0.00	0.00
G0106	285.56	139.50	G0154	0.00	0.00
G0107	13.47	3.50	G0155	0.00	0.00
G0108	0.00	60.41	G0156	0.00	0.00
G0109	0.00	35.88	G0159	0.00	0.00
G0110	161.64	51.99	G0160	0.00	0.00
G0111	67.35	19.41	G0161	0.00	0.00
G0112	70.72	112.04	G0163	0.00	1982.27
G0113	53.21	83.11	G0164	0.00	2000.94
G0114	68.02	61.14	G0165	0.00	1982.27
G0115	68.02	62.24	G0166	0.00	127.42
G0116	61.29	60.78	G0167	0.00	27.46
G0120	285.56	139.50	G0168	0.00	58.22
G0121	696.40	335.38	G0169	0.00	32.95
G0122	285.56	141.33	G0170	0.00	124.12
G0123	17.17	0.00	G0171	0.00	133.27
G0124	4.38	26.00	G0172	0.00	0.00
G0125	0.00	2186.20	J0120	0.00	0.00
G0126	0.00	2207.07	J0130	878.09	0.00
G0127	26.94	17.94	J0150	52.95	0.00
G0128	0.00	4.39	J0151	355.47	0.00
G0129	0.00	0.00	J0170	2.69	0.00
G0130	0.00	42.84	J0190	0.00	0.00
G0131	0.00	130.71	J0200	28.95	0.00
G0132	0.00	42.84	J0205	69.15	0.00
G0141	0.00	26.00	J0207	565.15	0.00
G0143	23.91	0.00	J0210	14.67	0.00

Code	Commercial	Medicare	Code	Commercial	Medicare
J0256	0.36	0.00	J0590	0.00	0.00
J0270	3.76	0.00	J0600	64.67	0.00
J0275	0.00	0.00	J0610	1.89	0.00
J0280	2.69	0.00	J0620	6.63	0.00
J0285	38.88	0.00	J0630	53.92	0.00
J0286	181.29	0.00	J0635	21.33	0.00
J0290	2.17	0.00	J0640	34.46	0.00
J0295	12.58	0.00	J0670	0.00	0.00
J0300	6.84	0.00	J0690	4.64	0.00
J0330	0.43	0.00	J0694	16.07	0.00
J0340	0.00	0.00	J0695	0.00	0.00
J0350	4345.76	0.00	J0696	22.63	0.00
J0360	14.82	0.00	J0697	16.84	0.00
J0380	2.15	0.00	J0698	20.86	0.00
J0390	26.97	0.00	J0702	8.35	0.00
J0395	305.02	0.00	J0704	5.53	0.00
J0400	0.00	0.00	J0710	3.07	0.00
J0456	37.31	0.00	J0713	11.27	0.00
J0460	1.01	0.00	J0715	12.11	0.00
J0470	46.58	0.00	J0720	14.26	0.00
J0475	0.00	0.00	J0725	5.31	0.00
J0476	116.27	0.00	J0730	0.75	0.00
J0500	3.50	0.00	J0735	85.97	0.00
J0510	0.00	0.00	J0740	1188.91	0.00
J0515	12.60	0.00	J0743	23.96	0.00
J0520	9.31	0.00	J0745	1.79	0.00
J0530	11.05	0.00	J0760	9.42	0.00
J0540	21.68	0.00	J0770	66.44	0.00
J0550	46.46	0.00	J0780	12.73	0.00
J0560	15.31	0.00	J0800	0.00	0.00
J0570	27.21	0.00	J0810	0.00	0.00
J0580	55.77	0.00	J0835	23.57	0.00
J0585	7.36	0.00	J0850	724.44	0.00

Code	Commercial	Medicare	Code	Commercial	Medicare
J0895	19.40	0.00	J1327	23.55	0.00
J0900	2.93	0.00	J1330	8.86	0.00
J0945	1.64	0.00	J1362	0.00	0.00
J0970	2.60	0.00	J1364	11.68	0.00
J1000	3.29	0.00	J1380	1.61	0.00
J1020	1.40	0.00	J1390	1.93	0.00
J1030	2.82	0.00	J1410	77.26	0.00
J1040	5.64	0.00	J1435	0.77	0.00
J1050	18.47	0.00	J1436	118.87	0.00
J1055	76.74	0.00	J1438	256.99	0.00
J1060	2.04	0.00	J1440	262.61	0.00
J1070	2.39	0.00	J1441	418.30	0.00
J1080	4.50	0.00	J1450	134.74	0.00
J1090	0.00	0.00	J1455	22.82	0.00
J1095	8.45	0.00	J1460	0.00	0.00
J1100	0.67	0.00	J1470	0.00	0.00
J1110	20.93	0.00	J1480	0.00	0.00
J1120	58.31	0.00	J1490	0.00	0.00
J1160	3.91	0.00	J1500	0.00	0.00
J1165	1.35	0.00	J1510	0.00	0.00
J1170	2.93	0.00	J1520	0.00	0.00
J1180	10.67	0.00	J1530	0.00	0.00
J1190	0.00	0.00	J1540	0.00	0.00
J1200	2.78	0.00	J1550	0.00	0.00
J1205	16.05	0.00	J1560	0.00	0.00
J1212	68.22	0.00	J1561	74.76	0.00
J1230	1.48	0.00	J1562	635.46	0.00
J1240	1.21	0.00	J1565	0.00	0.00
J1245	43.06	0.00	J1570	56.46	0.00
J1250	10.54	0.00	J1580	8.50	0.00
J1260	29.12	0.00	J1600	20.69	0.00
J1320	3.31	0.00	J1610	99.56	0.00
J1325	0.00	0.00	J1620	247.46	0.00

Code	Commercial	Medicare	Code	Commercial	Medicare
J1626	34.78	0.00	J1930	0.00	0.00
J1630	11.23	0.00	J1940	1.83	0.00
J1631	52.24	0.00	J1950	794.85	0.00
J1642	2.11	0.00	J1955	67.28	0.00
J1644	0.69	0.00	J1956	32.20	0.00
J1645	26.07	0.00	J1960	6.19	0.00
J1650	0.00	0.00	J1970	0.00	0.00
J1670	165.52	0.00	J1980	20.60	0.00
J1690	0.00	0.00	J1990	39.77	0.00
J1700	0.67	0.00	J2000	5.63	0.00
J1710	8.28	0.00	J2010	1.81	0.00
J1720	5.53	0.00	J2060	4.88	0.00
J1730	175.35	0.00	J2150	7.40	0.00
J1739	2.09	0.00	J2175	1.48	0.00
J1741	5.23	0.00	J2180	10.88	0.00
J1742	339.20	0.00	J2210	4.95	0.00
J1745	93.69	0.00	J2240	0.00	0.00
J1750	35.23	0.00	J2250	3.74	0.00
J1760	63.06	0.00	J2260	65.38	0.00
J1770	0.00	0.00	J2270	2.00	0.00
J1780	0.00	0.00	J2271	35.57	0.00
J1785	6.92	0.00	J2275	27.12	0.00
J1790	5.10	0.00	J2300	6.41	0.00
J1800	21.87	0.00	J2310	6.77	0.00
J1810	16.20	0.00	J2320	8.93	0.00
J1820	4.90	0.00	J2321	12.43	0.00
J1825	398.10	0.00	J2322	44.16	0.00
J1830	134.57	0.00	J2330	0.00	0.00
J1840	5.76	0.00	J2350	0.00	0.00
J1850	5.18	0.00	J2352	223.31	0.00
J1885	11.63	0.00	J2355	382.12	0.00
J1890	20.19	0.00	J2360	2.99	0.00
J1910	22.58	0.00	J2370	4.78	0.00

Code	Commercial	Medicare	Code	Commercial	Medicare
J2400	31.85	0.00	J2792	0.00	0.00
J2405	9.70	0.00	J2800	15.25	0.00
J2410	5.20	0.00	J2810	0.00	0.00
J2430	367.24	0.00	J2820	44.03	0.00
J2440	6.30	0.00	J2860	0.00	0.00
J2460	0.00	0.00	J2910	24.02	0.00
J2480	0.00	0.00	J2912	2.37	0.00
J2500	49.49	0.00	J2920	3.74	0.00
J2510	10.07	0.00	J2930	6.88	0.00
J2512	0.00	0.00	J2950	0.90	0.00
J2515	1.93	0.00	J2970	0.00	0.00
J2540	0.00	0.00	J2994	4471.58	0.00
J2543	8.00	0.00	J2995	188.08	0.00
J2545	208.80	0.00	J2996	513.98	0.00
J2550	2.28	0.00	J3000	11.12	0.00
J2560	4.47	0.00	J3010	2.58	0.00
J2590	1.42	0.00	J3030	69.62	0.00
J2597	9.42	0.00	J3070	6.21	0.00
J2640	0.00	0.00	J3080	0.00	0.00
J2650	0.00	0.00	J3105	3.38	0.00
J2670	24.11	0.00	J3120	3.35	0.00
J2675	3.48	0.00	J3130	6.69	0.00
J2680	27.96	0.00	J3140	0.00	0.00
J2690	9.16	0.00	J3150	2.22	0.00
J2700	2.80	0.00	J3230	5.23	0.00
J2710	1.25	0.00	J3240	0.00	0.00
J2720	1.44	0.00	J3245	654.15	0.00
J2725	92.31	0.00	J3250	4.62	0.00
J2730	137.58	0.00	J3260	23.40	0.00
J2760	53.38	0.00	J3265	2.88	0.00
J2765	3.20	0.00	J3270	0.00	0.00
J2780	2.88	0.00	J3280	7.98	0.00
J2790	182.38	0.00	J3301	1.40	0.00

Code	Commercial	Medicare	Code	Commercial	Medicare
J3302	0.60	0.00	J7120	23.10	0.00
J3303	4.47	0.00	J7130	0.00	0.00
J3305	112.64	0.00	J7190	1.59	0.00
J3310	10.54	0.00	J7191	3.50	0.00
J3320	39.59	0.00	J7192	2.21	0.00
J3350	135.88	0.00	J7194	0.80	0.00
J3360	1.42	0.00	J7196	0.00	0.00
J3364	92.87	0.00	J7197	1.61	0.00
J3365	779.56	0.00	J7198	0.00	0.00
J3370	19.77	0.00	J7199	0.00	0.00
J3390	38.80	0.00	J7300	0.00	0.00
J3400	23.33	0.00	J7310	7943.25	0.00
J3410	1.07	0.00	J7315	210.02	0.00
J3420	0.69	0.00	J7320	0.00	0.00
J3430	4.24	0.00	J7500	2.65	0.00
J3450	9.70	0.00	J7501	171.87	0.00
J3470	33.68	0.00	J7502	3.18	0.00
J3475	0.41	0.00	J7503	10.37	0.00
J3480	0.41	0.00	J7504	401.89	0.00
J3490	0.00	0.00	J7505	0.00	0.00
J3520	0.75	0.00	J7506	0.06	0.00
J3530	0.00	0.00	J7507	4.41	0.00
J3535	0.00	0.00	J7508	22.28	0.00
J3570	0.00	0.00	J7509	0.90	0.00
J7030	14.56	0.00	J7510	0.09	0.00
J7040	13.46	0.00	J7513	680.00	0.00
J7042	18.91	0.00	J7515	2.82	0.00
J7050	13.03	0.00	J7516	43.92	0.00
J7051	1.94	0.00	J7517	3.51	0.00
J7060	17.29	0.00	J7599	0.00	0.00
J7070	20.20	0.00	J7608	0.00	0.00
J7100	185.83	0.00	J7610	2.60	0.00
J7110	137.30	0.00	J7615	3.07	0.00

Appendix 6

Code	Commercial	Medicare	Code	Commercial	Medicare
J7618	0.00	0.00	J7670	2.43	0.00
J7619	0.00	0.00	J7672	2.11	0.00
J7620	0.77	0.00	J7675	2.90	0.00
J7625	1.31	0.00	J7680	0.00	0.00
J7627	0.00	0.00	J7681	0.00	0.00
J7628	0.00	0.00	J7682	75.88	0.00
J7629	0.00	0.00	J7683	0.37	0.00
J7630	1.31	0.00	J7684	0.37	0.00
J7631	0.65	0.00	J7699	0.00	0.00
J7635	0.00	0.00	J7799	0.00	0.00
J7636	0.00	0.00	J8499	0.00	0.00
J7637	0.00	0.00	J8510	3.40	0.00
J7638	0.00	0.00	J8520	3.79	0.00
J7639	60.97	0.00	J8521	11.96	0.00
J7640	0.00	0.00	J8530	3.40	0.00
J7642	0.00	0.00	J8560	74.12	0.00
J7643	0.00	0.00	J8600	3.31	0.00
J7644	0.00	0.00	J8610	5.61	0.00
J7645	2.45	0.00	J8999	0.00	0.00
J7648	0.00	0.00	J9000	65.27	0.00
J7649	0.00	0.00	J9001	201.14	0.00
J7650	0.00	0.00	J9015	988.51	0.00
J7651	0.00	0.00	J9020	102.20	0.00
J7652	0.00	0.00	J9031	266.76	0.00
J7653	0.00	0.00	J9040	516.39	0.00
J7654	0.00	0.00	J9045	159.03	0.00
J7655	4.04	0.00	J9050	166.60	0.00
J7658	0.00	0.00	J9060	0.00	0.00
J7659	0.00	0.00	J9062	335.04	0.00
J7660	0.00	0.00	J9065	89.71	0.00
J7665	0.00	0.00	J9070	9.92	0.00
J7668	0.00	0.00	J9080	18.90	0.00
J7669	0.00	0.00	J9090	39.70	0.00

Code	Commercial	Medicare	Code	Commercial	Medicare
J9091	79.41	0.00	J9218	112.59	0.00
J9092	159.31	0.00	J9230	17.83	0.00
J9093	10.24	0.00	J9245	579.45	0.00
J9094	19.46	0.00	J9250	0.77	0.00
J9095	40.84	0.00	J9260	10.93	0.00
J9096	81.71	0.00	J9265	341.34	0.00
J9097	163.46	0.00	J9266	2289.53	0.00
J9100	11.68	0.00	J9268	3074.51	0.00
J9110	46.73	0.00	J9270	151.31	0.00
J9120	21.19	0.00	J9280	241.01	0.00
J9130	23.27	0.00	J9290	813.93	0.00
J9140	39.57	0.00	J9291	1427.43	0.00
J9150	144.88	0.00	J9293	287.83	0.00
J9151	116.44	0.00	J9310	678.02	0.00
J9165	23.40	0.00	J9320	139.33	0.00
J9170	457.59	0.00	J9340	173.11	0.00
J9181	25.49	0.00	J9350	925.58	0.00
J9182	255.10	0.00	J9355	96.10	0.00
J9185	382.38	0.00	J9357	728.91	0.00
J9190	4.47	0.00	J9360	14.93	0.00
J9200	229.77	0.00	J9370	53.86	0.00
J9201	142.70	0.00	J9375	103.13	0.00
J9202	746.65	0.00	J9380	70.93	0.00
J9206	190.06	0.00	J9390	121.80	0.00
J9208	228.11	0.00	J9600	4199.27	0.00
J9209	58.89	0.00	J9999	0.00	0.00
J9211	475.01	0.00	K0001-UE	550.80	0.00
J9212	0.00	0.00	K0001-RR	73.95	48.19
J9213	55.83	0.00	K0001-NU	734.40	0.00
J9214	18.20	0.00	K0002-UE	674.48	0.00
J9215	14.88	0.00	K0002-NU	859.03	0.00
J9216	321.84	0.00	K0002-RR	108.38	72.19
J9217	944.69	0.00	K0003-NU	1378.28	0.00

Code	Commercial	Medicare	Code	Commercial	Medicare
K0003-UE	1034.03	0.00	K0018-RR	7.65	2.50
K0003-RR	121.13	79.05	K0018-UE	49.73	18.91
K0004-UE	1285.20	0.00	K0018-NU	77.78	25.19
K0004-RR	144.08	117.91	K0019-RR	6.38	1.51
K0004-NU	1713.60	0.00	K0019-UE	24.17	11.40
K0005-RR	198.90	163.11	K0019-NU	35.11	15.21
K0005-NU	2122.88	1631.14	K0020-UE	42.08	30.73
K0005-UE	1592.48	1223.34	K0020-NU	58.65	40.99
K0006-UE	1151.33	0.00	K0020-RR	5.10	4.11
K0006-NU	1527.45	0.00	K0021-UE	58.34	43.50
K0006-RR	167.66	110.65	K0021-NU	78.23	58.00
K0007-RR	195.08	157.49	K0021-RR	11.48	6.70
K0007-NU	1950.75	0.00	K0022-NU	58.01	44.31
K0007-UE	1909.95	0.00	K0022-UE	51.00	33.22
K0008	2371.50	0.00	K0022-RR	6.69	4.41
K0009	0.00	0.00	K0023-UE	91.80	62.27
K0010-NU	5495.25	0.00	K0023-RR	11.48	8.30
K0010-UE	4122.08	0.00	K0023-NU	171.23	83.02
K0010-RR	549.53	375.85	K0024-UE	151.09	73.72
K0011-RR	666.83	467.31	K0024-RR	20.15	9.84
K0011-NU	9033.38	0.00	K0024-NU	201.45	98.28
K0012	3887.48	0.00	K0025-NU	89.25	62.97
K0013	0.00	0.00	K0025-RR	8.93	6.20
K0014	0.00	0.00	K0025-UE	63.65	47.22
K0015-UE	161.93	120.23	K0026-NU	90.53	41.02
K0015-RR	45.90	16.04	K0026-RR	8.93	4.09
K0015-NU	216.75	160.31	K0026-UE	59.31	30.90
K0016-RR	15.30	9.65	K0027-RR	6.38	4.09
K0016-UE	103.43	76.08	K0027-UE	44.63	30.90
K0016-NU	137.70	101.44	K0027-NU	63.75	41.02
K0017-RR	6.38	4.50	K0028-UE	489.29	361.04
K0017-UE	44.63	33.82	K0028-RR	67.63	49.55
K0017-NU	58.65	45.09	K0028-NU	652.39	481.42

Code	Commercial	Medicare	Code	Commercial	Medicare
K0029-NU	59.67	43.89	K0040-RR	10.20	6.58
K0029-UE	45.08	32.93	K0041-UE	45.90	35.02
K0029-RR	5.30	4.37	K0041-NU	61.20	46.69
K0030	173.25	0.00	K0041-RR	6.38	4.68
K0031-RR	5.10	3.77	K0042-NU	42.08	32.14
K0031-UE	44.63	27.94	K0042-UE	31.88	24.10
K0031-NU	52.28	37.67	K0042-RR	3.83	3.20
K0032-RR	5.10	3.88	K0043-RR	2.55	1.72
K0032-UE	39.53	30.52	K0043-UE	16.58	12.93
K0032-NU	52.28	40.48	K0043-NU	25.50	17.23
K0033-RR	5.10	3.88	K0044-RR	2.55	1.47
K0033-NU	52.28	40.48	K0044-NU	19.13	14.68
K0033-UE	39.53	30.52	K0044-UE	14.03	11.01
K0034-NU	22.54	16.62	K0045-UE	51.00	37.47
K0034-RR	2.65	1.72	K0045-NU	67.58	49.95
K0034-UE	17.24	12.47	K0045-RR	6.38	5.15
K0035-UE	23.87	17.16	K0046-UE	16.58	12.93
K0035-NU	30.50	22.85	K0046-NU	25.50	17.23
K0035-RR	2.65	2.29	K0046-RR	2.55	1.72
K0036-RR	3.19	1.73	K0047-NU	91.80	67.48
K0036-UE	22.31	12.47	K0047-RR	8.93	6.77
K0036-NU	29.64	16.62	K0047-UE	70.13	50.60
K0037-UE	42.08	31.88	K0048-UE	133.88	80.94
K0037-NU	54.83	42.49	K0048-NU	167.66	103.61
K0037-RR	5.10	3.79	K0048-RR	19.13	11.66
K0038-NU	28.05	21.40	K0049-NU	38.25	26.82
K0038-UE	20.40	16.06	K0049-RR	3.83	2.69
K0038-RR	2.55	2.13	K0049-UE	29.33	20.10
K0039-NU	62.48	47.53	K0050-NU	39.53	28.68
K0039-RR	6.38	4.77	K0050-UE	31.88	21.52
K0039-UE	45.90	35.65	K0050-RR	3.83	2.86
K0040-NU	86.70	65.88	K0051-UE	48.45	34.80
K0040-UE	63.75	49.40	K0051-NU	63.75	46.42

Appendix 6

Code	Commercial	Medicare	Code	Commercial	Medicare
K0051-RR	6.38	4.66	K0062-RR	7.65	5.39
K0052-RR	14.03	8.15	K0063-RR	8.93	7.18
K0052-NU	144.08	81.56	K0063-NU	95.63	71.88
K0052-UE	115.26	61.16	K0063-UE	73.95	53.89
K0053-RR	11.48	8.99	K0064-RR	7.65	2.69
K0053-UE	102.00	67.51	K0064-NU	87.98	26.84
K0053-NU	127.50	90.01	K0064-UE	42.30	20.11
K0054-UE	90.53	69.23	K0065-UE	40.80	29.41
K0054-NU	119.85	92.32	K0065-RR	5.10	3.92
K0054-RR	11.48	9.23	K0065-NU	53.55	39.23
K0055-NU	130.05	83.90	K0066-NU	38.25	25.16
K0055-RR	15.30	8.39	K0066-RR	4.46	2.42
K0055-UE	102.00	62.94	K0066-UE	29.33	19.24
K0056-RR	15.30	8.39	K0067-NU	56.74	36.09
K0056-UE	102.00	62.94	K0067-UE	42.39	25.86
K0056-NU	130.05	83.90	K0067-RR	5.74	3.54
K0057-RR	19.13	10.96	K0068-UE	5.10	3.89
K0057-UE	114.75	82.17	K0068-NU	6.38	5.19
K0057-NU	159.38	109.58	K0069-UE	91.80	66.12
K0058-NU	71.40	53.26	K0069-NU	122.40	88.16
K0058-UE	54.83	39.94	K0070-UE	167.03	121.20
K0058-RR	6.38	5.33	K0070-NU	216.75	161.61
K0059-RR	3.83	2.79	K0071-UE	102.00	72.28
K0059-UE	29.33	20.99	K0071-NU	128.78	96.38
K0059-NU	39.53	27.98	K0072-NU	79.05	58.02
K0060-NU	34.43	24.48	K0072-UE	61.20	43.51
K0060-RR	3.83	2.45	K0073-UE	33.15	23.03
K0060-UE	26.78	18.35	K0073-RR	3.83	3.07
K0061-NU	47.18	34.73	K0073-NU	43.35	30.70
K0061-RR	5.10	3.48	K0074-NU	43.35	31.77
K0061-UE	36.98	26.07	K0074-RR	5.10	3.50
K0062-UE	54.83	40.36	K0074-UE	31.88	23.82
K0062-NU	73.95	53.84	K0075-UE	36.98	27.70

Code	Commercial	Medicare	Code	Commercial	Medicare
K0075-NU	48.45	36.91	K0091-UE	28.20	13.74
K0075-RR	5.74	4.16	K0092-RR	28.05	21.44
K0076-UE	22.95	16.92	K0092-NU	286.88	214.51
K0076-RR	3.51	2.27	K0092-UE	215.48	160.88
K0076-NU	29.33	22.54	K0093-RR	17.85	13.39
K0077-NU	71.40	51.92	K0093-NU	179.78	134.00
K0077-UE	52.28	38.93	K0093-UE	131.33	100.50
K0077-RR	7.01	5.19	K0094-UE	42.08	32.75
K0078-RR	1.15	0.84	K0094-NU	57.38	43.67
K0078-NU	12.75	8.47	K0094-RR	5.10	4.38
K0078-UE	8.61	6.34	K0095-RR	5.10	4.38
K0079-NU	71.60	52.51	K0095-UE	42.08	32.75
K0079-UE	23.87	26.23	K0095-NU	57.38	43.67
K0079-RR	7.96	5.48	K0096-UE	242.25	181.50
K0080-NU	186.97	138.35	K0096-NU	323.85	242.01
K0080-RR	19.89	14.68	K0096-RR	31.88	24.19
K0080-UE	141.88	104.54	K0097-NU	72.68	55.65
K0081-NU	49.73	35.89	K0097-RR	7.65	5.57
K0081-UE	39.53	26.91	K0097-UE	54.83	41.75
K0082	133.93	0.00	K0098-RR	2.55	2.39
K0083	167.08	0.00	K0098-UE	22.95	17.99
K0084	123.32	0.00	K0098-NU	30.60	24.01
K0085	222.77	0.00	K0099-NU	93.08	71.38
K0086	133.93	0.00	K0099-UE	70.13	53.54
K0087	133.93	0.00	K0099-RR	8.93	7.15
K0088	314.26	0.00	K0100-NU	114.75	78.01
K0089-NU	90.17	369.75	K0100-UE	89.25	59.05
K0089-UE	67.63	277.31	K0100-RR	14.03	7.84
K0090-NU	87.98	67.21	K0101-RR	45.90	38.50
K0090-UE	65.03	50.42	K0101-UE	483.23	0.00
K0090-RR	8.93	6.74	K0101-NU	652.80	0.00
K0091-RR	2.55	1.83	K0102-RR	5.10	3.83
K0091-NU	29.33	18.32	K0102-NU	49.73	38.25

Code	Commercial	Medicare	Code	Commercial	Medicare
K0102-UE	36.98	28.69	K0123	334.37	0.00
K0103-RR	6.63	4.95	K0137	3.85	2.13
K0103-NU	66.30	48.63	K0138	5.56	3.02
K0103-UE	45.90	35.61	K0139	3.83	3.22
K0104-RR	14.03	10.47	K0168	3.19	0.00
K0104-NU	136.43	104.81	K0169	2.23	0.00
K0104-UE	102.00	78.61	K0170	36.66	0.00
K0105-NU	114.75	87.72	K0171	11.16	0.00
K0105-UE	85.43	65.79	K0172	5.42	0.00
K0105-RR	11.48	8.76	K0173	13.07	0.00
K0106-RR	12.75	9.47	K0174	49.73	0.00
K0106-NU	123.68	94.54	K0175	28.05	0.00
K0106-UE	91.80	70.92	K0176	25.47	0.00
K0107-NU	119.85	91.72	K0177	4.46	0.00
K0107-RR	11.48	9.18	K0178	0.96	0.00
K0107-UE	89.25	68.79	K0179	5.42	0.00
K0108	0.00	0.00	K0180	2.23	0.00
K0109	0.00	0.00	K0181	8.61	0.00
K0112	314.93	235.36	K0182	0.64	0.34
K0113	191.25	143.56	K0183	94.99	0.00
K0114-NU	977.93	668.95	K0184	29.01	0.00
K0114-RR	99.45	66.91	K0185	47.18	0.00
K0114-UE	733.13	501.71	K0186	21.68	0.00
K0115-RR	99.45	76.72	K0187	48.45	0.00
K0115-UE	748.43	575.30	K0188	6.38	0.00
K0115-NU	998.33	767.04	K0189	18.17	0.00
K0116-NU	2084.63	1601.01	K0190	11.48	0.00
K0116-UE	1563.15	1200.77	K0191	38.89	0.00
K0116-RR	207.83	160.11	K0192	4.46	0.00
K0119	1.50	0.00	K0193	147.26	0.00
K0120	85.31	0.00	K0194	294.53	0.00
K0121	1.93	0.00	K0195	140.25	0.00
K0122	29.96	0.00	K0268	0.00	0.00

Code	Commercial	Medicare	Code	Commercial	Medicare
K0269	0.00	0.00	K0431	0.00	3.54
K0270	0.00	0.00	K0432	3.19	3.85
K0277	4.22	3.68	K0433	3.02	5.48
K0278	7.43	5.54	K0434	0.00	8.48
K0279	0.00	7.45	K0435	0.00	6.23
K0280	3.93	2.81	K0436	0.00	5.87
K0281	0.10	0.11	K0437	0.00	8.10
K0283	0.20	0.31	K0438	3.34	2.27
K0284	0.00	0.00	K0439	0.06	0.04
K0400	6.38	4.91	K0440	0.00	1549.67
K0401	0.00	0.00	K0441	0.00	1867.88
K0407	2.60	1.94	K0442	0.00	2098.73
K0408	3.83	4.36	K0443	0.00	2350.58
K0409	11.65	5.59	K0444	0.00	2602.42
K0410	2.23	1.91	K0445	0.00	1713.29
K0411	1.21	1.59	K0446	0.00	1678.97
K0412	2.40	0.00	K0447	0.00	860.48
K0415	0.00	0.00	K0448	0.00	0.00
K0416	0.00	0.00	K0449	0.00	18.13
K0417	0.00	0.00	K0450	0.00	0.00
K0418	7.15	0.00	K0451	7.33	0.00
K0419	0.00	15.15	K0452	0.00	0.00
K0420	0.00	41.98	K0455	0.00	0.00
K0421	0.00	3.79	K0456-RR	274.13	268.19
K0422	0.00	27.13	K0456-UE	2055.30	0.00
K0423	0.00	13.26	K0456-NU	2741.25	0.00
K0424	0.00	32.93	K0457-NU	155.55	133.15
K0425	0.00	4.07	K0457-RR	15.30	13.38
K0426	0.00	21.72	K0457-UE	116.66	99.86
K0427	0.00	24.88	K0458-UE	98.18	84.06
K0428	0.00	8.49	K0458-RR	12.75	11.22
K0429	4.40	4.50	K0458-NU	131.33	112.10
K0430	6.17	5.93	K0459-RR	22.95	19.70

Appendix 6

Code	Commercial	Medicare	Code	Commercial	Medicare
K0459-NU	230.78	196.93	K0532	0.00	0.00
K0459-UE	173.08	147.69	K0533	0.00	0.00
K0460	0.00	0.00	K0534	0.00	0.00
K0461	0.00	0.00	K0535	0.00	4.44
K0462	0.00	0.00	K0536	0.00	6.52
K0501	0.00	0.00	K0537	0.00	18.22
K0503	0.00	0.00	K0538-RR	0.00	0.00
K0504	0.00	0.00	K0539	0.00	0.00
K0505	0.00	0.00	K0540	0.00	0.00
K0506	0.00	0.00	L0100	637.82	477.51
K0507	0.00	0.00	L0110	159.06	119.15
K0508	0.00	0.00	L0120	7.27	22.01
K0509	0.00	0.00	L0130	180.73	135.31
K0511	0.45	0.00	L0140	70.76	53.09
K0512	0.00	0.00	L0150	30.36	89.63
K0513	0.00	0.00	L0160	149.18	129.89
K0514	41.59	0.00	L0170	714.32	534.87
K0515	0.00	0.00	L0172	140.57	105.29
K0516	0.00	0.00	L0174	304.73	227.83
K0518	0.00	0.00	L0180	153.00	307.31
K0519	0.00	0.00	L0190	548.89	410.84
K0520	0.00	0.00	L0200	572.16	428.29
K0521	0.00	0.00	L0210	49.09	36.73
K0522	0.00	0.00	L0220	135.79	101.58
K0523	0.00	0.00	L0300	192.53	144.15
K0524	0.00	0.00	L0310	364.65	273.40
K0525	0.00	0.00	L0315	291.34	218.10
K0526	0.00	0.00	L0317	395.25	295.88
K0527	0.26	0.00	L0320	136.34	309.87
K0528	0.26	0.00	L0330	507.77	380.17
K0529	0.00	2.42	L0340	723.24	541.44
K0530	0.00	0.00	L0350	1060.48	793.88
K0531	0.00	0.00	L0360	1569.84	1175.22

Code	Commercial	Medicare	Code	Commercial	Medicare
L0370	447.53	335.36	L0970	126.54	94.79
L0380	689.46	516.10	L0972	114.11	85.36
L0390	1577.49	1180.98	L0974	198.26	148.49
L0400	1717.74	1286.12	L0976	177.23	132.61
L0410	1968.60	1473.90	L0978	213.24	159.65
L0420	2088.45	1563.73	L0980	19.44	14.48
L0430	1484.42	1111.31	L0982	17.85	13.50
L0440	1241.21	929.16	L0984	66.30	49.65
L0500	150.45	112.47	L0999	0.00	0.00
L0510	304.73	228.60	L1000	2249.10	1683.83
L0515	202.73	151.79	L1010	74.27	55.66
L0520	133.88	341.76	L1020	95.63	71.69
L0530	459.00	343.60	L1025	138.02	103.42
L0540	148.16	370.07	L1030	70.44	52.76
L0550	1465.29	1096.99	L1040	86.38	64.70
L0560	1600.76	1198.49	L1050	92.12	69.05
L0565	1242.17	930.05	L1060	105.83	79.32
L0600	102.00	76.48	L1070	99.77	74.63
L0610	286.24	214.26	L1080	61.20	45.90
L0620	468.88	351.15	L1085	170.53	127.66
L0700	2239.54	1676.74	L1090	101.68	76.03
L0710	2313.49	1732.15	L1100	176.27	131.89
L0810	2857.59	2139.29	L1110	283.05	211.82
L0820	2393.18	1791.51	L1120	43.99	32.94
L0830	3473.74	2600.73	L1200	1735.59	1299.49
L0860	1349.59	1010.37	L1210	289.74	217.01
L0900	177.23	132.79	L1220	245.44	183.74
L0910	385.05	288.35	L1230	629.85	471.46
L0920	188.06	140.76	L1240	86.06	64.40
L0930	419.48	313.78	L1250	80.01	59.92
L0940	175.31	131.14	L1260	83.83	62.74
L0950	381.23	285.51	L1270	85.74	64.26
L0960	76.50	57.30	L1280	95.63	71.54

Code	Commercial	Medicare	Code	Commercial	Medicare
L1290	87.02	65.18	L1843	0.00	710.97
L1300	1850.34	1385.40	L1844	1412.70	1318.76
L1310	1904.21	1425.59	L1845	819.83	677.89
L1499	0.00	0.00	L1846	1106.06	880.55
L1500	2103.75	1575.37	L1847	0.00	455.74
L1510	1331.10	996.65	L1850	255.00	238.72
L1520	2527.37	1892.10	L1855	1217.31	911.38
L1600	142.80	106.88	L1858	1173.00	993.80
L1610	48.77	36.41	L1860	1188.62	889.96
L1620	148.54	111.12	L1870	1159.29	867.95
L1630	187.74	140.54	L1880	784.13	587.03
L1640	511.28	382.70	L1885	924.38	825.21
L1650	256.28	192.02	L1900	298.35	223.75
L1660	189.98	141.94	L1902	71.40	66.21
L1680	1349.91	1010.53	L1904	521.48	390.01
L1685	1317.08	986.52	L1906	91.16	99.74
L1686	1010.44	756.55	L1910	296.12	221.79
L1690	0.00	1532.26	L1920	387.60	289.94
L1700	1691.61	1266.53	L1930	262.01	196.20
L1710	1980.39	1482.63	L1940	547.93	410.17
L1720	1459.88	1092.88	L1945	1025.10	767.74
L1730	1253.64	938.68	L1950	825.24	617.76
L1750	218.03	163.18	L1960	613.91	459.72
L1755	1753.76	1313.10	L1970	788.27	590.16
L1800	52.28	55.17	L1980	406.73	304.38
L1810	97.54	81.68	L1990	493.74	369.70
L1815	91.16	80.35	L2000	1123.59	841.22
L1820	128.78	107.53	L2010	1024.14	766.85
L1825	29.33	45.60	L2020	1293.49	968.42
L1830	77.78	72.55	L2030	1122.00	840.19
L1832	612.00	504.24	L2035	70.13	138.13
L1834	782.85	643.81	L2036	2055.30	1538.76
L1840	910.35	762.59	L2037	1844.93	1381.40

Code	Commercial	Medicare	Code	Commercial	Medicare
L2038	1583.55	1185.78	L2240	92.76	69.36
L2039	0.00	1760.97	L2250	393.66	294.70
L2040	196.67	147.25	L2260	222.17	166.26
L2050	527.85	395.08	L2265	130.05	97.67
L2060	643.24	481.52	L2270	63.75	44.55
L2070	149.18	111.53	L2275	138.98	104.02
L2080	398.44	298.31	L2280	501.71	375.55
L2090	485.78	363.68	L2300	298.35	223.31
L2102	515.42	385.83	L2310	136.43	102.03
L2104	546.66	409.36	L2320	228.23	170.64
L2106	753.53	563.91	L2330	435.09	325.66
L2108	1099.05	886.15	L2335	251.81	188.42
L2112	516.69	386.95	L2340	495.02	370.68
L2114	642.92	481.40	L2350	987.17	739.02
L2116	650.25	590.44	L2360	57.38	42.91
L2122	908.44	680.21	L2370	284.33	212.91
L2124	1085.34	812.46	L2375	125.27	93.71
L2126	1215.08	993.14	L2380	136.43	102.10
L2128	1899.75	1422.15	L2385	148.54	111.09
L2132	893.78	669.04	L2390	121.13	90.78
L2134	1071.32	802.15	L2395	173.40	129.76
L2136	1310.06	980.82	L2397	124.63	93.22
L2180	129.73	97.13	L2405	56.42	69.08
L2182	101.68	76.02	L2415	204.00	96.25
L2184	137.38	102.74	L2425	201.77	113.58
L2186	166.71	124.86	L2430	0.00	113.58
L2188	331.82	248.40	L2435	191.25	137.26
L2190	96.90	72.43	L2492	112.84	84.58
L2192	394.93	295.72	L2500	256.28	261.65
L2200	52.59	39.43	L2510	804.53	602.44
L2210	74.59	55.74	L2520	510.32	382.07
L2220	90.84	67.92	L2525	1350.23	1011.00
L2230	85.11	63.64	L2526	758.63	568.07

Code	Commercial	Medicare	Code	Commercial	Medicare
L2530	260.42	194.87	L3000	251.18	0.00
L2540	468.24	350.64	L3001	147.90	0.00
L2550	318.11	238.19	L3002	122.40	0.00
L2570	527.53	395.04	L3003	150.45	0.00
L2580	514.14	384.91	L3010	195.08	0.00
L2600	227.59	170.33	L3020	247.35	0.00
L2610	269.03	201.42	L3030	247.35	0.00
L2620	295.80	221.75	L3040	43.99	0.00
L2622	339.79	254.34	L3050	40.80	0.00
L2624	366.88	274.64	L3060	79.05	0.00
L2627	1899.11	1421.79	L3070	24.23	0.00
L2628	1856.08	1389.53	L3080	9.88	0.00
L2630	274.44	205.37	L3090	15.30	0.00
L2640	372.30	278.72	L3100	25.50	0.00
L2650	132.92	99.53	L3140	73.95	0.00
L2660	206.55	154.58	L3150	61.84	0.00
L2670	189.02	141.48	L3160	19.13	0.00
L2680	173.40	129.79	L3170	32.51	0.00
L2750	93.08	69.33	L3201	73.31	0.00
L2755	0.00	103.52	L3202	72.04	0.00
L2760	67.26	50.39	L3203	70.13	0.00
L2770	68.53	51.21	L3204	70.13	0.00
L2780	75.23	56.13	L3206	72.99	0.00
L2785	35.06	26.29	L3207	74.27	0.00
L2795	94.35	70.47	L3208	38.89	0.00
L2800	118.58	88.47	L3209	55.14	0.00
L2810	86.70	64.77	L3211	58.65	0.00
L2820	102.00	72.02	L3212	81.92	0.00
L2830	103.91	77.92	L3213	98.81	0.00
L2840	48.45	36.23	L3214	105.19	0.00
L2850	68.53	51.35	L3215	133.88	0.00
L2860	0.00	0.00	L3216	161.93	0.00
L2999	0.00	0.00	L3217	175.63	0.00

Code	Commercial	Medicare	Code	Commercial	Medicare
L3218	31.88	0.00	L3440	54.83	0.00
L3219	150.45	0.00	L3450	44.63	0.00
L3221	180.41	0.00	L3455	18.70	0.00
L3222	199.22	0.00	L3460	32.19	0.00
L3223	44.63	0.00	L3465	22.95	0.00
L3224	0.00	48.77	L3470	56.10	0.00
L3225	0.00	56.11	L3480	38.25	0.00
L3230	234.60	0.00	L3485	25.50	0.00
L3250	456.45	0.00	L3500	28.05	0.00
L3251	62.79	0.00	L3510	26.14	0.00
L3252	249.90	0.00	L3520	42.71	0.00
L3253	62.48	0.00	L3530	12.75	0.00
L3254	0.00	0.00	L3540	47.18	0.00
L3255	0.00	0.00	L3550	7.65	0.00
L3257	45.26	0.00	L3560	10.20	0.00
L3260	25.50	0.00	L3570	42.08	0.00
L3265	27.73	0.00	L3580	62.48	0.00
L3300	31.88	0.00	L3590	48.45	0.00
L3310	63.75	0.00	L3595	14.03	0.00
L3320	168.94	0.00	L3600	79.05	0.00
L3330	273.27	0.00	L3610	127.50	0.00
L3332	19.13	0.00	L3620	79.05	0.00
L3334	18.81	0.00	L3630	96.90	0.00
L3340	45.90	0.00	L3640	31.88	0.00
L3350	29.01	0.00	L3649	0.00	0.00
L3360	21.68	0.00	L3650	64.39	48.13
L3370	26.14	0.00	L3660	110.93	83.42
L3380	44.94	0.00	L3670	122.40	91.78
L3390	62.48	0.00	L3675	0.00	126.55
L3400	59.93	0.00	L3700	75.23	56.65
L3410	101.36	0.00	L3710	133.88	100.33
L3420	32.51	0.00	L3720	708.90	530.83
L3430	81.60	0.00	L3730	977.29	731.61

Code	Commercial	Medicare	Code	Commercial	Medicare
L3740	1158.98	867.38	L3930	66.62	49.93
L3800	216.75	162.29	L3932	38.89	38.14
L3805	346.80	259.65	L3934	41.44	39.10
L3807	0.00	180.31	L3936	96.58	72.30
L3810	70.13	52.60	L3938	101.04	75.70
L3815	65.34	48.82	L3940	97.54	87.24
L3820	111.88	83.87	L3942	80.64	60.34
L3825	70.44	52.64	L3944	106.46	79.70
L3830	91.80	68.70	L3946	78.73	71.92
L3835	99.45	74.49	L3948	59.61	44.73
L3840	68.21	51.01	L3950	162.56	121.70
L3845	87.98	65.88	L3952	180.41	135.07
L3850	125.59	94.11	L3954	97.54	89.63
L3855	126.86	94.86	L3956	0.00	0.00
L3860	173.40	129.85	L3960	796.56	596.45
L3890	0.00	0.00	L3962	777.75	582.30
L3900	1402.82	1050.15	L3963	1807.95	1353.98
L3901	1741.97	1304.23	L3964	822.38	0.00
L3902	2640.53	1976.92	L3965	1313.25	0.00
L3904	3174.43	2376.67	L3966	1041.68	0.00
L3906	428.40	320.69	L3968	1154.19	0.00
L3907	550.80	412.26	L3969	842.78	0.00
L3908	51.00	48.63	L3970	325.44	0.00
L3910	253.41	304.42	L3972	303.45	0.00
L3912	97.54	76.97	L3974	187.43	0.00
L3914	78.41	69.57	L3980	335.01	250.90
L3916	137.70	103.08	L3982	404.81	302.97
L3918	85.11	63.61	L3984	373.26	279.34
L3920	106.14	79.48	L3985	633.68	474.35
L3922	96.90	79.36	L3986	607.54	454.90
L3924	115.71	86.53	L3995	35.38	26.54
L3926	100.73	75.35	L3999	0.00	0.00
L3928	45.58	47.24	L4000	1300.50	1057.49

Code	Commercial	Medicare	Code	Commercial	Medicare
L4010	743.33	556.61	L5200	3898.95	2918.93
L4020	954.02	714.36	L5210	2863.97	2144.11
L4030	559.41	418.74	L5220	3255.39	2437.17
L4040	452.31	338.54	L5230	4489.59	3361.34
L4045	363.38	272.06	L5250	6123.51	4584.57
L4050	457.41	342.40	L5270	6069.96	4544.41
L4055	295.80	221.71	L5280	6009.39	4498.96
L4060	351.90	263.58	L5300	3331.26	2494.02
L4070	311.74	233.40	L5310	4968.36	3719.79
L4080	112.20	83.89	L5320	4975.37	3724.90
L4090	100.09	74.89	L5330	6948.75	5202.47
L4100	115.39	86.51	L5340	7424.33	5558.69
L4110	94.03	70.33	L5400	1420.35	1063.44
L4130	549.53	411.48	L5410	493.11	369.18
L4205	0.00	0.00	L5420	1793.93	1343.08
L4210	0.00	0.00	L5430	592.88	444.63
L4350	72.68	74.14	L5450	480.68	359.99
L4360	247.35	229.65	L5460	643.56	481.81
L4370	209.10	156.57	L5500	1515.98	1134.83
L4380	85.43	89.08	L5505	2052.75	1536.85
L4392	19.13	18.61	L5510	1756.95	1286.40
L4394	17.85	13.58	L5520	1697.34	1270.66
L4396	144.08	132.74	L5530	2038.41	1526.18
L4398	97.58	61.11	L5535	2001.75	1498.40
L5000	596.38	446.44	L5540	2136.26	1599.28
L5010	1436.93	1075.73	L5560	2293.73	1717.34
L5020	2338.35	1751.07	L5570	2384.89	1785.43
L5050	2708.42	2027.81	L5580	2783.96	2084.36
L5060	3259.86	2440.49	L5585	3019.52	2260.73
L5100	2742.84	2053.61	L5590	2837.19	2124.11
L5105	4100.08	3069.56	L5595	4752.24	3557.80
L5150	4144.39	3102.91	L5600	5247.90	3928.86
L5160	4508.08	3374.97	L5610	2443.54	1829.38

Code	Commercial	Medicare	Code	Commercial	Medicare
L5611	1901.03	1423.63	L5654	391.43	293.03
L5613	2892.98	2165.42	L5655	322.58	234.37
L5614	4276.35	1339.71	L5656	437.33	327.76
L5616	1602.99	1200.06	L5658	429.68	321.28
L5617	614.55	447.06	L5660	680.85	509.40
L5618	331.50	248.49	L5661	717.83	537.71
L5620	327.68	245.65	L5662	623.48	467.12
L5622	427.76	320.33	L5663	813.45	608.87
L5624	429.68	321.24	L5664	784.13	586.61
L5626	562.59	421.29	L5665	604.35	452.43
L5628	569.93	426.62	L5666	82.88	61.86
L5629	374.85	280.81	L5667	1894.65	1418.74
L5630	529.76	396.55	L5668	118.58	89.23
L5631	518.93	388.23	L5669	1317.08	986.48
L5632	262.65	196.19	L5670	320.03	239.76
L5634	359.55	268.78	L5672	351.90	263.48
L5636	300.90	225.14	L5674	75.23	56.48
L5637	340.43	255.27	L5675	102.00	76.55
L5638	573.75	430.01	L5676	427.13	320.19
L5639	1323.45	990.66	L5677	581.40	435.66
L5640	754.80	565.00	L5678	47.18	35.08
L5642	731.85	547.45	L5680	359.55	268.94
L5643	1837.28	1375.27	L5682	738.23	552.59
L5644	697.43	521.89	L5684	57.38	42.52
L5645	942.23	705.01	L5686	59.93	45.14
L5646	646.43	484.13	L5688	72.68	53.97
L5647	938.40	702.86	L5690	116.03	86.46
L5648	776.48	581.74	L5692	156.83	117.41
L5649	2246.55	1682.30	L5694	214.20	160.30
L5650	576.30	431.36	L5695	192.53	144.10
L5651	1417.80	1061.12	L5696	218.03	163.49
L5652	515.10	385.23	L5697	94.35	70.93
L5653	687.23	514.25	L5698	123.68	92.17

Code	Commercial	Medicare	Code	Commercial	Medicare
L5699	220.58	164.75	L5840	2285.44	2994.85
L5700	3001.35	2419.76	L5845	3442.50	1423.01
L5701	4012.43	3004.33	L5846	4972.50	4331.17
L5702	4462.50	3838.90	L5850	116.03	113.03
L5704	555.90	465.25	L5855	312.38	272.88
L5705	1040.40	820.79	L5910	367.20	320.01
L5706	1012.99	805.26	L5920	643.88	468.82
L5707	1156.43	1093.04	L5925	332.78	296.89
L5710	371.43	317.80	L5930	3085.50	2689.40
L5711	610.29	461.37	L5940	571.20	443.21
L5712	456.45	380.74	L5950	912.77	687.45
L5714	457.73	369.59	L5960	1040.72	851.82
L5716	752.25	644.00	L5962	582.04	519.37
L5718	940.75	804.93	L5964	1075.46	827.51
L5722	1015.22	797.77	L5966	1385.93	1054.44
L5724	1785.00	1333.71	L5968	0.00	2885.05
L5726	2040.00	1537.08	L5970	238.43	179.46
L5728	2807.55	2102.51	L5972	410.55	311.41
L5780	1109.89	1011.63	L5974	274.13	205.91
L5785	612.00	459.07	L5975	0.00	368.07
L5790	865.09	635.33	L5976	660.45	494.84
L5795	1094.27	948.71	L5978	348.08	257.86
L5810	573.75	430.19	L5979	2700.45	2016.15
L5811	769.14	644.42	L5980	4217.70	3276.11
L5812	596.70	499.49	L5981	3274.20	2544.90
L5814	0.00	2948.53	L5982	682.13	510.81
L5816	692.33	751.44	L5984	621.24	503.36
L5818	943.50	848.54	L5985	260.10	225.62
L5822	1551.68	1504.67	L5986	747.15	559.92
L5824	1593.75	1355.04	L5987	0.00	5711.28
L5826	0.00	2494.89	L5988	0.00	1586.01
L5828	3327.75	2495.21	L5999	0.00	0.00
L5830	1946.93	1676.65	L6000	1404.41	1174.02

Code	Commercial	Medicare	Code	Commercial	Medicare
L6010	1466.89	1306.49	L6600	210.69	165.74
L6020	1499.72	1218.09	L6605	168.62	163.65
L6050	2227.74	1678.49	L6610	168.30	147.10
L6055	2828.27	2339.39	L6615	240.54	153.50
L6100	2270.78	1700.57	L6616	70.13	57.31
L6110	2412.30	1803.74	L6620	371.66	267.92
L6120	2575.50	2102.01	L6623	756.08	566.79
L6130	2549.36	2287.37	L6625	477.17	469.95
L6200	2794.80	2410.52	L6628	476.21	423.28
L6205	4056.41	3217.67	L6629	171.49	129.28
L6250	2996.25	2372.76	L6630	262.01	190.43
L6300	3968.12	3291.94	L6632	70.13	57.41
L6310	3576.38	2681.35	L6635	207.83	155.63
L6320	1804.44	1510.01	L6637	425.85	324.45
L6350	4462.50	3460.97	L6640	333.09	247.51
L6360	3243.60	2814.41	L6641	188.28	141.75
L6370	2215.95	1794.65	L6642	248.94	192.14
L6380	1262.25	1016.37	L6645	328.95	282.06
L6382	1702.13	1308.31	L6650	399.08	299.08
L6384	2316.68	1684.66	L6655	83.19	66.37
L6386	406.73	354.84	L6660	90.53	81.10
L6388	529.44	388.45	L6665	49.73	40.69
L6400	2284.16	2050.29	L6670	46.54	42.38
L6450	3243.92	2724.20	L6672	204.00	148.99
L6500	3169.65	2726.43	L6675	145.99	106.11
L6550	3769.54	3369.36	L6676	119.21	107.15
L6570	4512.54	3867.37	L6680	272.85	205.00
L6580	1893.38	1381.20	L6682	271.89	226.65
L6582	1622.44	1216.10	L6684	379.53	307.99
L6584	2433.98	1808.54	L6686	716.55	521.64
L6586	2005.89	1664.18	L6687	554.63	509.67
L6588	3375.56	2497.49	L6688	624.75	468.08
L6590	2689.61	2324.66	L6689	795.60	595.36

Code	Commercial	Medicare	Code	Commercial	Medicare
L6690	810.90	607.58	L6845	897.60	672.21
L6691	408.00	305.00	L6850	813.45	608.80
L6692	660.45	494.13	L6855	1034.03	774.33
L6693	0.00	2253.95	L6860	784.13	587.26
L6700	612.00	458.35	L6865	383.78	287.72
L6705	359.55	269.09	L6867	1133.48	848.89
L6710	406.73	304.96	L6868	283.05	211.85
L6715	404.18	302.92	L6870	280.50	210.01
L6720	1007.25	753.80	L6872	1111.80	832.18
L6725	487.05	364.94	L6873	552.08	413.34
L6730	776.79	564.63	L6875	916.73	686.78
L6735	351.90	263.28	L6880	595.43	445.55
L6740	459.00	343.26	L6890	200.18	150.29
L6745	419.48	314.07	L6895	659.18	493.40
L6750	414.38	310.45	L6900	1453.50	1334.64
L6755	413.10	309.57	L6905	1732.73	1297.30
L6765	432.23	323.43	L6910	1688.10	1263.84
L6770	416.93	311.78	L6915	738.23	553.15
L6775	493.43	369.43	L6920	0.00	5896.87
L6780	527.85	394.88	L6925	0.00	6807.85
L6790	532.95	399.26	L6930	0.00	5933.43
L6795	1461.15	1093.55	L6935	0.00	6935.29
L6800	1195.95	895.26	L6940	0.00	7752.42
L6805	401.63	300.63	L6945	0.00	9019.03
L6806	0.00	1284.03	L6950	0.00	8811.71
L6807	0.00	1164.35	L6955	0.00	10553.23
L6808	0.00	994.24	L6960	0.00	10643.72
L6809	437.33	327.85	L6965	0.00	12522.85
L6810	220.58	164.82	L6970	0.00	12887.15
L6825	1217.63	911.63	L6975	0.00	14120.23
L6830	1598.85	1196.55	L7010	0.00	3227.20
L6835	1392.30	1042.31	L7015	0.00	5128.25
L6840	967.73	724.11	L7020	0.00	3006.79

Code	Commercial	Medicare	Code	Commercial	Medicare
L7025	0.00	3034.30	L8110	24.86	0.00
L7030	0.00	4639.91	L8120	25.50	0.00
L7035	0.00	3107.47	L8130	38.25	0.00
L7040	0.00	2491.01	L8140	38.25	0.00
L7045	0.00	1428.18	L8150	33.15	0.00
L7170	0.00	5180.95	L8160	42.71	0.00
L7180	0.00	28864.46	L8170	42.71	0.00
L7185	0.00	5246.42	L8180	42.71	0.00
L7186	0.00	7815.87	L8190	172.13	0.00
L7190	0.00	6675.07	L8195	0.00	0.00
L7191	0.00	8167.13	L8200	172.13	0.00
L7260	0.00	1738.93	L8210	86.06	0.00
L7261	0.00	3165.53	L8220	25.50	0.00
L7266	0.00	874.82	L8230	26.78	0.00
L7272	0.00	1783.76	L8239	0.00	0.00
L7274	0.00	5075.00	L8300	98.49	74.53
L7360	267.75	200.93	L8310	156.83	117.67
L7362	295.80	221.38	L8320	62.48	47.24
L7364	470.48	352.10	L8330	58.65	43.63
L7366	633.68	474.28	L8400	19.13	13.91
L7499	0.00	0.00	L8410	24.23	18.30
L7500	0.00	0.00	L8415	25.50	18.94
L7510	0.00	0.00	L8417	0.00	59.68
L7520	0.00	0.00	L8420	22.95	17.18
L7900	376.13	425.78	L8430	26.78	19.56
L8000	43.35	32.26	L8435	19.13	18.58
L8010	71.40	53.59	L8440	49.73	36.95
L8015	0.00	47.69	L8460	79.05	58.89
L8020	237.15	177.26	L8465	57.38	43.10
L8030	372.30	278.76	L8470	7.65	5.90
L8035	0.00	2908.63	L8480	11.48	8.13
L8039	0.00	0.00	L8485	12.75	9.82
L8100	24.23	0.00	L8490	156.83	117.40

Code	Commercial	Medicare	Code	Commercial	Medicare
L8499	0.00	0.00	P9011	154.88	0.00
L8500	0.00	583.13	P9012	0.00	0.00
L8501	142.80	106.74	P9013	0.00	0.00
L8600	1235.16	551.76	P9016	0.00	0.00
L8603	0.00	348.43	P9017	0.00	0.00
L8610	0.00	517.18	P9018	0.00	0.00
L8612	0.00	537.26	P9019	0.00	0.00
L8613	0.00	227.21	P9020	0.00	0.00
L8614	0.00	15356.33	P9021	0.00	0.00
L8619	0.00	6591.54	P9022	0.00	0.00
L8630	0.00	297.69	P9023	0.00	0.00
L8641	0.00	309.29	P9603	0.00	0.00
L8642	0.00	250.87	P9604	8.51	0.00
L8658	0.00	269.68	P9612	56.17	0.00
L8670	0.00	442.66	P9615	0.00	0.00
L8699	0.00	0.00	Q0034	13.19	0.00
L9900	0.00	0.00	Q0035	21.28	25.63
M0064	62.97	22.70	Q0068	172.33	172.45
M0075	0.00	0.00	Q0081	76.59	0.00
M0076	0.00	0.00	Q0082	0.00	0.00
M0100	0.00	0.00	Q0083	141.27	0.00
M0300	0.00	0.00	Q0084	240.83	0.00
M0301	0.00	0.00	Q0085	0.00	0.00
M0302	0.00	0.00	Q0086	0.00	0.00
P2028	0.00	0.00	Q0091	0.00	31.49
P2029	0.00	0.00	Q0092	17.02	12.45
P2031	0.00	0.00	Q0111	17.02	5.90
P2033	0.00	0.00	Q0112	19.57	5.90
P2038	18.72	6.95	Q0113	0.00	7.47
P3000	23.83	7.15	Q0114	0.00	9.88
P3001	20.42	26.00	Q0115	0.00	13.68
P7001	45.95	0.00	Q0132	0.00	0.00
P9010	108.50	0.00	Q0136	20.42	0.00

Appendix 6

Code	Commercial	Medicare	Code	Commercial	Medicare
Q0144	47.33	0.00	Q1005	0.00	0.00
Q0156	260.41	0.00	Q9920	20.42	0.00
Q0157	127.65	0.00	Q9921	20.42	0.00
Q0160	1.72	0.00	Q9922	20.42	0.00
Q0161	2.06	0.00	Q9923	20.42	0.00
Q0163	0.09	0.00	Q9924	20.42	0.00
Q0164	0.92	0.00	Q9925	20.42	0.00
Q0165	1.36	0.00	Q9926	20.42	0.00
Q0166	72.76	0.00	Q9927	20.42	0.00
Q0167	5.55	0.00	Q9928	20.42	0.00
Q0168	10.86	0.00	Q9929	20.42	0.00
Q0169	0.44	0.00	Q9930	20.42	0.00
Q0170	0.19	0.00	Q9931	20.42	0.00
Q0171	0.12	0.00	Q9932	20.42	0.00
Q0172	0.48	0.00	Q9933	20.42	0.00
Q0173	0.65	0.00	Q9934	20.42	0.00
Q0174	0.92	0.00	Q9935	20.42	0.00
Q0175	0.97	0.00	Q9936	20.42	0.00
Q0176	1.09	0.00	Q9937	20.42	0.00
Q0177	0.29	0.00	Q9938	20.42	0.00
Q0178	0.27	0.00	Q9939	20.42	0.00
Q0179	38.92	0.00	Q9940	20.42	0.00
Q0180	112.33	0.00	R0070	86.80	0.00
Q0181	0.00	0.00	R0075	79.99	0.00
Q0183	0.00	0.00	R0076	78.29	0.00
Q0184	0.00	0.00	S0009	14.65	0.00
Q0185	0.00	0.00	S0010	357.42	0.00
Q0186	0.00	0.00	S0011	357.42	0.00
Q0187	0.00	0.00	S0012	114.07	0.00
Q1001	0.00	0.00	S0014	2.03	0.00
Q1002	0.00	0.00	S0016	28.53	0.00
Q1003	0.00	0.00	S0017	11.64	0.00
Q1004	0.00	0.00	S0020	0.00	0.00

Code	Commercial	Medicare	Code	Commercial	Medicare
S0021	0.00	0.00	S2054	0.00	0.00
S0023	2.06	0.00	S2055	0.00	0.00
S0024	24.51	0.00	S2109	0.00	0.00
S0028	5.41	0.00	S2190	0.00	0.00
S0029	190.62	0.00	S2204	0.00	0.00
S0030	35.50	0.00	S2205	0.00	0.00
S0032	6.57	0.00	S2206	0.00	0.00
S0034	44.93	0.00	S2207	0.00	0.00
S0039	27.95	0.00	S2208	0.00	0.00
S0040	0.00	0.00	S2209	0.00	0.00
S0071	3.74	0.00	S2210	0.00	0.00
S0072	74.51	0.00	S2300	0.00	0.00
S0073	11.51	0.00	S2350	0.00	0.00
S0074	10.14	0.00	S2351	0.00	0.00
S0077	16.54	0.00	S3645	0.00	0.00
S0078	91.91	0.00	S3650	0.00	0.00
S0080	168.07	0.00	S3652	0.00	0.00
S0081	0.00	0.00	S8035	0.00	0.00
S0090	12.53	0.00	S8040	0.00	0.00
S0096	0.00	0.00	S8048	0.00	0.00
S0097	281.66	0.00	S8049	0.00	0.00
S0098	0.00	0.00	S8060	0.00	0.00
S0601	0.00	0.00	S8092	0.00	0.00
S0605	0.00	0.00	S8095	0.00	0.00
S0610	0.00	0.00	S8096	0.00	0.00
S0612	0.00	0.00	S8110	0.00	0.00
S0620	0.00	0.00	S8200	0.00	0.00
S0621	0.00	0.00	S8205	0.00	0.00
S0800	0.00	0.00	S8260	0.00	0.00
S0810	0.00	0.00	S8300	0.00	0.00
S2050	0.00	0.00	S8950	0.00	0.00
S2052	0.00	0.00	S9001	0.00	0.00
S2053	0.00	0.00	S9022	0.00	0.00

Code	Commercial	Medicare	Code	Commercial	Medicare
S9023	0.00	0.00	S9991	0.00	0.00
S9024	0.00	0.00	S9992	0.00	0.00
S9033	0.00	0.00	S9994	0.00	0.00
S9055	0.00	0.00	S9996	0.00	0.00
S9056	0.00	0.00	S9999	0.00	0.00
S9075	0.00	0.00	V2020	78.36	55.40
S9085	0.00	0.00	V2025	0.00	0.00
S9090	0.00	0.00	V2100	75.66	34.60
S9122	0.00	0.00	V2101	52.01	36.47
S9123	0.00	0.00	V2102	75.32	51.31
S9124	0.00	0.00	V2103	50.66	30.05
S9125	0.00	0.00	V2104	64.17	33.29
S9126	0.00	0.00	V2105	51.34	36.23
S9127	0.00	0.00	V2106	49.99	40.21
S9128	0.00	0.00	V2107	54.04	38.24
S9129	0.00	0.00	V2108	55.39	39.59
S9140	0.00	0.00	V2109	62.15	43.81
S9141	0.00	0.00	V2110	60.80	43.23
S9455	0.00	0.00	V2111	63.50	45.07
S9460	0.00	0.00	V2112	70.25	49.19
S9465	0.00	0.00	V2113	78.36	55.44
S9470	0.00	0.00	V2114	85.11	60.06
S9472	0.00	0.00	V2115	102.68	65.36
S9473	0.00	0.00	V2116	82.41	58.10
S9474	0.00	0.00	V2117	116.86	67.56
S9475	0.00	0.00	V2118	91.87	64.80
S9480	0.00	0.00	V2199	0.00	0.00
S9485	0.00	0.00	V2200	103.35	45.30
S9524	0.00	0.00	V2201	70.25	49.37
S9527	0.00	0.00	V2202	82.41	58.10
S9528	0.00	0.00	V2203	64.85	45.70
S9543	0.00	0.00	V2204	64.85	47.77
S9990	0.00	0.00	V2205	78.36	51.66

Code	Commercial	Medicare	Code	Commercial	Medicare
V2206	78.36	55.50	V2317	149.96	106.39
V2207	78.36	50.49	V2318	183.74	129.62
V2208	75.66	52.99	V2319	62.15	43.88
V2209	81.06	57.05	V2320	64.85	46.30
V2210	89.17	62.92	V2399	0.00	0.00
V2211	91.87	65.26	V2410	112.13	79.23
V2212	106.73	67.38	V2430	145.91	95.48
V2213	83.76	68.07	V2499	0.00	0.00
V2214	122.94	73.99	V2500	129.70	71.82
V2215	106.73	75.10	V2501	174.28	109.39
V2216	114.84	81.33	V2502	143.21	134.76
V2217	109.43	76.87	V2503	175.63	124.12
V2218	107.74	89.37	V2510	143.21	98.05
V2219	55.39	39.35	V2511	208.05	140.87
V2220	44.58	31.91	V2512	235.07	166.45
V2299	0.00	0.00	V2513	205.69	139.75
V2300	139.15	57.67	V2520	125.64	92.15
V2301	108.08	67.97	V2521	226.97	160.44
V2302	116.19	72.46	V2522	221.56	156.14
V2303	85.79	56.74	V2523	174.28	133.06
V2304	83.76	59.37	V2530	243.18	197.07
V2305	97.27	68.80	V2531	306.00	432.63
V2306	99.97	70.83	V2599	0.00	0.00
V2307	95.92	67.07	V2600	0.00	0.00
V2308	86.46	70.29	V2610	0.00	0.00
V2309	93.89	76.57	V2615	0.00	0.00
V2310	111.12	75.66	V2623	1122.68	793.15
V2311	110.78	78.73	V2624	56.07	53.78
V2312	109.77	79.17	V2625	463.39	327.03
V2313	130.71	88.42	V2626	249.94	176.29
V2314	133.75	94.97	V2627	1550.95	1138.54
V2315	159.42	105.43	V2628	380.98	268.83
V2316	140.50	98.84	V2629	0.00	0.00

Code	Commercial	Medicare	Code	Commercial	Medicare
V2630	0.00	0.00	V5100	1816.08	0.00
V2631	0.00	0.00	V5110	409.35	0.00
V2632	0.00	0.00	V5120	1587.43	0.00
V2700	58.09	38.71	V5130	1688.75	0.00
V2710	78.36	56.66	V5140	1756.30	0.00
V2715	15.54	10.28	V5150	1875.19	0.00
V2718	35.13	25.23	V5160	490.08	0.00
V2730	27.02	18.63	V5170	1304.39	0.00
V2740	16.89	9.27	V5180	1103.77	0.00
V2741	13.17	8.89	V5190	1290.21	0.00
V2742	12.83	8.86	V5200	405.98	0.00
V2743	19.59	11.32	V5210	1417.20	0.00
V2744	20.27	14.50	V5220	1361.81	0.00
V2750	24.32	16.87	V5230	1407.74	0.00
V2755	20.27	14.68	V5240	420.16	0.00
V2760	22.97	14.16	V5299	0.00	0.00
V2770	25.67	17.24	V5336	0.00	0.00
V2780	17.56	11.07	V5362	0.00	0.00
V2781	0.00	0.00	V5363	0.00	0.00
V2785	0.00	0.00	V5364	0.00	0.00
V2799	0.00	0.00			
V5008	60.80	0.00			
V5010	79.71	0.00			
V5011	124.29	0.00			
V5014	149.96	0.00			
V5020	69.91	0.00			
V5030	1103.77	0.00			
V5040	838.97	0.00			
V5050	970.02	0.00			
V5060	810.60	0.00			
V5070	450.56	0.00			
V5080	1132.14	0.00			
V5090	402.60	0.00			

Appendix 7:

Companies Accepting HCPCS Level II Codes

Note: These companies have indicated that they process HCPCS Level II codes. Companies are listed in alphabetic order.

ACS CLAIMS SERVICE
PO BOX 257
MECHANICSBURG, PA 17055-0257
TEL: (717) 795-9997
FAX: (717) 795-8516

PO BOX 296
DALLAS, TX 75221-0296
TEL: (214) 826-8148
FAX: (214) 826-8239
TOLL FREE: (800) 456-9653

ADMINISTRATION SYSTEMS RESEARCH CORP
3033 ORCHARD VISTA DR SE
GRAND RAPIDS, MI 49546-7000
PO BOX 6392
GRAND RAPIDS, MI 49516-6392
TEL: (616) 957-1751
FAX: (616) 957-8986
TOLL FREE: (800) 968-2449

ADMINISTRATIVE CONSULTANTS, INC
92 BROOKSIDE RD
WATERBURY, CT 06708-1402
PO BOX 1471
WATERBURY, CT 06721-1471
TEL: (203) 756-8061
FAX: (203) 754-3941

ADMINISTRATIVE SERVICES
3301 E ROYALTON RD
BROADVIEW HEIGHTS, OH 44147-2886
TEL: (440) 526-2730
FAX: (440) 526-1608
TOLL FREE: (800) 634-8816

ADMINISTRATIVE SERVICES, INC
7990 SW 117TH AVE, STE 133
MIAMI, FL 33183-3815
PO BOX 839000
MIAMI, FL 33283-9000
TEL: (305) 595-4040
FAX: (305) 596-6820
TOLL FREE: (800) 749-1858

ADMIRAL INSURANCE CO
1255 CALDWELL RD
CHERRY HILL, NJ 08034-3220
PO BOX 5725
CHERRY HILL, NJ 08034-0524
TEL: (856) 429-9200
FAX: (856) 428-3390

ADVANCED BENEFIT ADMINISTRATORS
6420 SW MACADAM AVE, STE 380
PORTLAND, OR 97201-3519
TEL: (503) 245-3770
FAX: (503) 245-4122
TOLL FREE: (800) 443-6531

6420 SW MACADAM AVE, STE 380
PORTLAND, OR 97201-3519
TEL: (503) 245-3770
FAX: (503) 245-4122
TOLL FREE: (800) 443-6531

6420 SW MACADAM AVE, STE 380
PORTLAND, OR 97201-3519
TEL: (503) 245-3770
FAX: (503) 245-4122
TOLL FREE: (800) 443-6531

6420 SW MACADAM AVE, STE 380
PORTLAND, OR 97201-3519
TEL: (503) 245-3770
FAX: (503) 245-4122
TOLL FREE: (800) 443-6531

6420 SW MACADAM AVE, STE 380
PORTLAND, OR 97201-3519
TEL: (503) 245-3770
FAX: (503) 245-4122
TOLL FREE: (800) 443-6531

6420 SW MACADAM AVE, STE 380
PORTLAND, OR 97201-3519
TEL: (503) 245-3770
FAX: (503) 245-4122
TOLL FREE: (800) 443-6531

6420 SW MACADAM AVE, STE 380
PORTLAND, OR 97201-3519
TEL: (503) 245-3770
FAX: (503) 245-4122
TOLL FREE: (800) 443-6531

6420 SW MACADAM AVE, STE 380
PORTLAND, OR 97201-3519
TEL: (503) 245-3770
FAX: (503) 245-4122
TOLL FREE: (800) 443-6531

ADVANCED INSURANCE SERVICES & BENEFITS
600 JEFFERSON AVE
MEMPHIS, TN 38105-4912
PO BOX 19
MEMPHIS, TN 38101-0019
TEL: (901) 544-2344
FAX: (901) 544-2328
TOLL FREE: (800) 772-1352

AEARO CO
90 MECHANIC ST, STE 1
SOUTHBRIDGE, MA 01550-2562
TEL: (508) 764-5705
FAX: (508) 764-5648

AETNA HEALTH CARE

HOUSTON, TX
PO BOX 851
HOUSTON, TX 77001-0851
TEL: (713) 350-2150
FAX: (713) 663-0731
TOLL FREE: (800) 876-7778

AETNA LIFE & CASUALTY
151 FARMINGTON AVE
HARTFORD, CT 06156-0002
PO BOX 150417
HARTFORD, CT 06115-0417
TEL: (860) 273-0123
TOLL FREE: (800) 872-3862

AETNA / U.S. HEALTHCARE
1385 E SHAW
FRESNO, CA 93710-7901
TEL: (559) 241-1000
FAX: (559) 241-1226
TOLL FREE: (800) 756-7039

4630 WOODLANDS CORP BLVD
TAMPA, FL 33614
PO BOX 31450
TAMPA, FL 33631-3450
TEL: (813) 775-0000
TOLL FREE: (800) 344-3496

11675 GREAT OAKS WY
ALPHARETTA, GA 30022-2421
TEL: (770) 346-1000
TOLL FREE: (800) 323-9930

1000 MIDDLE ST
MIDDLETOWN, CT 06457-4621
TEL: (860) 636-8300
FAX: (860) 638-6599
TOLL FREE: (800) 445-3184

FRESNO, CA
PO BOX 24019
FRESNO, CA 93779-4019
TEL:
FAX: (781) 902-3871
TOLL FREE: (800) 323-9930

1425 UNION MEETING RD
BLUE BELL, PA 19422-1965
PO BOX 1125
BLUE BELL, PA 19422-0770
TEL: (215) 775-4800
TOLL FREE: (800) 872-3862

55 LANE RD, STE 1
FAIRFIELD, NJ 07004-1098
TEL: (973) 575-5600
FAX: (973) 244-3911
TOLL FREE: (800) 852-0629

7600A LEESBURG PIKE, STE 300
FALLS CHURCH, VA 22043-2000
TEL: (703) 903-7100
FAX: (703) 903-0316
TOLL FREE: (800) 231-8415

AETNA / U.S. HEALTHCARE CO
7601 ORA GLEN DR
GREENBELT, MD 20770-3647
TEL: (301) 441-1600
FAX: (301) 489-5284
TOLL FREE: (800) 635-3121
IN-STATE: (800) 635-3121

AIG CLAIM SERVICES, INC
PO BOX 25477
TAMPA, FL 33622-5477
TEL: (813) 218-3000
FAX: (813) 272-1122
IN-STATE: (800) 647-4767

120 S CENTRAL AVE, STE 300
CLAYTON, MO 63105-1705
TEL: (314) 719-4000
FAX: (314) 863-5939
TOLL FREE: (888) 745-7819

120 S CENTRAL AVE, STE 300
CLAYTON, MO 63105-1705
TEL: (314) 719-4000
FAX: (314) 863-5939
TOLL FREE: (888) 745-7819

625 LIBERTY AVE, STE 900
PITTSBURGH, PA 15222-3134
TEL: (412) 393-3960
FAX: (412) 393-0921
TOLL FREE: (800) 892-9779
IN-STATE: (800) 258-7152

70 PINE ST - 5TH FL
NEW YORK, NY 10270-0002
TEL: (212) 770-7000
FAX: (212) 943-1125

625 LIBERTY AVE, STE 900
PITTSBURGH, PA 15222-3134
TEL: (412) 393-3960
FAX: (412) 393-0921
TOLL FREE: (800) 892-9779
IN-STATE: (800) 258-7152

ALL RISK ADMINISTRATORS
PO BOX 66237
SAINT PETERSBURG BEACH, FL 33736-6237
TEL: (727) 367-3315
FAX: (727) 367-4510
TOLL FREE: (800) 338-4485

ALLIED GROUP INSURANCE CO
3820 109TH ST, DEPT 5573
DES MOINES, IA 50391-5573
TEL: (612) 896-1774
FAX: (612) 896-6640
TOLL FREE: (800) 862-6024

ALPHA DATA SYSTEMS, INC
1545 W MOCKINGBIRD LN, STE 6000
DALLAS, TX 75235-5060
TEL: (214) 638-1485
TOLL FREE: (800) 342-5248

ALTIUS
10421 S JORDAN GTWY, STE 400
SOUTH JORDAN, UT 84095-3918
PO BOX 95950
SOUTH JORDAN, UT 84095-0950
TEL: (801) 355-1234

AMERICAN COMMERCIAL LINES

1701 E MARKET ST
JEFFERSONVILLE, IN 47130-4717
PO BOX 610
JEFFERSONVILLE, IN 47131-0610
TEL: (812) 288-0100
FAX: (812) 288-1720
TOLL FREE: (800) 548-7689

AMERICAN FAMILY INSURANCE

PO BOX 59173
MINNEAPOLIS, MN 55459-0173
TEL: (612) 933-4446
FAX: (612) 933-7268
TOLL FREE: (800) 374-1111

AMERICAN HEALTH CARE PROVIDERS, INC

4601 SAUK TRL, STE 1
RICHTON PARK, IL 60471-1274
PO BOX 7000
RICHTON PARK, IL 60471-7000
TEL: (708) 503-5000
FAX: (708) 503-5001
TOLL FREE: (800) 242-7460

4601 SAUK TRL, STE 1
RICHTON PARK, IL 60471-1274
PO BOX 7000
RICHTON PARK, IL 60471-7000
TEL: (708) 503-5000
FAX: (708) 503-5001
TOLL FREE: (800) 242-7460

4601 SAUK TRL, STE 1
RICHTON PARK, IL 60471-1274
PO BOX 7000
RICHTON PARK, IL 60471-7000
TEL: (708) 503-5000
FAX: (708) 503-5001
TOLL FREE: (800) 242-7460

AMERICAN HERITAGE LIFE INSURANCE CO

1776 AMERICAN HERITAGE LIFE DR
JACKSONVILLE, FL 32224-6688
TEL: (904) 992-1776
FAX: (904) 992-2695
TOLL FREE: (800) 535-8086

AMERICAN LIFE INSURANCE CO

208 S LA SALLE ST, STE 2070
CHICAGO, IL 60604-1189
TEL: (312) 372-5722
FAX: (312) 372-5727

AMERICAN MEDICAL & LIFE INSURANCE CO

35 N BROADWAY
HICKSVILLE, NY 11801-4236
TEL: (516) 822-8700
FAX: (516) 931-1010
TOLL FREE: (800) 822-0004

AMERICAN MINING INSURANCE CO, INC

3490 INDEPENDENCE DR
BIRMINGHAM, AL 35209-5604
PO BOX 660988
BIRMINGHAM, AL 35266-0988
TEL: (205) 870-3535
FAX: (205) 823-6177
TOLL FREE: (800) 448-5621

3490 INDEPENDENCE DR
BIRMINGHAM, AL 35209-5604
PO BOX 660988
BIRMINGHAM, AL 35266-0988
TEL: (205) 870-3535
FAX: (205) 823-6177
TOLL FREE: (800) 448-5621

3490 INDEPENDENCE DR
BIRMINGHAM, AL 35209-5604
PO BOX 660988
BIRMINGHAM, AL 35266-0988
TEL: (205) 870-3535
FAX: (205) 823-6177
TOLL FREE: (800) 448-5621

3490 INDEPENDENCE DR
BIRMINGHAM, AL 35209-5604
PO BOX 660988
BIRMINGHAM, AL 35266-0988
TEL: (205) 870-3535
FAX: (205) 823-6177
TOLL FREE: (800) 448-5621

3490 INDEPENDENCE DR
BIRMINGHAM, AL 35209-5604
PO BOX 660988
BIRMINGHAM, AL 35266-0988
TEL: (205) 870-3535
FAX: (205) 823-6177
TOLL FREE: (800) 448-5621

3490 INDEPENDENCE DR
BIRMINGHAM, AL 35209-5604
PO BOX 660988
BIRMINGHAM, AL 35266-0988
TEL: (205) 870-3535
FAX: (205) 823-6177
TOLL FREE: (800) 448-5621

3490 INDEPENDENCE DR
BIRMINGHAM, AL 35209-5604
PO BOX 660988
BIRMINGHAM, AL 35266-0988
TEL: (205) 870-3535
FAX: (205) 823-6177
TOLL FREE: (800) 448-5621

3490 INDEPENDENCE DR
BIRMINGHAM, AL 35209-5604
PO BOX 660988
BIRMINGHAM, AL 35266-0988
TEL: (205) 870-3535
FAX: (205) 823-6177
TOLL FREE: (800) 448-5621

3490 INDEPENDENCE DR
BIRMINGHAM, AL 35209-5604
PO BOX 660988
BIRMINGHAM, AL 35266-0988
TEL: (205) 870-3535
FAX: (205) 823-6177
TOLL FREE: (800) 448-5621

AMERICAN NATIONAL INSURANCE CO

ONE MOODY PLZ, FL 18
GALVESTON, TX 77550-7960
PO BOX 1520
GALVESTON, TX 77553-1520
TEL: (409) 763-4661
FAX: (409) 766-6694
TOLL FREE: (800) 899-6805

AMERICAN PIONEER LIFE

411 N BAYLEN ST
PENSACOLA, FL 32501-3901
PO BOX 130
PENSACOLA, FL 32591-0130
TEL: (850) 469-8220
FAX: (850) 433-1186
TOLL FREE: (800) 999-2224

AMERICAN POSTAL WORKERS UNION HEALTH PLAN

12345 NEW COLUMBIA PIKE
SILVER SPRING, MD 20904
PO BOX 967-0967
SILVER SPRING, MD 20910
TEL: (301) 622-1700
FAX: (301) 622-6074
TOLL FREE: (800) 222-2798
IN-STATE: (800) 222-2798

AMERICAN REPUBLIC INSURANCE CO

601 6TH AVE
DES MOINES, IA 50309-1605
PO BOX 1
DES MOINES, IA 50334-0001
TEL: (515) 245-2000
FAX: (515) 245-4282
TOLL FREE: (800) 247-2190

AMERICAN RESOURCES INSURANCE CO

1111 HILLCREST RD
MOBILE, AL 36695-3952
PO BOX 91149
MOBILE, AL 36691-1149
TEL: (334) 639-0985
FAX: (334) 633-2944
TOLL FREE: (800) 826-6570

AMERICAN SERVICE LIFE INSURANCE CO

9151 GRAPEVINE HWY
NORTH RICHLAND HILLS, TX
   76180-5605
PO BOX 982017
NORTH RICHLAND HILLS, TX
   76182-8017
FAX: (817) 255-8101
TOLL FREE: (800) 733-8880
IN-STATE: (800) 733-1110

AMERICAN TRUST ADMINISTRATORS, INC

7101 COLLEGE BLVD, STE 1505
SHAWNEE MISSION, KS 66210-
   2082
PO BOX 87
SHAWNEE MISSION, KS 66201-
   0087
TEL: (913) 451-4900
FAX: (913) 451-0598
TOLL FREE: (800) 843-4121

AMERICAN UNION LIFE INSURANCE CO

303 E WASHINGTON ST
BLOOMINGTON, IL 61701-4040
PO BOX 2814
BLOOMINGTON, IL 61702-2814
TEL: (309) 829-1061
FAX: (309) 827-0303

303 E WASHINGTON ST
BLOOMINGTON, IL 61701-4040
PO BOX 2814
BLOOMINGTON, IL 61702-2814
TEL: (309) 829-1061
FAX: (309) 827-0303

303 E WASHINGTON ST
BLOOMINGTON, IL 61701-4040
PO BOX 2814
BLOOMINGTON, IL 61702-2814
TEL: (309) 829-1061
FAX: (309) 827-0303

AMERIHEALTH HMO, INC

PHILADELPHIA, PA
PO BOX 41574
PHILADELPHIA, PA 19101-1574
TEL: (302) 652-6500
FAX: (302) 777-6444
TOLL FREE: (800) 444-6282

PHILADELPHIA, PA
PO BOX 41574
PHILADELPHIA, PA 19101-1574
TEL: (302) 652-6500
FAX: (302) 777-6444
TOLL FREE: (800) 444-6282

PHILADELPHIA, PA
PO BOX 41574
PHILADELPHIA, PA 19101-1574
TEL: (302) 652-6500
FAX: (302) 777-6444
TOLL FREE: (800) 444-6282

AMWAY CORP

7575 E FULTON ST E
ADA, MI 49355-0001
TEL: (616) 787-6000
FAX: (616) 787-6177
TOLL FREE: (800) 528-5748

7575 E FULTON ST E
ADA, MI 49355-0001
TEL: (616) 787-6000
FAX: (616) 787-6177
TOLL FREE: (800) 528-5748

7575 E FULTON ST E
ADA, MI 49355-0001
TEL: (616) 787-6000
FAX: (616) 787-6177
TOLL FREE: (800) 528-5748

7575 E FULTON ST E
ADA, MI 49355-0001
TEL: (616) 787-6000
FAX: (616) 787-6177
TOLL FREE: (800) 528-5748

7575 E FULTON ST E
ADA, MI 49355-0001
TEL: (616) 787-6000
FAX: (616) 787-6177
TOLL FREE: (800) 528-5748

7575 E FULTON ST E
ADA, MI 49355-0001
TEL: (616) 787-6000
FAX: (616) 787-6177
TOLL FREE: (800) 528-5748

7575 E FULTON ST E
ADA, MI 49355-0001
TEL: (616) 787-6000
FAX: (616) 787-6177
TOLL FREE: (800) 528-5748

7575 E FULTON ST E
ADA, MI 49355-0001
TEL: (616) 787-6000
FAX: (616) 787-6177
TOLL FREE: (800) 528-5748

7575 E FULTON ST E
ADA, MI 49355-0001
TEL: (616) 787-6000
FAX: (616) 787-6177
TOLL FREE: (800) 528-5748

7575 E FULTON ST E
ADA, MI 49355-0001
TEL: (616) 787-6000
FAX: (616) 787-6177
TOLL FREE: (800) 528-5748

7575 E FULTON ST E
ADA, MI 49355-0001
TEL: (616) 787-6000
FAX: (616) 787-6177
TOLL FREE: (800) 528-5748

7575 E FULTON ST E
ADA, MI 49355-0001
TEL: (616) 787-6000
FAX: (616) 787-6177
TOLL FREE: (800) 528-5748

7575 E FULTON ST E
ADA, MI 49355-0001
TEL: (616) 787-6000
FAX: (616) 787-6177
TOLL FREE: (800) 528-5748

7575 E FULTON ST E
ADA, MI 49355-0001
TEL: (616) 787-6000
FAX: (616) 787-6177
TOLL FREE: (800) 528-5748

7575 E FULTON ST E
ADA, MI 49355-0001
TEL: (616) 787-6000
FAX: (616) 787-6177
TOLL FREE: (800) 528-5748

7575 E FULTON ST E
ADA, MI 49355-0001
TEL: (616) 787-6000
FAX: (616) 787-6177
TOLL FREE: (800) 528-5748

ANTHEM BLUE CROSS - BLUE SHIELD
2400 MARKET ST
YOUNGSTOWN, OH 44507-1426
PO BOX 0701
YOUNGSTOWN, OH 44507-0701
TEL: (330) 492-2151
TOLL FREE: (800) 442-1832

ANTHEM BLUE CROSS - BLUE SHIELD OF CONNECTICUT
370 BASSETT RD
NORTH HAVEN, CT 06473-4202
PO BOX 533
NORTH HAVEN, CT 06473-0533
TEL: (203) 239-4911
FAX: (203) 985-7834
TOLL FREE: (800) 922-4670

AON SELECT
110 GIBRALTAR RD, STE 116
HORSHAM, PA 19044-2371
TEL: (215) 443-0404
FAX: (215) 443-0435

ARIZONA PHYSICIANS, IPA, INC
3141 N 3RD AVE
PHOENIX, AZ 85013-4345
TEL: (602) 274-6102
FAX: (602) 664-5466
IN-STATE: (800) 348-4058

ARIZONA PUBLIC SERVICE CO
STA 8482
PHOENIX, AZ 85004
PO BOX 53970
PHOENIX, AZ 85072-3970
TEL: (602) 250-3578
FAX: (602) 250-2453

ARKANSAS BEST CORP
3801 OLD GREENWOOD RD
FORT SMITH, AR 72903-5937
PO BOX 10048
FORT SMITH, AR 72917-0048
TEL: (501) 785-6178
FAX: (501) 785-6011

ARTHUR J. GALLAGAR & CO
2345 GRAND BLVD, STE 800
KANSAS CITY, MO 64108-2671
PO BOX 419115
KANSAS CITY, MO 64141-6115
TEL: (816) 421-7788
FAX: (816) 472-5517
TOLL FREE: (800) 279-7500

ASH GROVE CEMENT CO
8900 INDIAN CREEK PKY, STE 600
OVERLAND PARK, KS 66210-1518
PO BOX 25900
OVERLAND PARK, KS 66225-5900
TEL: (913) 451-8900
FAX: (913) 451-8324
TOLL FREE: (800) 545-1822

ASSOCIATED ADMINISTRATORS, INC
2929 NW 31ST AVE
PORTLAND, OR 97210-1799
PO BOX 5096
PORTLAND, OR 97208-5096
TEL: (503) 223-3185
FAX: (503) 727-7444
TOLL FREE: (800) 888-9603

ASSOCIATION PLAN ADMINISTRATORS, INC
2858 W MARKET ST, STE N
AKRON, OH 44333-4035
PO BOX 5427
AKRON, OH 44334-0427
TEL: (330) 867-9050
FAX: (330) 867-7029
TOLL FREE: (800) 624-2564

ASSOCIATION & SOCIETY INSURANCE CORP
11300 ROCKVILLE PIKE, STE 500
ROCKVILLE, MD 20852-3008
PO BOX 2510
ROCKVILLE, MD 20847-2510
TEL: (301) 816-0045
FAX: (301) 816-1125
TOLL FREE: (800) 638-2610

ASSUMPTION MUTUAL LIFE INSURANCE CO
770 MAIN ST
MONCTON, NB E1C-8L1
PO BOX 160
MONCTON, NB E1C-8L1
TEL: (506) 853-6040
FAX: (506) 853-5459
TOLL FREE: (800) 455-7337

770 MAIN ST
MONCTON, NB E1C-8L1
PO BOX 160
MONCTON, NB E1C-8L1
TEL: (506) 853-6040
FAX: (506) 853-5459
TOLL FREE: (800) 455-7337

770 MAIN ST
MONCTON, NB E1C-8L1
PO BOX 160
MONCTON, NB E1C-8L1
TEL: (506) 853-6040
FAX: (506) 853-5459
TOLL FREE: (800) 455-7337

770 MAIN ST
MONCTON, NB E1C-8L1
PO BOX 160
MONCTON, NB E1C-8L1
TEL: (506) 853-6040
FAX: (506) 853-5459
TOLL FREE: (800) 455-7337

770 MAIN ST
MONCTON, NB E1C-8L1
PO BOX 160
MONCTON, NB E1C-8L1
TEL: (506) 853-6040
FAX: (506) 853-5459
TOLL FREE: (800) 455-7337

770 MAIN ST
MONCTON, NB E1C-8L1
PO BOX 160
MONCTON, NB E1C-8L1
TEL: (506) 853-6040
FAX: (506) 853-5459
TOLL FREE: (800) 455-7337

770 MAIN ST
MONCTON, NB E1C-8L1
PO BOX 160
MONCTON, NB E1C-8L1
TEL: (506) 853-6040
FAX: (506) 853-5459
TOLL FREE: (800) 455-7337

770 MAIN ST
MONCTON, NB E1C-8L1
PO BOX 160
MONCTON, NB E1C-8L1
TEL: (506) 853-6040
FAX: (506) 853-5459
TOLL FREE: (800) 455-7337

770 MAIN ST
MONCTON, NB E1C-8L1
PO BOX 160
MONCTON, NB E1C-8L1
TEL: (506) 853-6040
FAX: (506) 853-5459
TOLL FREE: (800) 455-7337

770 MAIN ST
MONCTON, NB E1C-8L1
PO BOX 160
MONCTON, NB E1C-8L1
TEL: (506) 853-6040
FAX: (506) 853-5459
TOLL FREE: (800) 455-7337

ATLANTIC MUTUAL / CENTENNIAL INSURANCE CO
628 HEBORN AVE- BLDG 2
GLASTONBURY, CT 06033-6510
PO BOX 6510
GLASTONBURY, CT 06033-6510
TEL: (860) 657-9966
FAX: (860) 657-7962
TOLL FREE: (800) 289-2299

628 HEBORN AVE- BLDG 2
GLASTONBURY, CT 06033-6510
PO BOX 6510
GLASTONBURY, CT 06033-6510
TEL: (860) 657-9966
FAX: (860) 657-7962
TOLL FREE: (800) 289-2299

628 HEBORN AVE- BLDG 2
GLASTONBURY, CT 06033-6510
PO BOX 6510
GLASTONBURY, CT 06033-6510
TEL: (860) 657-9966
FAX: (860) 657-7962
TOLL FREE: (800) 289-2299

628 HEBORN AVE- BLDG 2
GLASTONBURY, CT 06033-6510
PO BOX 6510
GLASTONBURY, CT 06033-6510
TEL: (860) 657-9966
FAX: (860) 657-7962
TOLL FREE: (800) 289-2299

AUTOMOBILE MECHANICS LOCAL NO 701
500 W PLAINFIELD RD, STE 100
COUNTRYSIDE, IL 60525-3582
TEL: (708) 482-0110
FAX: (708) 482-9140
TOLL FREE: (800) 704-6270

AUTOMOTIVE PETROLEUM & ALLIED
300 S GRAND AVE, STE 232
SAINT LOUIS, MO 63103-2430
TEL: (314) 531-3052
FAX: (314) 531-5285

BABB, INC
850 RIDGE AVE
PITTSBURGH, PA 15212-6095
TEL: (412) 237-2020
FAX: (412) 322-1756
TOLL FREE: (800) 245-6102
IN-STATE: (800) 892-1015

BASHAS' SUPERMARKETS
22402 S BASHA RD
CHANDLER, AZ 85248-4908
PO BOX 488
CHANDLER, AZ 85244-0488
TEL: (480) 895-9350
TOLL FREE: (800) 755-7292

BELLSOUTH ADMINISTRATORS
CORPORATE TWO - 5615
   CORPORATE BLVD
METAIRIE, LA 70808-2568
PO BOX 8570
METAIRIE, LA 70011-8570
TEL: (504) 849-1459
FAX: (504) 849-1347
TOLL FREE: (800) 366-2475

BENEFIT ADMINISTRATORS, INC
1111 S GLENSTONE, STE 2-203
SPRINGFIELD, MO 65804-0300
PO BOX 10868
SPRINGFIELD, MO 65808-0868
TEL: (417) 866-8913
FAX: (417) 866-2103
TOLL FREE: (800) 375-8913

BENEFIT CLAIMS PAYERS, INC
1717 W NORTHERN AVE, STE
   200
PHOENIX, AZ 85021-5478
PO BOX 37400
PHOENIX, AZ 85069-7400
TEL: (602) 861-6868
FAX: (602) 861-6878
TOLL FREE: (800) 266-6868

BENEFIT COORDINATORS CORP
111 RYAN CT
PITTSBURGH, PA 15205-1310
TEL: (412) 276-1111
FAX: (412) 276-6650
TOLL FREE: (800) 685-6100

BENEFIT MANAGEMENT, INC
628 W BROADWAY ST, STE 100
NORTH LITTLE ROCK, AR 72201-4120
PO BOX 5989
NORTH LITTLE ROCK, AR 72119-5989
TEL: (501) 375-5500
FAX: (501) 375-4718

BENEFIT PLAN ADMINISTRATORS, INC
101 S JEFFERSON ST
ROANOKE, VA 24011-1322
PO BOX 11746
ROANOKE, VA 24022-1746
TEL: (540) 345-2721
FAX: (540) 342-0282
TOLL FREE: (800) 277-8973

101 S JEFFERSON ST
ROANOKE, VA 24011-1322
PO BOX 11746
ROANOKE, VA 24022-1746
TEL: (540) 345-2721
FAX: (540) 342-0282
TOLL FREE: (800) 277-8973

101 S JEFFERSON ST
ROANOKE, VA 24011-1322
PO BOX 11746
ROANOKE, VA 24022-1746
TEL: (540) 345-2721
FAX: (540) 342-0282
TOLL FREE: (800) 277-8973

101 S JEFFERSON ST
ROANOKE, VA 24011-1322
PO BOX 11746
ROANOKE, VA 24022-1746
TEL: (540) 345-2721
FAX: (540) 342-0282
TOLL FREE: (800) 277-8973

101 S JEFFERSON ST
ROANOKE, VA 24011-1322
PO BOX 11746
ROANOKE, VA 24022-1746
TEL: (540) 345-2721
FAX: (540) 342-0282
TOLL FREE: (800) 277-8973

101 S JEFFERSON ST
ROANOKE, VA 24011-1322
PO BOX 11746
ROANOKE, VA 24022-1746
TEL: (540) 345-2721
FAX: (540) 342-0282
TOLL FREE: (800) 277-8973

101 S JEFFERSON ST
ROANOKE, VA 24011-1322
PO BOX 11746
ROANOKE, VA 24022-1746
TEL: (540) 345-2721
FAX: (540) 342-0282
TOLL FREE: (800) 277-8973

BENEFIT PLANNERS, INC
2111 WEST AVE
SAN ANTONIO, TX 78201-2822
PO BOX 690450
SAN ANTONIO, TX 78269-0450
TEL: (210) 699-1872
FAX: (210) 697-3108
TOLL FREE: (800) 292-5386

194 S MAIN ST
BOERNE, TX 78006-2399
TEL: (210) 699-1872
FAX: (210) 697-3108
TOLL FREE: (800) 292-5386

BENEFIT & RISK MANAGEMENT SERVICES
3610 AMERICAN RIVER DR, STE 100
SACRAMENTO, CA 95864-5999
TEL: (916) 974-2626
FAX: (916) 974-2653
TOLL FREE: (800) 959-4767

BENICORP INSURANCE CO
7702 WOODLAND DR, STE 200
INDIANAPOLIS, IN 46278-1717
PO BOX 68917
INDIANAPOLIS, IN 46268-0917
TEL: (317) 290-1205
FAX: (317) 216-7877
TOLL FREE: (800) 837-1205

BERWANGER OVERMYER ASSOCIATES
2245 N BANK DR
COLUMBUS, OH 43220-5438
PO BOX 20945
COLUMBUS, OH 43220-0945
TEL: (614) 457-7000
FAX: (614) 457-1507
TOLL FREE: (800) 837-0503
IN-STATE: (800) 837-0503

BLUE CROSS - BLUE SHIELD
450 RIVERCHASE PKY E
BIRMINGHAM, AL 35244-2858
PO BOX 995
BIRMINGHAM, AL 35298-0995
TEL: (205) 988-2100
FAX: (205) 988-2949

2444 W LAS PALMARITAS DR
PHOENIX, AZ 85021-4883
PO BOX 2924
PHOENIX, AZ 85062-2924
TEL: (602) 864-4400
FAX: (602) 864-4242
TOLL FREE: (800) 232-2345

26 CORPORATE HILL DR
LITTLE ROCK, AR 72205-4538
PO BOX 2181
LITTLE ROCK, AR 72203-2181
TEL: (501) 228-8600
FAX: (501) 228-8716
TOLL FREE: (800) 605-8301

237 MILLSAP RD, STE 1
FAYETTEVILLE, AR 72703-6252
TEL: (501) 527-2310
FAX: (501) 527-2323
TOLL FREE: (888) 847-1900

3501 OLD GREENWOOD RD, STE 5
FORT SMITH, AR 72903-5975
TEL: (501) 648-1635
FAX: (501) 648-6322
TOLL FREE: (800) 299-4060

100 GREENWOOD AVE, STE C
HOT SPRINGS, AR 71913-4441
TEL: (501) 620-2620
FAX: (501) 620-2650
TOLL FREE: (800) 588-5733

901 ARKANSAS BLVD
TEXARKANA, AR 71854-2201
TEL: (870) 773-2584
FAX: (870) 779-9138
TOLL FREE: (800) 470-9621

1920 N COLLEGE AVE
EL DORADO, AR 71730-3251
TEL: (870) 862-5461
FAX: (870) 862-4472
TOLL FREE: (800) 843-1329

1800 W 73RD ST
PINE BLUFF, AR 71603-8328
TEL: (870) 536-1223
FAX: (870) 543-2915
TOLL FREE: (800) 236-0369

1110 W B ST, STE 6
RUSSELLVILLE, AR 72801-3506
TEL: (501) 968-4713
FAX: (501) 968-7799
TOLL FREE: (800) 462-8917

105 E MATTHEWS AVE, STE B
JONESBORO, AR 72401-3127
TEL: (870) 935-4871
FAX: (870) 974-5713
TOLL FREE: (800) 299-4124

21555 OXNARD ST
WOODLAND HILLS, CA 91367-4943
PO BOX 4239
WOODLAND HILLS, CA 91365-4239
TEL: (818) 703-2345
FAX: (818) 703-2848
TOLL FREE: (800) 999-3643

700 BROADWAY
DENVER, CO 80203-3440
PO BOX 173690
DENVER, CO 80217-3690
TEL: (303) 831-2131
TOLL FREE: (800) 433-5447

ONE BRANDYWINE GTWY
WILMINGTON, DE 19801-1173
PO BOX 1991
WILMINGTON, DE 19899-1991
TEL: (302) 421-3000
FAX: (302) 421-2089
TOLL FREE: (800) 633-2563
IN-STATE: (800) 292-7865

532 RIVERSIDE AVE
JACKSONVILLE, FL 32202-4918
PO BOX 1798
JACKSONVILLE, FL 32231-1798
TEL: (904) 791-6111
FAX: (904) 791-8738

2357 WARM SPRINGS RD
COLUMBUS, GA 31904-5668
PO BOX 9907
COLUMBUS, GA 31908-9907
TEL: (706) 571-5371
FAX: (706) 571-5487
TOLL FREE: (800) 241-7475

3350 PEACHTREE RD NE
ATLANTA, GA 30326-1048
PO BOX 4445
ATLANTA, GA 30302-4445
TEL: (404) 842-8000
FAX: (404) 842-8010
TOLL FREE: (800) 441-2273

818 KEEAUMOKU ST
HONOLULU, HI 96814-2365
PO BOX 860
HONOLULU, HI 96808-0860
TEL: (808) 948-5110
FAX: (808) 948-6555
IN-STATE: (800) 790-4672

670 PONAHAWAI ST, STE 121
HILO, HI 96720-2660
TEL: (808) 935-5441
FAX: (808) 935-5444

75-166 KALANI ST, STE 202
KAILUA-KONA, HI 96740-1857
TEL: (808) 329-5291
FAX: (808) 329-5293

4366 KUKUI GROVE ST, STE 103
LIHUE, HI 96766-2006
TEL: (808) 245-3393
FAX: (808) 245-3596

33 LONO AVE, STE 350
KAHULUI, HI 96732-1608
TEL: (808) 871-6295
FAX: (808) 871-7429

220 VIRGINIA AVE
INDIANAPOLIS, IN 46204-3632
TEL: (317) 287-7778
TOLL FREE: (800) 331-1476

1201 ZENITH DR
SIOUX CITY, IA 51103-5216
PO BOX 1677
SIOUX CITY, IA 51102-1677
TEL: (712) 277-3081
FAX: (712) 279-8450
TOLL FREE: (800) 245-6105

1133 SW TOPEKA BLVD
TOPEKA, KS 66629-0001
PO BOX 239
TOPEKA, KS 66601-0239
TEL: (785) 291-4180
FAX: (785) 291-8465
TOLL FREE: (800) 432-3990
IN-STATE: (800) 234-0495

1133 SW TOPEKA AVE
TOPEKA, KS 66629-0001
PO BOX 3518
TOPEKA, KS 66601-3518
TEL: (785) 291-4010
FAX: (785) 291-8848
TOLL FREE: (800) 332-0028

9901 LINN STATION RD
LOUISVILLE, KY 40223-3838
PO BOX 37690
LOUISVILLE, KY 40233-7690
TEL: (502) 423-2011
FAX: (502) 423-2627
TOLL FREE: (800) 880-2583

9901 LINN STATION RD
LOUISVILLE, KY 40233-3838
PO BOX 37180
LOUISVILLE, KY 40233-7180
TEL: (513) 872-8100
FAX: (513) 872-8174
TOLL FREE: (800) 442-1832

TWO GANNETT DR
SOUTH PORTLAND, ME 04106-6909
TEL: (207) 822-8282
FAX: (207) 822-7375
TOLL FREE: (800) 482-0966
IN-STATE: (800) 822-6011

611 CASCADE W PKY SE
GRAND RAPIDS, MI 49546-2107
PO BOX 894
GRAND RAPIDS, MI 49518-0894
TEL: (616) 957-5057
FAX: (616) 957-3476
TOLL FREE: (800) 968-2583

25925 TELEGRAPH RD
SOUTHFIELD, MI 48034-2518
PO BOX 5097
SOUTHFIELD, MI 48086-5097
TEL: (248) 354-7450
FAX: (248) 799-6972
TOLL FREE: (800) 637-2227
IN-STATE: (800) 821-6886

600 E LAFAYETTE BLVD
DETROIT, MI 48226-2998
PO BOX 2888
DETROIT, MI 48231-2888
TEL: (313) 225-8000
FAX: (313) 225-6239
TOLL FREE: (800) 637-2227

PO BOX 64179
SAINT PAUL, MN 55164-0179
TEL: (651) 662-8501
FAX: (651) 456-1004
TOLL FREE: (800) 382-2000

620 NORTH ST, STE 200
JACKSON, MS 39202-3140
PO BOX 1043
JACKSON, MS 39215-1043
TEL: (601) 932-3704
FAX: (601) 939-7035
TOLL FREE: (800) 222-8046
IN-STATE: (800) 222-8046

560 N PARK AVE
HELENA, MT 59601-2702
TEL: (406) 791-4000
FAX: (406) 727-9355
TOLL FREE: (800) 447-7828

404 FULLER AVE
HELENA, MT 59601-5092
PO BOX 4309
HELENA, MT 59604-4309
TEL: (406) 444-8200
FAX: (406) 442-6946
TOLL FREE: (800) 447-7828

7261 MERCY RD
OMAHA, NE 68180-0001
PO BOX 3248
OMAHA, NE 68180-3248
TEL: (402) 390-1820
FAX: (402) 392-2141
TOLL FREE: (800) 642-8980

1811 W 2ND ST, STE 105
GRAND ISLAND, NE 68803-5400
TEL: (308) 381-6130
TOLL FREE: (800) 373-9109

1233 LINCOLN MALL
LINCOLN, NE 68508-2847
TEL: (402) 458-4800
TOLL FREE: (800) 562-6394

3000 GOFFS FALLS RD
MANCHESTER, NH 03111-0001
TEL: (603) 695-7000
FAX: (603) 695-7304
TOLL FREE: (800) 225-2666

3 PENN PLZ E
NEWARK, NJ 07105-2200
PO BOX 247, DEPT V
NEWARK, NJ 07101-0247
TEL: (973) 466-4000
TOLL FREE: (800) 355-2583

PO BOX 27630
ALBUQUERQUE, NM 87125-
  7630
TEL: (505) 291-3500
FAX: (505) 291-3541
TOLL FREE: (800) 835-8699

622 3RD AVE
NEW YORK, NY 10017-6707
PO BOX 345
NEW YORK, NY 10150-0341
TEL: (212) 476-1000
TOLL FREE: (800) 261-5962

12 RHOADS DR- UTICA
  BUSINESS PARK
UTICA, NY 13502-6398
TEL: (315) 798-4200
FAX: (315) 792-9752
TOLL FREE: (800) 765-5226

165 COURT ST
ROCHESTER, NY 14647-0001
TEL: (716) 454-1700
FAX: (716) 238-4400
TOLL FREE: (800) 847-1200

800 S DUKE ST
DURHAM, NC 27701-3902
PO BOX 2291
DURHAM, NC 27702-2291
TEL: (919) 489-7431
FAX: (919) 765-4837
TOLL FREE: (800) 222-2783
IN-STATE: (800) 222-5028

4510 13TH AVE SW
FARGO, ND 58121-0001
TEL: (701) 282-1100
FAX: (701) 277-2005
TOLL FREE: (800) 874-2656
IN-STATE: (800) 342-4718

1351 WILLIAM HOWARD TAFT
  RD
CINCINNATI, OH 45206-1775
PO BOX 37180
CINCINNATI, OH 45222-0180
TEL: (513) 872-8100
FAX: (513) 872-8174
TOLL FREE: (800) 442-1832

6740 N HIGH ST
WORTHINGTON, OH 43085-
  7500
PO BOX 425
WORTHINGTON, OH 43085-
  0425
TEL: (614) 438-3500
FAX: (513) 872-8174
TOLL FREE: (800) 467-4663

9901 LINN STATION RD
LOUISVILLE, KY 40233-3838
PO BOX 37180
LOUISVILLE, KY 40233-7180
TEL: (513) 872-8100
FAX: (513) 872-8174
TOLL FREE: (800) 442-1832

1215 S BOULDER AVE, RM 205
TULSA, OK 74119-2800
PO BOX 3283
TULSA, OK 74102-3283
TEL: (918) 560-3500
TOLL FREE: (800) 942-5837

1215 S BOULDER AVE, RM 205
TULSA, OK 74119-2800
PO BOX 21128
TULSA, OK 74121-1128
TEL: (405) 841-9777
FAX: (405) 841-9629
TOLL FREE: (800) 722-5675

400 COUNTRY CLUB RD, STE 120
EUGENE, OR 97401-6041
TEL: (541) 342-3317
TOLL FREE: (800) 228-0978

1221 W HAMILTON ST
ALLENTOWN, PA 18102-4370
TEL: (610) 820-2700
FAX: (610) 820-2663
TOLL FREE: (800) 958-5558

PO BOX 363628
SAN JUAN, PR 00936-3628
TEL: (787) 749-4949
FAX: (787) 749-4190

444 WESTMINSTER ST
PROVIDENCE, RI 02903-3279
TEL: (401) 459-1000
FAX: (401) 351-2050
TOLL FREE: (800) 637-3718

I-20 E AT ALPINE RD
COLUMBIA, SC 29219-0001
TEL: (803) 788-3860
FAX: (803) 736-3420
TOLL FREE: (800) 868-2500
IN-STATE: (800) 288-2227

85 N DANNY THOMAS BLVD
MEMPHIS, TN 38103-2398
PO BOX 98
MEMPHIS, TN 38101-0098
TEL: (901) 544-2111
FAX: (901) 544-2440
TOLL FREE: (800) 222-7212

901 S CENTRAL EXPY
RICHARDSON, TX 75080-7399
PO BOX 655730
RICHARDSON, TX 75080
TEL: (972) 766-6900
FAX: (972) 766-6060
TOLL FREE: (800) 521-2227

4150 PINNACLE, STE 203
EL PASO, TX 79902-1035
TEL: (915) 496-6600
FAX: (915) 496-6719
TOLL FREE: (888) 585-6799

2890 COTTONWOOD PKY
SALT LAKE CITY, UT 84121-7035
PO BOX 30270
SALT LAKE CITY, UT 84130-0270
TEL: (801) 333-2000
FAX: (801) 333-6523
TOLL FREE: (800) 624-6519

4723 HARRISON BLVD, STE 101
OGDEN, UT 84403-4399
TEL: (801) 476-9140
FAX: (801) 476-9138
TOLL FREE: (800) 638-0050

363 N UNIVERSITY AVE, STE 101
PROVO, UT 84601-8421
TEL: (801) 375-2090
TOLL FREE: (800) 624-6519

249 E TABERNACLE ST, STE 102
SAINT GEORGE, UT 84770-2951
TEL: (435) 673-0111
TOLL FREE: (800) 662-0876

PO BOX 186
MONTPELIER, VT 05601-0186
TEL: (802) 223-6131
FAX: (802) 223-1077
TOLL FREE: (800) 457-6648
IN-STATE: (800) 247-2583

2015 STAPLES MAIL RD
RICHMOND, VA 23230-2521
PO BOX 27401
RICHMOND, VA 23279-7401
TEL: (804) 354-7000
FAX: (804) 354-7600
TOLL FREE: (800) 451-1527

1800 NINTH AVE
SEATTLE, WA 98101-1322
PO BOX 21267
SEATTLE, WA 98111-3267
TEL: (206) 464-3600
FAX: (206) 389-5669
TOLL FREE: (800) 732-9326
IN-STATE: (800) 322-1737

7600 EVERGREEN WY
EVERETT, WA 98203-6413
TEL: (425) 348-8160
FAX: (425) 348-8167
TOLL FREE: (800) 328-7273
IN-STATE: (800) 548-8385

1101 S BOONE ST
ABERDEEN, WA 98520-6736
TEL: (360) 532-9320

1501 MARKET ST
TACOMA, WA 98402-3326
TEL: (253) 597-6500

401 W MICHIGAN ST
MILWAUKEE, WI 53203-2896
PO BOX 2025
MILWAUKEE, WI 53201-2025
TEL: (414) 226-5000
FAX: (414) 226-5040
TOLL FREE: (800) 558-1584

2270 EASTRIDGE CTR
EAU CLAIRE, WI 54701-3409
TEL: (715) 836-1200
TOLL FREE: (800) 848-3308

BLUE CROSS - BLUE SHIELD
823 MAIN ST
STEVENS POINT, WI 54481-2621
TEL: (715) 345-1500

BLUE CROSS - BLUE SHIELD
145 S PIONEER RD
FOND DU LAC, WI 54935-3871
TEL: (414) 923-4141
TOLL FREE: (800) 822-7442

BLUE CROSS - BLUE SHIELD
19 W MAIN ST
EVANSVILLE, WI 53536-2106
TEL: (608) 882-4317
TOLL FREE: (800) 535-7011

BLUE CROSS - BLUE SHIELD
PO BOX 2266
CHEYENNE, WY 82003-2266
TEL: (307) 634-1393
FAX: (307) 778-8582
TOLL FREE: (800) 442-2376
IN-STATE: (800) 442-2376

BLUE CROSS - BLUE SHIELD OF ILLINOIS
75 EXECUTIVE DR, STE 300
AURORA, IL 60504-7947
PO BOX 2037
AURORA, IL 60507-2037
TEL: (630) 978-7878
FAX: (630) 978-8460
TOLL FREE: (800) 538-8833

BLUE CROSS - BLUE SHIELD OF NEBRASKA
2401 S 73RD ST, STE 2
OMAHA, NE 68124-2307
PO BOX 241739
OMAHA, NE 68124-5739
TEL: (402) 392-2800
FAX: (402) 392-2761
TOLL FREE: (800) 843-2373

BLUE CROSS OF CALIFORNIA
40 NE ST
WOODLAND, CA 95695-3130
PO BOX 769028
WOODLAND, CA 95776-9028
TEL: (916) 636-2100
FAX: (916) 636-2314
TOLL FREE: (800) 999-3643

40 NE ST
WOODLAND, CA 95695-3130
PO BOX 769028
WOODLAND, CA 95776-9028
TEL: (916) 636-2100
FAX: (916) 636-2314
TOLL FREE: (800) 999-3643

BLUE RIDGE ADMINISTRATORS
1650 STATE FARM BLVD
CHARLOTTESVILLE, VA 22911-8609
PO BOX 1067
CHARLOTTESVILLE, VA 22902-1067
TEL: (804) 977-0000
FAX: (804) 979-1047
TOLL FREE: (800) 677-1867

BLUE SHIELD OF CALIFORNIA
129 N GUILD AVE
CHICO, CA 95240-0843
PO BOX 272530
CHICO, CA 95927-2530
TEL: (209) 367-2800
TOLL FREE: (800) 444-2595
IN-STATE: (800) 633-0337

129 N GUILD AVE
CHICO, CA 95240-0843
PO BOX 272560
CHICO, CA 95927-2560
TEL: (209) 367-2800
TOLL FREE: (800) 334-9894
IN-STATE: (800) 633-0337

129 N GUILD AVE
CHICO, CA 95240-0843
PO BOX 272550
CHICO, CA 95927-2550
TEL: (209) 367-2800
TOLL FREE: (800) 444-1409
IN-STATE: (800) 633-0337

129 N GUILD AVE
CHICO, CA 95240-0843
PO BOX 272510
CHICO, CA 95927-2510
TEL: (209) 367-2800
TOLL FREE: (800) 824-8839
IN-STATE: (800) 633-0337

40 N EAST ST
WOODLAND, CA 95776-5900
PO BOX 769028
WOODLAND, CA 95776-9028
TOLL FREE: (800) 688-0327

129 N GUILD AVE
CHICO, CA 95240-0843
PO BOX 272570
CHICO, CA 95927-2570
TEL: (209) 367-2800
TOLL FREE: (800) 241-4896
IN-STATE: (800) 633-0337

PO BOX 1505
RED BLUFF, CA 96080-1505
TOLL FREE: (800) 622-0632

BLUE SHIELD OF NORTHEASTERN NEW YORK
187 WOLF RD
ALBANY, NY 12205-1158
PO BOX 15013
ALBANY, NY 12212-5013
TEL: (518) 453-5700
TOLL FREE: (800) 888-1238

BOON-CHAPMAN
7600 CHEVY CHASE DR, STE 300
AUSTIN, TX 78752-1566
PO BOX 9201
AUSTIN, TX 78766-9201
TEL: (512) 454-2681
FAX: (512) 459-1552
TOLL FREE: (800) 252-9653

BPS INC
145 N CHURCH ST, STE 300, BTC-80
SPARTANBURG, SC 29306-5163
PO BOX 1227
SPARTANBURG, SC 29304-1227
TEL: (864) 585-4338
FAX: (864) 573-7709
TOLL FREE: (800) 868-7526

BROKERAGE CONCEPTS, INC
651 ALLENDALE RD
KING OF PRUSSIA, PA 19406-1467
PO BOX 60608
KING OF PRUSSIA, PA 19406-0608
TEL: (610) 337-2600
FAX: (610) 491-4992
TOLL FREE: (800) 220-2600

BROKERAGE SERVICES, INC
11200 LOOMAS BLVD NE
ALBUQUERQUE, NM 87112-5580
PO BOX 11020
ALBUQUERQUE, NM 87192-0020
TEL: (505) 292-5533
FAX: (505) 293-7725
TOLL FREE: (800) 274-5533

BUFFALO ROCK CO, INC
103 OXMOOR RD
BIRMINGHAM, AL 35209-5915
PO BOX 10048
BIRMINGHAM, AL 35202-0048
TEL: (205) 942-3435
FAX: (205) 940-7768

103 OXMOOR RD
BIRMINGHAM, AL 35209-5915
PO BOX 10048
BIRMINGHAM, AL 35202-0048
TEL: (205) 942-3435
FAX: (205) 940-7768

103 OXMOOR RD
BIRMINGHAM, AL 35209-5915
PO BOX 10048
BIRMINGHAM, AL 35202-0048
TEL: (205) 942-3435
FAX: (205) 940-7768

BUNZL DISTRIBUTION USA, INC
701 EMERSON RD, STE 500
SAINT LOUIS, MO 63141-6754
PO BOX 419111
SAINT LOUIS, MO 63141-9111
TEL: (314) 997-5959
FAX: (314) 997-0247

BUSINESS ADMINISTRATORS & CONSULTANTS, INC
6331 E LIVINGSTON AVE
REYNOLDSBURG, OH 43068-2756
PO BOX 107
REYNOLDSBURG, OH 43068-0107
TEL: (614) 863-8780
FAX: (614) 863-9137
TOLL FREE: (800) 521-2654

C & O EMPLOYEES' HOSPITAL ASSOCIATION
511 MAIN ST, 2ND FL
CLIFTON FORGE, VA 24422-1166
TEL: (540) 862-5728
FAX: (540) 862-3552

511 MAIN ST, 2ND FL
CLIFTON FORGE, VA 24422-1166
TEL: (540) 862-5728
FAX: (540) 862-3552

511 MAIN ST, 2ND FL
CLIFTON FORGE, VA 24422-1166
TEL: (540) 862-5728
FAX: (540) 862-3552

511 MAIN ST, 2ND FL
CLIFTON FORGE, VA 24422-1166
TEL: (540) 862-5728
FAX: (540) 862-3552

511 MAIN ST, 2ND FL
CLIFTON FORGE, VA 24422-1166
TEL: (540) 862-5728
FAX: (540) 862-3552

511 MAIN ST, 2ND FL
CLIFTON FORGE, VA 24422-1166
TEL: (540) 862-5728
FAX: (540) 862-3552

CAHABA GOVERNMENT BENEFIT ADMINISTRATORS
PO BOX 830140
BIRMINGHAM, AL 35283-0140
TEL: (205) 985-0191
FAX: (205) 981-4965
TOLL FREE: (800) 292-8855

CALIFORNIA MOTOR CAR DEALERS ASSOCIATION
420 CULVER BLVD
PLAYA DEL REY, CA 90293-7706
TEL: (310) 306-6232
FAX: (310) 822-6733
TOLL FREE: (800) 445-8290
IN-STATE: (800) 262-6232

CAM ADMINISTRATIVE SERVICES, INC
25800 NORTHWESTERN HWY, STE 700
SOUTHFIELD, MI 48075-8410
PO BOX 5131
SOUTHFIELD, MI 48086-5131
TEL: (248) 827-1050
FAX: (248) 827-2112
TOLL FREE: (800) 732-8906

CAPITAL DISTRICT PHYSICIANS' HEALTH PLAN, INC
17 COLUMBIA CIR
ALBANY, NY 12203-5190
TEL: (518) 862-3700
FAX: (518) 452-0003
TOLL FREE: (800) 777-CARE

CAPITAL HEALTH PLAN
2140 CENTERVILLE PL
TALLAHASSEE, FL 32308-4418
PO BOX 15349
TALLAHASSEE, FL 32317-5349
TEL: (850) 383-3377
FAX: (850) 383-3441
TOLL FREE: (800) 390-1434

CAPITOL BLUE CROSS
2500 ELMERTON AVE
HARRISBURG, PA 17110-9764
TEL: (717) 541-7000
FAX: (717) 541-6072
TOLL FREE: (800) 958-5558

CARE AMERICA HEALTH PLANS
6300 CANOGA AVE
WOODLAND HILLS, CA 91367-2580
PO BOX 946
WOODLAND HILLS, CA 91365-0946
TEL: (818) 228-5050
FAX: (818) 228-5103
TOLL FREE: (800) 827-2273

CARE CHOICES HEALTH PLANS
522 4TH ST, STE 250
SIOUX CITY, IA 51101-1748
TEL: (712) 252-2344
FAX: (712) 294-7018
TOLL FREE: (800) 535-6252

CAREMARK MEDICAL & DENTAL PLAN
2211 SANDERS RD
NORTHBROOK, IL 60062-6126
TEL: (847) 559-4700
FAX: (847) 559-3905

CARETON HEALTH CARE
PO BOX 22987
KNOXVILLE, TN 37933-0987
TEL: (865) 470-7470
FAX: (423) 778-4620
TOLL FREE: (800) 976-7747

CARILION HEALTH PLANS
110 W CAMPBELL AVE SW
ROANOKE, VA 24011-1220
PO BOX 1531
ROANOKE, VA 24007-1531
TEL: (540) 857-5262
FAX: (540) 343-0748

CARITEN HEALTHCARE
1021 W OAKLAND AVE, STE 300
JOHNSON CITY, TN 37604-2192
TEL: (423) 952-3180
FAX: (423) 952-3188

CARNEGIE-MELLON UNIVERSITY
143 N CRAIG ST
PITTSBURGH, PA 15213-1555
TEL: (412) 268-4747
FAX: (412) 268-1524

CAROLINA BENEFIT ADMINISTRATORS

291 S PINE ST
SPARTANBURG, SC 29302-2626
PO BOX 3257
SPARTANBURG, SC 29304-3257
TEL: (864) 573-6937
FAX: (864) 582-2265
TOLL FREE: (800) 476-2295

CARPENTERS COMBINED FUNDS

495 MANSFIELD AVE- 1ST FL
PITTSBURGH, PA 15205-4376
TEL: (412) 922-5330
FAX: (412) 922-3420
IN-STATE: (800) 242-2539

CELTIC LIFE INSURANCE CO

200 S WACKER DR, STE 900
CHICAGO, IL 60606-5849
PO BOX 06410
CHICAGO, IL 60606-0410
TEL: (312) 332-5401
TOLL FREE: (800) 477-7870

CEMARA ADMINISTRATORS INC

3450 N ROCK RD, STE 605
WICHITA, KS 67226-1356
PO BOX 8902
WICHITA, KS 67208-0902
TEL: (316) 631-3939
FAX: (316) 631-3788
TOLL FREE: (800) 285-1551

CEMETERY WORKERS WELFARE FUND

2409 38TH AVE
LONG ISLAND CITY, NY 11101-3512
TEL: (718) 729-7400
FAX: (718) 729-0253

CENTRAL DATA SERVICES, INC

503 MARTINDALE ST, 5TH FL
PITTSBURGH, PA 15212-5746
TEL: (412) 321-6172
FAX: (412) 237-1444

CENTRAL ILLINOIS CARPENTERS

2400 N MAIN ST, STE 100
EAST PEORIA, IL 61611-1735
TEL: (309) 699-7200
FAX: (309) 699-7032

CENTRAL PENNSYLVANIA TEAMSTERS HEALTH & WELFARE FUND

1055 SPRING ST
READING, PA 19610-1747
PO BOX 15224
READING, PA 19612-5224
TEL: (610) 320-5500
FAX: (610) 320-9209
TOLL FREE: (800) 331-0420
IN-STATE: (800) 422-8330

CENTURY FURNITURE

401 11TH ST NW
HICKORY, NC 28601-4750
PO BOX 608
HICKORY, NC 28603-0608
TEL: (828) 328-1851
FAX: (828) 328-2176

CHAMPUS

PO BOX 7031
CAMDEN, SC 29020-7031
TEL: (843) 665-7822
TOLL FREE: (800) 403-3950

PO BOX 870001
SURFSIDE BEACH, SC 29587-0001
TEL: (843) 650-6100
TOLL FREE: (800) 930-2929

PO BOX 870026
SURFSIDE BEACH, SC 29587-8726
TEL: (843) 650-6100
TOLL FREE: (800) 225-4816

PO BOX 7031
CAMDEN, SC 29020-7031
TEL: (843) 665-7822
TOLL FREE: (800) 403-3950

PO BOX 870001
SURFSIDE BEACH, SC 29587-0001
TEL: (843) 650-6100
TOLL FREE: (800) 930-2929

PO BOX 870027
SURFSIDE BEACH, SC 29587-8727
TEL: (843) 650-6100
TOLL FREE: (800) 225-4816

PO BOX 7011
CAMDEN, SC 29020-7011
TOLL FREE: (800) 578-1294

PO BOX 7011
CAMDEN, SC 29020-7011
TOLL FREE: (800) 578-1294

PO BOX 7011
CAMDEN, SC 29020-7011
TOLL FREE: (800) 578-1294

PO BOX 7031
CAMDEN, SC 29020-7031
TEL: (843) 665-7822
TOLL FREE: (800) 403-3950

PO BOX 7031
CAMDEN, SC 29020-7031
TEL: (843) 665-7822
TOLL FREE: (800) 403-3950

1717 W BROADWAY
MADISON, WI 53713-1895
PO BOX 7985
MADISON, WI 53707-7985
TEL: (608) 259-4848
TOLL FREE: (800) 578-1294

PO BOX 870001
SURFSIDE BEACH, SC 29587-0001
TEL: (843) 650-6100
TOLL FREE: (800) 930-2929

PO BOX 870028
SURFSIDE BEACH, SC 29587-8728
TEL: (843) 665-7822
TOLL FREE: (800) 225-4816

PO BOX 7021
CAMDEN, SC 29020-7021
TEL: (843) 665-7822
TOLL FREE: (800) 493-1613

PO BOX 7021
CAMDEN, SC 29020-7021
TEL: (843) 665-7822
TOLL FREE: (800) 493-1613

PO BOX 870029
SURFSIDE BEACH, SC 29587-8729
TEL: (843) 665-7822
TOLL FREE: (800) 225-4816

PO BOX 870026
SURFSIDE BEACH, SC 29587-8726
TEL: (843) 650-6100
TOLL FREE: (800) 225-4816

PO BOX 7021
CAMDEN, SC 29020-7021
TEL: (843) 665-7822
TOLL FREE: (800) 493-1613

PO BOX 7031
CAMDEN, SC 29020-7031
TEL: (843) 665-7822
TOLL FREE: (800) 403-3950

PO BOX 7011
CAMDEN, SC 29020-7011
TOLL FREE: (800) 578-1294

PO BOX 7011
CAMDEN, SC 29020-7011
TOLL FREE: (800) 578-1294

PO BOX 7011
CAMDEN, SC 29020-7011
TOLL FREE: (800) 578-1294

PO BOX 7021
CAMDEN, SC 29020-7021
TEL: (843) 665-7822
TOLL FREE: (800) 493-1613

PO BOX 870029
SURFSIDE BEACH, SC 29587-8729
TEL: (843) 665-7822
TOLL FREE: (800) 225-4816

PO BOX 7031
CAMDEN, SC 29020-7031
TEL: (843) 665-7822
TOLL FREE: (800) 403-3950

PO BOX 7021
CAMDEN, SC 29020-7021
TEL: (843) 665-7822
TOLL FREE: (800) 493-1613

PO BOX 870029
SURFSIDE BEACH, SC 29587-8729
TEL: (843) 665-7822
TOLL FREE: (800) 225-4816

PO BOX 870027
SURFSIDE BEACH, SC 29587-8727
TEL: (843) 650-6100
TOLL FREE: (800) 225-4816

1717 W BROADWAY
MADISON, WI 53713-1895
PO BOX 8999
MADISON, WI 53708-8999
TEL: (608) 221-4711
FAX: (608) 223-3611
TOLL FREE: (800) 406-2832

PO BOX 870033
SURFSIDE BEACH, SC 29587-8733
TEL: (843) 650-6100
TOLL FREE: (800) 225-4816

PO BOX 7011
CAMDEN, SC 29020-7011
TOLL FREE: (800) 578-1294

PO BOX 7011
CAMDEN, SC 29020-7011
TOLL FREE: (800) 578-1294

PO BOX 870032
SURFSIDE BEACH, SC 29587-8732
TEL: (843) 650-6100
TOLL FREE: (800) 225-4816

PO BOX 7011
CAMDEN, SC 29020-7011
TOLL FREE: (800) 578-1294

PO BOX 7021
CAMDEN, SC 29020-7021
TOLL FREE: (800) 493-1613

PO BOX 870031
SURFSIDE BEACH, SC 29587-8731
TEL: (843) 650-6100
TOLL FREE: (800) 225-4816

PO BOX 7021
CAMDEN, SC 29020-7021
TEL: (843) 665-7822
TOLL FREE: (800) 493-1613

PO BOX 8929
MADISON, WI 53708-8929
TOLL FREE: (800) 404-0110

PO BOX 7011
CAMDEN, SC 29020-7011
TOLL FREE: (800) 578-1294

1717 W BROADWAY
MADISON, WI 53713-1895
PO BOX 7985
MADISON, WI 53707-7985
TEL: (608) 259-4848
TOLL FREE: (800) 578-1294

PO BOX 7011
CAMDEN, SC 29020-7011
TOLL FREE: (800) 578-1294

PO BOX 7031
CAMDEN, SC 29020-7031
TEL: (843) 665-7822
TOLL FREE: (800) 403-3950

PO BOX 870031
SURFSIDE BEACH, SC 29587-8731
TEL: (843) 650-6100
TOLL FREE: (800) 225-4816

PO BOX 7031
CAMDEN, SC 29020-7031
TEL: (843) 665-7822
TOLL FREE: (800) 403-3950

PO BOX 7021
CAMDEN, SC 29020-7021
TEL: (843) 665-7822
TOLL FREE: (800) 493-1613

PO BOX 870032
SURFSIDE BEACH, SC 29587-8732
TEL: (843) 650-6100
TOLL FREE: (800) 225-4816

PO BOX 7011
CAMDEN, SC 29020-7011
TOLL FREE: (800) 578-1294

1717 W BROADWAY
MADISON, WI 53713-1895
PO BOX 7985
MADISON, WI 53707-7985
TEL: (608) 259-4848
TOLL FREE: (800) 578-1294

PO BOX 7021
CAMDEN, SC 29020-7021
TOLL FREE: (800) 493-1613

PO BOX 7011
CAMDEN, SC 29020-7011
TOLL FREE: (800) 578-1294

PO BOX 8929
MADISON, WI 53708-8929
TEL:
TOLL FREE: (800) 404-0110

PO BOX 7021
CAMDEN, SC 29020-7021
TEL: (843) 665-7822
TOLL FREE: (800) 493-1613

PO BOX 7021
CAMDEN, SC 29020-7021
TEL: (843) 665-7822
TOLL FREE: (800) 493-1613

PO BOX 870026
SURFSIDE BEACH, SC 29587-8726
TEL: (843) 650-6100
TOLL FREE: (800) 225-4816

CHER BUMPS & ASSOCIATES
6100 N ROBINSON, STE 204
OKLAHOMA CITY, OK 73118-7494
PO BOX 548805
OKLAHOMA CITY, OK 73154-8805
TEL: (405) 840-6022
FAX: (405) 858-7361
TOLL FREE: (888) 840-8924

CHOICECARE HEALTH PLANS, INC
655 EDEN PARK DR, STE 400
CINCINNATI, OH 45202-6056
PO BOX 3188
CINCINNATI, OH 45201-3188
TEL: (513) 784-5200
FAX: (513) 784-5310
TOLL FREE: (800) 543-7158

CHURCHILL ADMINISTRATIVE PLANS, INC
270 SYLVAN AVE
ENGLEWOOD CLIFFS, NJ 07632-2521
TEL: (201) 871-8400

CIGNA CORPORATION
600 E TAYLOR
SHERMAN, TX 75090-2881
PO BOX 9328
SHERMAN, TX 75091-9328
TEL: (903) 892-8167
FAX: (903) 892-6271
TOLL FREE: (800) 525-5803
IN-STATE: (800) 238-8801

600 E TAYLOR
SHERMAN, TX 75090-2881
PO BOX 9025
SHERMAN, TX 75091-9025
TEL: (903) 892-8167
FAX: (903) 892-6271
TOLL FREE: (800) 525-5803
IN-STATE: (800) 238-8801

600 E TAYLOR
SHERMAN, TX 75090-2881
PO BOX 9303
SHERMAN, TX 75091-9303
TEL: (903) 892-8167
FAX: (903) 892-6271
TOLL FREE: (800) 525-5803
IN-STATE: (800) 238-8801

600 E TAYLOR
SHERMAN, TX 75090-2881
PO BOX 9305
SHERMAN, TX 75091-9305
TEL: (903) 892-8167
FAX: (903) 892-6271
TOLL FREE: (800) 525-5803
IN-STATE: (800) 238-8801

600 E TAYLOR
SHERMAN, TX 75090-2881
PO BOX 9338
SHERMAN, TX 75091-9338
TEL: (903) 892-8167
FAX: (903) 892-6271
TOLL FREE: (800) 525-5803
IN-STATE: (800) 238-8801

1601 CHESTNUT ST- TWO LIBERTY PL
PHILADELPHIA, PA 19192-1550
TEL: (215) 761-1000

1630 E SHAW AVE, STE 106
FRESNO, CA 93710-8107
PO BOX 24005
FRESNO, CA 93779-4005
TEL: (559) 222-2500
TOLL FREE: (800) 841-4143

9740 APPALOOSA RD
SAN DIEGO, CA 92131-1601
TEL: (858) 693-4600
FAX: (858) 693-4881
TOLL FREE: (800) 822-2994

4025 W MINERAL KING AVE
VISALIA, CA 93277-1666
TEL: (559) 738-2050
TOLL FREE: (800) 272-2471

900 COTTAGE GROVE RD
HARTFORD, CT 06152-1315
TEL: (860) 726-6000
TOLL FREE: (800) 832-3211

2220 PARKLAKE DR NE, STE 100
ATLANTA, GA 30345-2815
PO BOX 49400
ATLANTA, GA 30359-1400
TEL: (770) 723-7894
FAX: (770) 723-7890
TOLL FREE: (800) 942-2471
IN-STATE: (800) 526-7431

TWO VANTAGE WY
NASHVILLE, TN 37228-1504
PO BOX 1465
NASHVILLE, TN 37202-1465
TEL: (615) 244-5650
FAX: (615) 782-4651
IN-STATE: (800) 627-2782

ONE CIGNA DR
BOURBONNAIS, IL 60914-4475
TEL: (815) 929-6000
FAX: (815) 935-3499
TOLL FREE: (800) 654-8777

PO BOX 3310 STA DR
ALBUQUERQUE, NM 87190-3310
TOLL FREE: (800) 525-5803

1000 POLARIS PKY
COLUMBUS, OH 43240-2008
PO BOX 182331
COLUMBUS, OH 43218-2331
TEL: (614) 785-1310
FAX: (614) 786-7777

PO BOX 2300
PITTSBURGH, PA 15230-2300
TEL: (412) 490-7812
TOLL FREE: (800) 338-7691

Appendix 7

3838 N CAUSEWAY BLVD #2800-
   B
METAIRIE, LA 70002-8319
TEL: (504) 832-1994
FAX: (504) 831-7499
TOLL FREE: (800) 238-8801

8310 N CAPITOL TX HWY, STE
   175
AUSTIN, TX 78731
TEL: (512) 894-4207

600 E TAYLOR
SHERMAN, TX 75090-2881
PO BOX 9336
SHERMAN, TX 75091-9336
TEL: (903) 892-8167
FAX: (903) 892-6271
TOLL FREE: (800) 525-5803
IN-STATE: (800) 238-8801

5100 N BROOKLINE- 9TH FL
OKLAHOMA CITY, OK 73112-
   3623
TEL: (405) 943-7711
TOLL FREE: (800) 832-3211
IN-STATE:

600 E TAYLOR
SHERMAN, TX 75090-2881
PO BOX 9337
SHERMAN, TX 75091-9337
TEL: (903) 892-8167
FAX: (903) 892-6271
TOLL FREE: (800) 525-5803
IN-STATE: (800) 238-8801

600 E TAYLOR
SHERMAN, TX 75090-2881
PO BOX 2546
SHERMAN, TX 75091-2546
TEL: (903) 892-8167
FAX: (903) 892-6271
TOLL FREE: (800) 525-5803
IN-STATE: (800) 238-8801

CIGNA HEALTHCARE
2 COLLEGE PARK DR
HOOKSETT, NH 03106-1636
TEL: (603) 225-5077
FAX: (603) 268-7981
TOLL FREE: (800) 531-3121
IN-STATE: (800) 531-3121

2 COLLEGE PARK DR
HOOKSETT, NH 03106-1636
TEL: (603) 225-5077
FAX: (603) 268-7981
TOLL FREE: (800) 531-3121
IN-STATE: (800) 531-3121

CINCINNATI INSURANCE CO
3150 HOLCOMB BRIDGE RD,
   STE 350
NORCROSS, GA 30071-1312
PO BOX 920338
NORCROSS, GA 30010-0338
TEL: (770) 662-8753
FAX: (770) 417-4635

3150 HOLCOMB BRIDGE RD,
   STE 350
NORCROSS, GA 30071-1312
PO BOX 920338
NORCROSS, GA 30010-0338
TEL: (770) 662-8753
FAX: (770) 417-4635

3150 HOLCOMB BRIDGE RD,
   STE 350
NORCROSS, GA 30071-1312
PO BOX 920338
NORCROSS, GA 30010-0338
TEL: (770) 662-8753
FAX: (770) 417-4635

3150 HOLCOMB BRIDGE RD,
   STE 350
NORCROSS, GA 30071-1312
PO BOX 920338
NORCROSS, GA 30010-0338
TEL: (770) 662-8753
FAX: (770) 417-4635

CITIZENS INSURANCE CO OF AMERICA
645 W GRAND RIVER AVE
HOWELL, MI 48843-2185
TEL: (517) 546-2160
FAX: (517) 546-1667
TOLL FREE: (800) 388-1300

CITY OF AMARILLO GROUP HEALTH PLAN
909 E 7TH
AMARILLO, TX 79186-0001
PO BOX 1971
AMARILLO, TX 79105-1971
TEL: (806) 378-4235
FAX: (806) 378-9488

CITY OF EULESS EMPLOYEE BENEFITS PLAN
201 N ECTOR DR
EULESS, TX 76039-3543
TEL: (817) 685-1475
FAX: (817) 685-1819

CITY PUBLIC SERVICE GROUP HEALTH PLAN
145 NAVARRO ST
SAN ANTONIO, TX 78205-2986
PO BOX 1771
SAN ANTONIO, TX 78296-1771
TEL: (210) 978-2900
FAX: (210) 978-3351

CIVIL SERVICE EMPLOYEES INSURANCE CO
2720 GATEWAY OAKS DR, STE
   300
SACRAMENTO, CA 95833-4305
PO BOX 13506
SACRAMENTO, CA 95853-3506
TEL: (916) 564-5126
FAX: (800) 332-0262
TOLL FREE: (800) 282-6848

2720 GATEWAY OAKS DR, STE
   300
SACRAMENTO, CA 95833-4305
PO BOX 13506
SACRAMENTO, CA 95853-3506
TEL: (916) 564-5126
FAX: (800) 332-0262
TOLL FREE: (800) 282-6848

2720 GATEWAY OAKS DR, STE
   300
SACRAMENTO, CA 95833-4305
PO BOX 13506
SACRAMENTO, CA 95853-3506
TEL: (916) 564-5126
FAX: (800) 332-0262
TOLL FREE: (800) 282-6848

2720 GATEWAY OAKS DR, STE
   300
SACRAMENTO, CA 95833-4305
PO BOX 13506
SACRAMENTO, CA 95853-3506
TEL: (916) 564-5126
FAX: (800) 332-0262
TOLL FREE: (800) 282-6848

2720 GATEWAY OAKS DR, STE 300
SACRAMENTO, CA 95833-4305
PO BOX 13506
SACRAMENTO, CA 95853-3506
TEL: (916) 564-5126
FAX: (800) 332-0262
TOLL FREE: (800) 282-6848

2720 GATEWAY OAKS DR, STE 300
SACRAMENTO, CA 95833-4305
PO BOX 13506
SACRAMENTO, CA 95853-3506
TEL: (916) 564-5126
FAX: (800) 332-0262
TOLL FREE: (800) 282-6848

2720 GATEWAY OAKS DR, STE 300
SACRAMENTO, CA 95833-4305
PO BOX 13506
SACRAMENTO, CA 95853-3506
TEL: (916) 564-5126
FAX: (800) 332-0262
TOLL FREE: (800) 282-6848

2720 GATEWAY OAKS DR, STE 300
SACRAMENTO, CA 95833-4305
PO BOX 13506
SACRAMENTO, CA 95853-3506
TEL: (916) 564-5126
FAX: (800) 332-0262
TOLL FREE: (800) 282-6848

CLAIMSWARE, INC
PO BOX 6125
GREENVILLE, SC 29606-6125
TEL: (864) 234-8200
FAX: (864) 234-8202
TOLL FREE: (800) 992-8088

CNA
6575 W LOOP S, STE 570
HOUSTON, TX 77401-3509
TEL: (512) 660-5920
FAX: (512) 660-5930
TOLL FREE: (800) 999-0972

CNA FINANCIAL CORP
CNA PLZ- 333 S WABASH AVE, FL 1
CHICAGO, IL 60604-1040
TEL: (312) 822-5000
FAX: (312) 822-6419
TOLL FREE: (800) 262-4473

COAST BENEFITS
3850 S VALLEY VIEW BLVD
LAS VEGAS, NV 89103-2904
PO BOX 80040
LAS VEGAS, NV 89180-0040
TEL: (702) 889-1155
FAX: (702) 889-1284

COLLIN COUNTY COURTHOUSE
210 S MCDONALD ST, STE 612
MCKINNEY, TX 75069-5667
TEL: (972) 548-4604

COLUMBIA UNIVERSAL LIFE INSURANCE CO
11211 TAYLOR DRAPER LN, STE 200
AUSTIN, TX 78759-3971
PO BOX 200225
AUSTIN, TX 78720-0225
TEL: (512) 345-3200
FAX: (512) 343-7599
TOLL FREE: (800) 880-1370

COMCAR INDUSTRIES, INC
111 HAVENDALE BLVD
AUBURNDALE, FL 33823-4509
PO BOX 67
AUBURNDALE, FL 33823-0067
TEL: (863) 967-1101
FAX: (863) 551-1442
TOLL FREE: (800) 524-1101

COMMUNITY HEALTH PLAN OF OHIO
1915 TAMARACK RD
NEWARK, OH 43055-1300
TEL: (740) 348-1400
FAX: (740) 348-1500
TOLL FREE: (800) 806-2756

COMPDENT CORP
100 MANSELL CT E, STE 400
ROSWELL, GA 30076-4859
PO BOX 769729
ROSWELL, GA 30076-9729
TEL: (770) 552-7101
FAX: (770) 998-6871
TOLL FREE: (800) 295-6279

100 MANSELL CT E, STE 400
ROSWELL, GA 30076-4859
PO BOX 769729
ROSWELL, GA 30076-9729
TEL: (770) 552-7101
FAX: (770) 998-6871
TOLL FREE: (800) 295-6279

100 MANSELL CT E, STE 400
ROSWELL, GA 30076-4859
PO BOX 769729
ROSWELL, GA 30076-9729
TEL: (770) 552-7101
FAX: (770) 998-6871
TOLL FREE: (800) 295-6279

100 MANSELL CT E, STE 400
ROSWELL, GA 30076-4859
PO BOX 769729
ROSWELL, GA 30076-9729
TEL: (770) 552-7101
FAX: (770) 998-6871
TOLL FREE: (800) 295-6279

100 MANSELL CT E, STE 400
ROSWELL, GA 30076-4859
PO BOX 769729
ROSWELL, GA 30076-9729
TEL: (770) 552-7101
FAX: (770) 998-6871
TOLL FREE: (800) 295-6279

100 MANSELL CT E, STE 400
ROSWELL, GA 30076-4859
PO BOX 769729
ROSWELL, GA 30076-9729
TEL: (770) 552-7101
FAX: (770) 998-6871
TOLL FREE: (800) 295-6279

100 MANSELL CT E, STE 400
ROSWELL, GA 30076-4859
PO BOX 769729
ROSWELL, GA 30076-9729
TEL: (770) 552-7101
FAX: (770) 998-6871
TOLL FREE: (800) 295-6279

100 MANSELL CT E, STE 400
ROSWELL, GA 30076-4859
PO BOX 769729
ROSWELL, GA 30076-9729
TEL: (770) 552-7101
FAX: (770) 998-6871
TOLL FREE: (800) 295-6279

100 MANSELL CT E, STE 400
ROSWELL, GA 30076-4859
PO BOX 769729
ROSWELL, GA 30076-9729
TEL: (770) 552-7101
FAX: (770) 998-6871
TOLL FREE: (800) 295-6279

100 MANSELL CT E, STE 400
ROSWELL, GA 30076-4859
PO BOX 769729
ROSWELL, GA 30076-9729
TEL: (770) 552-7101
FAX: (770) 998-6871
TOLL FREE: (800) 295-6279

100 MANSELL CT E, STE 400
ROSWELL, GA 30076-4859
PO BOX 769729
ROSWELL, GA 30076-9729
TEL: (770) 552-7101
FAX: (770) 998-6871
TOLL FREE: (800) 295-6279

100 MANSELL CT E, STE 400
ROSWELL, GA 30076-4859
PO BOX 769729
ROSWELL, GA 30076-9729
TEL: (770) 552-7101
FAX: (770) 998-6871
TOLL FREE: (800) 295-6279

COMPUSYS OF ALABAMA
PO BOX 11708
MONTGOMERY, AL 36111-0708
TEL: (334) 279-0110
FAX: (334) 279-0087
TOLL FREE: (888) 481-5826

COMPUSYS OF ARIZONA
531 E BETHANY HOME RD, STE 106
PHOENIX, AZ 85012-1283
TEL: (602) 234-0497
FAX: (602) 234-2182

4727 N 16TH ST, STE 102
PHOENIX, AZ 85016-4603
TEL: (602) 234-0593

3109 N 24TH ST, BLDG B
PHOENIX, AZ 85016-7313
TEL: (602) 956-3516
FAX: (602) 956-1943

COMPUSYS OF COLORADO, INC
10620 E BETHANY DR- BLDG 7
AURORA, CO 80014-2602
TEL: (303) 745-0147
FAX: (303) 745-7010

COMPUSYS OF NEW MEXICO
1200 SAN PEDRO NE
ALBUQUERQUE, NM 87110-6726
PO BOX 11399
ALBUQUERQUE, NM 87192-0399
TEL: (505) 262-1921
FAX: (505) 266-0922
TOLL FREE: (800) 926-5581

COMPUSYS OF TEXAS
12324 HYMEADOW DR, BLDG 4
AUSTIN, TX 78750-0001
TEL: (512) 250-9020
FAX: (512) 250-9487
TOLL FREE: (800) 933-7472

COMPUTER SCIENCE CORP
800 N PEARL ST
ALBANY, NY 12204-1898
PO BOX 4444
ALBANY, NY 12204-0444
TEL: (518) 447-9200
FAX: (518) 447-9240
IN-STATE: (800) 522-5518

CONSECO INSURANCE GROUP
PO BOX 1250
ROCKFORD, IL 61105-1250
TEL: (815) 965-8955
FAX: (815) 720-2990
TOLL FREE: (800) 659-7374

CONSOLIDATED ASSOCIATION OF RAILROAD EMPLOYEES CARE
4912 MIDWAY DR
TEMPLE, TX 76502-1519
PO BOX 6130
TEMPLE, TX 76503-6130
TEL: (254) 773-1330
FAX: (254) 774-8029
TOLL FREE: (800) 334-1330

CONTINENTAL GENERAL INSURANCE CO
8901 INDIAN HILLS DR
OMAHA, NE 68114-4071
PO BOX 247007
OMAHA, NE 68124-7007
TEL: (402) 397-3200
FAX: (402) 952-4771
TOLL FREE: (800) 545-8905
IN-STATE: (800) 397-3200

CONTINENTAL LIFE & ACCIDENT
304 N MAIN ST
ROCKFORD, IL 61101-1095
PO BOX 1300
ROCKFORD, IL 61105-1300
TEL: (815) 987-5000
FAX: (815) 720-2998
TOLL FREE: (800) 221-3770

COOPERATIVE BENEFIT ADMINISTRATORS
PO BOX 6249
LINCOLN, NE 68506-0249
TEL: (402) 483-9200
FAX: (402) 483-9201

CORESOURCE
6100 FAIRVIEW RD, STE 1000
CHARLOTTE, NC 28210-9916
TEL: (704) 552-0900
FAX: (704) 552-8635
TOLL FREE: (800) 327-5462
IN-STATE: (800) 821-0345

CORESOURCE, INC
4940 CAMPBELL BLVD, STE 200
BALTIMORE, MD 21236-5978
TEL: (410) 931-5060
FAX: (410) 931-3653
TOLL FREE: (800) 624-7130

229 HUBER VILLAGE BLVD
WESTERVILLE, OH 43081-5325
PO BOX 6118
WESTERVILLE, OH 43086-6118
TEL: (614) 890-0070
FAX: (614) 794-0736
TOLL FREE: (800) 282-3920

940 W VALLEY RD
WAYNE, PA 19087-1894
PO BOX 6994
WAYNE, PA 19087-6994
TEL: (610) 687-5924
FAX: (610) 687-1959
TOLL FREE: (800) 345-1166

CORESTAR
146 INDUSTRIAL PARK
JACKSON, MN 56143-9511
TEL: (507) 847-5740
FAX: (507) 847-2358
TOLL FREE: (800) 274-6965

146 INDUSTRIAL PARK
JACKSON, MN 56143-9511
TEL: (507) 847-5740
FAX: (507) 847-2358
TOLL FREE: (800) 274-6965

CORPORATE DIVERSIFIED SERVICES
2401 S 73RD ST, STE 1
OMAHA, NE 68124-2307
PO BOX 2835
OMAHA, NE 68103-2835
TEL: (402) 393-3133
FAX: (402) 398-3773
TOLL FREE: (800) 642-4089

CORVEL CORP
3745 CENTER POINT RD NE, STE B
CEDAR RAPIDS, IA 52402-2926
TEL: (319) 378-0606
FAX: (319) 378-0614

1860 E 54TH ST
DAVENPORT, IA 52807-2763
TEL: (319) 441-1599
FAX: (319) 441-1609

1701 48TH ST, STE 275
WEST DES MOINES, IA 50266-6703
TEL: (515) 225-9668
FAX: (515) 225-9772

5414 GLENN AVE
SIOUX CITY, IA 51106-3829
TEL: (712) 266-0325
FAX: (712) 266-0328

918 WILLIAMS ST
GREAT BEND, KS 67530-5027
TEL: (316) 793-7257
FAX: (316) 793-7561

7500 COLLEGE BLVD, STE 750
OVERLAND PARK, KS 66210-4096
TEL: (913) 498-1887
FAX: (913) 498-1885

PO BOX 1006
TOPEKA, KS 66601-1006
TEL: (785) 296-1954
FAX: (785) 296-6995

245 N WACO, STE 225
WICHITA, KS 67202-1155
TEL: (316) 264-2900
FAX: (316) 264-2977

ONE PLAZA E- 101
   PROSPEROUS PL, STE 325
LEXINGTON, KY 40509-1881
TEL: (606) 543-1403
FAX: (606) 543-8403

12910 SHELBYVILLE RD, STE 236
LOUISVILLE, KY 40243-1595
TEL: (502) 244-5300
FAX: (502) 344-8855

320 HARRISON ST
PADUCAH, KY 42001-0717
TEL: (270) 575-0676
FAX: (270) 575-1077

412 N 4TH ST, STE 230
BATON ROUGE, LA 70802-5523
TEL: (225) 388-0888
FAX: (225) 388-0890

477 CONGRESS ST, STE 1005
PORTLAND, ME 04101-3406
TEL: (207) 874-9558
FAX: (207) 772-8614

132 HOLIDAY CT, STE 205
ANNAPOLIS, MD 21401-7005
TEL: (410) 573-5120
FAX: (410) 573-5179

6 N PARK DR, STE 106
HUNT VALLEY, MD 21030-1877
TEL: (410) 403-3700
FAX: (410) 403-3725

2053 DAY RD, STE 300
HAGERSTOWN, MD 21740-1233
TEL: (301) 791-0006
FAX: (301) 791-1886

1300 PICCARD DR, STE 110
ROCKVILLE, MD 20850-4303
TEL: (301) 548-6600
FAX: (301) 548-6430

289 GREAT RD, UNIT 304
ACTON, MA 01720-4770
TEL: (978) 266-9136
FAX: (978) 266-9167

330 WHITNEY AVE, STE 440
HOLYOKE, MA 01040-2751
TEL: (413) 534-8275
FAX: (413) 532-8824

38705 SEVEN MILE RD, STE 230
LIVONIA, MI 48152-2632
TEL: (734) 432-1500
FAX: (734) 432-1510

1500 E BELTLINE SE, STE 240
GRAND RAPIDS, MI 49506-4361
TEL: (616) 977-0705
FAX: (616) 977-0713

2147 COMMONS PKY, STE B
OKEMOS, MI 48864-3987
TEL: (517) 381-1531
FAX: (517) 381-1534

5750 NEW KING ST, STE 200
TROY, MI 48007-2696
TEL: (248) 267-9348
FAX:

111 N MAIN ST, STE 203
AUSTIN, MN 55912-3474
TEL: (507) 433-7364
FAX: (507) 433-2486

1100 HWY 210 W
BRAINERD, MN 56401-3283
TEL: (218) 829-8544
FAX: (218) 829-8551

332 W SUPERIOR ST, STE 505
DULUTH, MN 55802-1801
TEL: (218) 722-1500
FAX: (218) 723-8866

PO BOX 230
GRAND RAPIDS, MN 55744-
0230
TEL: (218) 326-5613
FAX: (218) 326-8583

108 E WALNUT ST
MANKATO , MN 56001-3655
TEL: (507) 388-4486
FAX: (507) 388-4481

MARKETPLACE CTR - 1915 HIGH
ST, STE 102
ROCHESTER, MN 55901
TEL: (507) 252-5542
FAX: (507) 252-5557

26 6TH AVE N, STE 240
SAINT CLOUD, MN 56303-3601
TEL: (320) 252-5150
FAX: (320) 252-2535

1380 ENERGY LN, STE 205
SAINT PAUL, MN 55108-5269
TEL: (651) 642-1717
FAX: (651) 642-0142

14231 SEAWAY RD
GULFPORT, MS 39503-4628
TEL: (228) 214-1540
FAX: (228) 214-1542

795 WOODLANDS PKY, STE 108
RIDGELAND, MS 39157-5217
TEL: (601) 977-8922
FAX: (601) 977-9123

2800 FORUM BLVD, STE 1
COLUMBIA, MO 65203-5468
TEL: (573) 447-1501
FAX: (573) 447-1507

4817 S GOLD RD
SPRINGFIELD, MO 65619
TEL: (417) 823-0322
FAX: (417) 823-3073

1066 EXECUTIVE PKY, STE 104
SAINT LOUIS, MO 63141-6340
TEL: (314) 205-9300
FAX: (314) 205-9304

PO BOX 595
LAUREL, MT 59044-0595
TEL: (406) 248-2686
FAX: (406) 245-2780

443 1/2 MAIN ST
KALISPELL, MT 59901-4872
TEL: (406) 755-7901
FAX: (406) 755-7979

36 S LAST CHANCE GULCH, STE
L9
HELENA, MT 59601-4126
TEL: (406) 248-2686
FAX: (406) 248-2780

5601 S 27TH ST, STE 204
LINCOLN, NE 68512-1666
TEL: (402) 423-8787
FAX: (402) 423-8829

440 REGENCY PARKWAY DR, STE
14
OMAHA, NE 68114-3790
TEL: (402) 393-0400
FAX: (402) 393-0500

3900 PARADISE RD, STE 182
LAS VEGAS, NV 89109-0928
TEL: (702) 699-7020
FAX: (702) 699-7005

ONE BEDFORD FARMS, STE 105
BEDFORD, NH 03110-6524
TEL: (603) 625-0184
FAX: (603) 625-0185

4350 HADDONFIELD RD, STE
300
PENNSAUKEN, NJ 08109-3377
TEL: (856) 661-9670
FAX: (856) 661-9671

325 COLUMBIA TPKE, STE 104
FLORHAM PARK, NJ 07932-1212
TEL: (973) 377-0110
FAX: (973) 377-8022

7510 MONTGOMERY BLVD NE,
STE 103
ALBUQUERQUE, NM 87109-
1500
TEL: (505) 830-0222
FAX: (505) 830-0200

3 LEAR JET LN
LATHAM , NY 12110-2314
TEL: (518) 220-9080
FAX: (518) 220-9514

5500 MAIN ST, STE 203
WILLIAMSVILLE, NY 14221-6737
TEL: (716) 565-3124
FAX: (716) 565-3128

150 MOTOR PKY, STE 104
HAUPPAUGE, NY 11788-5167
TEL: (631) 952-2200
FAX: (631) 952-2255

370 LEXINGTON AVE, STE 1512
NEW YORK, NY 10017-6503
TEL: (212) 983-7107
FAX: (212) 983-7108

31 ERIE CANAL DR, STE F-1
ROCHESTER, NY 14626-4602
TEL: (716) 723-6417
FAX: (716) 723-6448

225 GREENFIELD PKY, STE 101
LIVERPOOL , NY 13088-6666
TEL: (315) 451-8670
FAX: (315) 451-8675

2 WILLIAM ST, STE 305
WHITE PLAINS, NY 10601-1910
TEL: (914) 285-1201
FAX: (877) 531-3187

15720 JOHN J DELANEY DR, STE
202
CHARLOTTE, NC 28277-1479
TEL: (704) 543-1382
FAX: (704) 543-1385

1840 EASTCHESTER DR, STE 102
HIGH POINT, NC 27265-1496
TEL: (336) 841-3025
FAX: (336) 841-3026

3125 POPLARWOOD CT, STE 202
RALEIGH, NC 27604-1020
TEL: (919) 790-2260
FAX: (919) 790-1522

1626 HARBOUR DR, BLDG A
WILMINGTON, NC 28401-7716
TEL: (910) 790-2260
FAX: (910) 790-1522

1321 23RD ST S, STE A
FARGO, ND 58103-3724
TEL: (701) 293-6204
FAX: (701) 293-9666

4221 MALSBARY RD, STE 106
CINCINNATI, OH 45242-5521
PO BOX 429365
CINCINNATI, OH 45242-9395
TEL: (513) 794-4040
FAX: (513) 794-0782

6902 PEARL RD, STE 200
CLEVELAND, OH 44130-3621
TEL: (440) 885-7377
FAX: (440) 885-2197

57 E WILSON BRIDGE RD
COLUMBUS, OH 43085-2301
TEL: (614) 848-3530
FAX: (614) 848-3626

4210 W SYLVANIA, STE 205
TOLEDO, OH 43632-4501
TEL: (419) 244-6455
FAX: (419) 244-6499

50 PENN PL, STE 504
OKLAHOMA CITY, OK 73118
TEL: (405) 843-3532
FAX: (405) 843-3552

6450 S LEWIS, STE 225
TULSA, OK 74136-1045
TEL: (918) 747-3505
FAX: (918) 747-3546

10260 SW GREENBERG RD, STE
    1165
PORTLAND, OR 97223-5521
TEL: (503) 244-2093
FAX: (503) 244-2189

5000 TILGHMAN ST, STE 245
ALLENTOWN, PA 18104-9121
TEL: (610) 391-1567
FAX: (610) 391-0280

5010 RITTER RD, STE 108
MECHANICSBURG, PA 17055-
    4828
TEL: (717) 796-0992
FAX: (717) 796-0994

VALLEY FORGE CORPORATE
    CTR- 1000 MADISON AVE
NORRISTOWN, PA 19403-2426
TEL: (610) 676-0200
FAX: (610) 676-0100

FOSTER PLZ 7- 661 ANDERSEN
    DR
PITTSBURGH, PA 15220-2746
TEL: (412) 922-4077
FAX: (412) 922-4285

321 SPRUCE ST, STE 801
SCRANTON, PA 18503-1400
TEL: (570) 346-3337
FAX: (570) 346-3889

1210 NORTHBROOK DR, STE 410
TREVOSE, PA 19053-8428
TEL: (215) 953-5060
FAX: (215) 953-5065

416 PONCE DE LEON AVE
HATO REY, PR 00918-3418
TEL: (787) 641-2333
FAX: (787) 641-2330

140 STONERIDGE DR, STE 150
COLUMBIA, SC 29210-8268
TEL: (803) 376-5065
FAX: (803) 376-5070

150 EXECUTIVE CENTER DR, STE
    129
GREENVILLE, SC 29615-4505
TEL: (864) 281-7890
FAX: (864) 281-7892

1470 BEN SAWYER BLVD, STE 13
MOUNT PLEASANT, SC 29464-
    4593
TEL: (843) 856-3902
FAX: (843) 856-3906

405 NW 8TH AVE, STE 310
ABERDEEN, SD 57401-2700
TEL: (605) 229-7455
FAX: (605) 229-7465

2040 W MAIN ST, STE 302
RAPID CITY, SD 57702-2447
TEL: (605) 394-8874
FAX: (605) 394-8975

3904 W TECHNOLOGY CIR
SIOUX FALLS, SD 57106-4200
TEL: (605) 361-1360
FAX: (605) 361-1370

9041 EXECUTIVE PARK DR, STE
    100
KNOXVILLE, TN 37923-4603
TEL: (865) 692-0009
FAX: (865) 692-0010

3150 LENOX PARK BLVD, STE
    117
MEMPHIS, TN 37027-4299
TEL: (901) 818-0451
FAX: (901) 818-0429

7000 EXECUTIVE CENTER DR,
    STE 250
BRENTWOOD, TN 37027-3247
TEL: (615) 371-8828
FAX: (615) 371-8560

3721 EXECUTIVE CENTER DR,
    STE 201
AUSTIN, TX 78731-1639
TEL: (512) 418-0020
FAX: (512) 418-1208

14901 QUORUM DR, STE 635
DALLAS, TX 75240-6768
TEL: (972) 239-1391
FAX: (972) 386-5133

4110 RIO BRAVO, STE 115
EL PASO, TX 79902-1026
TEL: (915) 533-8777
FAX: (915) 533-8797

801 CHERRY ST, STE 2400
FORT WORTH, TX 76102-6824
TEL: (817) 348-0000
FAX: (817) 348-9999

10777 WESTHEIMER, STE 350
HOUSTON, TX 77042-3457
TEL: (713) 977-8880
FAX: (713) 977-0229

8200 NASHVILLE AVE- BLDG C-
    STE 1
LUBBOCK, TX 79423-1906
TEL: (806) 798-2777
FAX: (806) 798-2655

100 SAVANNAH, STE 655
MCALLEN, TX 78503-1237
TEL: (956) 994-0011
FAX: (956) 994-9909

1100 NE LOOP, STE 410
SAN ANTONIO, TX 78209
TEL: (210) 824-5052
FAX: (210) 824-4740

6095 S FASHION BLVD, STE 160
MURRAY, UT 84107-7386
TEL: (801) 269-8723
FAX: (801) 269-0096

15-17 COTTAGE ST, STE 4
BARRE, VT 05641-3700
TEL: (802) 476-9836
FAX: (207) 772-8614

PO BOX 1250
ABINGDON, VA 24212-1250
TEL: (540) 676-0503
FAX: (540) 676-0722

Appendix 7

11350 RANDOM HILLS RD, STE 420
FAIRFAX, VA 22030-7449
TEL: (703) 385-5646
FAX: (703) 385-0180

1910 WILLIAM ST, STE 201
FREDERICKSBURG, VA 22401-5128
TEL: (540) 372-9868
FAX: (540) 372-2042

4860 COX RD, STE 210
GLEN ALLEN, VA 23060-9248
PO BOX 2910
GLEN ALLEN, VA 23058
TEL: (804) 273-1999
FAX: (804) 273-9817

2727 ELECTRIC RD, STE 208
ROANOKE, VA 24018-3500
TEL: (540) 725-8600
FAX: (540) 725-9906

860 GREENBRIER CIR, STE 405
CHESAPEAKE, VA 23320-2640
TEL: (757) 366-0184
FAX: (757) 366-8643

4164 MERIDIAN, STE 302
BELLINGHAM, WA 98226-5583
TEL: (360) 647-2404
FAX: (360) 671-6498

411 HOSPITAL WY, STE 104
BREWSTER, WA 98812
TEL: (509) 689-3612
FAX:

10828 GRAVELLY LAKE DR, STE 10
TACOMA, WA 98499-1334
TEL: (353) 581-0434
FAX: (353) 581-0569

4303 MACCORKLE AVE SE
CHARLESTON, WV 25304-2503
TEL: (304) 925-0493
FAX: (304) 925-0497

1600 SHAWANO AVE, STE 203E
GREEN BAY, WI 54303-3255
TEL: (920) 498-2999
FAX: (920) 498-1895

PO BOX 1568
WAUSAU, WI 54402-1568
TEL: (715) 355-0922
FAX: (715) 355-0923

COUNTY OF LOS ANGELES
1436 GOODRICH BLVD
COMMERCE, CA 90022-5111
TEL: (213) 738-2279

COVENANT ADMINISTRATORS, INC
11330 LAKEFIELD DR, STE 100
ATLANTA, GA 30097-1578
PO BOX 740042
ATLANTA, GA 30374-0042
TEL: (678) 258-8000
FAX: (770) 239-3989
TOLL FREE: (800) 374-6101
IN-STATE: (888) 239-3909

CPIC LIFE
PO BOX 3007
LODI, CA 95241-1911
TEL: (209) 367-3415
FAX: (209) 367-3450
TOLL FREE: (800) 642-5599
IN-STATE: (800) 537-0666

CRAWFORD & CO
4341 B ST, STE 301
ANCHORAGE, AK 99503-5927
TEL: (907) 561-5222
FAX: (907) 561-7383
IN-STATE: (888) 549-5222

DAKOTACARE
1323 S MINNESOTA AVE
SIOUX FALLS, SD 57105-0624
TEL: (605) 334-4000
FAX: (605) 336-0270
TOLL FREE: (800) 628-3778
IN-STATE: (800) 325-5598

DC CHARTERED HEALTH PLAN, INC
820 FIRST ST NE, LOWR LL100
WASHINGTON, DC 20002-8036
TEL: (202) 408-4710
FAX: (202) 408-4730
TOLL FREE: (800) 799-4710

DCA HEALTHCARE MANAGEMENT GROUP
3405 ANNAPOLIS LN N, STE 100
PLYMOUTH, MN 55447-5326
TEL: (612) 541-7500
FAX: (612) 541-5999
TOLL FREE: (800) 284-4464

DELMARVA HEALTH PLAN, INC
301 BAY ST, STE 401
EASTON, MD 21601-2797
PO BOX 2410
EASTON, MD 21601-2410
TEL: (410) 822-7223
FAX: (410) 822-8152
TOLL FREE: (800) 334-3427
IN-STATE: (800) 334-3427

301 BAY ST, STE 401
EASTON, MD 21601-2797
PO BOX 2410
EASTON, MD 21601-2410
TEL: (410) 822-7223
FAX: (410) 822-8152
TOLL FREE: (800) 334-3427
IN-STATE: (800) 334-3427

DISTRICT 6 HEALTH FUND
18 E 31ST ST
NEW YORK, NY 10016-6702
TEL: (212) 696-5545
FAX: (212) 696-5556
TOLL FREE: (800) 331-1070

DIVERSIFIED GROUP ADMINISTRATORS
311 S CENTRAL AVE
CANONSBURG, PA 15317-1637
PO BOX 330
CANONSBURG, PA 15317-0330
TEL: (724) 746-8700
FAX: (724) 746-8508
TOLL FREE: (800) 221-8490
IN-STATE: (800) 222-2322

EASTERN BENEFIT SYSTEMS OF CENTENNIAL FINANCIAL GROUP
200 FREEWAY DR E
EAST ORANGE, NJ 07018
TEL: (973) 676-6100
FAX: (973) 676-6794
TOLL FREE: (800) 524-0227
IN-STATE: (800) 772-3610

EAU CLAIRE HEALTH PROTECTION PLAN
3430 OAKWOOD MALL DR
EAU CLAIRE, WI 54701
PO BOX 1060
EAU CLAIRE, WI 54702
TEL: (715) 835-6174
FAX: (715) 838-0220
TOLL FREE: (800) 835-6174

EDUCATORS MUTUAL LIFE INSURANCE CO
202 N PRINCE ST
LANCASTER, PA 17603
PO BOX 83888
LANCASTER, PA 17608-3888
TEL: (717) 397-2751
FAX: (717) 397-1821
TOLL FREE: (800) 233-0307

202 N PRINCE ST
LANCASTER, PA 17603
PO BOX 83888
LANCASTER, PA 17608-3888
TEL: (717) 397-2751
FAX: (717) 397-1821
TOLL FREE: (800) 233-0307

202 N PRINCE ST
LANCASTER, PA 17603
PO BOX 83888
LANCASTER, PA 17608-3888
TEL: (717) 397-2751
FAX: (717) 397-1821
TOLL FREE: (800) 233-0307

202 N PRINCE ST
LANCASTER, PA 17603
PO BOX 83888
LANCASTER, PA 17608-3888
TEL: (717) 397-2751
FAX: (717) 397-1821
TOLL FREE: (800) 233-0307

ELCA BOARD OF PENSIONS
800 MARQUETTE AVE, STE 1050
MINNEAPOLIS, MN 55402
PO BOX 59093
MINNEAPOLIS, MN 55459-0093
TEL: (612) 333-7651
FAX: (612) 334-5399
TOLL FREE: (800) 352-2876

ELECTRONIC DATA SYSTEMS
PO BOX 15508
SACRAMENTO, CA 65852
TEL: (916) 636-1100
FAX: (916) 636-1056
IN-STATE: (800) 541-5555

EMERALD HEALTH NETWORK, INC
1100 SUPERIOR AVE, STE 1600
CLEVELAND, OH 44114
PO BOX 94808
CLEVELAND, OH 44101-4808
TEL: (216) 479-2030
FAX: (216) 241-4158
TOLL FREE: (800) 683-6830

EMPIRE BLUE CROSS - BLUE SHIELD
11 CORPORATE WOODS BLVD
ALBANY, NY 12211
PO BOX 11800
ALBANY, NY 12211-0800
TEL: (518) 367-4737
FAX: (518) 367-5373

EMPLOYEE BENEFIT PLAN ADMINISTRATORS
210 MAIN ST
MANCHESTER, CT 06040
TEL: (860) 643-6401
FAX: (860) 643-6818
TOLL FREE: (800) 848-2129

EMPLOYEE BENEFIT SYSTEMS CORP
1701 MOUNT PLEASANT ST, STE 1
BURLINGTON, IA 52601-2776
PO BOX 1053
BURLINGTON, IA 52601-1053
TEL: (319) 752-3200
FAX: (319) 754-4480
TOLL FREE: (800) 373-1327

EQUITABLE PLAN SERVICES, INC
12312 SAINT ANDREWS DR
OKLAHOMA CITY, OK 73120
PO BOX 770466
OKLAHOMA CITY, OK 73177-0466
TEL: (405) 755-2929
FAX: (405) 755-1185
TOLL FREE: (800) 749-2631

ERISA ADMINISTRATIVE SERVICES, INC
1429 SECOND ST
SANTA FE, NM 87505
TEL: (505) 988-4974
FAX: (505) 988-8943

12325 HYMEADOW DR- BLDG 4
AUSTIN, TX 78750-0001
TEL: (512) 250-9397
FAX: (512) 335-7298
TOLL FREE: (800) 933-7472

2156 W 2200 S
SALT LAKE CITY, UT 84119-1326
TEL: (801) 973-1001
FAX: (801) 973-1007

2156 W 2200 S
SALT LAKE CITY, UT 84119-1326
PO BOX 30101
SALT LAKE CITY, UT 84130-0101
TEL: (801) 973-1001
FAX: (801) 973-1007

2156 W 2200 S
SALT LAKE CITY, UT 84119-1326
PO BOX 30261
SALT LAKE CITY, UT 84130-0261
TEL: (801) 973-1001
FAX: (801) 973-1007

2156 W 2200 S
SALT LAKE CITY, UT 84119-1326
PO BOX 30058
SALT LAKE CITY, UT 84130-0058
TEL: (801) 973-1001
FAX: (801) 973-1007

2156 W 2200 S
SALT LAKE CITY, UT 84119-1326
PO BOX 30021
SALT LAKE CITY, UT 84130-0021
TEL: (801) 973-8010
FAX: (801) 973-1007
TOLL FREE: (800) 943-6203

FAMILY HEALTH PLAN OF MICHIGAN, INC
901 N MACOMB ST
MONROE, MI 48161
TEL: (734) 457-5370
FAX: (734) 457-5506
TOLL FREE: (800) 322-8966

FARM BUREAU MUTUAL INSURANCE CO
194 E COMMERCIAL
WEISER, ID 83672
TEL: (208) 549-1414
FAX: (208) 549-1433

FARM BUREAU MUTUAL INSURANCE CO OF IDAHO
444 E 5TH N
BURLEY, ID 83318-3462
TEL: (208) 678-0431
FAX: (208) 678-5368

PO BOX 4848
POCATELLO, ID 83205-4848
TEL: (208) 232-7914
FAX: (208) 233-9388

FEDERATED MUTUAL INSURANCE CO
2701 N ROCKY PT DR, STE 1200
TAMPA, FL 33607
PO BOX 31716
TAMPA, FL 33631-3716
TEL: (813) 287-0155
FAX: (813) 287-0785
TOLL FREE: (888) 507-0852
IN-STATE: (800) 237-8292

FIDELITY SECURITY LIFE INSURANCE CO
PO BOX 418131
KANSAS CITY, MO 64141-9131
TEL: (816) 756-1060
FAX: (816) 968-0560
TOLL FREE: (800) 821-7303

FIRST HEALTH
3200 HIGHLAND AVE
DOWNERS GROVE, IL 60515
TEL: (800) 962-7809
TOLL FREE: (800) 554-4954

FIRST HEALTH SERVICES CORP
4411 BUSINESS PARK BLVD, STE 16
ANCHORAGE, AK 99503
TEL: (907) 561-5650
FAX: (907) 563-1082
IN-STATE: (800) 770-5650

FIRST INTEGRATED HEALTH
19191 S VERMONT, STE 700
TORRANCE, CA 90590
PO BOX 5279
TORRANCE, CA 90510-5279
TEL: (310) 532-8887
FAX: (310) 532-2824
TOLL FREE: (800) 433-3554

FORTIS BENEFITS INSURANCE CO
1950 SPECTRUM CIR, STE B100
MARIETTA, GA 30067-6052
FAX: (770) 916-0905
TOLL FREE: (800) 955-1586

FOX-EVERETT, INC
3780 I-55 N FRONTAGE RD, STE 200
JACKSON, MS 39211
PO BOX 23096
JACKSON, MS 39225-3096
TEL: (601) 981-6000
FAX: (601) 718-5399

FRINGE BENEFIT COORDINATORS
1239 NW 10TH AVE
GAINESVILLE, FL 32601-4154
TEL: (352) 372-2028
FAX: (352) 372-9805
IN-STATE: (800) 654-1452

GALLATIN MEDICAL CLINICS
10720 PARAMOUNT BLVD
DOWNEY, CA 90241-3306
PO BOX 868
DOWNEY, CA 90241
TEL: (562) 923-6511
FAX: (562) 861-6884

GARDNER & WHITE
8902 N MERIDIAN ST, STE 202
INDIANAPOLIS, IN 46260
PO BOX 40619
INDIANAPOLIS, IN 46240-0619
TEL: (317) 581-1580
FAX: (317) 587-0780
TOLL FREE: (800) 347-5737

GEM INSURANCE CO
930 N FINANCE CENTER DR
TUCSON, AZ 85710
PO BOX 115
TUCSON, AZ 85702-0115
FAX: (888) 359-5304
TOLL FREE: (800) 888-7164

930 N FINANCE CENTER DR
TUCSON, AZ 85710
PO BOX 115
TUCSON, AZ 85702-0115
FAX: (888) 359-5304
TOLL FREE: (800) 888-7164

930 N FINANCE CENTER DR
TUCSON, AZ 85710
PO BOX 115
TUCSON, AZ 85702-0115
FAX: (888) 359-5304
TOLL FREE: (800) 888-7164

930 N FINANCE CENTER DR
TUCSON, AZ 85710
PO BOX 115
TUCSON, AZ 85702-0115
FAX: (888) 359-5304
TOLL FREE: (800) 888-7164

GENERAL AMERICAN LIFE INSURANCE CO
719 TEACO RD
KENNETT, MO 63857-3749
PO BOX 14490
KENNETT, MO 63178
TEL: (314) 843-8700
FAX: (314) 525-5740
TOLL FREE: (800) 633-8989

GEORGIA BANKERS ASSOCIATION INSURANCE
50 HURT PLZ, STE 1050
ATLANTA, GA 30303-2916
TEL: (404) 522-1501
FAX: (404) 522-9848

GERBER LIFE INSURANCE CO
66 CHURCH ST
WHITE PLAINS, NY 10601-1901
TEL: (914) 761-4404
FAX: (914) 761-4772
TOLL FREE: (800) 253-3074

GILBERT-MAGILL CO
920 MAIN ST, STE 1800
KANSAS CITY, MO 64105
PO BOX 410249
KANSAS CITY, MO 64141-0249
TEL: (816) 474-3535
FAX: (816) 842-5795
TOLL FREE: (800) 522-2460

GMAC INSURANCE
500 W 5TH ST
WINSTON-SALEM, NC 27152
PO BOX 3199
WINSTON-SALEM, NC 27102-
3199
TEL: (336) 770-2000
FAX: (336) 770-2122
TOLL FREE: (800) 642-0506

500 W 5TH ST
WINSTON-SALEM, NC 27152
PO BOX 3199
WINSTON-SALEM, NC 27102-
3199
TEL: (336) 770-2000
FAX: (336) 770-2122
TOLL FREE: (800) 642-0506

500 W 5TH ST
WINSTON-SALEM, NC 27152
PO BOX 3199
WINSTON-SALEM, NC 27102-
3199
TEL: (336) 770-2000
FAX: (336) 770-2122
TOLL FREE: (800) 642-0506

500 W 5TH ST
WINSTON-SALEM, NC 27152
PO BOX 3199
WINSTON-SALEM, NC 27102-
3199
TEL: (336) 770-2000
FAX: (336) 770-2122
TOLL FREE: (800) 642-0506

GOLDEN RULE LIFE INSURANCE CO
712 11TH ST
LAWRENCEVILLE, IL 62439-2395
TEL: (618) 943-8000
FAX: (618) 943-8031

7440 WOODLAND DR
INDIANAPOLIS, IN 46278-1719
TEL: (317) 297-4123
FAX: (317) 298-4410
IN-STATE: (800) 265-7791

GOLDEN STATE MUTUAL LIFE INSURANCE CO
4844 TELEGRAPH AVE
OAKLAND, CA 94609
PO BOX 3087
OAKLAND, CA 94609-0087
TEL: (510) 547-8101
FAX: (510) 547-0743
TOLL FREE: (800) 225-5476

1244 SOLANO AVE
VALLEJO, CA 94590
TEL: (707) 644-6606
FAX: (707) 644-6615
TOLL FREE: (800) 225-5476

7100 BOLING DR, STE 250
SACRAMENTO, CA 95823
TEL: (916) 399-1132
FAX: (916) 399-0193
TOLL FREE: (800) 225-5476

242 E AIRPORT DR, STE 100
SAN BERNARDINO, CA 92408
TEL: (909) 884-9224
FAX: (909) 383-7116
TOLL FREE: (800) 225-5476

5141 S CRENSHAW BLVD
LOS ANGELES, CA 90043
PO BOX 512332
LOS ANGELES, CA 90051-0332
TEL: (323) 296-6565
FAX: (323) 296-3319
TOLL FREE: (800) 225-5476

212 W 24TH ST, STE C
NATIONAL CITY, CA 72050
TEL: (619) 477-0146
FAX: (619) 477-7739
TOLL FREE: (800) 225-5476

1225 E 5TH ST
WINSTON-SALEM, NC 27101
TEL: (336) 723-0546
FAX: (336) 723-1873
TOLL FREE: (800) 225-5476

4410 N TRYON ST
CHARLOTTE, NC 28213-6921
TEL: (704) 598-4853
FAX: (704) 598-0232
TOLL FREE: (800) 225-5476

221 ATLANTIC AVE
ROCKY MOUNT, NC 27801
TEL: (252) 442-7011
FAX: (252) 442-7581
TOLL FREE: (800) 225-5476

9730 S WESTERN AVE, STE 834
EVERGREEN PARK, IL 60805-
2814
TEL: (708) 422-0444
FAX: (708) 422-1972
TOLL FREE: (800) 225-5476

15565 NORTHLAND DR, STE 605
WEST SOUTHFIELD, MI 48075
TEL: (248) 552-1113
FAX: (248) 552-1912
TOLL FREE: (800) 225-5476

6060 N CENTRAL EXPY, STE 718
DALLAS, TX 75206
TEL: (214) 361-9320
FAX: (214) 891-9720
TOLL FREE: (800) 225-5476

4801 ALMEDA RD
HOUSTON, TX 77004
TEL: (713) 526-4361
FAX: (713) 522-0321
TOLL FREE: (800) 225-5476

211 N ROSS ST
TYLER, TX 75702
TEL: (903) 593-4251
FAX: (903) 593-6895
TOLL FREE: (800) 225-5476

1460 INTERSTATE HWY 10 E
BEAUMONT, TX 77703
TEL: (409) 838-4969
FAX: (409) 838-3058
TOLL FREE: (800) 225-5476

2001 BEACH ST, STE 514
FORT WORTH, TX 76103
TEL: (817) 534-2777
FAX: (817) 534-1562
TOLL FREE: (800) 225-5476

GRAND VALLEY CORP
829 FOREST HILLS AVE SE
GRAND RAPIDS, MI 49546-2325
TEL: (616) 949-2410
FAX: (616) 949-4978

GRAY INSURANCE CO
3601 N I-10 SERVICE RD W
METAIRIE, LA 70002
PO BOX 6202
METAIRIE, LA 70009
TEL: (504) 888-7790
FAX: (504) 887-5658

GREAT-WEST LIFE & ANNUITY
1740 TECHNOLOGY DR, STE 300
SAN JOSE, CA 95110-1315
PO BOX 1120
SAN JOSE, CA 95108
TEL: (408) 453-2130
FAX: (408) 453-7963
TOLL FREE: (800) 685-1050

1511 N WEST SHORE BLVD, STE 850
TAMPA, FL 33607
PO BOX 31251
TAMPA, FL 33631-3251
FAX: (813) 281-0019
TOLL FREE: (800) 333-5251

4055 VALLEY VIEW LN, STE 400
DALLAS, TX 75244
TEL: (972) 458-0990
FAX:
TOLL FREE: (800) 685-3020

1802 DEL RANGE BLVD, STE 200
CHEYENNE, WY 82001
TOLL FREE: (800) 288-9575

1775 SHERMAN ST, STE 3000
DENVER, CO 80203
PO BOX 950
DENVER, CO 80201
TEL: (303) 839-1710
FAX: (303) 790-1998
TOLL FREE: (800) 685-2020

455 MARKET ST, STE 2000
SAN FRANCISCO, CA 94105-2435
TEL: (415) 777-4646
FAX: (415) 957-9842
TOLL FREE: (800) 685-1040

HORSHAM, PA
PO BOX 1000
HORSHAM, PA 19044-1000
TEL:
FAX: (215) 674-9517
TOLL FREE: (800) 685-4010

GROCER'S INSURANCE GROUP
6605 SE LAKE RD
PORTLAND, OR 97222
PO BOX 22146
PORTLAND, OR 97269
TEL: (503) 833-1600
FAX: (503) 833-1699
TOLL FREE: (800) 777-3602

GROUP BENEFIT SERVICES, INC
6 N PARK, STE 310
HUNT VALLEY, MD 21030
TEL: (410) 832-1300
FAX: (410) 832-1315
TOLL FREE: (800) 638-6085

GROUP BENEFITS UNLIMITED
1000 PLAZA DR, STE 300
CHAMBERSBURG, IL 60173
TEL: (847) 330-6000
FAX: (847) 330-9400
TOLL FREE: (800) 772-0666

GROUP HEALTH COOPERATIVE
5615 W SUNSET HWY
SPOKANE, WA 99224
PO BOX 204
SPOKANE, WA 99210-0204
TEL: (509) 838-9100
FAX: (509) 458-0368
TOLL FREE: (800) 767-4670
IN-STATE: (800) 838-9100

GROUP HEALTH MANAGERS
26205 FIVE-MILE RD
REDFORD, MI 48239-3154
TEL: (313) 535-7100
FAX: (313) 535-8472
TOLL FREE: (800) 992-2508

GROUP HEALTH PLAN OF SAINT LOUIS
111 CORPORATE OFFICE DR, STE 400
EARTH CITY, MO 63045
TEL: (314) 453-1700
FAX: (314) 506-1958
TOLL FREE: (800) 743-3901

111 CORPORATE OFFICE DR, STE 400
EARTH CITY, MO 63045
TEL: (314) 453-1700
FAX: (314) 506-1555
TOLL FREE: (800) 743-3901

GROUP INSURANCE PLAN CHATTANOOGA
1500 N DALE MABRY HWY E 6
TAMPA, FL 33607
PO BOX 31601
TAMPA, FL 33631-3601
TEL: (813) 871-4664
FAX: (813) 871-4601

GROUP SERVICES & ADMINISTRATION, INC
3113 CLASSEN BLVD
OKLAHOMA CITY, OK 73118-3818
TEL: (405) 528-4400
FAX: (405) 528-5558
TOLL FREE: (800) 475-4445

3113 CLASSEN BLVD
OKLAHOMA CITY, OK 73118-3818
TEL: (405) 528-4400
FAX: (405) 528-5558
TOLL FREE: (800) 475-4445

3113 CLASSEN BLVD
OKLAHOMA CITY, OK 73118-3818
TEL: (405) 528-4400
FAX: (405) 528-5558
TOLL FREE: (800) 475-4445

3113 CLASSEN BLVD
OKLAHOMA CITY, OK 73118-3818
TEL: (405) 528-4400
FAX: (405) 528-5558
TOLL FREE: (800) 475-4445

3113 CLASSEN BLVD
OKLAHOMA CITY, OK 73118-3818
TEL: (405) 528-4400
FAX: (405) 528-5558
TOLL FREE: (800) 475-4445

GUARANTEE LIFE INSURANCE CO
530 RIVER OAKS W
CALUMET CITY, IL 60409
TEL: (708) 868-4232
FAX: (708) 891-8886
TOLL FREE: (800) 323-8764

GUARDIAN LIFE INSURANCE CO OF AMERICA
777 E MAGNESIUM
SPOKANE, WA 99208
PO BOX 2467
SPOKANE, WA 99210
TEL: (509) 468-6000
FAX: (509) 468-6420
TOLL FREE: (800) 695-4542

GULF GUARANTY EMPLOYEE BENEFIT SERVICES, INC
4785 I-55 N, STE 106
JACKSON, MS 39206
PO BOX 14977
JACKSON, MS 39236-4977
TEL: (601) 981-9505
FAX: (601) 981-6805
TOLL FREE: (800) 890-7337

GULFCO LIFE INSURANCE CO
660 N MAIN
MARKSVILLE, LA 71351
PO BOX 157
MARKSVILLE, LA 71351-0157
TEL: (318) 253-7564
FAX: (318) 253-4903

H.E.R.E.I.U. WELFARE FUNDS
711 N COMMONS DR
AURORA, IL 60504
PO BOX 6020
AURORA, IL 60598
TEL: (630) 236-5100
FAX: (630) 236-4394

HARRINGTON BENEFIT SERVICES
3041 MORSE CROSSING
COLUMBUS, OH 43219
TEL: (614) 470-7000
FAX: (614) 470-7171
TOLL FREE: (800) 848-4623
IN-STATE: (800) 848-2664

HARRIS METHODIST HEALTH PLAN
1301 PENNSYLVANIA
FORT WORTH, TX 76104
PO BOX 90100
FORT WORTH, TX 76011
TEL: (817) 878-5800
FAX: (817) 462-7235
TOLL FREE: (800) 633-8598

HAWAII MEDICAL SERVICE ASSOCIATION
818 KEEAUMOKU ST
HONOLULU, HI 96814
PO BOX 860
HONOLULU, HI 96808-0860
TEL: (808) 948-5110
FAX: (808) 948-6811

818 KEEAUMOKU ST
HONOLULU, HI 96814
PO BOX 860
HONOLULU, HI 96808-0860
TEL: (808) 948-5110
FAX: (808) 948-6811

818 KEEAUMOKU ST
HONOLULU, HI 96814-2365
PO BOX 860
HONOLULU, HI 96808-0860
TEL: (808) 948-6111
FAX: (808) 948-6555
TOLL FREE: (800) 776-4672

818 KEEAUMOKU ST
HONOLULU, HI 96814
PO BOX 860
HONOLULU, HI 96808-0860
TEL: (808) 948-5110
FAX: (808) 948-6811

HEALTH ALLIANCE MEDICAL PLANS
102 E MAIN ST
URBANA, IL 61801
TEL: (217) 337-8100
FAX: (217) 337-8008
TOLL FREE: (800) 851-3379

HEALTH ALLIANCE PLAN OF MICHIGAN
2850 W GRAND BLVD
DETROIT, MI 48202-2692
TEL: (313) 872-8100
TOLL FREE: (800) 422-4641
IN-STATE: (800) 367-3292

HEALTH AMERICA
2575 INTERSTATE DR
HARRISBURG, PA 17110
TEL: (412) 553-7300
FAX: (412) 553-7384
TOLL FREE: (800) 788-6445

HEALTH CARE ADMINISTRATORS
2401 CHANDLER RD, STE 300
MUSKOGEE, OK 74403
PO BOX 1309
MUSKOGEE, OK 74402
TEL: (918) 687-1261
FAX: (918) 682-7984
TOLL FREE: (800) 749-1422

HEALTH CARE ADMINISTRATORS, INC
415 N 26TH ST, STE 101
LAFAYETTE, IN 47904
PO BOX 6108
LAFAYETTE, IN 47903-6108
TEL: (765) 474-5455
FAX: (765) 448-7799
TOLL FREE: (888) 448-7447

HEALTH CARE SERVICE CORP
300 E RANDOLPH ST
CHICAGO, IL 60601
PO BOX 1364
CHICAGO, IL 60690
TEL: (312) 938-6000
TOLL FREE: (800) 892-2803

300 E RANDOLPH ST
CHICAGO, IL 60601
PO BOX 1364
CHICAGO, IL 60690
TEL: (312) 938-6000
TOLL FREE: (800) 892-2803

300 E RANDOLPH ST
CHICAGO, IL 60601
PO BOX 1364
CHICAGO, IL 60690
TEL: (312) 938-6000
TOLL FREE: (800) 892-2803

HEALTH FIRST

278 BARKS RD W
MARION, OH 43302
PO BOX 1820
MARION, OH 43301-1820
TEL: (740) 387-6355
FAX: (740) 383-3840
TOLL FREE: (800) 858-1472

HEALTH FIRST, INC

821 E SE LOOP 323, II
AMERICAN CTR, STE 200
TYLER, TX 75701
PO BOX 130217
TYLER, TX 75713
TEL: (903) 581-2600
FAX: (903) 509-5726
TOLL FREE: (800) 477-2287
IN-STATE: (800) 477-2287

HEALTH GUARD

280 GRANITE RUN DR, STE 105
LANCASTER, PA 17601-6810
TEL: (717) 560-9049
FAX: (717) 560-9413
TOLL FREE: (800) 269-4606

HEALTH NET

21600 OXIDE ST
WOODLAND HILLS, CA 91367
PO BOX 9103
WOODLAND HILLS, CA 91409
TEL: (818) 676-6775
FAX: (818) 676-8755
TOLL FREE: (800) 522-0088

2300 MAIN ST, STE 700
KANSAS CITY, MO 64108
TEL: (816) 221-8400
FAX: (816) 221-7709
TOLL FREE: (800) 468-1442

2300 MAIN ST, STE 700
KANSAS CITY, MO 64108
TEL: (816) 221-8400
FAX: (816) 221-7709
TOLL FREE: (800) 468-1442

HEALTH NET HMO, INC

44 VANTAGE WY, STE 300
NASHVILLE, TN 37241
PO BOX 20000
NASHVILLE, TN 37202
TEL: (615) 291-7022
FAX: (615) 401-4647
TOLL FREE: (800) 881-9466
IN-STATE: (800) 314-3258

HEALTH PARTNERS

8100 34TH AVE S
BLOOMINGTON, MN 55425
PO BOX 1309
BLOOMINGTON, MN 55440
TEL: (612) 883-6000
FAX: (612) 883-6100
TOLL FREE: (800) 828-1159

HEALTH PLAN

52160 NATIONAL RD E
SAINT CLAIRSVILLE, OH 43950
TEL: (740) 695-7605
FAX: (740) 695-8103
TOLL FREE: (800) 624-6961

52160 NATIONAL RD E
SAINT CLAIRSVILLE, OH 43950
TEL: (740) 695-7605
FAX: (740) 695-8103
TOLL FREE: (800) 624-6961

HEALTH PLAN OF NEVADA, INC

2724 TENAYA
LAS VEGAS, NV 89128
PO BOX 15645
LAS VEGAS, NV 89114
TEL: (702) 242-7444
FAX: (702) 242-9038

HEALTH PLAN OF THE REDWOODS

3033 CLEVELAND AVE
SANTA ROSA, CA 95403
TEL: (707) 544-2273
FAX: (707) 525-4261
IN-STATE: (800) 248-2070

HEALTH RISK MANAGEMENT

5250 LOVERS LN
KALAMAZOO, MI 49002
PO BOX 4022
KALAMAZOO, MI 49003-4022
TEL: (616) 567-7364
FAX: (616) 382-1525
TOLL FREE: (800) 253-0966
IN-STATE: (800) 632-5674

10900 HAMPSHIRE AVE S
MINNEAPOLIS, MN 55438-2306
TEL: (952) 829-3500
FAX: (952) 829-3622
TOLL FREE: (800) 824-3882

HEALTH SERVICES MEDICAL CORP

8278 WILLETT PKY
BALDWINSVILLE, NY 13027
TEL: (315) 638-2133
FAX: (315) 638-0985
TOLL FREE: (800) 388-3264

HEALTHCARE AMERICA PLANS, INC

453 S WEBB RD, STE 200
WICHITA, KS 67207
PO BOX 780008
WICHITA, KS 67278-0008
TEL: (316) 687-1600
TOLL FREE: (800) 475-4274

HEALTHCARE PARTNERS MEDICAL GROUP, INC

1149 W 190TH ST, STE 101
TORRANCE, CA 90248
PO BOX 6099
TORRANCE, CA 90504
TEL: (310) 965-1100
FAX: (310) 352-6219

HELLER ASSOCIATES

2755 BRISTOL ST, STE 250
COSTA MESA, CA 92626-5985
TEL: (714) 549-7052
FAX: (714) 549-4816
IN-STATE: (800) 552-2929

HERITAGE INSURANCE MANAGERS, INC

PO BOX 659570
SAN ANTONIO, TX 78265-9570
TEL: (210) 829-7467
FAX: (210) 822-4113
TOLL FREE: (800) 456-7480

HGSA ADMINISTRATORS — MEDICARE PART B CARRIER

1800 CENTER ST
CAMP HILL, PA 17011
PO BOX 890125
CAMP HILL, PA 17089-0125
TEL: (717) 763-5700
FAX: (717) 760-9296

HMA, INC

1600 W BROADWAY RD, STE 385
COTTONWOOD, AZ 85282
PO BOX 2069
COTTONWOOD, AZ 86326
TEL: (480) 921-8944
FAX: (480) 894-5230
TOLL FREE: (800) 448-3585

1600 W BROADWAY RD, STE 385
COTTONWOOD, AZ 85282
PO BOX 2069
COTTONWOOD, AZ 86326
TEL: (480) 921-8944
FAX: (480) 894-5230
TOLL FREE: (800) 448-3585

1600 W BROADWAY RD, STE 385
COTTONWOOD, AZ 85282
PO BOX 2069
COTTONWOOD, AZ 86326
TEL: (480) 921-8944
FAX: (480) 894-5230
TOLL FREE: (800) 448-3585

1600 W BROADWAY RD, STE 385
COTTONWOOD, AZ 85282
PO BOX 2069
COTTONWOOD, AZ 86326
TEL: (480) 921-8944
FAX: (480) 894-5230
TOLL FREE: (800) 448-3585

HMO COLORADO, INC

700 BROADWAY
DENVER, CO 80273
TEL: (303) 831-0801
FAX: (303) 861-9018
TOLL FREE: (800) 544-3879
IN-STATE: (800) 533-5643

HMO NEW MEXICO, INC

12800 INDIAN SCHOOL NE
ALBUQUERQUE, NM 87112
PO BOX 11968
ALBUQUERQUE, NM 87192-0168
TEL: (505) 291-6945
FAX: (505) 237-5310
TOLL FREE: (800) 423-1630
IN-STATE: (800) 423-1630

12800 INDIAN SCHOOL NE
ALBUQUERQUE, NM 87112
PO BOX 11968
ALBUQUERQUE, NM 87192-0168
TEL: (505) 291-6945
FAX: (505) 237-5310
TOLL FREE: (800) 423-1630
IN-STATE: (800) 423-1630

12800 INDIAN SCHOOL NE
ALBUQUERQUE, NM 87112
PO BOX 11968
ALBUQUERQUE, NM 87192-0168
TEL: (505) 291-6945
FAX: (505) 237-5310
TOLL FREE: (800) 423-1630
IN-STATE: (800) 423-1630

HOLY CROSS RESOURCES, INC

ST MARY'S LOURDES HALL, 3575 MOREAU CT
SOUTH BEND, IN 46628-4320
TEL: (219) 283-4600
FAX: (219) 283-4709
TOLL FREE: (800) 348-2616

HOMETOWN HEALTH PLAN

240 S ROCKS, STE 123
RENO, NV 89502
TEL: (775) 982-3000
FAX: (775) 982-3160
TOLL FREE: (800) 336-0123
IN-STATE: (800) 336-0123

100 LILLIAN GISH BLVD, STE 301
MASSILLON, OH 44647
TEL: (330) 837-6880
FAX: (330) 837-6869
IN-STATE: (800) 426-9013

HUMA MEMORIAL SISTERS OF CHARITY

9494 SOUTHWEST FWY, STE 300
HOUSTON, TX 77074
TEL: (713) 430-1400
FAX: (713) 778-2375
TOLL FREE: (800) 776-2885

HUMANA, INC

500 W MAIN ST
LOUISVILLE, KY 40202-1438
TEL: (502) 580-1000
FAX: (502) 580-3127
TOLL FREE: (800) 448-6262
IN-STATE: (800) 486-2620

500 W MAIN ST
LOUISVILLE, KY 40202-1438
TEL: (502) 580-1000
FAX: (502) 580-3127
TOLL FREE: (800) 448-6262
IN-STATE: (800) 486-2620

500 W MAIN ST
LOUISVILLE, KY 40202-1438
TEL: (502) 580-1000
FAX: (502) 580-3127
TOLL FREE: (800) 448-6262
IN-STATE: (800) 486-2620

500 W MAIN ST
LOUISVILLE, KY 40202-1438
TEL: (502) 580-1000
FAX: (502) 580-3127
TOLL FREE: (800) 448-6262
IN-STATE: (800) 486-2620

500 W MAIN ST
LOUISVILLE, KY 40202-1438
TEL: (502) 580-1000
FAX: (502) 580-3127
TOLL FREE: (800) 448-6262
IN-STATE: (800) 486-2620

500 W MAIN ST
LOUISVILLE, KY 40202-1438
TEL: (502) 580-1000
FAX: (502) 580-3127
TOLL FREE: (800) 448-6262
IN-STATE: (800) 486-2620

500 W MAIN ST
LOUISVILLE, KY 40202-1438
TEL: (502) 580-1000
FAX: (502) 580-3127
TOLL FREE: (800) 448-6262
IN-STATE: (800) 486-2620

500 W MAIN ST
LOUISVILLE, KY 40202-1438
TEL: (502) 580-1000
FAX: (502) 580-3127
TOLL FREE: (800) 448-6262
IN-STATE: (800) 486-2620

500 W MAIN ST
LOUISVILLE, KY 40202-1438
TEL: (502) 580-1000
FAX: (502) 580-3127
TOLL FREE: (800) 448-6262
IN-STATE: (800) 486-2620

500 W MAIN ST
LOUISVILLE, KY 40202-1438
TEL: (502) 580-1000
FAX: (502) 580-3127
TOLL FREE: (800) 448-6262
IN-STATE: (800) 486-2620

500 W MAIN ST
LOUISVILLE, KY 40202-1438
TEL: (502) 580-1000
FAX: (502) 580-3127
TOLL FREE: (800) 448-6262
IN-STATE: (800) 486-2620

500 W MAIN ST
LOUISVILLE, KY 40202-1438
TEL: (502) 580-1000
FAX: (502) 580-3127
TOLL FREE: (800) 448-6262
IN-STATE: (800) 486-2620

500 W MAIN ST
LOUISVILLE, KY 40202-1438
TEL: (502) 580-1000
FAX: (502) 580-3127
TOLL FREE: (800) 448-6262
IN-STATE: (800) 486-2620

10450 HOLMES RD, STE 100
KANSAS CITY, MO 64131
TEL: (816) 941-8900
FAX: (816) 942-6782

500 W MAIN ST
LOUISVILLE, KY 40202-1438
TEL: (502) 580-1000
FAX: (502) 580-3127
TOLL FREE: (800) 448-6262
IN-STATE: (800) 486-2620

500 W MAIN ST
LOUISVILLE, KY 40202-1438
TEL: (502) 580-1000
FAX: (502) 580-3127
TOLL FREE: (800) 448-6262
IN-STATE: (800) 486-2620

500 W MAIN ST
LOUISVILLE, KY 40202-1438
TEL: (502) 580-1000
FAX: (502) 580-3127
TOLL FREE: (800) 448-6262
IN-STATE: (800) 486-2620

500 W MAIN ST
LOUISVILLE, KY 40202-1438
TEL: (502) 580-1000
FAX: (502) 580-3127
TOLL FREE: (800) 448-6262
IN-STATE: (800) 486-2620

500 W MAIN ST
LOUISVILLE, KY 40202-1438
TEL: (502) 580-1000
FAX: (502) 580-3127
TOLL FREE: (800) 448-6262
IN-STATE: (800) 486-2620

500 W MAIN ST
LOUISVILLE, KY 40202-1438
TEL: (502) 580-1000
FAX: (502) 580-3127
TOLL FREE: (800) 448-6262
IN-STATE: (800) 486-2620

111 W PLEASANT ST
MILWAUKEE, WI 53212
PO BOX 12359
MILWAUKEE, WI 53212-0359
TEL: (414) 223-3300
FAX: (414) 223-7777
TOLL FREE: (800) 289-0260

500 W MAIN ST
LOUISVILLE, KY 40202-1438
TEL: (502) 580-1000
FAX: (502) 580-3127
TOLL FREE: (800) 448-6262
IN-STATE: (800) 486-2620

IDAHO FARM BUREAU MUTUAL INSURANCE CO
435 LINCOLN
AMERICAN FALLS, ID 83211
PO BOX 239
AMERICAN FALLS, ID 83211
TEL: (208) 226-5066
FAX: (208) 226-7929

225 W GRAND AVE
ARCO, ID 83213
PO BOX 824
ARCO, ID 83213-0824
TEL: (208) 527-3431
FAX: (208) 527-3432

124 N OAK ST
BLACKFOOT, ID 83221
PO BOX 668
BLACKFOOT, ID 83221-0668
TEL: (208) 785-2410
FAX: (208) 785-2422

6426 KOOTENAI ST
BONNERS FERRY, ID 83805
PO BOX 1387
BONNERS FERRY, ID 83805-1387
TEL: (208) 267-5502
FAX: (208) 267-5503

6912 N GOVERNMENT WY
DALTON GARDENS, ID 83815-8747
TEL: (208) 772-6662
FAX: (208) 772-2553

906 S WASHINGTON
EMMETT, ID 83617
PO BOX 156
EMMETT, ID 83617-0156
TEL: (208) 365-5382
FAX: (208) 365-2465

131 3RD AVE E
GOODING, ID 83330-1101
TEL: (208) 934-8405
FAX: (208) 934-8406

IDAHO FARM BUREAU MUTUAL INSURANCE CO
345 MAIN
GRAND VIEW, ID 83624
PO BOX 428
GRAND VIEW, ID 83624-0428
TEL: (208) 834-2766
FAX: (208) 834-2526

IDAHO FARM BUREAU MUTUAL INSURANCE CO
711 N MAIN
HAILEY, ID 83313
PO BOX 609
HAILEY, ID 83333-0609
TEL: (208) 788-3529
FAX: (208) 788-3619

118 W IDAHO AVE
HOMEDALE, ID 83628
PO BOX 1197
HOMEDALE, ID 83628-1197
TEL: (208) 337-4041
FAX: (208) 337-4042

1655 HOLLIPARK
IDAHO FALLS, ID 83401
PO BOX 2948
IDAHO FALLS, ID 83403-2948
TEL: (208) 522-2652
FAX: (208) 522-2675

200 E AVE A
JEROME, ID 83338
PO BOX C
JEROME, ID 83338
TEL: (208) 324-4378
FAX: (208) 324-4393

2007 14TH AVE
LEWISTON, ID 83501-3019
TEL: (208) 743-5533
FAX: (208) 743-5535

34 N MAIN
MALAD, ID 83252
TEL: (208) 766-2259
FAX: (208) 766-4211

470 WASHINGTON ST
MONTPELIER, ID 83254
TEL: (208) 847-0851
FAX: (208) 847-0856

150 126TH ST, STE C
OROFINO, ID 83544
TEL: (208) 476-4722
FAX: (208) 476-7348

235 N MAIN
PAYETTE, ID 83661
TEL: (208) 642-4414
FAX: (208) 642-4415

200 W ALAMEDA
POCATELLO, ID 83201
PO BOX 4848
POCATELLO, ID 83205
TEL: (208) 233-9442
FAX: (208) 233-4167

IDAHO FARM BUREAU MUTUAL INSURANCE CO
170 S 2ND E
SODA SPRINGS, ID 83276
PO BOX 506
SODA SPRINGS, ID 83276-0506
TEL: (208) 547-3315
FAX: (208) 547-3316

IDAHO FARM BUREAU MUTUAL INSURANCE CO
325 E MAIN
SAINT ANTHONY, ID 83445
PO BOX 528
SAINT ANTHONY, ID 83445-0528
TEL: (208) 624-3171
FAX: (208) 624-3173

414 MAIN AVE
SAINT MARIES, ID 83861
TEL: (208) 245-5568
FAX: (208) 245-5569

IHC HEALTH PLANS
4646 W LAKE PARK BLVD
SALT LAKE CITY, UT 84120
TEL: (801) 442-5000
FAX: (801) 442-5003
TOLL FREE: (800) 538-5038
IN-STATE: (800) 442-5038

4646 W LAKE PARK BLVD
SALT LAKE CITY, UT 84120
TEL: (801) 442-5000
FAX: (801) 442-5003
TOLL FREE: (800) 538-5038
IN-STATE: (800) 442-5038

4646 W LAKE PARK BLVD
SALT LAKE CITY, UT 84120
TEL: (801) 442-5000
FAX: (801) 442-5003
TOLL FREE: (800) 538-5038
IN-STATE: (800) 442-5038

ILLINOIS MASONIC COMMUNITY HEALTH PLAN
836 W WELLINGTON
CHICAGO, IL 60657
TEL: (773) 296-7167
FAX: (773) 296-5598

INSURANCE CO OF THE WEST
11455 EL CAMINO REAL
SAN DIEGO, CA 92130
PO BOX 85563
SAN DIEGO, CA 92186-5563
TEL: (858) 350-2400
FAX: (858) 350-2543
TOLL FREE: (800) 877-1111

INSURANCE MANAGEMENT ADMINISTRATORS OF LOUISIANA
1325 BARKSDALE BLVD, STE 300
BOSSIER CITY, LA 71111
PO BOX 71120
BOSSIER CITY, LA 71171
TEL: (318) 747-0577
FAX: (318) 747-5074

INSURANCE MANAGEMENT ASSOCIATES, INC
250 N WATER ST, STE 600
WICHITA, KS 67202
PO BOX 2992
WICHITA, KS 67201
TEL: (316) 267-9221
FAX: (316) 266-6385
TOLL FREE: (800) 288-6732

INSURANCE & PERSONNEL SERVICES
2121 N WEBB RD
GRAND ISLAND, NE 68803
PO BOX 2160
GRAND ISLAND, NE 68802
TEL: (308) 384-8700
FAX: (308) 384-8423

INSURERS ADMINISTRATIVE CORP
2101 W PEORIA AVE, STE 100
PHOENIX, AZ 85029
PO BOX 39119
PHOENIX, AZ 85069-9119
TEL: (602) 870-1400
FAX: (602) 395-0496
TOLL FREE: (800) 843-3106

INSUREX BENEFITS ADMINISTRATORS
1835 UNION AVE, STE 400
MEMPHIS, TN 38104
PO BOX 41779
MEMPHIS, TN 38174
TEL: (901) 725-6435
FAX: (901) 725-6437

Appendix 7

INTEGRATED HEALTH SERVICES
235 ELM ST NE
ALBUQUERQUE, NM 87102
PO BOX 30278
ALBUQUERQUE, NM 87190
TEL: (505) 222-8260
FAX: (505) 242-7114

INTER VALLEY HEALTH PLAN
300 S PARK AVE
POMONA, CA 91766
PO BOX 6002
POMONA, CA 91769-6002
TEL: (909) 623-6333
FAX: (909) 622-2907
TOLL FREE: (800) 251-8191

INTERACTIVE MEDICAL SYSTEMS, INC
5621 DEPARTURE DR, STE 117
RALEIGH, NC 27616
PO BOX 19108
RALEIGH, NC 27619
TEL: (919) 877-9933
FAX: (919) 877-0615

4505 FALLS OF NEUSE, STE 550
RALEIGH, NC 27609
PO BOX 19108
RALEIGH, NC 27619
TEL: (919) 877-9933

5621 DEPARTURE DR, STE 117
RALEIGH, NC 27616
PO BOX 19108
RALEIGH, NC 27619
TEL: (919) 877-9933
FAX: (919) 877-0615

5621 DEPARTURE DR, STE 117
RALEIGH, NC 27616
PO BOX 19108
RALEIGH, NC 27619
TEL: (919) 877-9933
FAX: (919) 877-0615

5621 DEPARTURE DR, STE 117
RALEIGH, NC 27616
PO BOX 19108
RALEIGH, NC 27619
TEL: (919) 877-9933
FAX: (919) 877-0615

INTERCARE BENEFIT SYSTEMS, INC
5500 GREENWOOD PLZ BLVD
ENGLEWOOD, CO 80111
PO BOX 3559
ENGLEWOOD, CO 80155
TEL: (303) 770-5710
FAX: (303) 770-2743
TOLL FREE: (800) 426-7453

INTERCONTINENTAL CORP
135 N PENNSYLVANIA ST, STE 770
INDIANAPOLIS, IN 46204
TEL: (317) 238-5700
FAX: (317) 637-6634
TOLL FREE: (800) 962-6831

INTERGROUP OF ARIZONA
930 N FINANCE CTR DR
TUCSON, AZ 85710
TEL: (520) 751-6111
FAX: (520) 290-5176
TOLL FREE: (800) 289-2818

INTERMOUNTAIN ADMINISTRATORS, INC
2806 S GARFIELD ST
MISSOULA, MT 59801
PO BOX 3018
MISSOULA, MT 59806-3018
TEL: (406) 721-2222
FAX: (406) 721-2252
TOLL FREE: (800) 877-1122

J.P. FARLEY CORP
22021 BROOKPARK RD, STE 100
CLEVELAND, OH 44126
PO BOX 268000
CLEVELAND, OH 44126-8000
TEL: (440) 734-6800
FAX: (440) 734-1668
TOLL FREE: (800) 634-0173

JARDINE GROUP SERVICES CORP
13 CORNELL RD
LATHAM, NY 12110
TEL: (518) 782-3000
FAX: (518) 782-3157
TOLL FREE: (800) 366-5273

JEFFERSON LIFE INSURANCE CO
9304 FOREST LN N, STE 256
DALLAS, TX 75243
PO BOX 749008
DALLAS, TX 75374-9008
TEL: (214) 340-8995
FAX: (214) 340-6114
TOLL FREE: (800) 343-5542

JEFFERSON-PILOT LIFE INSURANCE CO
100 N GREEN ST
GREENSBORO, NC 27401
PO BOX 21008
GREENSBORO, NC 27420
TEL: (336) 691-3000
FAX: (336) 691-4500
TOLL FREE: (800) 458-1419
IN-STATE: (800) 792-2268

JENSEN ADMINISTRATIVE SERVICES
4885 S 9TH E, STE 202
SALT LAKE CITY, UT 84117-5725
TEL: (801) 266-3256
FAX: (801) 266-4383
TOLL FREE: (800) 345-3248

4885 S 9TH E, STE 202
SALT LAKE CITY, UT 84117-5725
TEL: (801) 266-3256
FAX: (801) 266-4383
TOLL FREE: (800) 345-3248

4885 S 9TH E, STE 202
SALT LAKE CITY, UT 84117-5725
TEL: (801) 266-3256
FAX: (801) 266-4383
TOLL FREE: (800) 345-3248

4885 S 9TH E, STE 202
SALT LAKE CITY, UT 84117-5725
TEL: (801) 266-3256
FAX: (801) 266-4383
TOLL FREE: (800) 345-3248

JFP BENEFIT MANAGEMENT
100 S JACKSON ST, STE 200
JACKSON, MI 49201
PO BOX 189
JACKSON, MI 49204-0189
TEL: (517) 784-0535
FAX: (517) 784-0821
IN-STATE: (800) 589-7660

JM FAMILY ENTERPRISES
8019 BAYBERRY RD
JACKSONVILLE, FL 32256-7411
TEL: (904) 443-6650
FAX: (904) 443-6670
TOLL FREE: (800) 736-3936

JOHN ALDEN LIFE INSURANCE CO
1005 MAIN ST
BOISE, ID 83702
PO BOX 1599
BOISE, ID 83702-1599
TEL: (208) 368-7770
FAX: (208) 336-1050
TOLL FREE: (800) 328-4316

1005 MAIN ST
BOISE, ID 83702
PO BOX 1599
BOISE, ID 83702-1599
TEL: (208) 368-7770
FAX: (208) 336-1050
TOLL FREE: (800) 328-4316

1005 MAIN ST
BOISE, ID 83702
PO BOX 1599
BOISE, ID 83702-1599
TEL: (208) 368-7770
FAX: (208) 336-1050
TOLL FREE: (800) 328-4316

1005 MAIN ST
BOISE, ID 83702
PO BOX 1599
BOISE, ID 83702-1599
TEL: (208) 368-7770
FAX: (208) 336-1050
TOLL FREE: (800) 328-4316

1005 MAIN ST
BOISE, ID 83702
PO BOX 1599
BOISE, ID 83702-1599
TEL: (208) 368-7770
FAX: (208) 336-1050
TOLL FREE: (800) 328-4316

1005 MAIN ST
BOISE, ID 83702
PO BOX 1599
BOISE, ID 83702-1599
TEL: (208) 368-7770
FAX: (208) 336-1050
TOLL FREE: (800) 328-4316

1005 MAIN ST
BOISE, ID 83702
PO BOX 1599
BOISE, ID 83702-1599
TEL: (208) 368-7770
FAX: (208) 336-1050
TOLL FREE: (800) 328-4316

1005 MAIN ST
BOISE, ID 83702
PO BOX 1599
BOISE, ID 83702-1599
TEL: (208) 368-7770
FAX: (208) 336-1050
TOLL FREE: (800) 328-4316

1005 MAIN ST
BOISE, ID 83702
PO BOX 1599
BOISE, ID 83702-1599
TEL: (208) 368-7770
FAX: (208) 336-1050
TOLL FREE: (800) 328-4316

1005 MAIN ST
BOISE, ID 83702
PO BOX 1599
BOISE, ID 83702-1599
TEL: (208) 368-7770
FAX: (208) 336-1050
TOLL FREE: (800) 328-4316

1005 MAIN ST
BOISE, ID 83702
PO BOX 1599
BOISE, ID 83702-1599
TEL: (208) 368-7770
FAX: (208) 336-1050
TOLL FREE: (800) 328-4316

1005 MAIN ST
BOISE, ID 83702
PO BOX 1599
BOISE, ID 83702-1599
TEL: (208) 368-7770
FAX: (208) 336-1050
TOLL FREE: (800) 328-4316

1005 MAIN ST
BOISE, ID 83702
PO BOX 1599
BOISE, ID 83702-1599
TEL: (208) 368-7770
FAX: (208) 336-1050
TOLL FREE: (800) 328-4316

1005 MAIN ST
BOISE, ID 83702
PO BOX 1599
BOISE, ID 83702-1599
TEL: (208) 368-7770
FAX: (208) 336-1050
TOLL FREE: (800) 328-4316

1005 MAIN ST
BOISE, ID 83702
PO BOX 1599
BOISE, ID 83702-1599
TEL: (208) 368-7770
FAX: (208) 336-1050
TOLL FREE: (800) 328-4316

1005 MAIN ST
BOISE, ID 83702
PO BOX 1599
BOISE, ID 83702-1599
TEL: (208) 368-7770
FAX: (208) 336-1050
TOLL FREE: (800) 328-4316

1005 MAIN ST
BOISE, ID 83702
PO BOX 1599
BOISE, ID 83702-1599
TEL: (208) 368-7770
FAX: (208) 336-1050
TOLL FREE: (800) 328-4316

1005 MAIN ST
BOISE, ID 83702
PO BOX 1599
BOISE, ID 83702-1599
TEL: (208) 368-7770
FAX: (208) 336-1050
TOLL FREE: (800) 328-4316

1005 MAIN ST
BOISE, ID 83702
PO BOX 1599
BOISE, ID 83702-1599
TEL: (208) 368-7770
FAX: (208) 336-1050
TOLL FREE: (800) 328-4316

1005 MAIN ST
BOISE, ID 83702
PO BOX 1599
BOISE, ID 83702-1599
TEL: (208) 368-7770
FAX: (208) 336-1050
TOLL FREE: (800) 328-4316

1005 MAIN ST
BOISE, ID 83702
PO BOX 1599
BOISE, ID 83702-1599
TEL: (208) 368-7770
FAX: (208) 336-1050
TOLL FREE: (800) 328-4316

JOHNSON INSURANCE
176 MCSWAIN DR
COLUMBIA, SC 29169
PO BOX 21308
COLUMBIA, SC 29221-1308
TEL: (803) 739-0001
FAX: (803) 739-2200

KAISER PERMANENTE
711 KAPIOLANI BLVD
HONOLULU, HI 96814
PO BOX 31000
HONOLULU, HI 96849-5086
TEL: (808) 597-5340
FAX: (808) 597-5300
TOLL FREE: (800) 596-5955
IN-STATE: (800) 596-5955

500 NE MULTNOMAH, STE 100
PORTLAND, OR 97232
TEL: (503) 813-2800
FAX: (503) 813-2710
TOLL FREE: (800) 813-2000

KEENAN & ASSOCIATES
2105 S BASCOM AVE, STE 310
CAMPBELL, CA 95008
TEL: (408) 377-3338
FAX: (408) 371-1796
TOLL FREE: (800) 334-6554

3610 CENTRAL, STE 400
RIVERSIDE, CA 92506
TEL: (909) 788-0330
FAX: (909) 788-8013
TOLL FREE: (800) 654-8347

KENTUCKY FARM BUREAU MUTUAL INSURANCE CO
2909 RING RD
ELIZABETHTOWN, KY 42701
PO BOX 958
ELIZABETHTOWN, KY 42702-0958
TEL: (270) 765-4400
FAX: (270) 765-7956
TOLL FREE: (800) 782-3811

KEYSTONE MERCY HEALTH PLAN
200 STEVENS DR, STE 350
LESTER, PA 19113
TEL: (215) 937-7300
FAX: (215) 937-5300
IN-STATE: (800) 521-6007

KITSAP PHYSICIANS SERVICE
400 WARREN AVE
BREMERTON, WA 98337
PO BOX 339
BREMERTON, WA 98337
TEL: (360) 377-5576
FAX: (360) 415-6514
TOLL FREE: (800) 552-7114

KLAIS & CO
1867 W MARKET ST
AKRON, OH 44313
TEL: (330) 867-8443
FAX: (330) 867-0827
TOLL FREE: (800) 331-1096

LANCER CLAIM SERVICE CORP
333 CITY BLVD W
ORANGE, CA 92868
PO BOX 7048
ORANGE, CA 92863
TEL: (714) 939-0700
FAX: (714) 978-8023
TOLL FREE: (800) 821-0540
IN-STATE: (800) 645-5324

LANDMARK HEALTH CARE
1750 HOWE AVE, STE 300
SACRAMENTO, CA 95825-3369
TEL: (916) 646-3477
FAX: (916) 929-8350
TOLL FREE: (800) 638-4557

LEWER AGENCY, INC
4534 WORNALL RD
KANSAS CITY, MO 64111
TEL: (816) 753-4390
FAX: (816) 561-6840
TOLL FREE: (800) 821-7715

LIFE INSURANCE CO OF GEORGIA
4850 E STREET RD
LANGHORNE, PA 19053
PO BOX 3013
LANGHORNE, PA 19047
TOLL FREE: (800) 877-7756

4850 E STREET RD
LANGHORNE, PA 19053
PO BOX 3013
LANGHORNE, PA 19047
TOLL FREE: (800) 877-7756

LOCALS 302 & 612 INTERNATIONAL
2815 SECOND AVE, STE 300
SEATTLE, WA 98121
PO BOX 34684
SEATTLE, WA 98124
TEL: (206) 441-7574
FAX: (206) 441-9110
TOLL FREE: (800) 331-6158
IN-STATE: (800) 732-1121

M-PLAN
8802 N MERIDIAN ST, STE 100
INDIANAPOLIS, IN 46260-5371
TEL: (317) 571-5300
FAX: (317) 705-3119
TOLL FREE: (800) 878-8802

MANAGED HEALTH, INC
25 BROADWAY, STE 900
NEW YORK, NY 10004
FAX: (212) 801-1799
TOLL FREE: (888) 260-1010

MARSH USE INC
1000 RIDGEWAY LOOP RD
MEMPHIS, TN 38120
PO BOX 171377
MEMPHIS, TN 38120
TEL: (901) 761-1550
FAX: (901) 684-3858

MASSACHUSETTS MUTUAL LIFE INSURANCE CO
1350 MAIN ST
SPRINGFIELD, MA 01103
PO BOX 51130
SPRINGFIELD, MA 01151-5130
TEL: (413) 788-8411
TOLL FREE: (800) 288-8630

MAYO HEALTH PLAN
21 1ST ST SW, STE 401
ROCHESTER, MN 55902
TEL: (507) 284-8274
FAX: (507) 284-0528
TOLL FREE: (800) 635-6671

MCCREARY CORPORATION
700 CENTRAL PKY
STUART, FL 34994-3985
TEL: (561) 287-7650
FAX: (561) 287-1387
TOLL FREE: (800) 431-2221

MED-PAY, INC
1650 E BATTLEFIELD, STE 300
SPRINGFIELD, MO 65804
PO BOX 10909
SPRINGFIELD, MO 65808
TEL: (417) 886-6886
FAX: (417) 886-2276
TOLL FREE: (800) 777-9087

MEDICAID FISCAL AGENTS
301 TECHNA CENTER DR
MONTGOMERY, AL 36117
TEL: (334) 215-0111
FAX: (334) 215-4298
IN-STATE: (800) 688-7989

500 E MARCHAM, STE 400
LITTLE ROCK, AR 72201
PO BOX 8036
LITTLE ROCK, AR 72203-2501
TEL: (501) 374-6608
FAX: (501) 374-0549
IN-STATE: (800) 457-4454

PO BOX 2941
HARTFORD, CT 06104-2941
TEL: (860) 832-9259
IN-STATE: (800) 842-8440

NEW CASTLE, DE
PO BOX 907
NEW CASTLE, DE 19720
TEL: (302) 454-7154
FAX: (302) 454-7603
IN-STATE: (800) 999-3371

201 S GRAND AVE E- PRESCOTT BLOOM BLDG
SPRINGFIELD, IL 62794
PO BOX 19105
SPRINGFIELD, IL 62793
TEL: (217) 782-5567
FAX: (217) 524-7194

PO BOX 3571
TOPEKA, KS 66601
TOLL FREE: (800) 933-6593

275 E MAIN ST, 6WA
FRANKFORT, KY 40621-0001
TEL: (502) 564-4321

8591 UNITED PLAZA BLVD, STE 340
BATON ROUGE, LA 70809
PO BOX 91024
BATON ROUGE, LA 70821-9024
TEL: (504) 237-3200
TOLL FREE: (800) 473-2783

BUREAU OF MED SVCS- 249 WESTERN AVE
AUGUSTA, ME 04333-0001
TEL: (207) 287-3081
IN-STATE: (800) 321-5557

201 W PRESTON ST, RM SS18
BALTIMORE, MD 21201
PO BOX 1935
BALTIMORE, MD 21203
TEL: (410) 767-5503
FAX: (410) 333-7118
TOLL FREE: (800) 445-1159

5 MIDDLESEX AVE
SOMERVILLE, MA 02145
PO BOX 9101
SOMERVILLE, MA 02145-9101
TEL: (617) 625-0120
FAX: (617) 576-4087
TOLL FREE: (800) 325-5231

111 E CAPITOL ST, STE 400
JACKSON, MS 39201
PO BOX 23077
JACKSON, MS 38225-3077
TEL: (601) 960-2800
FAX: (601) 960-2807
TOLL FREE: (800) 884-3222

PO BOX 5600
JEFFERSON CITY, MO 65102
TEL: (573) 751-2896
TOLL FREE: (800) 392-0938

34 N LAST CHANCE GULCH
HELENA, MT 59601
TEL: (406) 449-7693
FAX: (406) 442-4402
IN-STATE: (800) 624-3958

701 E JEFFERSON
PHOENIX, AZ 85084
PO BOX 25520
PHOENIX, AZ 85002-9949
TEL: (602) 417-4000
FAX: (602) 253-5472
TOLL FREE: (800) 523-0231

301 CENTENNIAL MALL S
LINCOLN, NE 68508
PO BOX 95026
LINCOLN, NE 68509-5026
TEL: (402) 471-9147
FAX: (402) 471-9092
TOLL FREE: (800) 430-3244

7 EAGLE SQ, STE 4
CONCORD, NH 03301
PO BOX 2001
CONCORD, NH 03302
TEL: (603) 224-1747
FAX: (603) 225-7964
IN-STATE:

3705 QUAKERBRIDGE RD, STE 101
TRENTON, NJ 08619-1209
TEL: (609) 584-0200
FAX: (609) 584-8270
TOLL FREE: (800) 776-6334

1720 RANDOLPH RD, STE A
ALBUQUERQUE, NM 87106
PO BOX 25700
ALBUQUERQUE, NM 87125
TEL: (505) 246-9988
FAX: (505) 246-8485
IN-STATE: (800) 282-4477

4905 WATEREDGE DR
RALEIGH, NC 27606
TEL: (919) 851-8888
FAX: (919) 851-4014
TOLL FREE: (800) 688-6696

600 E BLVD AVE
BISMARCK, ND 58505-0261
TEL: (701) 328-2321
FAX: (701) 328-1544
TOLL FREE: (800) 755-2604

201 NW 63RD, STE 100
OKLAHOMA CITY, OK 73116-
8210
TEL: (405) 841-3400
FAX: (405) 841-3510

515 HEALTH & WELFARE BLDG-
7TH AND FORSTER ST
HARRISBURG, PA 17120
PO BOX 2675
HARRISBURG, PA 17105-2675
TEL: (717) 787-1870
FAX: (717) 787-4639
TOLL FREE: (800) 537-8862

600 NEW LONDON AVE
CRANSTON, RI 02920-3037
TEL: (401) 462-3575

700 GOVERNORS DR- KNIEP
BLDG
PIERRE, SD 57501-2291
TEL: (605) 945-5006
FAX: (605) 773-5246
IN-STATE: (800) 452-7691

729 CHURCH ST- 3RD FL
NASHVILLE, TN 37243
TEL: (615) 255-8313
FAX: (615) 254-7728
IN-STATE: (800) 821-8186

288 N 1460 W
SALT LAKE CITY, UT 84116
PO BOX 143106
SALT LAKE CITY, UT 84114-3106
TEL: (801) 538-6451
FAX: (801) 538-6952
TOLL FREE: (800) 662-9651
IN-STATE: (800) 662-9651

6406 BRIDGE RD
MADISON, WI 53784-1846
TEL: (608) 221-4746

MEDICAL MUTUAL OF OHIO

3737 W SALVANIA AVE
TOLEDO, OH 43623-4422
PO BOX 943
TOLEDO, OH 43656-0001
TEL: (419) 473-6403
FAX: (419) 473-6200
TOLL FREE: (800) 700-2583

6715 TIPPECANOE RD - BLDG C,
STE 201
CANFIELD, OH 44406-8180
TEL: (330) 702-2890
TOLL FREE: (800) 458-6813

2060 E 9TH ST
CLEVELAND, OH 44115
PO BOX 6018
CLEVELAND, OH 44101
TEL: (216) 522-8622
FAX: (216) 694-2910
TOLL FREE: (800) 233-2058

2060 READING RD, STE 300
CINCINNATI, OH 45202-1455
TEL: (513) 684-8100
TOLL FREE: (800) 272-1660

MEDICARE — PART A

400 E COURT AVE
DES MOINES, IA 50309-2017
TEL: (515) 471-7300
FAX: (515) 471-7222

400 E COURT AVE
DES MOINES, IA 50309-2017
TEL: (515) 471-7300
FAX: (515) 471-7222

400 E COURT AVE
DES MOINES, IA 50309-2017
TEL: (515) 471-7300
FAX: (515) 471-7222

400 E COURT AVE
DES MOINES, IA 50309-2017
TEL: (515) 471-7300
FAX: (515) 471-7222

400 E COURT AVE
DES MOINES, IA 50309-2017
TEL: (515) 471-7300
FAX: (515) 471-7222

400 E COURT AVE
DES MOINES, IA 50309-2017
TEL: (515) 471-7300
FAX: (515) 471-7222

400 E COURT AVE
DES MOINES, IA 50309-2017
TEL: (515) 471-7300
FAX: (515) 471-7222

400 E COURT AVE
DES MOINES, IA 50309-2017
TEL: (515) 471-7300
FAX: (515) 471-7222

400 E COURT AVE
DES MOINES, IA 50309-2017
TEL: (515) 471-7300
FAX: (515) 471-7222

400 E COURT AVE
DES MOINES, IA 50309-2017
TEL: (515) 471-7300
FAX: (515) 471-7222

400 E COURT AVE
DES MOINES, IA 50309-2017
TEL: (515) 471-7300
FAX: (515) 471-7222

MEDICARE — PART A
INTERMEDIARIES
2444 W LAS PAMARITAS DR
PHOENIX, AZ 85021
PO BOX 13466
PHOENIX, AZ 85002-3466
TEL: (602) 864-4100
FAX: (602) 864-4653

601 S GAINES ST
LITTLE ROCK, AR 72201
PO BOX 2181
LITTLE ROCK, AR 72203-2181
TEL: (501) 378-2000
FAX: (501) 378-2576
TOLL FREE: (800) 813-8868

21555 OXNARD ST
VAN NUYS, CA 91367
PO BOX 70000
VAN NUYS, CA 91470
TEL: (818) 703-2345
FAX: (818) 703-2848
TOLL FREE: (800) 234-0111

2357 WARM SPRINGS RD
COLUMBUS, GA 31904
PO BOX 9907
COLUMBUS, GA 31908
TEL: (706) 571-5371
FAX: (706) 571-5431

450 COLUMBUS BLVD
HARTFORD, CT 06103
PO BOX 150450
HARTFORD, CT 06115-0450
TEL: (860) 702-6669
FAX: (860) 702-6587

8115 KNUE RD
INDIANAPOLIS, IN 46250
PO BOX 37630
INDIANAPOLIS, IN 46250
TEL: (317) 841-4400
FAX: (317) 841-4691
TOLL FREE: (800) 999-7608

400 E COURT AVE
DES MOINES, IA 50309-2017
TEL: (515) 471-7300
FAX: (515) 471-7222

1133 SW TOPEKA BLVD
TOPEKA, KS 66601
TEL: (785) 291-7000
FAX: (785) 291-6924

3535 BLUE CROSS RD
SAINT PAUL, MN 55122
PO BOX 64560
SAINT PAUL, MN 55164
TEL: (651) 662-8000
FAX: (651) 662-2745
TOLL FREE: (800) 382-2000

4305 13TH AVE SW
FARGO, ND 58103
TEL: (701) 277-2655
FAX: (701) 277-2196

450 COLUMBUS BLVD
HARTFORD, CT 06103
PO BOX 150450
HARTFORD, CT 06115
TEL: (860) 702-6669
FAX: (860) 702-6587

1064 FLINT DR
JACKSON, MS 39208
PO BOX 23046
JACKSON, MS 39225-3046
TEL: (601) 936-0105
FAX: (601) 932-9233

450 COLUMBUS BLVD
HARTFORD, CT 06103
PO BOX 150450
HARTFORD, CT 06115-0450
TEL: (860) 702-6669
FAX: (860) 702-6587

1133 SW TOPEKA BLVD
TOPEKA, KS 66601
TEL: (785) 291-7000
FAX: (785) 291-6924

340 N LAST CHANCE GULCH
HELENA, MT 59601-5012
PO BOX 4309
HELENA, MT 59604-4309
TEL: (406) 791-4000
FAX: (406) 791-4119
TOLL FREE: (800) 447-7828

1800 CENTER ST
CAMP HILL, PA 17011
PO BOX 890089
CAMP HILL, PA 17089-0089
TEL: (717) 763-3151
FAX: (717) 763-3544

532 RIVERSIDE AVE- 17TH &
    18TH FLS
JACKSONVILLE, FL 32202
PO BOX 2711
JACKSONVILLE, FL 32231
TEL: (904) 355-8899
FAX: (904) 791-8296
IN-STATE: (800) 333-7586

HWY 79, 346 HOLMER RD
MINDEN, LA 71055
TEL: (318) 377-7387
TOLL FREE: (800) 772-1213

730 CHESTNUT ST
CHATTANOOGA, TN 37402-
    1790
TEL: (423) 755-5950

7261 MERCY RD
OMAHA, NE 68124-2349
PO BOX 24563
OMAHA, NE 68124-0563
TEL: (402) 390-1850
FAX: (402) 398-3640

1133 SW TOPEKA BLVD
TOPEKA, KS 66601
TEL: (785) 291-7000
FAX: (785) 291-6924

3000 GOFFS FALLS RD
MANCHESTER, NH 03111
TEL: (603) 695-7204
FAX: (603) 695-7741

33 WASHINGTON ST, FL 2
NEWARK, NJ 07102
PO BOX 1236
NEWARK, NJ 07101
TEL: (973) 456-2112
FAX: (973) 456-2086

ONE WORLD TRADE CENTER
SYRACUSE, NY 10048
PO BOX 4846
SYRACUSE, NY 13221-4846
TEL: (315) 442-4400
FAX: (315) 442-4815
TOLL FREE: (800) 442-8430

1901 MAIN ST
BUFFALO, NY 14208
PO BOX 80
BUFFALO, NY 14240
TEL: (716) 887-6900
FAX: (716) 887-7912
TOLL FREE: (800) 252-6550
IN-STATE: (800) 695-2583

Appendix 7

4305 13TH AVE SW
FARGO, ND 58103-3309
PO BOX 6706
FARGO, ND 58108-6706
TEL: (701) 277-2655
FAX: (701) 277-2196

4361 ERWIN SIMPSON RD
MASON, OH 45040
TEL: (513) 872-8100
FAX: (513) 852-4562

1215 S BOULDER AVE
TULSA, OK 74119
PO BOX 3404
TULSA, OK 74101
TEL: (918) 560-2090
FAX: (918) 560-3506

450 COLUMBUS BLVD
HARTFORD, CT 06103
PO BOX 150450
HARTFORD, CT 06115
TEL: (860) 702-6669
FAX: (860) 702-6587

444 WESTMINSTER ST
PROVIDENCE, RI 02903
TEL: (401) 455-0177
FAX: (401) 459-1709
TOLL FREE: (800) 662-5170

3000 GOFFS FALLS RD
MANCHESTER, NH 03111
TEL: (603) 695-7204
FAX: (603) 695-7741

450 COLUMBUS BLVD
HARTFORD, CT 06103
PO BOX 150450
HARTFORD, CT 06115
TEL: (860) 702-6669
FAX: (860) 702-6587

PO BOX 16788
COLUMBUS, OH 43216-6788
TEL: (614) 277-6100
FAX: (614) 277-6802
TOLL FREE: (800) 282-0530

4000 HOUSE AVE
CHEYENNE, WY 82001
PO BOX 908
CHEYENNE, WY 82003
TEL: (307) 432-2860
FAX: (307) 632-1654
IN-STATE: (800) 442-2376

MEDICARE — PART B CARRIERS
1149 S BROADWAY

LOS ANGELES, CA 90015
PO BOX 54905
LOS ANGELES, CA 90054
TEL: (213) 742-3996
FAX: (213) 741-6803
TOLL FREE:

402 OTTERSON DR
CHICO, CA 95928
TEL: (530) 896-7025
FAX: (530) 896-7182

425 N 21ST ST
CAMP HILL, PA 17011
PO BOX 890101
CAMP HILL, PA 17089-0101
TEL: (717) 972-8699

532 RIVERSIDE AVE, 17TH FL
JACKSONVILLE, FL 32202
PO BOX 2360
JACKSONVILLE, FL 32231
TEL: (904) 634-4994
FAX: (904) 791-8378
IN-STATE: (800) 333-7586

8115 KNUE RD
INDIANAPOLIS, IN 46250
TEL: (317) 845-2992
FAX: (317) 841-4691
TOLL FREE: (800) 999-7608

1133 SW TOPEKA BLVD
TOPEKA, KS 66629
PO BOX 239
TOPEKA, KS 66601
TEL: (785) 291-4003
FAX: (785) 291-8532

1133 SW TOPEKA AVE
TOPEKA, KS 66629
PO BOX 239
TOPEKA, KS 66601
TEL: (785) 291-4003
FAX: (785) 291-8532

444 WESTMINSTER ST
PROVIDENCE, RI 02903
TEL: (401) 272-3131

4305 16TH AVE S
FARGO, ND 58103-3373
PO BOX 6701
FARGO, ND 58103
TOLL FREE: (800) 444-4606
IN-STATE: (800) 332-6681

701 NW 63RD ST
OKLAHOMA CITY, OK 73116
TEL: (405) 843-9379

1133 SW TOPEKA AVE
TOPEKA, KS 66629
PO BOX 239
TOPEKA, KS 66601
TEL: (785) 291-4003
FAX: (785) 291-8532

1901 MAIN ST, STE 1
BUFFALO, NY 14208
PO BOX 80
BUFFALO, NY 14240-0080
TEL: (716) 887-6900
TOLL FREE: (800) 950-0051

PO BOX 16786
COLUMBUS, OH 43216-6786
TEL: (614) 277-1199
FAX: (614) 277-6805
TOLL FREE: (800) 282-0530

3400 S PARK PL
COLUMBUS, OH 43123
PO BOX 57
COLUMBUS, OH 43216-0057
FAX: (614) 249-4467
TOLL FREE: (800) 282-0530
IN-STATE: (800) 848-0106

4305 13TH AVE SW
FARGO, ND 58103
TEL: (701) 277-2655
FAX: (701) 282-1002
TOLL FREE: (800) 874-2656
IN-STATE: (800) 247-2267

300 ARBOR LK DR, STE 1300
COLUMBIA, SC 29223
PO BOX 100190
COLUMBIA, SC 29202
TEL: (803) 788-5568
FAX: (803) 691-2188

2890 COTTONWOOD PKY
SALT LAKE CITY, UT 84121
PO BOX 30269
SALT LAKE CITY, UT 84030
TEL: (801) 333-2440
FAX: (801) 333-6505
IN-STATE: (800) 426-3477

3400 S PARK PL
COLUMBUS, OH 43123
PO BOX 57
COLUMBUS, OH 43216-0057
TEL:
FAX: (614) 249-4467
TOLL FREE: (800) 282-0530
IN-STATE: (800) 848-0106

PO BOX 1787
MADISON, WI 53701-1787
TEL: (608) 221-3218
IN-STATE: (800) 944-0051

MENNONITE MUTUAL AID ASSOCIATION
1110 N MAIN ST
GOSHEN, IN 46528
PO BOX 483
GOSHEN, IN 46526-0483
TEL: (219) 533-9511
FAX: (219) 533-5264
TOLL FREE: (800) 348-7468

MICHIGAN FARM BUREAU MUTUAL INSURANCE CO
7373 W SAGINAW
LANSING, MI 48917
PO BOX 30100
LANSING, MI 48909
TEL: (517) 323-7000
FAX: (517) 323-6793
TOLL FREE: (800) 292-2680

MID-SOUTH INSURANCE CO
4317 RAMSEY ST
FAYETTEVILLE, NC 28303
PO BOX 2547
FAYETTEVILLE, NC 28311
TEL: (910) 822-1020
FAX: (910) 822-3018
TOLL FREE: (800) 822-9993

MIDWEST SECURITY ADMINISTRATORS
1150 SPRINGHURST DR, STE 140
GREEN BAY, WI 54304
PO BOX 19035
GREEN BAY, WI 54307-9035
TEL: (920) 496-2500

MIDWEST SECURITY INSURANCE CO
2700 MIDWEST DR
ONALASKA, WI 54650
TEL: (608) 783-7130
FAX: (608) 783-8581
TOLL FREE: (800) 542-6642

2700 MIDWEST DR
ONALASKA, WI 54650
TEL: (608) 783-7130
FAX: (608) 783-8581
TOLL FREE: (800) 542-6642

2700 MIDWEST DR
ONALASKA, WI 54650
TEL: (608) 783-7130
FAX: (608) 783-8581
TOLL FREE: (800) 542-6642

2700 MIDWEST DR
ONALASKA, WI 54650
TEL: (608) 783-7130
FAX: (608) 783-8581
TOLL FREE: (800) 542-6642

2700 MIDWEST DR
ONALASKA, WI 54650
TEL: (608) 783-7130
FAX: (608) 783-8581
TOLL FREE: (800) 542-6642

MILLENNIUM CARE ADMINISTRATORS (DBA MCA ADMINISTRATORS)
5900 ROCHE DR- 5TH FL
COLUMBUS, OH 43229
PO BOX 18245
COLUMBUS, OH 43218-0245
TEL: (614) 888-1212
FAX: (614) 888-2240
TOLL FREE: (800) 229-6786
IN-STATE: (800) 524-4426

MILLETTE ADMINISTRATORS, INC
4619 MAIN ST, STE A
MOSS POINT, MS 39563
TEL: (228) 475-8687
TOLL FREE: (800) 456-8647

NALC HEALTH BENEFIT PLAN
20547 WAVERLY CT
ASHBURN, VA 20149-0001
TEL: (703) 729-4677
FAX: (703) 729-0076
TOLL FREE: (800) 548-8484

NAPUS HEALTH BENEFIT PLAN
550 12TH ST SW
WASHINGTON, DC 20065
TEL: (202) 479-8000
FAX: (202) 479-3520
TOLL FREE: (800) 424-7474

NATIONAL HEALTH PLANS
1005 W ORANGEBURG, STE B
MODESTO, CA 95350-4163
PO BOX 5356
MODESTO, CA 95352
TEL: (209) 527-3350
FAX: (209) 527-6773
TOLL FREE: (800) 468-8600

NATIONAL TRAVELERS LIFE INSURANCE CO
5700 WESTOWN PKY
WEST DES MOINES, IA 50266
PO BOX 9197
WEST DES MOINES, IA 50266-9197
TEL: (515) 221-0101
FAX: (515) 327-5830
TOLL FREE: (800) 232-5818

NATIONWIDE LIFE INSURANCE CO
ONE NATIONWIDE PLZ
COLUMBUS, OH 43215
PO BOX 2399
COLUMBUS, OH 43216-2399
TEL: (614) 249-7111
FAX: (614) 249-7705
TOLL FREE: (800) 772-9956

NORTHEAST MEDICAL CENTER
920 CHURCH ST N
CONCORD, NC 28025
TEL: (704) 783-3000
FAX: (704) 783-1487
TOLL FREE: (800) 842-6868

NORTHWEST WASHINGTON MEDICAL BUREAU
333 E GILKEY RD
BURLINGTON, WA 98233-2823
TEL: (360) 755-4000
FAX: (360) 755-4567
TOLL FREE: (800) 659-7229

NYL CARE
2425 WEST LOOP S, STE 1000
HOUSTON, TX 77027
PO BOX 56228
HOUSTON, TX 77027-0228
TEL: (713) 624-5000
FAX: (713) 354-7002
TOLL FREE: (800) 833-5318

ODS HEALTH PLAN
601 SW 2ND AVE
PORTLAND, OR 97204-3156
PO BOX 40384
PORTLAND, OR 97240
TEL: (503) 228-6554
FAX: (503) 243-5105
TOLL FREE: (800) 852-5195

OLYMPIC HEALTH MANAGEMENT
PO BOX 5348
BELLINGHAM, WA 98227
TEL: (360) 647-9080
FAX: (360) 734-6199
TOLL FREE: (800) 533-3941

PACIFIC INDEMNITY CO
801 S FIGUROA ST
LOS ANGELES, CA 90017
PO BOX 30850
LOS ANGELES, CA 90030-0850
TEL: (213) 612-0880
FAX: (213) 612-5731
TOLL FREE: (800) 262-4459

PACIFICARE HEALTH SYSTEMS, INC
HILLSBORO, OR
PO BOX 3007
HILLSBORO, OR 97123
TEL: (503) 533-6300
FAX: (503) 533-6335
TOLL FREE: (800) 922-1444

PAN AMERICAN LIFE INSURANCE CO
601 POYDRAS ST
NEW ORLEANS, LA 70130
PO BOX 60219
NEW ORLEANS, LA 70130
TEL: (504) 566-1300
FAX: (504) 523-8584
TOLL FREE: (800) 227-3417

PARTNERS NATIONAL HEALTH PLANS
2085 FRONTIS PLZ BLVD
WINSTON-SALEM, NC 27114
PO BOX 17268
WINSTON-SALEM, NC 27116
TEL: (336) 760-4822
FAX: (336) 760-3198
TOLL FREE: (800) 942-5695
IN-STATE: (800) 942-5695

2085 FRONTIS PLZ BLVD
WINSTON-SALEM, NC 27114
PO BOX 17268
WINSTON-SALEM, NC 27116
TEL: (336) 760-4822
FAX: (336) 760-3198
TOLL FREE: (800) 942-5695
IN-STATE: (800) 942-5695

2085 FRONTIS PLZ BLVD
WINSTON-SALEM, NC 27114
PO BOX 17268
WINSTON-SALEM, NC 27116
TEL: (336) 760-4822
FAX: (336) 760-3198
TOLL FREE: (800) 942-5695
IN-STATE: (800) 942-5695

PAULA INSURANCE CO
1780 E BULLARD, STE 101
FRESNO, CA 93710
PO BOX 40009
FRESNO, CA 93755-0009
TEL: (559) 439-3330
FAX: (559) 439-3505

PEER REVIEW ORGANIZATIONS
40600 ANN ARBOR RD, STE 200
PLYMOUTH, MI 48170-4486
TEL: (734) 459-0900

PERSONAL INSURANCE ADMINISTRATORS
PO BOX 5004
THOUSAND OAKS, CA 91359
TEL: (805) 777-0032
FAX: (805) 777-0033
TOLL FREE: (800) 468-4343

PERSONALCARE HEALTH MANAGEMENT
210 BOX DR
CHAMPAIGN, IL 61820-7399
TEL: (217) 366-1226
FAX: (217) 366-5410
TOLL FREE: (800) 431-1211

210 BOX DR
CHAMPAIGN, IL 61820-7399
TEL: (217) 366-1226
FAX: (217) 366-5410
TOLL FREE: (800) 431-1211

PHARMACIST MUTUAL
808 U.S. HWY 18 W
ALGONA, IA 50511
PO BOX 370
ALGONA, IA 50511-0370
TEL: (515) 295-2461
FAX: (515) 295-9306
TOLL FREE: (800) 247-5930

PHICO
ONE PHICO DR
MECHANICSBURG, PA 17055
PO BOX 85
MECHANICSBURG, PA 17055-0085
TEL: (717) 691-1600
FAX: (717) 766-2837
TOLL FREE: (800) 627-4626

PHS HEALTH PLANS
ONE FAR MILL CROSSING
SHELTON, CT 06484
PO BOX 904
SHELTON, CT 06484-0944
TEL: (203) 381-6400
FAX: (203) 225-4000
IN-STATE: (800) 848-4747

ONE FAR MILL CROSSING
SHELTON, CT 06484
PO BOX 904
SHELTON, CT 06484-0944
TEL: (203) 381-6400
FAX: (203) 225-4000
IN-STATE: (800) 848-4747

ONE FAR MILL CROSSING
SHELTON, CT 06484
PO BOX 904
SHELTON, CT 06484-0944
TEL: (203) 381-6400
FAX: (203) 225-4000
IN-STATE: (800) 848-4747

PHYSICIANS BENEFITS TRUST
1440 N NORTHWEST HWY
PARK RIDGE, IL 60068-1400
TEL:
FAX: (312) 541-4589
TOLL FREE: (800) 621-0748

PHYSICIANS HEALTH PLAN OF NORTHERN INDIANA, INC
8101 W JEFFERSON BLVD
FORT WAYNE, IN 46804
PO BOX 2359
FORT WAYNE, IN 46801-2359
TEL: (219) 432-6690
FAX: (219) 432-0493
TOLL FREE: (800) 982-6257

PLAN OF BLUE CROSS - BLUE SHIELD OF MONTANA
404 FULLER AVE
GREAT FALLS, MT 59403
PO BOX 5004
GREAT FALLS, MT 59403
TEL: (406) 447-8600
TOLL FREE: (800) 447-7828

PREFERRED HEALTH NETWORK
1099 WINTERSON RD
LINTHICUM HEIGHTS, MD 21090
TEL: (410) 850-7461
TOLL FREE: (800) 422-1996

PREFERRED HEALTH SYSTEMS INSURANCE CO
8535 E 21ST ST N
WICHITA, KS 67206
PO BOX 49288
WICHITA, KS 67201-9288
TEL: (316) 609-2345
FAX: (316) 609-2346
TOLL FREE: (800) 660-8114

8535 E 21ST ST N
WICHITA, KS 67206
PO BOX 49218
WICHITA, KS 67201-9218
TEL: (316) 609-2390
FAX: (316) 609-2327
TOLL FREE: (800) 660-8114

PREMERA BLUE CROSS
7001 220TH ST SW
MOUNTLAKE TERRACE, WA 98043-2160
PO BOX 327
MOUNTLAKE TERRACE, WA 98111
TEL: (425) 670-4700
FAX: (425) 670-5457
TOLL FREE: (800) 527-6675

3900 E SPRAGUE
SPOKANE, WA 99202-4847
PO BOX 3048
SPOKANE, WA 99220-3048
TEL: (509) 536-4700
FAX: (509) 536-4771
TOLL FREE: (800) 835-3510
IN-STATE: (800) 572-0778

7001 220TH ST SW
MOUNTLAKE TERRACE, WA 98043-2160
PO BOX 327
MOUNTLAKE TERRACE, WA 98111
TEL: (425) 670-4700
FAX: (425) 670-5457
TOLL FREE: (800) 527-6675

3900 E SPRAGUE
SPOKANE, WA 99202-4847
PO BOX 3048
SPOKANE, WA 99220-3048
TEL: (509) 536-4700
FAX: (509) 536-4771
TOLL FREE: (800) 835-3510
IN-STATE: (800) 572-0778

PRESBYTERIAN HEALTH PLAN / FHP OF NEW MEXICO
PO BOX 27489
ALBUQUERQUE, NM 87125
TEL: (505) 923-5799
FAX: (505) 923-5277
TOLL FREE: (800) 356-2884
IN-STATE: (800) 356-2219

PRIME HEALTH OF ALABAMA
1400 UNIVERSITY BLVD S
MOBILE, AL 36609
PO BOX 851239
MOBILE, AL 36685-1239
TEL: (334) 342-0022
FAX: (334) 380-3236
TOLL FREE: (800) 544-9449

PRINCIPAL FINANCIAL GROUP
1245 CORPORATE BLVD, STE 200
AURORA, IL 60504-9955
TEL: (630) 978-5100
FAX: (630) 978-5117

1245 CORPORATE BLVD, STE 200
AURORA, IL 60504-9955
TEL: (630) 978-5100
FAX: (630) 978-5117

1245 CORPORATE BLVD, STE 200
AURORA, IL 60504-9955
TEL: (630) 978-5100
FAX: (630) 978-5117

620 S GLENSTONE AVE, STE 300
SPRINGFIELD, MO 65802
PO BOX 2593
SPRINGFIELD, MO 65801-2593
TEL: (417) 877-0085
TOLL FREE: (800) 422-5002

1245 CORPORATE BLVD, STE 200
AURORA, IL 60504-9955
TEL: (630) 978-5100
FAX: (630) 978-5117

620 S GLENSTONE AVE, STE 300
SPRINGFIELD, MO 65802
PO BOX 2593
SPRINGFIELD, MO 65801-2593
TEL: (417) 877-0085
TOLL FREE: (800) 422-5002

PRIORITY HEALTH
1111 E HERNDON, STE 202
FRESNO, CA 93720-3100
PO BOX 25790
FRESNO, CA 93729-8790
TEL: (559) 435-8366
FAX: (559) 435-9718
TOLL FREE: (800) 350-8366

PROFESSIONAL ADMINISTRATION GROUP
PO BOX 13391
OVERLAND PARK, KS 66282-3391
TEL: (913) 327-7108
FAX: (913) 451-4762

PROFESSIONAL ADMINISTRATORS, INC
3751 MAGUIRE BLVD, STE 100
ORLANDO, FL 32803
PO BOX 140415
ORLANDO, FL 32814-0415
TEL: (407) 896-0521
FAX: (407) 897-6976
TOLL FREE: (800) 741-0521
IN-STATE: (800) 432-2686

PROFESSIONAL BENEFIT ADMINISTRATORS, INC
15 SPINNING WHEEL RD, STE 210
OAK BROOK, IL 60521
PO BOX 4687
OAK BROOK, IL 60522-4687
TEL: (630) 655-3755
FAX: (630) 655-3781

PROFESSIONAL RISK MANAGEMENT
2101 WEBSTER ST, STE 900
OAKLAND, CA 94612
TEL: (510) 452-9300
FAX: (510) 452-1479

PROTECTED HOME MUTUAL LIFE INSURANCE CO
30 E STATE ST
SHARON, PA 16146
TEL: (724) 981-1520
FAX: (724) 981-2682
TOLL FREE: (800) 223-8821
IN-STATE: (800) 222-8894

PROVIDENCE HEALTH PLANS
1501 FOURTH AVE, STE 600
SEATTLE, WA 98101
TEL: (206) 215-9000
TOLL FREE: (800) 443-0996

PRUDENTIAL HEALTH CARE PLAN, INC
HOUSTON, TX
PO BOX 4804
HOUSTON, TX 77210
TEL: (918) 624-4600
FAX: (918) 624-5050
TOLL FREE: (800) 345-8310

7700 CHEVY CHASE DR- BLDG 1, STE 500
AUSTIN, TX 78752
TEL: (512) 323-0440
FAX:
TOLL FREE: (800) 621-2645

PRUDENTIAL HEALTHCARE OF CALIFORNIA
5800 CANOGA AVE
WOODLAND HILLS, CA 91367
TEL: (818) 992-2000
FAX:
TOLL FREE: (800) 433-3150

PUBLIC EMPLOYEES HEALTH PROGRAM
560 E 200 S
SALT LAKE CITY, UT 84102-2020
TEL: (801) 366-7500
FAX: (801) 366-7596
TOLL FREE: (800) 933-7347

PYRAMID LIFE INSURANCE CO
6201 JOHNSON DR
SHAWNEE MISSION, KS 66202
PO BOX 772
SHAWNEE MISSION, KS 66201-0772
TEL: (913) 722-1110
FAX: (913) 722-3567
TOLL FREE: (800) 444-0321

QUEEN'S ISLAND CARE/QUEEN'S HEALTH PLAN
500 ALA MOANA BLVD, STE 200
HONOLULU, HI 96813
PO BOX 37549
HONOLULU, HI 96837
TEL: (808) 522-7500
FAX: (808) 522-8642
TOLL FREE: (800) 856-4668

RAYTHEON CO
141 SPRING ST
LEXINGTON, MA 02421
TEL: (781) 862-6600
FAX: (781) 860-2172
TOLL FREE: (800) 843-4121

REGENCE BLUE CROSS - BLUE SHIELD
201 HIGH ST SE
SALEM, OR 97308
PO BOX 12625
SALEM, OR 97309
TEL: (503) 585-0581
FAX: (503) 588-4350
TOLL FREE: (800) 228-0978

REGENCE BLUE CROSS - BLUE SHIELD
100 SW MARKET ST
PORTLAND, OR 97207
PO BOX 900
PORTLAND, OR 97207-0900
TEL: (503) 274-0761
FAX: (503) 375-4293
TOLL FREE: (800) 643-4512
IN-STATE: (800) 228-0978

100 SW MARKET ST
PORTLAND, OR 97207
PO BOX 900
PORTLAND, OR 97207-0900
TEL: (503) 274-0761
FAX: (503) 375-4293
TOLL FREE: (800) 643-4512
IN-STATE: (800) 228-0978

REGENCE BLUE CROSS - BLUE SHIELD
100 SW MARKET ST
PORTLAND, OR 97201
PO BOX 100
PORTLAND, OR 97207-0100
TEL: (503) 225-5227
TOLL FREE: (800) 452-7278

201 HIGH ST SE
SALEM, OR 97308
PO BOX 12625
SALEM, OR 97309
TEL: (503) 585-0581
FAX: (503) 588-4350
TOLL FREE: (800) 228-0978

REGENCE BLUE CROSS - BLUE SHIELD
100 SW MARKET ST
PORTLAND, OR 97207
PO BOX 900
PORTLAND, OR 97207-0900
TEL: (503) 274-0761
FAX: (503) 375-4293
TOLL FREE: (800) 643-4512
IN-STATE: (800) 228-0978

REGENCE BLUE CROSS - BLUE SHIELD
201 HIGH ST SE
SALEM, OR 97308
PO BOX 12625
SALEM, OR 97309
TEL: (503) 585-0581
FAX: (503) 588-4350
TOLL FREE: (800) 228-0978

REGENCE BLUE CROSS - BLUE SHIELD
100 SW MARKET ST
PORTLAND, OR 97207
PO BOX 900
PORTLAND, OR 97207-0900
TEL: (503) 274-0761
FAX: (503) 375-4293
TOLL FREE: (800) 643-4512
IN-STATE: (800) 228-0978

REGENCE BLUE SHIELD
1800 9TH AVE, STE 200
SEATTLE, WA 98101
PO BOX 91005
SEATTLE, WA 98111-9105
TEL: (206) 340-6600
FAX: (206) 389-6719
TOLL FREE: (800) 222-6129

REGENCE BLUE SHIELD OF IDAHO
1602 21ST AVE
LEWISTON, ID 83501
PO BOX 1106
LEWISTON, ID 83501-1106
TEL: (208) 746-2671
FAX: (208) 798-2090
TOLL FREE: (800) 632-2022

REGENCY EMPLOYEE BENEFITS
330 SUPERIOR MALL
PORT HURON, MI 48060
PO BOX 610609
PORT HURON, MI 48061-0609
TEL: (810) 987-7711
FAX: (810) 987-7603
TOLL FREE: (800) 369-3718

REINSURANCE MANAGEMENT, INC
9485 REGENCY SQUARE BLVD, STE 220
JACKSONVILLE, FL 32225
TEL: (904) 727-5088
FAX: (904) 727-7892
TOLL FREE: (800) 830-3856

RESOURCE PARTNER
180 E BROAD ST
COLUMBUS, OH 43215
PO BOX 189
COLUMBUS, OH 43216-0189
TEL: (614) 220-5001
FAX: (614) 220-5033
TOLL FREE: (800) 848-6181

RISK MANAGEMENT RESOURCES, INC
11161 ANDERSON ST, STE 200
LOMA LINDA, CA 92354-2825
PO BOX 1770
LOMA LINDA, CA 92354-0570
TEL: (909) 824-4386
FAX: (909) 824-4775

RIVERBEND GOVERNMENT BENEFITS ADMINISTRATOR
730 CHESTNUT ST
CHATTANOOGA, TN 37402
TEL: (423) 755-5783
FAX: (423) 752-6518

RMSCO, INC
115 CONTINUM DR
LIVERPOOL, NY 13088
PO BOX 6309
LIVERPOOL, NY 13217
TEL: (315) 474-8200
FAX: (315) 476-8440

ROBERT, BOUCK & ASSOCIATES
126 N 30TH ST, STE 205
QUINCY, IL 62301
TEL: (217) 223-8354
FAX: (217) 223-8621

ROBERT S. WEISS & CO
SILVER HILLS BUS CTR- 500 S BROAD ST
MERIDEN, CT 06450
PO BOX 1034
MERIDEN, CT 06450-1034
TEL: (203) 235-6882
FAX: (203) 639-7422
TOLL FREE: (800) 466-7900

ROCKFORD HEALTH PLANS
3401 N PERRYVILLE RD
ROCKFORD, IL 61114
TEL: (815) 654-3600
FAX: (815) 282-0634
TOLL FREE: (800) 331-0424

ROCKY MOUNTAIN HMO
2775 CROSSROADS BLVD
GRAND JUNCTION, CO 81506
PO BOX 10600
GRAND JUNCTION, CO 81502
TEL: (970) 244-7760
FAX: (970) 244-7880
TOLL FREE: (800) 843-0719
IN-STATE: (800) 843-0719

ROYAL STATE GROUP
819 S BERETANIA ST, STE 100
HONOLULU, HI 96813
TEL: (808) 539-1600
FAX: (808) 538-1458

ROYAL & SUNALLIANCE

801 N BRAND BLVD, STE 500
GLENDALE, CA 91203
PO BOX 29035
GLENDALE, CA 91209-9035
TEL: (818) 241-5212
FAX: (818) 543-6393
TOLL FREE: (800) 252-0431

80 WOLF RD, STE 606
ALBANY, NY 12212
TEL: (315) 426-4000
TOLL FREE: (800) 553-2556

300 E LOMBARD ST, STE 700
BALTIMORE, MD 21202
TEL: (410) 685-5844
FAX: (410) 637-1699
TOLL FREE: (800) 482-4446

25 NEW CHARDON ST
BOSTON, MA 02114
PO BOX 8088
BOSTON, MA 02114-8808
TEL: (617) 742-7750
FAX: (617) 557-4252
TOLL FREE: (800) 367-7036
IN-STATE: (800) 367-7036

80 WOLF RD, STE 606
ALBANY, NY 12212
TEL: (315) 426-4000
TOLL FREE: (800) 553-2556

80 WOLF RD, STE 606
ALBANY, NY 12212
TEL: (315) 426-4000
TOLL FREE: (800) 553-2556

255 E 5TH ST, STE 2100
CINCINNATI, OH 45202
TEL: (513) 421-2183
FAX: (513) 357-9580
TOLL FREE: (800) 843-5772

SAFECO INSURANCE CO OF AMERICA

2055 SUGARLOAF CIR
DULUTH, GA 30097
TEL: (678) 417-3000
FAX: (770) 879-3333
TOLL FREE: (800) 241-2279

3637 S GEYER RD
SAINT LOUIS, MO 63127
PO BOX 66783
SAINT LOUIS, MO 63166
TEL: (314) 957-4500
FAX: (314) 957-4630
TOLL FREE: (800) 843-1487

330 N BRAND BLVD, STE 900
GLENDALE, CA 91203
PO BOX 29082
GLENDALE, CA 91029-9082
TEL: (818) 956-4200
FAX: (818) 956-4259
TOLL FREE: (800) 826-8921

5901 E GALBRAITH RD, STE 2
CINCINNATI, OH 45236
PO BOX 36177
CINCINNATI, OH 45236-0177
TEL: (513) 745-5861
FAX: (513) 745-5810
TOLL FREE: (800) 543-7138

SAN DIEGO ELECTRICAL HEALTH & WELFARE TRUST

SAN DIEGO, CA
PO BOX 231219
SAN DIEGO, CA 92194-1219
TEL: (858) 569-6322
FAX: (858) 573-0830
TOLL FREE: (800) 632-2569

SEABURY & SMITH

2615 NORTHGATE DR
IOWA CITY, IA 52245
PO BOX 1520
IOWA CITY, IA 52244-1520
TEL: (319) 351-2667
FAX: (319) 351-0603
TOLL FREE: (800) 562-4023

SECURITY HEALTH PLAN OF WISCONSIN, INC

1515 SAINT JOSEPH AVE
MARSHFIELD, WI 54449
PO BOX 8000
MARSHFIELD, WI 54449-8000
TEL: (715) 221-9555
FAX: (715) 221-9500
TOLL FREE: (800) 472-2363

SELF INSURED SERVICES CO

300 SECURITY BLDG
DUBUQUE, IA 52001
PO BOX 389
DUBUQUE, IA 52004-0389
TEL: (319) 583-7344
FAX: (319) 583-0439

SENTRY INSURANCE MUTUAL CO

3 CARLISLE RD
WESTFORD, MA 01886
PO BOX 584
WESTFORD, MA 01886-0584
TEL: (978) 392-7000
FAX: (978) 392-7033
TOLL FREE: (800) 225-1390

1800 N POINT DR
STEVENS POINT, WI 54481
TEL: (715) 346-6000
FAX: (715) 346-6161
TOLL FREE: (800) 638-8763

SHELTER INSURANCE COMPANIES

1817 W BROADWAY
COLUMBIA, MO 65218-0001
TEL: (573) 445-8441
FAX: (573) 445-3199
TOLL FREE: (800) 743-5837

1817 W BROADWAY
COLUMBIA, MO 65218-0001
TEL: (573) 445-8441
FAX: (573) 445-3199
TOLL FREE: (800) 743-5837

1817 W BROADWAY
COLUMBIA, MO 65218-0001
TEL: (573) 445-8441
FAX: (573) 445-3199
TOLL FREE: (800) 743-5837

1817 W BROADWAY
COLUMBIA, MO 65218-0001
TEL: (573) 445-8441
FAX: (573) 445-3199
TOLL FREE: (800) 743-5837

1817 W BROADWAY
COLUMBIA, MO 65218-0001
TEL: (573) 445-8441
FAX: (573) 445-3199
TOLL FREE: (800) 743-5837

1817 W BROADWAY
COLUMBIA, MO 65218-0001
TEL: (573) 445-8441
FAX: (573) 445-3199
TOLL FREE: (800) 743-5837

1817 W BROADWAY
COLUMBIA, MO 65218-0001
TEL: (573) 445-8441
FAX: (573) 445-3199
TOLL FREE: (800) 743-5837

1817 W BROADWAY
COLUMBIA, MO 65218-0001
TEL: (573) 445-8441
FAX: (573) 445-3199
TOLL FREE: (800) 743-5837

1817 W BROADWAY
COLUMBIA, MO 65218-0001
TEL: (573) 445-8441
FAX: (573) 445-3199
TOLL FREE: (800) 743-5837

1817 W BROADWAY
COLUMBIA, MO 65218-0001
TEL: (573) 445-8441
FAX: (573) 445-3199
TOLL FREE: (800) 743-5837

1817 W BROADWAY
COLUMBIA, MO 65218-0001
TEL: (573) 445-8441
FAX: (573) 445-3199
TOLL FREE: (800) 743-5837

1817 W BROADWAY
COLUMBIA, MO 65218-0001
TEL: (573) 445-8441
FAX: (573) 445-3199
TOLL FREE: (800) 743-5837

SIGMA ADMINISTRATORS
111 E 5600 S, STE 305
SALT LAKE CITY, UT 84107
PO BOX 57767
SALT LAKE CITY, UT 84157-0767
TEL: (801) 263-3300
FAX: (801) 263-3319

SIGNA HEALTHCARE
100 FRONT ST, STE 300
WORCESTER , MA 01608
TEL: (508) 799-2642
FAX: (508) 849-4299
TOLL FREE: (800) 244-1870
IN-STATE: (800) 922-8380

SILVER STATE MEDICAL ADMINISTRATORS
2720 N TENAYA WY
LAS VEGAS, NV 89128
PO BOX 15392
LAS VEGAS, NV 89114-5392
TEL: (702) 242-7800
FAX: (800) 869-2477

SOUTHERN BENEFIT ADMINISTRATORS, INC
2001 CALDWELL DR
GOODLETTSVILLE, TN 37072
PO BOX 1449
GOODLETTSVILLE, TN 37070-1449
TEL: (615) 859-0131
FAX: (615) 859-0818
TOLL FREE: (800) 831-4914

SOUTHERN CALIFORNIA PIPE TRADES TRUST FUND
501 SHATTO PL- 5TH FL
LOS ANGELES, CA 90020-1713
TEL: (213) 385-6161
FAX: (213) 487-3640
IN-STATE: (800) 595-7473

SOUTHERN GROUP ADMINISTRATORS, INC
200 S MARSHALL ST
WINSTON-SALEM, NC 27101-5251
TEL: (336) 723-7111
FAX: (336) 722-4748
TOLL FREE: (800) 334-8159

SOUTHERN GUARANTY INSURANCE CO
PO BOX 235004
MONTGOMERY, AL 36123-5004
TEL: (334) 270-6000
FAX: (334) 270-6115
TOLL FREE: (800) 633-5606

PO BOX 235004
MONTGOMERY, AL 36123-5004
TEL: (334) 270-6000
FAX: (334) 270-6115
TOLL FREE: (800) 633-5606

PO BOX 235004
MONTGOMERY, AL 36123-5004
TEL: (334) 270-6000
FAX: (334) 270-6115
TOLL FREE: (800) 633-5606

PO BOX 235004
MONTGOMERY, AL 36123-5004
TEL: (334) 270-6000
FAX: (334) 270-6115
TOLL FREE: (800) 633-5606

SOUTHERN HEALTH PLAN, INC
600 JEFFERSON AVE
CHATTANOOGA, TN 38101
PO BOX 180150
CHATTANOOGA, TN 37404
TEL: (901) 544-2636
FAX: (901) 544-2440
TOLL FREE: (800) 527-9206

SOUTHERN HEALTH SERVICES
9881 MAYLAND DR
RICHMOND, VA 23233-1411
PO BOX 85603
RICHMOND, VA 23285-5603
TEL: (804) 747-3700
FAX: (804) 747-8723
TOLL FREE: (800) 627-4872

SOUTHERN INSURANCE MANAGEMENT ASSOCIATION
1812 UNIVERSITY BLVD
TUSCALOOSA, AL 35401
PO BOX 1520
TUSCALOOSA, AL 35403-1520
TEL: (205) 345-3505
TOLL FREE: (800) 476-9928

SOUTHWEST ADMINISTRATORS
1000 S FREEMONT AVE- BLDG A9 WEST
ALHAMBRA, CA 91803
PO BOX 1121
ALHAMBRA, CA 91802-1121
TEL: (626) 284-4792

SPECIAL AGENTS MUTUAL BENEFIT ASSOCIATION

11301 OLD GEORGETOWN RD
ROCKVILLE, MD 20852-2800
TEL: (301) 984-1440
FAX: (301) 984-6224
TOLL FREE: (800) 638-6589

SPECTARA

2811 LORD BALTIMORE DR
BALTIMORE, MD 21244-2644
TEL: (410) 265-6033
FAX: (410) 944-5118
TOLL FREE: (800) 638-6265
IN-STATE: (800) 638-6265

2811 LORD BALTIMORE DR
BALTIMORE, MD 21244-2644
TEL: (410) 265-6033
FAX: (410) 944-5118
TOLL FREE: (800) 638-6265
IN-STATE: (800) 638-6265

2811 LORD BALTIMORE DR
BALTIMORE, MD 21244-2644
TEL: (410) 265-6033
FAX: (410) 944-5118
TOLL FREE: (800) 638-6265
IN-STATE: (800) 638-6265

2811 LORD BALTIMORE DR
BALTIMORE, MD 21244-2644
TEL: (410) 265-6033
FAX: (410) 944-5118
TOLL FREE: (800) 638-6265
IN-STATE: (800) 638-6265

ST. FRANCIS HOME CARE

414 PETTIGRU ST
GREENVILLE, SC 29601
PO BOX 9312
GREENVILLE, SC 29605
TEL: (864) 233-5300
FAX: (864) 233-4873

ST. LOUIS LABOR HEALTH INSTITUTE

300 S GRANDE BLVD
SAINT LOUIS, MO 63103-2430
TEL: (314) 658-5627
FAX: (314) 652-5022
TOLL FREE: (800) 466-5688

STANDARD LIFE & ACCIDENT INSURANCE CO

ONE MOODY PLZ
GALVESTON, TX 77550
PO BOX 1800
GALVESTON, TX 77553-1800
TEL: (405) 290-1000
FAX: (409) 766-6663
TOLL FREE: (800) 827-2524

STANTON GROUP

3405 ANNAPOLIS LN N, STE 100
PLYMOUTH, MN 55447
TEL: (763) 278-4000
FAX: (763) 278-4601
TOLL FREE: (800) 284-4464

STATE FARM INSURANCE CO

2980 S PRIEST DR
TEMPE, AZ 85282
TEL: (484) 636-3100
FAX: (484) 784-3870

304 N HERSHEY
BLOOMINGTON, IL 61702
PO BOX 2700
BLOOMINGTON, IL 61710
TEL: (309) 664-7000
TOLL FREE: (800) 538-4643

8900 AMBERGLEN BLVD
AUSTIN, TX 78729
TEL: (512) 918-4000
FAX: (512) 918-5298

STATE OF NEW YORK INSURANCE DEPARTMENT LIQUIDATION BUREAU

123 WILLIAM ST
NEW YORK, NY 10038-3804
TEL: (212) 341-6400
FAX: (212) 341-6104

TAYLOR EMPLOYEES HEALTH & DENTAL PLAN

1725 ROE CREST
NORTH MANKATO, MN 56002
PO BOX 3728
NORTH MANKATO, MN 56002-3728
TEL: (507) 625-2828
FAX: (507) 625-7742
TOLL FREE: (800) 345-6954

1725 ROE CREST
NORTH MANKATO, MN 56002
PO BOX 3728
NORTH MANKATO, MN 56002-3728
TEL: (507) 625-2828
FAX: (507) 625-7742
TOLL FREE: (800) 345-6954

1725 ROE CREST
NORTH MANKATO, MN 56002
PO BOX 3728
NORTH MANKATO, MN 56002-3728
TEL: (507) 625-2828
FAX: (507) 625-7742
TOLL FREE: (800) 345-6954

1725 ROE CREST
NORTH MANKATO, MN 56002
PO BOX 3728
NORTH MANKATO, MN 56002-3728
TEL: (507) 625-2828
FAX: (507) 625-7742
TOLL FREE: (800) 345-6954

1725 ROE CREST
NORTH MANKATO, MN 56002
PO BOX 3728
NORTH MANKATO, MN 56002-3728
TEL: (507) 625-2828
FAX: (507) 625-7742
TOLL FREE: (800) 345-6954

1725 ROE CREST
NORTH MANKATO, MN 56002
PO BOX 3728
NORTH MANKATO, MN 56002-3728
TEL: (507) 625-2828
FAX: (507) 625-7742
TOLL FREE: (800) 345-6954

1725 ROE CREST
NORTH MANKATO, MN 56002
PO BOX 3728
NORTH MANKATO, MN 56002-3728
TEL: (507) 625-2828
FAX: (507) 625-7742
TOLL FREE: (800) 345-6954

1725 ROE CREST
NORTH MANKATO, MN 56002
PO BOX 3728
NORTH MANKATO, MN 56002-
3728
TEL: (507) 625-2828
FAX: (507) 625-7742
TOLL FREE: (800) 345-6954

1725 ROE CREST
NORTH MANKATO, MN 56002
PO BOX 3728
NORTH MANKATO, MN 56002-
3728
TEL: (507) 625-2828
FAX: (507) 625-7742
TOLL FREE: (800) 345-6954

1725 ROE CREST
NORTH MANKATO, MN 56002
PO BOX 3728
NORTH MANKATO, MN 56002-
3728
TEL: (507) 625-2828
FAX: (507) 625-7742
TOLL FREE: (800) 345-6954

1725 ROE CREST
NORTH MANKATO, MN 56002
PO BOX 3728
NORTH MANKATO, MN 56002-
3728
TEL: (507) 625-2828
FAX: (507) 625-7742
TOLL FREE: (800) 345-6954

1725 ROE CREST
NORTH MANKATO, MN 56002
PO BOX 3728
NORTH MANKATO, MN 56002-
3728
TEL: (507) 625-2828
FAX: (507) 625-7742
TOLL FREE: (800) 345-6954

1725 ROE CREST
NORTH MANKATO, MN 56002
PO BOX 3728
NORTH MANKATO, MN 56002-
3728
TEL: (507) 625-2828
FAX: (507) 625-7742
TOLL FREE: (800) 345-6954

1725 ROE CREST
NORTH MANKATO, MN 56002
PO BOX 3728
NORTH MANKATO, MN 56002-
3728
TEL: (507) 625-2828
FAX: (507) 625-7742
TOLL FREE: (800) 345-6954

1725 ROE CREST
NORTH MANKATO, MN 56002
PO BOX 3728
NORTH MANKATO, MN 56002-
3728
TEL: (507) 625-2828
FAX: (507) 625-7742
TOLL FREE: (800) 345-6954

TEACHERS PROTECTIVE MUTUAL LIFE INSURANCE CO
116-118 N PRINCE ST
LANCASTER, PA 17603
PO BOX 597
LANCASTER, PA 17608-0597
TEL: (717) 394-7156
FAX: (717) 394-7024
TOLL FREE: (800) 555-3122

116-118 N PRINCE ST
LANCASTER, PA 17603
PO BOX 597
LANCASTER, PA 17608-0597
TEL: (717) 394-7156
FAX: (717) 394-7024
TOLL FREE: (800) 555-3122

116-118 N PRINCE ST
LANCASTER, PA 17603
PO BOX 597
LANCASTER, PA 17608-0597
TEL: (717) 394-7156
FAX: (717) 394-7024
TOLL FREE: (800) 555-3122

116-118 N PRINCE ST
LANCASTER, PA 17603
PO BOX 597
LANCASTER, PA 17608-0597
TEL: (717) 394-7156
FAX: (717) 394-7024
TOLL FREE: (800) 555-3122

116-118 N PRINCE ST
LANCASTER, PA 17603
PO BOX 597
LANCASTER, PA 17608-0597
TEL: (717) 394-7156
FAX: (717) 394-7024
TOLL FREE: (800) 555-3122

THE ALLIANCE
650 S CHERRY ST, STE 300
DENVER, CO 80246
TEL: (303) 333-6767
FAX: (303) 322-3830
TOLL FREE: (800) 996-2447

THE WHEELER COMPANIES
200 CAHABA PARK CIR, STE 250
BIRMINGHAM, AL 35242
PO BOX 43350
BIRMINGHAM, AL 35243-0350
TEL: (205) 995-8688
FAX: (205) 980-9047
TOLL FREE: (800) 741-8688

TOWER LIFE INSURANCE CO
TOWER LIFE BLDG, 310 S ST
   MARY ST, STE 400
SAN ANTONIO, TX 78205-3164
TEL: (210) 554-4400
FAX: (210) 554-4401
TOLL FREE: (800) 880-4576

TRIGON
PO BOX 27280
RICHMOND, VA 23261
TEL: (804) 358-1551
FAX: (804) 354-4340
IN-STATE: (800) 451-1527

TRIGON ADMINISTRATORS
7130 GLEN FOREST DR
RICHMOND, VA 23226
PO BOX 85631
RICHMOND, VA 23285-5631
TEL: (804) 673-5900
FAX: (804) 673-5400
TOLL FREE: (800) 368-8002

TRINITY UNIVERSAL INSURANCE CO
PO BOX 655028
DALLAS, TX 75265-5028
TEL: (214) 360-8000
FAX: (214) 360-8076
TOLL FREE: (800) 777-2249

TRUSTMARK INSURANCE
8324 S AVE
BOARDMAN, OH 44513
TEL: (330) 758-2212
FAX: (330) 758-3242
TOLL FREE: (800) 544-7312

8324 S AVE
BOARDMAN, OH 44513
TEL: (330) 758-2212
FAX: (330) 758-3242
TOLL FREE: (800) 544-7312

8324 S AVE
BOARDMAN, OH 44513
TEL: (330) 758-2212
FAX: (330) 758-3242
TOLL FREE: (800) 544-7312

400 FIELD DR
LAKE FOREST, IL 60045-2586
TEL: (847) 615-1500
FAX: (847) 615-3910

8324 S AVE
BOARDMAN, OH 44513
TEL: (330) 758-2212
FAX: (330) 758-3242
TOLL FREE: (800) 544-7312

8324 S AVE
BOARDMAN, OH 44513
TEL: (330) 758-2212
FAX: (330) 758-3242
TOLL FREE: (800) 544-7312

8324 S AVE
BOARDMAN, OH 44513
TEL: (330) 758-2212
FAX: (330) 758-3242
TOLL FREE: (800) 544-7312

8324 S AVE
BOARDMAN, OH 44513
TEL: (330) 758-2212
FAX: (330) 758-3242
TOLL FREE: (800) 544-7312

8324 S AVE
BOARDMAN, OH 44513
TEL: (330) 758-2212
FAX: (330) 758-3242
TOLL FREE: (800) 544-7312

8324 S AVE
BOARDMAN, OH 44513
TEL: (330) 758-2212
FAX: (330) 758-3242
TOLL FREE: (800) 544-7312

8324 S AVE
BOARDMAN, OH 44513
TEL: (330) 758-2212
FAX: (330) 758-3242
TOLL FREE: (800) 544-7312

8324 S AVE
BOARDMAN, OH 44513
TEL: (330) 758-2212
FAX: (330) 758-3242
TOLL FREE: (800) 544-7312

8324 S AVE
BOARDMAN, OH 44513
TEL: (330) 758-2212
FAX: (330) 758-3242
TOLL FREE: (800) 544-7312

8324 S AVE
BOARDMAN, OH 44513
TEL: (330) 758-2212
FAX: (330) 758-3242
TOLL FREE: (800) 544-7312

UNICARE
3820 AMERICAN DR
PLANO, TX 75070-6126
TEL: (972) 599-6500
TOLL FREE: (800) 332-2060

UNICARE LIFE & HEALTH
3179 TEMPLE AVE, STE 200
POMONA, CA 91768
PO BOX 60004
POMONA, CA 91716
TEL: (909) 444-6000
FAX: (909) 444-6161

3200 GREENFIELD RD
DEARBORN, MI 48120
PO BOX 4479
DEARBORN, MI 48126
TEL: (313) 336-5550
TOLL FREE: (800) 332-2060
IN-STATE: (800) 843-8184

7025 ALBERTPICK RD- 5TH FL
SCHAUMBURG, IL 27409
PO BOX 4046
SCHAUMBURG, IL 60168
TEL: (336) 665-1888
FAX: (336) 605-6406
TOLL FREE: (800) 597-6735

UNION LABOR LIFE INSURANCE CO
161 FORBES RD, STE 204
BRAINTREE, MA 02184-2606
TEL: (781) 848-7474
FAX: (781) 849-6113
TOLL FREE: (800) 248-0029

111 MASSACHUSETTS AVE NW
WASHINGTON, DC 20001
TEL: (202) 682-0900
FAX: (202) 682-8795

UNITED CHAMBERS ADMINISTRATORS
1805 HIGH PT DR
NAPERVILLE, IL 60563
PO BOX 3058
NAPERVILLE, IL 60566
TEL: (630) 505-3100
FAX: (630) 577-2915
TOLL FREE: (800) 323-3529

UNITED FARM FAMILY MUTUAL INSURANCE
9135 BROADWAY
MERRILLVILLE, IN 46410
TEL: (219) 756-9650
FAX: (219) 756-9669
TOLL FREE: (800) 477-6767

UNITED GOVERNMENT SERVICES
401 W MICHIGAN ST
MILWAUKEE, WI 53203
TEL: (414) 226-5000
FAX: (414) 226-5226
TOLL FREE: (800) 558-1584

UNITED HERITAGE MUTUAL LIFE INSURANCE CO
1212 12TH AVE RD
NAMPA, ID 83686
PO BOX 48
NAMPA, ID 83653-0048
TEL: (208) 466-7856
FAX: (208) 466-0825
TOLL FREE: (800) 657-6351

USI ADMINISTRATORS
7402 HODGSON MEMORIAL DR, STE 210
SAVANNAH, GA 31406
PO BOX 9888
SAVANNAH, GA 31412-0088
TEL: (912) 691-1551
FAX: (912) 352-8935
TOLL FREE: (800) 631-3441

ONE HUNTINGTON
QUANDRANGLE, STE 4N
MELVILLE, NY 11747-4414
PO BOX 8911
MELVILLE, NY 11747-8911
TEL: (631) 694-4900
FAX: (631) 694-5650

VALERO HEALTHCARE ADMISSION
2269 S UNIVERSITY DR, STE 308
FORT LAUDERDALE, FL 33324
TEL: (210) 370-2769
TOLL FREE: (800) 531-7911
IN-STATE: (800) 292-7816

VIA CHRISTI ST. JOSEPH MEDICAL CENTER
3600 E HARRY ST
WICHITA, KS 67218-3784
TEL: (316) 685-1111
TOLL FREE: (800) 851-0051

VIACHRISTI ST. FRANCIS
929 N ST FRANCIS ST
WICHITA, KS 67214
TEL: (316) 268-5192
FAX: (316) 268-6985
TOLL FREE: (800) 362-0070

VIRGINIA SURETY CO
4850 STREET RD
TREVOSE, PA 19049
TEL: (215) 953-3000
FAX: (215) 953-3156
TOLL FREE: (800) 523-6599
IN-STATE: (800) 523-5758

4850 STREET RD
TREVOSE, PA 19049
TEL: (215) 953-3000
FAX: (215) 953-3156
TOLL FREE: (800) 523-6599
IN-STATE: (800) 523-5758

WARD NORTH AMERICA, INC
3330 ARCTIC BLVD, STE 206
ANCHORAGE, AK 99503
TEL: (907) 561-1725
FAX: (907) 562-6595

WAUSAU INSURANCE CO
200 WESTWOOD DR
WAUSAU, WI 54401-7881
PO BOX 8017
WAUSAU, WI 54402-8017
TEL: (715) 845-5211
FAX: (715) 847-7569
TOLL FREE: (800) 826-9781

WEA INSURANCE GROUP
45 NOB HILL RD
MADISON, WI 53713
PO BOX 7338
MADISON, WI 53707
TEL: (608) 276-4000
FAX: (608) 276-9119
TOLL FREE: (800) 279-4000

WESTCHESTER TEAMSTERS HEALTH & WELFARE
160 S CENTRAL AVE
ELMSFORD, NY 10523-3521
TEL: (914) 592-9330
FAX: (914) 592-1519

WEYCO, INC
PO BOX 30132
LANSING, MI 48909
TEL: (517) 349-7010
FAX: (517) 349-7335
TOLL FREE: (800) 748-0003

WILLSE & ASSOCIATES
100 S CHARLES- TWR 2, STE 9
BALTIMORE, MD 21201
PO BOX 1196
BALTIMORE, MD 21297
TEL: (410) 347-1925
FAX: (410) 347-1924
TOLL FREE: (800) 423-9791

WISCONSIN SHEETMETAL HEALTH
PO BOX 3500
MADISON, WI 53704
TEL: (608) 277-0477
TOLL FREE: (800) 779-7577

ZENITH ADMINISTRATORS, INC
6801 E WASHINGTON BLVD
COMMERCE, CA 90040
PO BOX 22041
COMMERCE, CA 90022-2041
TEL: (323) 722-7171
FAX: (323) 728-2982

2873 N DIRKSEN PKY, STE 200
SPRINGFIELD, IL 62702
TEL: (217) 753-4531
FAX: (217) 753-3953
TOLL FREE: (800) 538-6466

Appendix 8:
Durable Medical Equipment

Reference List

The first column is an alphabetic list of various generic categories of equipment on which national coverage decisions have been made by the Health Care Financing Administration (HCFA). The second column notes the coverage status of each equipment category. The section mark (§) refers to the appropriate section in the Medicare Coverage Issues Manual.

Item — Coverage Status

Air cleaners — Not covered-environmental control equipment; not primarily medical in nature

Air conditioners — Not covered-environmental control equipment; not primarily medical in nature

Air-fluidized bed (E0194) — (See §60-19.)

Alternating pressure pads, mattresses and lamb's wool pads (E0180-E0199, E0371-E0373) — Covered if patient has, or is highly susceptible to, decubitus ulcers, and patient's physician has specified that he or she will be supervising its use in connection with the course of treatment

Audible/visible signal pacemaker monitor (E0610-E0615) — (See "Self-contained pacemaker monitor.")

Augmentative communication device (V5336) — (See "Communicator.")

Bathtub lifts (E0625) — Not covered-convenience item; not primarily medical in nature

Bathtub seats (E0245) — Not covered-comfort or convenience item; hygienic equipment; not primarily medical in nature

Bead bed — (See §60-19.)

Bed baths (home type) — Not covered-hygienic equipment; not primarily medical in nature

Bed boards (E0273, E0315) — Not covered-not primarily medical in nature

Bed lifter (bed elevator) — Not covered-not primarily medical in nature

Bed pans (autoclavable hospital type) (E0275, E0276) — Covered if patient is bed confined

Bed side rails (E0305, E0310) — (See "Hospital beds," §60-18.)

Beds-lounge (power or manual) — Not covered-not a hospital bed; comfort or convenience item; not primarily medical in nature

Beds-oscillating (E0270) — Not covered-institutional equipment; inappropriate for home use

Bidet toilet seat (E0244) — (See "Toilet seats.")

Blood glucose analyzer-reflectance colorimeter — Not covered-unsuitable for home use (See §60-11.)

Blood glucose monitor (E0607, E0609) — Covered if patient meets certain conditions (See §60-11.)

Braille teaching texts — Not covered-educational equipment; not primarily medical in nature

Canes (E0100, E0105) — Covered if patient's condition impairs ambulation. (See §60-3.)

Carafes — Not covered-convenience item; not primarily medical in nature

Catheters — Not covered-nonreusable disposable supply

Note: Noncovered catheters are classified as medical supplies of an expendable nature. Covered catheters include items classified as prosthetic devices (see Medicare Carriers Manual section 2130, Medicare Coverage Issues Manual sections 35-78, 35-81, 50-32, 60-14, 65-9 and 65-10.)

Commodes (E0160-E0175) — Covered if patient is confined to bed or room

Note: The term "room confined" means that leaving the room is medically contraindicated. The accessibility of bathroom facilities generally would not be a factor in this determination. However, confinement of a patient to his or her home where there are no toilet facilities may be equated to room confinement. Moreover, payment also may be made if a patient's medical condition confines him or her to a floor of his/her home and there is no bathroom located on that floor. (See "Hospital beds" in §60-18 for definition of bed confinement.) —

Communicator — Not covered-convenience item; not primarily medical in nature

Continuous passive motion (CPM) devices (E0935) — Covered for patients who have received a total knee replacement. Use of the device must commence within two days following surgery. In addition, coverage is limited to the three-week period following surgery during which the device is used in the patient's home.

There is insufficient evidence to justify coverage of these devices for longer periods of time or for other applications. —

Continuous positive airway pressure (CPAP) (E0452, E0601, K0183-K0189, K0193, K0194) — (See §60-17.)

Crutches (E0110-E0116) — Covered if patient's condition impairs ambulation

Cushion lift power seat (E0621-E0635) — (See "Seat lifts.")

Dehumidifiers (room or central heating system type) — Not covered-environmental control equipment; not primarily medical in nature

Diathermy machines (standard and pulsed wave types) — Not covered-inappropriate for home use (See §35-41.)

Digital electronic pacemaker monitor (E0610, E0615) — (See "Self-contained pacemaker monitor.")

Disposable sheets and bags — Not covered-nonreusable disposable supplies

Elastic stockings (A4490-A4495, A4500-A4510) — Not covered-nonreusable supply; not rental-type items

Electric air cleaners — Not covered--(See "Air cleaners.")

Electric hospital beds (E0250-E0270) — (See "Hospital beds" §60-18.)

Electrostatic machines — Not covered--(See "Air cleaners" and "Air conditioners.")

Elevators — Not covered-convenience item; not primarily medical in nature

Emesis basins — Not covered-convenience item; not primarily medical in nature

Esophageal dilator — Not covered-physician instrument; inappropriate for patient use

Exercise equipment — Not covered-not primarily medical in nature

Fabric supports — Not covered-nonreusable supplies; not rental-type item

Face masks (oxygen) (A4619-A4621) — Covered if oxygen is covered (See §60-4.)

Face masks (surgical) — Not covered-nonreusable disposable items

Flowmeter (E1353) — (See "Medical oxygen regulators.")

Fluidic breathing assister (E0500) — (See "IPPB machines.")

Fomentation device (E0210-E0239) — (See "Heating pads.")

Gel flotation pads and mattresses (E0196) — (See "Alternating pressure pads and mattresses.")

Grab bars (E0910, E0940) — Not covered-self-help device; not primarily medical in nature

Heat and massage foam cushion pad (E0186, E0187, E0196, E0272) — Not covered-not primarily medical in nature; personal comfort item

Heating and cooling plants — Not covered-environmental control equipment; not primarily medical in nature

Heating pads (E0210, E0215-E0217, E0238) — Covered if the contractor's medical staff determines that the patient's medical condition is one for which the application of heat in the form of a heating pad is therapeutically effective

Heat lamps (E0200, E0205) — Covered if the contractor's medical staff determines that the patient's medical condition is one for which the application of heat in the form of a heat lamp is therapeutically effective

Hospital beds (E0250-E0270, E0290-E0297) — (See §60-18.)

Hot packs — (See "Heating pads.")

Humidifiers (oxygen) (E0550-E0560) — (See "Oxygen humidifiers.")

Humidifiers (room or central heating system types) — Not covered-environmental control equipment; not medical in nature

Hydraulic lift (E0630) — (See "Patient lifts.")

Incontinence pads (A5149) — Not covered-nonreusable supply; hygienic item

Infusion pumps (B9000-B9006, E0781-E0791, E1520, K0284, K0417) — For external and implantable pumps, see §60-14. If the pump is used with an enteral or parenteral nutritional therapy system, see §§65-10 through 65-10.2 for special coverage rules

Injectors (hypodermic jet pressure powered devices for injection of insulin) (A4210) — Not covered-effectiveness not adequately demonstrated

IPPB machines (E0500) — Covered if patient's ability to breathe is severely impaired

Iron lungs (E0460) — (See "Ventilators.")

Irrigating kit (A4320-A4355, A4397, A4398) — Not covered-nonreusable supply; hygienic equipment

Lamb's wool pads (E0188-E0189) — Covered under same conditions as alternating pressure pads and mattresses

Leotards — Not covered--(See "Pressure leotards.")

Lymphedema pumps (segmental and nonsegmental therapy types) (E0650-E0673) — Covered (See §60-16.)

Massage devices — Not covered-personal comfort items; not primarily medical in nature

Mattress (E0184-E0187, E0196, E0271, E0272, E0277) — Covered only when hospital bed is medically necessary (Separate charge for replacement mattress should not be allowed when hospital bed with mattress is rented.) (See §60-18.)

Medical oxygen regulators (E1353) — Covered if patient's ability to breathe is severely impaired (See §60-4.)

Mobile geriatric chair — (See "Rolling chairs.")

Motorized wheelchairs — (See "Wheelchairs (power operated).")

Muscle stimulators (E0720, E0730, E0740-E0745, E0751, E0753) — Covered for certain conditions (See §35-77.)

Nebulizers (E0570-E0585, K0168-K0182) — Covered if patient's ability to breathe is severely impaired

Oscillating beds (E0270) — Not covered-institutional equipment; inappropriate for home use

Overbed tables (E0274, E0315) — Not covered-convenience item; not primarily medical in nature

Oxygen (E0424-E0444) — Covered if the oxygen has been prescribed for use in connection with medically necessary durable medical equipment (See §60-4.)

Oxygen humidifiers (E0550-E0560) — Covered if a medical humidifier has been prescribed for use in connection with medically necessary durable medical equipment for purposes of moisturizing oxygen (See §60-4.)

Oxygen regulators (medical) (E1353) — (See "Medical oxygen regulators.")

Oxygen tents (E0455) — (See §60-4.)

Paraffin bath units (portable) (A4265, E0235) — (See "Portable paraffin bath units.")

Paraffin bath units (standard) — Not covered-institutional equipment; inappropriate for home use

Parallel bars — Not covered-support exercise equipment; primarily for institutional use; in the home setting other devices (e.g., a walker) satisfy the patient's need

Patient lifts (E0621-E0635) — Covered if contractor's medical staff determines that the patient's condition is such that periodic movement is necessary to affect improvement or to arrest or retard deterioration in his or her condition

Percussors (E0480) — Covered for mobilizing respiratory tract secretions in patients with chronic obstructive lung disease, chronic bronchitis, or emphysema, when patient or operator of powered percussor has received appropriate training by a physician or therapist, and no one competent to administer manual therapy is available

Portable oxygen systems (E0430, E0435):

1. Regulated (adjustable flow rate) — Covered under the conditions specified in §60-4. Refer all claims to medical staff for this determination

2. Preset (flow rate not adjustable) — Not covered-emergency, first-aid, or precautionary equipment; essentially not therapeutic in nature

Portable paraffin bath units (A4265, E0235) — Covered when the patient has undergone a successful trial period of paraffin therapy ordered by a physician and the patient's condition is expected to be relieved by long-term use of this modality

Portable room heaters — Not covered-environmental control equipment; not primarily medical in nature

Portable whirlpool pumps — Not covered-not primarily medical in nature; personal comfort items

Postural drainage boards (E0606) — Covered if patient has a chronic pulmonary condition

Preset portable oxygen units — Not covered-emergency, first-aid, or precautionary equipment; essentially not therapeutic in nature

Pressure leotards — Not covered-nonreusable supply, not rental-type item

Pulse tachometer — Not covered-not reasonable or necessary for monitoring pulse of homebound patient with or without a cardiac pacemaker

Quad-canes (E0100-E0105) — (See "Walkers.")

Raised toilet seats (E0244) — Not covered-convenience item; hygienic equipment; not primarily medical in nature

Reflectance colorimeters — (See "Blood glucose analyzer.")

Respirators (E0450-E0460) — (See "Ventilators.")

Rolling chairs (E1031) — Covered if the contractor's medical staff determines that the patient's condition is such that there is a medical need for this item, and it has been prescribed by the patient's physician in lieu of a wheelchair. Coverage is limited to those rollabout chairs having casters of at least 5 inches in diameter and specifically designed to meet the needs of ill, injured or otherwise impaired individuals.

Coverage is denied for the wide range of chairs with smaller casters, as are found in general use in homes, offices and institutions for many purposes not related to the care or treatment of ill or injured persons. This type of chair is not primarily medical in nature.

Safety roller (E0147) — (See §60-15.)

Sauna baths — Not covered-not primarily medical in nature; personal comfort items

Seat lifts (E0621-E0635) — Covered under the conditions specified in §60-8. Refer all to medical staff for this determination.

Self-contained pacemaker monitor (E0610, E0615) — Covered when prescribed by a physician for a patient with a cardiac pacemaker (See §§50-1C and 60-7.)

Sitz bath (E0160-E0162) — Covered if the contractor's medical staff determines that the patient has an infection or injury of the perineal area and the item has been prescribed by the patient's physician as a part of his or her planned regimen of treatment in the patient's home.

Spare tanks of oxygen — Not covered-convenience or precautionary supply

Speech teaching machine — Not covered-education equipment; not primarily medical in nature

Stairway elevators — Not covered. (See "Elevators.")

Standing table — Not covered-convenience item; not primarily medical in nature

Steam packs (E0225, E0239) — These packs are covered under the same conditions as a heating pad (See "Heating pads.")

Suction machine (E0600) — Covered if the contractor's medical staff determines that the machine specified in the claim is medically required and appropriate for home use without technical or professional supervision

Support hose — Not covered--(See "Fabric supports.")

Surgical leggings — Not covered-nonreusable supply; not rental-type item

Telephone alert systems — Not covered-these are emergency communications systems and do not serve a diagnostic or therapeutic purpose

Telephone arms — Not covered-convenience item; not medical in nature

Toilet seats — Not covered-not medical equipment

Traction equipment (E0840-E0948) — Covered if patient has orthopedic impairment requiring traction equipment that prevents ambulation during the period of use (consider covering devices usable during ambulation [e.g., cervical traction collar, under the brace provision])

Trapeze bars (E0910-E0940) — Covered if patient is bed confined and the patient needs a trapeze bar to sit up because of respiratory condition, to change body position for other medical reasons or to get in and out of bed

Treadmill exerciser — Not covered-exercise equipment; not primarily medical in nature

Ultraviolet cabinet (E0690) — Covered for selected patients with generalized intractable psoriasis. Using appropriate consultation, the contractor should determine whether medical and other factors justify treatment at home rather than at alternative sites (e.g., outpatient department of a hospital)

Urinals (autoclavable hospital type) (E0325, E0326) — Covered if patient is bed confined

Vaporizers (E0605) — Covered if patient has a respiratory illness

Ventilators (E0450, E0453, E0460) — Covered for treatment of neuromuscular diseases, thoracic restrictive diseases and chronic respiratory failure consequent to chronic obstructive pulmonary disease. Includes both positive and negative pressure types

Walkers (E0130-E0147) — Covered if patient's condition impairs ambulation (See also §60-15.)

Water and pressure pads and mattresses (A4640, —

E0176-E0199) — (See "Alternating pressure pads and mattresses.")

Wheelchairs (E0950-E1298, K0001) — Covered if patient's condition is such that without the use of a wheelchair, he or she would otherwise be bed or chair-confined. An individual may qualify for a wheelchair and still be considered bed-confined

Wheelchairs (power operated) and wheelchairs with other special features (E1050-E1110, E1170-E1298, K0002-K0109, K0195) — Covered if patient's condition is such that a wheelchair is medically necessary and the patient is unable to operate the wheelchair manually. Claims for a power wheelchair or a wheelchair with other special features should be referred for medical consultation. Payment for special features is limited to those that are medically required because of the patient's condition (See §60-5 for power operated wheelchairs and §60-6 for specially sized wheelchairs.)

Note: A power-operated vehicle that may appropriately be used as a wheelchair can be covered (See §60-5 for coverage details.) —

Whirlpool bath equipment (standard) (E1300, E1310) — Covered if patient is homebound and has a condition for which the whirlpool bath can be expected to provide substantial therapeutic benefit justifying its cost. When the patient is not homebound but has such a condition, payment is restricted to the cost of providing the services elsewhere (e.g., an outpatient department of a participating hospital, if that alternative is less costly). In all cases, refer claim to medical staff for a determination

Whirlpool pumps — Not covered--(See "Portable whirlpool pumps.")

White cane — Not covered--(See §60-3.)

Source: Health Care Financing Administration, Medicare Coverage Issues Manual, section 60-9.

Index

Aggrastat, J3245
A-hydroCort, J1720
Aimsco Ultra Thin syringe, 1 cc or 1/2 cc, each, A4206
Air ambulance (see also Ambulance)
Air bubble detector, dialysis, E1530
Air fluidized bed, E0194
Airlife Brand Misty-Neb Nebulizer, E0580
Air pressure pad/mattress, E0176, E0186, E0197
Air travel and nonemergency transportation, A0140
Aircast, L4350–L4380
Aircast air stirrup ankle brace, L1906
Akineton, J0190
Alarm, pressure, dialysis, E1540
Alatrofloxacin mesylate, J0200
Albumarc, P9041-P9042
Albumin, human, P9041-P9042
Albuterol
  inhalation solution
    concentrated, J7618
    unit dose, J7619
Alcohol, A4244
Alcohol wipes, A4245
Aldesleukin, J9015
Aldomet, J0210
Alferon N, J9215
Algiderm, alginate dressing, A6196–A6199
Alginate dressing, A6196–A6199
Alglucerase, J0205
Algosteril, alginate dressing, A6196–A6199
Alkaban-AQ, J9360
Alkaline battery for blood glucose monitor, A4254
Alkeran, J8600
Allkare protective barrier wipe, box of 100, A5119
Allogenic cord blood harvest, S2140
Allograft
  cellular, C1859-C1863
    DuraDerm, C1858-C1863
    tissue, C1865-C1868
  small intestine, S2052
  small intestine and liver, S2053
Alpha 1-proteinase inhibitor, human, J0256
Alteplase recombinant, J2997

Alternating pressure mattress/pad, A4640, E0180, E0181, E0277
  pump, E0182
  replacement pad, A4640
Alveoloplasty, D7310–D7320
Amalgam dental restoration, D2110–D2161
Ambicor penile prosthesis, C1007
Ambulance, A0021–A0999
  air, A0436
  disposable supplies, A0382–A0398
  oxygen, A0422
Ambulation device, E0100–E0159
Amcort, J3302
A-methaPred, J2920, J2930
Amifostine, J0207
Amikacin sulfate, S0072
Aminaid, enteral nutrition, B4154
Aminocaproic acid, S0017
Aminophylline/Aminophyllin, J0280
Amiodarone hydrochloride, J0282
Amirosyn-RF, parenteral nutrition, B5000
Amitriptyline HCl, J1320
Ammonia test paper, A4774
Amobarbital, J0300
Amphocin, J0285
Amphotec, J0286
Amphotericin B, J0285
  B lipid complex, J0286
Ampicillin sodium, J0290
  sodium/sulbactam sodium, J0295
Amplatz renal dilator set, C8543
Amputee
  adapter, wheelchair, E0959
  prosthesis, L5000–L7510, L7520, L7900, L8400–L8465
  stump sock, L8470–L8490
  wheelchair, E1170–E1190, E1200, K0100
AMS 700 penile prosthesis, C1007
AMS sphincter 800 urinary prosthesis, C3500
Amygdalin, J3570
Amytal, J0300
Anabolin LA 100, J2320–J2322
Analgesia, dental, D9230
Ancef, J0690
Anchorsew, C1811
Ancure endograft delivery system, C1117
Andrest 90-4, J0900
Andro-Cyp, J1070–J1090
Andro-Estro 90-4, J0900

Asparaginase, J9020
Assessment
  audiologic, V5008–V5020
  cardiac output, M0302
  speech, V5362–V5364
Astramorph, J2275
Atgam, J7504
Atherectomy catheter and burr, C1043
Atherectomy system, peripheral, C1500
Ativan, J2060
Atrial pacing catheter, C1055
Atropine
  inhalation solution
    concentrated, J7635
    unit dose, J7636
  sulfate, J0460
Attends, adult diapers, A4335
Audiologic assessment, V5008–V5020
Auricular prosthesis, D5914, D5927
Aurothioglucose, J2910
Authentic Mick TP brachytherapy
  needle, C1700
Autoclix lancet device, A4258
Auto-Glide folding walker, E0143
Autolance lancet device, A4258
Autolet lancet device, A4258
Autolet Lite lancet device, A4258
Autolet Mark II lancet device, A4258
Avonex, J1825
Azathioprine, J7500, J7501
Azithromycin dihydrate, Q0144
Azithromycin injection, J0456
Aztreonam, S0073

Back supports, L0500–L0960
Baclofen, J0475, J0476
  intrathecal refill kit, C9008-C9010
  intrathecal screening kit, C9007
Bacterial sensitivity study, P7001
Bactocill, J2700
Bag
  drainage, A4357
  irrigation supply, A4398
  spacer, for metered dose inhaler,
    A4627
  urinary, A5112, A4358
Baker, spinal orthosis, L0370
BAL in oil, J0470
Balken, fracture frame, E0946

Bandages, A4460
  Orthoflex™ Elastic Plaster Bandages,
    A4580
  Specialist™ Plaster Bandages, A4580
Banflex, J2360
Bard
  10F Dual Lumen ureteral catheter,
    C2601
  Composix Mesh, C6001-C6006
  FasLata allograft tissue, C1865-C1868
  Inlay Double Pigtail ureteral stent,
    C5280
  Memotherm colorectal stent, C5131-
    C5133
  Memotherm-Flex biliary stent, C5001-
    C5003
  Reconix ePTFE reconstruction patch,
    C6034-C6041
  Sperma Tex Mesh, C1864
  UroForce balloon dilatation catheter,
    C1938
Barium enema, G0106
  cancer screening, G0120
Base of tongue somnoplasty coagulating
  electrode, C1321
Baseball finger splint, A4570
Basiliximab, Q2019
Bathtub
  heat unit, E0249
  stool or bench, E0245
  transfer rail, E0246
  wall rail, E0241, E0242
Battery, K0082–K0087, L7360, L7364
  blood glucose monitor, A4254
  charger, E1066, K0088–K0089,
    L7362, L7366
  TENS, A4630
  ventilator, A4611–A4613
  wheelchair, A4631
Bayer chemical reagent strips, box of
  100 glucose/ketone urine test
  strips, A4250
BCG live, intravesical, J9031
BCW 600, manual wheelchair, K0007
BCW Power, power wheelchair, K0014
BCW recliner, manual wheelchair, K0007
B-D alcohol swabs, box, A4245
B-D disposable insulin syringes, up to
  1cc, per syringe, A4206
B-D lancets, per box of 100, A4258
Bebax, foot orthosis, L3160
Becaplermin gel, S0157

Index

Bock, hand prosthesis, L6875, L6880
Bock Dynamic, foot prosthesis, L5972
Bock, Otto *see* Otto Bock
Body jacket
    lumbar-sacral orthosis (spinal),
        L0500–L0565, L0600, L0610
    scoliosis, L1300, L1310
Body sock, L0984
Body Wrap
    foam positioners, E0191
    therapeutic overlay, E0199
Bond or cement, ostomy, skin, A4364
Bonnie, Sliding Rail catheter, C1981
Boot
    pelvic, E0944
    surgical, ambulatory, L3260
Boston type spinal orthosis, L1200
Botulinum toxin type A, J0585
Brachytherapy
    radioelements, Q3001
    seed, C1800-C1806
Brachytherapy Needle, C1701
Brachytherapy Seed, C1805
Brake attachment, wheeled walker,
    E0159
Breast and pelvic exam, G0101
Breast prosthesis, L8000–L8035, L8600
    adhesive skin support, A4280
Breast pump, all types, E0602
Breathing circuit, A4618
Brethine, J3105
Bricanyl subcutaneous, J3105
Bridge
    recement, D6930
    repair, by report, D6980
Brompheniramine maleate, J0945
Broncho-Cath endobronchial tubes, with
    CPAP system, E0601
Bronkephrine, J0590
Buck's, traction
    frame, E0870
    stand, E0880
Bupivicaine, S0020
Bus, nonemergency transportation,
    A0110
Butorphanot tartrate nasal spray, S0012
BX Velocity Balloon-Expandable Stent
    with Raptor Over-the-Wire delivery
    system, C5038
Bypass Speedy catheter, C1981

Cabergoline, Q2001
Caine (-1, -2), J2000

Calcijex, J0635
Calcimar, J0630
Calcitonin-salmon, J0630
Calcitriol, J0635
Calcium
    disodium edetate, J0600
    disodium versenate, J0600
    EDTA, J0600
    gluconate, J0610
    glycerophosphate and calcium lactate,
        J0620
    lactate and calcium glycerophosphate,
        J0620
    leucovorin, J0640
Calibrator solution, A4256
Calphosan, J0620
CAMP
    lumbosacral support, L0910, L0920,
        L0940, L0950
    thoracolumbar support, L0300
Camptosar, J9206
Cancer screening
    barium enema, G0122
    breast exam, G0101
    cervical exam, G0101
    colorectal, G0104–G0106,
        G0120–G0122
Cane, E0100, E0105
    accessory, A4636, A4637
    Easy-Care quad, E0105
    quad canes, E0105
    Quadri-Poise, E0105
    wooden canes, E0100
Canister
    disposable, used with suction pump,
        A7000
    non-disposable, used with suction
        pump, A7001
Cannula
    fistula, set (for dialysis), A4730
    nasal, A4615
    tracheostomy, A4623
Capecitabine, oral, J8520, J8521
Carbocaine with Neo-Cobefrin, J0670
Carbon filter, A4680
Carboplatin, J9045
Cardia event, recorder implantable,
    E0616
Cardiokymography, Q0035
Cardiovascular services, M0300–M0302
Carelet safety lancet, A4258

Carex
adjustable bath/shower stool, E0245
aluminum crutches, E0114
cane, E0100
folding walker, E0135
shower bench, E0245
Carmustine, J9050
Carnitor, J1955
Carries susceptibility test, D0425
Carticel, C1059
Casec, enteral nutrition, B4155
Cash, spinal orthosis, L0370
Cast
diagnostic, dental, D0470
hand restoration, L6900–L6915
materials, special, A4590
padding, (not separately reimbursable
from the casting procedure or
casting supplies codes)
Delta-Rol™ Cast Padding
Sof-Rol™ Cast Padding
Specialist™ 100 Cotton Cast
Padding
Specialist™ Cast Padding
plaster, A4580, L2102, L2122
supplies, A4580, A4590
Delta-Cast™ Elite™ Casting
Material, A4590
Delta-Lite™ Conformable Casting
Tape, A4590
Delta-Lite™ C-Splint™ Fibreglass
Immobilizer, A4590
Delta-Lite™ "S" Fibreglass Casting
Tape, A4590
Flashcast™ Elite™ Casting Material,
A4590
Orthoflex™ Elastic Plaster
Bandages, A4580
Orthoplast™ Splints (and
Orthoplast™ II Splints), A4590
Specialist™ Plaster Bandages,
A4580
Specialist™ Plaster Roll Immobilizer,
A4580
Specialist™ Plaster Splints, A4580
synthetic, L2104, L2124
thermoplastic, L2106, L2126
Caster, wheelchair, E0997, E0998,
K0099
Catheter, A4300–A4365

Catheter
ablation, C1003, C1056, C1104
Biosense Webster Celsius ablation,
C2012-C2015
Blazer II XP, C2020
Navi-Star diagnostic/ablation,
C2016-C2017
anchoring device, A4333, A4334
percutaneous, A5200
Arrow-Trerotola percutaneous
thrombolytic device, C2200
balloon, C1030, C1031, C1072
balloon dilatation, C1810
Bard
10F dual lumen ureteral, C2601
UroForce balloon dilatation, C1938
cap, disposable (dialysis), A4860
Clinicath Peripherally Inserted central
(PICC), C2598, C2599
Clinicath Peripherally Inserted midline
(PICC) C2597
Constellation diagnostic, C2001
Cordis Maxi LD PTA balloon, C1942
Cordis PowerFlex PTA balloon, C1940
coronary, C1034, C1061
coronary angioplasty balloon, C1981
CrossSail coronary dilatation, C1943
diagnostic, C1047, C1054, C1107
electrophysiology
Cordis deflectable tip (quadrapolar),
C2011
EP deflectable tip, C2004-C2006
Irvine Luma-Cath 7F steerable
electrophysiology, C2009
Irvine Luma-Cath fixed curve
electrophysiology, C2007,
C2008
EP Medsystems
deflectable electrophysiology,
C2019
SilverFlex electrophysiology, non-
deflectable, C2021
external collection device,
A4327–A4330, A4348
implantable intraspinal, E0785
Flexima Biliary Drainage, C2609
Gold Probe Single-Use
Electrohemostasis, C2600
imaging, C1033, C1038
indwelling, A4338–A4346
indwelling, insertion of, G0002
insertion tray, A4354

Index

Catheter — *continued*
  intermittent, with insertion supplies,
    A4353
  intracardiac, C1035
  intracardiac echocardiography, C1035
  irrigation supplies, A4319, A4355
  Irvine Inquiry steerable
    electrophysiology 5F, C2002,
    C2003
  joint supportive device, A4464
  Jupiter PTA balloon dilatation, C1941
  lubricant, A4332
  male, external, A4324, A4325
  Ninja PTCA dilatation, Raptor PTCA
    dilatation, C1939
  Opti-Plast Centurion 5.5F PTA, shaft
    length 50cm to 120cm, C1933
  Opti-Plast XL 5.5F PTA, shaft length
    75 cm to 120cm, C1933
  Oratec
    SpineCath Intradiscal, C2607
    SpineCath XL Intradiscal, C2606
  Orbiter ST steerable electrode, C2000
  oropharyngeal suction, A4628
  percutaneous transluminal coronary
    angioplasty, C1930
  percutaneous transluminal coronary
    angioplasty guide, C1101
  peripheral dilatation, C1074
  Polaris T, C2018
  Scimed 6F Wiseguide guide, C2608
  SciMed Remedy coronary balloon
    dilatation infusion (20mm),
    C1932
  Spectranetics
    concentric laser, C2602-C2604
    extreme laser, C2605
  starter set, A4329
  Synergy balloon dilatation, C1937
  Talon Balloon Dilatation, C1931
  thrombectomy, C1051, C1054
  trachea (suction), A4624
  transesophageal, C1055
  Ultraverse 3.5F Balloon dilatation,
    C1934
  Uromax Ultra High Pressure balloon
    dilatation with Hydroplus
    coating, C1936
  Veripath Peripheral Guiding Catheter,
    C2151
  WorkHorse PTA balloon, C1935
Catheter, Mariner CS catheter, C1025

Catheterization, specimen collection,
  P9612, P9615
Cefadyl, J0710
Cefazolin sodium, J0690
Cefizox, J0715
Cefonicid sodium, J0695
Cefotaxime sodium, J0698
Cefotetan disodium, S0074
Cefoxitin, J0694
Ceftazidime, J0713
Ceftizoxime sodium, J0715
Ceftriaxone sodium, J0696
Ceftoperazone, S0021
Cefuroxime sodium, J0697
Celestone phosphate, J0704
Cellular therapy, M0075
Cel-U-Jec, J0704
Cement, ostomy, A4364
Cenacort
  A-40, J3301
  Forte, J3302
Centrifuge, A4650
Cephalin floculation, blood, P2028
Cephalothin sodium, J1890
Cephapirin sodium, J0710
Cerebral blood flow studies, xenon,
  S9023
Ceredase, J0205
Cerezyme, J1785
Certified nurse assistant, S9122
Cerubidine, J9150
Cervical
  collar, L0120, L0130, L0140, L0150
  halo, L0810–L0830
  head harness/halter, E0942
  helmet, L0100, L0110
    Softop, leather protective, L0110
  orthosis, L0100–L0200
  pillow, E0943
  traction equipment, not requiring
    frame, E0855
Cervical cap contraceptive, A4261
Cervical-thoracic-lumbar-sacral orthosis
  (CTLSO), L0700, L0710, L1000
Chair
  adjustable, dialysis, E1570
  lift, E0627
  rollabout, E1031
  sitz bath, E0160–E0162
Challenger manual wheelchair, K0009
Champion 1000 manual wheelchair,
  K0004

Champion 30000, manual wheelchair, K0005
Chealamide, J3520
CheckMate Plus blood glucose monitor, E0607
Chelation therapy, M0300
Chemical endarterectomy, M0300
Chemistry and toxicology tests, P2028–P3001
Chemotherapy
    administration, Q0083–Q0085 (hospital reporting only)
    dental, D4381
    drug, oral, not otherwise classified, J7150, J8999, J9999
    drugs (see also drug by name), J9000–J9999
Chemstrip bG, box of 50 blood glucose test strips, A4253
Chemstrip K, box of 100 ketone urine test strips, A4250
Chemstrip UGK, box of 100 glucose/ketone urine test strips, A4250
Chest compression vest, S8200
    system generator and hoses, S8205
Chest shell (cuirass), E0457
Chest wrap, E0459
Chin
    cup, cervical, L0150
    strap (for CPAP device), K0186
Chlor-100, J0730
Chloramphenicol sodium succinate, J0720
Chlordiazepoxide HCl, J1990
Chloromycetin sodium succinate, J0720
Chloroprocaine HCl, J2400
Chloroquine HCl, J0390
Chlorothiazide sodium, J1205
Chlorpheniramine maleate, J0730
Chlor-Pro (10), J0730
Chlorpromazine HCl, J3230, Q0171–Q0172
Chlorprothixene, J3080
Chlortrimeton, J0730
Choice PTCA guidewire, C3551
Chondrocytes, cultured autologous, C1059
Chopart prosthetic
    ankle, L5050, L5060
    below knee, L5100
Chorex (-5, -10), J0725
Chorignon, J0725

Chorionic gonadotropin, J0725
Choron 10, J0725
Chromic phosphate, Q3011
Chronimed Comfort insulin infusion set
    23", A4230
    43", A4230
Chubby, Sliding Rail catheter, C1981
Chux's, A4554
Cida
    exostatic cervical collar, L0140, L0150
    form fit collar, L0120
Cidofovir, J0740
Cilastatin sodium, imipenem, J0743
Cimetidine hydrochloride, S0023
Ciprofloxacin, S0024
Cisplatin, J9060, J9062
Cladribine, J9065
Claforan, J0698
Clamp
    dialysis, A4910, A4918, A4920
    external urethral, A4356
Clavicle
    splint, L3650, L3660
    support
        2-buckle closure, L3660
        4-buckle closure, L3660
Cleaning solvent, Nu-Hope
    4 oz bottle, A4455
    16 oz bottle, A4455
Cleanser, wound, A6260
Cleansing agent, dialysis equipment, A4790
Clevis, hip orthosis, L2570, L2600, L2610
Clinical trials
    lodging costs, S9994
    meals, S9996
    phase II, S9990
    phase III, S9991
    transportation costs, S9992
Clindamycin phosphate, S0077
Clonidine, J0735
Clotting time tube, A4771
Clubfoot wedge, L3380
Cobex, J3420
Cochlear prosthetic implant, L8614
    replacement, L8619
Codeine phosphate, J0745
Codimal-A, J0945
Cogentin, J0515
Colchicine, J0760
Colistimethate sodium, J0770

Coronary artery bypass surgery, direct — *continued*
with coronary venous grafts, only
single, S2207
Corset, spinal orthosis, L0970–L0976
Corticotropin, J0800
Cortisone acetate, J0810
Cortone acetate, J0810
Cortrosyn, J0835
Corvert, J1742
Cosmegen, J9120
Cosyntropin, J0835
Cotranzine, J0780
Counseling for control of dental disease,
D1310, D1320
Cover, wound
alginate dressing, A6196–A6198
collagen dressing, A6021–A6024
foam dressing, A6209–A6214
hydrocolloid dressing, A6234–A6239
hydrogel dressing, A6242–A6248
specialty absorptive dressing,
A6251–A6256
Coyote
20mm, Coyote 9/15/25mm catheter,
C1981
dilatation catheter
20mm/30mm/40mm, C1930
CPAP (continuous positive airway
pressure) device, E0601
chin strap, K0186
compressor, K0269
filter, K0188–K0189
headgear, K0185
humidifier, K0268
nasal application accessories, K0183,
K0184
tubing, K0187
Cradle, bed, E0280
Criticare HN, enteral nutrition, B4153
Cromolyn sodium, inhalation solution,
unit dose, J7631
Crowns, D2710–D2810, D2930–D2933,
D4249, D6720–D6792
Crutches, E0110–E0116
accessories, A4635–A4637, K0102
aluminum, E0114
forearm, E0111
Ortho-Ease, E0111
underarm, other than wood, pair,
E0114
Quikfit Custom Pack, E0114
Red Dot, E0114

Crutches — *continued*
underarm, wood, single, E0113
Ready-for-use, E0113
wooden, E0112
Cryoprecipitate, each unit, P9012
Cryosurgical ablation
tumerous tissue, liver, S2210
Crysticillin (300 A.S., 600 A.S.), J2510
CSTA, C1004
CTLSO, L1000–L1120, L0700, L0710
Cuirass, E0457
Culture sensitivity study, P7001
Curasorb, alginate dressing,
A6196–A6199
Cushion, wheelchair, E0962–E0965,
E0977
Geo-Matt, E0964
High Profile Therapeutic Dry
Flotation, 4-inch, E0965
Low Profile Therapeutic Dry
Flotation, 2-inch, E0963
Custom Masterhinge™ Hip Hinge 3,
L2999
Cyanocobalamin cobalt, C1079, C1089,
Q3012
Cyberpmocs meirpcubermetoc
gemeratpr. C1048
Cycler dialysis machine, E1594
Cyclophosphamide, J9070–J9092
lyophilized, J9093–J9097
oral, J8530
Cyclosporine, J7502, J7515, J7516
Cylinder tank carrier, K0104
Cytarabine, J9110
Cytarabine 100, J9100
CytoGam, J0850
Cytomegalovirus immune globulin
(human), J0850
Cytopathology, screening, G0123,
G0124, G0141, G0143–G0148
Cytosar-U, J9100
Cytovene, J1570
Cytoxan, J8530, J9070–J9097

Dacarbazine, J9130, J9140
Daclizumab, J7513
Dactinomycin, J9120
Dalalone, J1100
L.A., J1095
Dalfopristin, C1024, J2270
Dalteparin sodium, J1645
Daunorubicin citrate, J9151
HCl, J9150

Dental procedures — *continued*
  diagnostic, D0120–D0999
  endodontics, D3110–D3999
  implant services, D6010–D6199
  maxillofacial, D5911–D5999
  oral and maxillofacial surgery,
    D7110–D7999
  orthodontic, D8010–D8999
  periodontic, D4210–D4999
  preventive, D1110–D1550
  prosthodontic, fixed, D6210–D6999
  prosthodontic, removable,
    D5110–D5899
  restorative, D2110–D2999
Dentures, D5110–D5899
DepAndro
  100, J1070
  200, J1080
Dep-Androgyn, J1060
DepMedalone
  40, J1030
  80, J1040
Depo
  -Medrol, J1020, J1030, J1040
  -Provera, J1050, J1055
  -Testadiol, J1060
  -Testosterone, J1070, J1080, J1090
Depo-estradiol cypionate, J1000
Depogen, J1000
Depoject, J1030, J1040
Depopred
  -40, J1030
  -80, J1040
Depotest, J1070, J1080
Depotestogen, J1060
Derata injection device, A4210
Dermal tissue, Q0183–Q0185
Desferal mesylate, J0895
Desmopressin acetate, J2597
Detector, blood leak, dialysis, E1560
Dexacen-4, J1100
Dexamethasone
  acetate, J1095
  inhalation solution
    concentrated, J7637
    unit dose, J7638
  sodium phosphate, J1100
Dexasone, J1100
Dexasone L.A., J1095
Dexferrum (iron dextran), J1750
Dexone, J1100
Dexrazoxane HCl, J1190
Dextran, J7100, J7110

Dextrose, S5010-S5014
  saline (normal), J7042
  water, J7060, J7070
Dextrostick, A4772
D.H.E. 45, J1110
Diabetes supplies
  alcohol swabs, per box, A4245
  battery for blood glucose monitor,
    A4254
  bent needle set for insulin pump
    infusion, A4231
  blood glucose monitor, E0607
  blood glucose test strips, box of 50,
    A4253
  injection device, needle-free, A4210
  insulin, J1820
  insulin pump, external, E0784
  lancet device, A4258
  lancets, box of 100, A4259
  non needle cannula for insulin
    infusion, A4232
  syringe, disposable, per syringe,
    A4206
  urine glucose/ketone test strips, box
    of 100, A4250
Diabetic management program
  follow-up visit to MD provider, S9141
  follow-up visit to non-MD provider,
    S9140
  group session, S9455
  nurse visit, S9460
Diagnostic
  dental services, D0100–D0999
  radiology services, R0070–R0076
Dialet lancet device, A4258
Dialysate
  concentrate additives, A4765
  solution, A4700, A4705
  testing solution, A4760
Dialysis
  air bubble detector, E1530
  bath conductivity, meter, E1550
  blood leak detector, E1560
  CAPD supply kit, A4900
  CCPD supply kit, A4901
  equipment, E1510–E1702
  filter, A4680
  fluid barrier, E1575
  forceps, A4910
  heparin infusion pump, E1520
  home equipment repair, A4890
  kit, A4820, A4900, A4901, A4905,
    A4914

Dialysis — *continued*
measuring cylinder, A4921
peritoneal, A4300, A4900, A4901,
A4905, E1592, E1594, E1630,
E1640
pressure alarm, E1540
replacement parts for equipment,
E1640
shunt, A4740
supplies, A4650–A4927
thermometer, A4910
tourniquet, A4910
unipuncture control system, E1580
Dialyzer, artificial kidney, A4690
holder, A4919
Diamox, J1120
Diaper, A4335, S8402
Diascan blood glucose monitor, E0609
Diazepam, J3360
Diazoxide, J1730
Dibent, J0500
Didronel, J1436
Diethylstilbestrol diphosphate, J9165
Diflucan injection, J1750
Digital subtraction angiography, S9022
Digi-Voice blood glucose monitor,
E0609
Digoxin, J1160
Dihydrex, J1200
Dihydroergotamine mesylate, J1110
Dilantin, J1165
Dilaudid, J1170
Dilocaine, J2000
Dilomine, J0500
Dilor, J1180
Dimenhydrinate, J1240
Dimercaprol, J0470
Dimethyl sulfoxide (DMSO), J1212
Dinate, J1240
Dioval (XX, 40), J0970, J1380, J1390
Diphenacen-50, J1200
Diphenhydramine HCl, J1200, Q0163
Dipyridamole, J1245
Disarticulation
lower extremities, prosthesis,
L5000–L5999
upper extremities, prosthesis,
L6000–L6692
Discrete Technology, Over-the-Wire /
Rapid Exchange coronary stent
system, C5030-C5032

Disetronic
glass cartridge syringe for insulin
pump, each, A4232
insulin infusion set with bent needle,
with or without wings, each,
A4231
Disetronic H-Tron insulin pump, E0784
Diskard head halter, E0940
Diskectomy, lumbar, S2350, S2351
single interspace, S2350
Disotate, J3520
Di-Spaz, J0500
Disposable
diapers, A4335
supplies, ambulance, A0382–A0398
underpads, A4554
Ditate-DS, J0900
Diuril sodium, J1205
D-med 80, J1040
DMSO, J1212
Dobutamine HCl, J1250
Dobutrex, J1250
Docetaxel, J9170
Dolasetron mesylate, J1260, Q0180
Dolophine HCl, J1230
Dome, J9130
and mouthpiece (for nebulizer),
A7016
Dommanate, J1240
Don-Joy
cervical support collar, L0150
deluxe knee immobilizer, L1830
rib belt, L0210
wrist forearm splint, L3984
Donor cadaver
harvesting multivisceral organs, with
allografts, S2055
Dornase alpha, inhalation solution, unit
dose, J7639
Dorrance prosthesis
hand, L6825
hook, L6700–L6780
Dorsiwedge™ Night Splint, A4570,
L2999, L4398
Double bar
"AK," knee-ankle-foot orthosis, L2020,
L2030
"BK," ankle-foot orthosis, L1990
Doxil, J9001
Doxorubicin HCl, J9000
Drainage
bag, A4347, A4357, A4358
board, postural, E0606

Index

Index

Folex, J9260
    PFS, J9260
Foley catheter, A4312–A4316,
    A4338–A4346
Follutein, J0725
Fomepizole, Q2008
Fomivirsen sodium, intraocular, J1452
Foot, cast boot
    Specialist™ Closed-Back Cast Boot,
        L3260
    Specialist™ Gaitkeeper™ Boot, L3260
    Specialist™ Open-Back Cast Boot,
        L3260
    Specialist™ Toe Insert for Specialist™
        Closed-Back Cast Boot and
        Specialist™ Health/Post
        Operative Shoe, A9270
Foot, insoles/heel cups
    Specialist™ Heel Cups, L3485
    Specialist™ Insoles, L3510
Foot, soles
    Masterfoot™ Walking Cast Sole,
        L3649
    Solo™ Cast Sole, L3540
Footdrop splint, L4398
Footplate, E0175, E0970
Footwear, orthopedic, L3201–L3265
Forceps, dialysis, A4910
Forearm crutches, E0110, E0111
Fortaz, J0713
Fortex, alginate dressing, A6196–A6199
Foscarnet sodium, J1455
Foscavir, J1455
Fosphenytoin, Q2009
Fosphenytoin sodium, S0078
Four Poster, fracture frame, E0946
Four-pronged finger splint, A4570
Fracture
    bedpan, E0276
    frame, E0920, E0930, E0946-E0948
    orthosis, L2102-L2136, L3980-L3986
    orthotic additions, L2180-L2192,
        L3995
    Specialist™ Pre-Formed Humeral
        Fracture Brace, L3980
Fragmin, J1645
Frames (spectacles), V2020, V2025
    sales tax, S9999
FreAmine HBC, parenteral nutrition,
    B5100
Frejka, hip orthosis, L1600
    replacement cover, L1610
FUDR, J9200
Fungizone, J0285

Furomide MD, J1940
Furosemide, J1940

Gadolinium, A4647
Gait analysis, S9033
Gallium ga 67, Q3002
Gamastan, J1460–J1561
Gamma globulin, J1460–J1561
Gammar, J1561
Gamulin RH, J2790
Ganciclovir
    implant, J7310
    sodium, J1570
Garamycin, J1580
Gas system
    compressed, E0424, E0425
    gaseous, E0430, E0431, E0441, E0443
    liquid, E0434–E0440, E0442, E0444
Gastrostomy/jejunostomy tubing, B4084
Gastrostomy tube, B4084, B4085
Gauze (see also Bandage),
        A6216–A6230, A6263, A6264,
        A6266
    elastic, A6263, A6405
    impregnated, A6222–A6230, A6266
    nonelastic, A6264, A6406
    nonimpregnated, A6216, A6221,
        A6402, A6406
    pads, A6216–A6230, A6402–A6404
        Johnson & Johnson, A6402
        Kendall, A6402
        Moore, A6402
Gel
    conductive, A4558
    pressure pad, E0178, E0185, E0196
Gem DR implantable defibrillator, C1363
Gemcitabine HCl, J9201
Gemtuzumab ozogamicin, C9004
GemZar, J9201
Generator
    prosthesis, C1048
Genmould™ Creamy Plaster, A4580
Gentamicin (sulfate), J1580
Gentran, J7100, J7110
Geo-Matt
    therapeutic overlay, E0199
    wheelchair cushion, E0964
Geronimo PR, power wheelchair, K0011
Gerval Protein, enteral nutrition, B4155
Gesterol
    50, J2675
    L.A. 250, J1741
Gingival procedures, D4210–D4240

Handgrip (cane, crutch, walker), A4636
Harness, E0942, E0944, E0945
Harvard pressure clamp, dialysis, A4920
Harvesting multivisceral organs, cadaver
    donor, S2055
Harvey arm abduction orthosis, L3960
Headgear (for CPAP device), K0185
Hearing devices, L8614, V5008–V5299
Heat
    application, E0200–E0239
    lamp, E0200, E0205
    pad, E0210, E0215, E0217, E0218,
        E0238, E0249
    units, E0239
        Hydroacollator, mobile, E0239
        Thermalator T-12-M, E0239
Heater (nebulizer), E1372
Heating pad, Dunlap, E0210
Heel
    elevator, air, E0370
    pad, L3480, L3485
    protector, E0191
    shoe, L3430–L3485
    stabilizer, L3170
Helicopter, ambulance (see also
    Ambulance), A0040
Helmet, cervical, L0100, L0110
Hemalet lancet device, A4258
Hemin, Q2011
Hemi-wheelchair, E1083–E1086
Hemipelvectomy prosthesis, L5280,
    L5340
Hemodialysis
    kit, A4820
    machine, E1590
Hemodialyzer, portable, E1635
Hemofil M, J7190
Hemophilia clotting factor, J7190–J7198
Hemophilia clotting factor, NOC, J7199
Hemostats, A4850
Hemostix, A4773
Heparin
    for dialysis, A4800
    infusion pump (for dialysis), E1520
    lock flush, J1642
    sodium, J1644
HepatAmine, parenteral nutrition, B5100
Hepatic-aid, enteral nutrition, B4154
Hepatitis B immune globulin, C9105
Hep-Lock (U/P), J1642
Herceptin, J9355
Hernia mesh, C6001-C6006

Hexadrol phosphate, J1100
Hexalite, A4590
Hexapolar, octapolar, quadrapolar),
    C2010
Hexior power wheelchair, K0014
High Profile therapeutic dry flotation
    cushion, E0965
Hip
    Custom Masterhinge™ Hip Hinge 3,
        L2999
    disarticulation prosthesis, L5250,
        L5270, L5330
    Masterhinge™ Hip Hinge 3, L2999
    orthosis (HO), L1600-L1686
Hip-knee-ankle-foot orthosis (HKAFO),
    L2040–L2090
Histaject, J0945
Histerone (-50, -100), J3140
Histrelin acetate, Q2020
Hi-Torque guide wire, C1365-C1367
Hi-Torque Whisper coronary guide wire,
    C3552
HIV-1 antibody testing, S3645
HKAFO, L2040–L2090
HN2, J9230
Hole cutter tool, A4421
Hollister
    belt adapter, A4421
    closed pouch, A5051, A5052
    colostomy/ileostomy kit, A4421,
        A5061
    drainable pouches, A5061
        with flange, A5063
    medical adhesive, A4364
    pediatric ostomy belt, A4367
    remover, adhesive, A4455
    replacement filters, A4421
    stoma cap, A5055
    skin barrier, A4362, A5122, A5123
    skin cleanser, A4335
    skin conditioning creme, A4335
    skin gel protective dressing wipes,
        A5119
    stoma cap, A5055
    two-piece pediatric ostomy system,
        A5054, A5063, A5073, A5123
    urostomy pouch, A5071, A5072
Home health
    aide, S9122
        home health setting, G0156
    services of
        clinical social worker, G0155
        occupational therapist, G0152

Home health — *continued*
  services of — *continued*
    physical therapist, G0151
    skilled nurse, G0154
    speech/language pathologist,
      G0153
Home health care
  administration of medication, IM
    epidurally or subcutaneously,
      S9543
  certified nurse assistant, S9122
  home health aide, S9122
  nursing care, S9123, S9124
Home uterine monitor, S9001
Hosmer
  baby mitt, L6870
  child hand, mechanical, L6872
  forearm lift, assist unit only, L6635
  gloves, above hands, L6890, L6895
  hand prosthesis, L6868
  hip orthotic joint, post-op, L1685
  hook
    #5, L6705
    #5X, L6710
    #5XA, L6715
    child, L6755, L6765
    small adult, L6770
    stainless steel #8, L6735
      with neoprene, L6780
    with
      neoprene fingers, #8X, L6740
      neoprene fingers, #88X, L6745
      plastisol, #10P, L6750
    work, #3, L6700
      for use with tools, #7, L6725
      with lock, #6, L6720
      with wider opening, L6730
  passive hand, L6868
  soft, passive hand, L6865
Hospice care, S9126
Hot water bottle, E0220
H-Tron insulin pump, E0784
Houdini security suit, E0700
Hoyer patient lifts, E0621, E0625, E0630
Hudson
  adult multi-vent "venturi" style mask,
    A4620
  nasal cannula, A4615
  oxygen supply tubing, A4616
  UC-BL type shoe insert, L3000
Humalog, J1820
Human insulin, J1820
Humatrope, S5022

Humidifier, E0550–E0560, K0268
Humulin insulin, J1820
Hyaluronate, J7315
Hyaluronidase, J3470
Hyate, J7191
Hybolin
  decanoate, J2321
  improved, J0340
Hycamtin, J9350
Hydeltra-TBA, J1690
Hydeltrasol, J2640
Hydralazine HCl, J0360
Hydrate, J1240
Hydraulic patient lift, E0630
Hydrochlorides of opium alkaloids,
  J2480
Hydrocollator, E0225, E0239
Hydrocolloid dressing, A6234–A6241
Hydrocortisone
  acetate, J1700
  sodium phosphate, J1710
  sodium succinate, J1720
Hydrocortone
  acetate, J1700
  phosphate, J1710
Hydrogel dressing, A6242–A6248
Hydrolyser 6F/7F Mechanical
  Thrombectomy catheter, C1054
Hydromorphone, J1170
Hydroxyprogesterone caproate, J1739,
  J1741
Hydroxyzine HCl, J3410
  pamoate, Q0177–Q0178
Hylan G-F 20, J7320
Hylutin, J1741
Hyoscyamine sulfate, J1980
Hyperbaric oxygen chamber, topical,
  A4575
Hyperstat IV, J1730
Hypertonic saline solution, J7130
Hypo-Let lancet device, A4258
HypRho-D, J2790
Hyprogest 250, J1741
Hyrexin-50, J1200
Hyzine-50, J3410

Ibutilide fumarate, J1742
  injection, S0096
Ice cap or collar, E0230
Idamycin, J9211
Idarubicin HCl, J9211
Ifex, J9208

Ifosfamide, J9208
IL-2, J9015
Iletin insulin, J1820
Ilfeld, hip orthosis, L1650
Ilotycin Gluceptate, J1362
Imagyn Medical Technologies IsoStar
    prostate brachytherapy needle,
    C1702
Imiglucerase, J1785
Imipramine HCl, J3270
Imitrex, J3030
Immune globulin IV, J1561, J1562,
    J1563
Immunosuppressive drug, not otherwise
    classified, J7599
Implant
    access system, A4301
    aqueous shunt, L8612
    breast, L8600
    cochlear, L8614, L8619
    collagen, urinary tract, L8603
    contraceptive, A4260
    dental, D3460, D5925,
        D6030–D6999, D7270–D7272,
        D7850
    ganciclovir, J7310
    goserelin acetate, J9202
    hallux, L8642
    infusion pump, E0782, E0783
    injectable bulking agent, urinary tract,
        L8606
    intraocular lens, C1006
    joint, L8630, L8641, L8658
    lacrimal duct, A4262, A4263
    maintenance procedures, D6080,
        D6100
    maxillofacial, D5913–D5937
    medication pellet(s), subcutaneous,
        S2190
    metacarpophalangeal joint, L8630
    metatarsal joint, L8641
    neurostimulator, electrodes/leads,
        E0753
    neurostimulator, pulse generator or
        receiver, E0755–E0756
    not otherwise specified, L8699
    ocular, L8610
    ossicular, L8613
    osteogenesis stimulator, E0749
    penile, C1007
    percutaneous access system, A4301
    removal, dental, D6100
    repair, dental, D6090

Implant — continued
    vascular access portal, A4300
    vascular graft, L8670
    Zoladex, J9202
Impregnated gauze dressing,
    A6222–A6230
Imuran, J7500, J7501
Inapsine, J1790
Incontinence
    appliances and supplies,
        A4310–A4421, A5071–A5075,
        A5102–A5114, K0280, K0281
    treatment system, E0740
Incontinence lines, S8405
Inderal, J1800
Indium/111
    capromab pendetide, A9507
    oxyquinoline, C1091
    pentetate disodium, C1092
InDura Intraspinal Catheter, C1025
Indwelling catheter insertion, G0002
Infergen, J9212
Infliximab injection, J1745
Infusion pump
    ambulatory, with administrative
        equipment, E0781
    epoprostenol, K0455
    heparin, dialysis, E1520
    implantable, E0782, E0783
    implantable, non-programmable,
        C1336-C1337
    implantable, programmable, C3800
    implantable, refill kit, A4220
    insulin, E0784
    mechanical, reusable, E0779, E0780
    supplies, A4221, A4222,
        A4230–A4232
    Versa-Pole IV, E0776
    therapy, other than chemotherapeutic
        drugs, Q0081
Infusion pump rental, S5025
Infusion system for pain, C1368
Inhalation solution (see also drug name),
    J7610–J7799
Injectable bulking agent, urinary tract,
    L8606
Injections (see also drug name),
    J0120–J7506
    contrast material, during MRI, A4643
    dental service, D9610, D9630
    supplies for self-administered, A4211
Inlay/onlay dental restoration,
    D2510–D2664

Innovar, J1810
Inos dual chamber pacemaker, C4308
Insert, convex, for ostomy, A5093
Insertion
    indwelling catheter, G0002
    midline central venous catheter,
        S9528
    peripherally inserted central venous
        catheter (PICC), S9527
    tray, A4310–A4316
Insulin, J1820
Insulin pump, external, E0784
Intal, J7630
Integrity dual chamber pacemaker,
    C4300-C4301
Interferon
    Alfa, J9212–J9215
    Alfacon-1, J9212
    Beta-1a, J1825
    Beta-1b, J1830
    Gamma, J9216
Intergrilin injection, J1327
Intermittent
    peritoneal dialysis system, E1592
    positive pressure breathing (IPPB)
        machine, E0500
Internal receiver, neurostimulation
    system, C1369
Interphalangeal joint, prosthetic implant,
    L8658
Interscapular thoracic prosthesis
    endoskeletal, L6570
    upper limb, L6350–L6370
InterStim Therapy 3080/3086 Lead,
    C1378
IntraCoil Peripheral Stent, C5039-C5040
Intraocular lens, C3851
Intraocular lenses, V2630–V2632,
    Q1001–Q1005
    new technology
        category 1, Q1001
        category 2, Q1002
        category 3, Q1003
        category 4, Q1004
        category 5, Q1005
Intraoral radiographs, D0210–D0240
IntraStent, biliary stent, C5011-C5013
Intrauterine copper contraceptive, J7300
Intron A, J9214
Iobenguane sulfate I-131, A9508, C1045
Iodinated I-131 albumin, C9100
Iodine swabs/wipes, A4247

IPD
    supply kit, A4905
    system, E1592
IPPB machine, E0500
Ipratropium bromide
    0.2%, J7645
    inhalation solution, unit dose, J7644
Irinotecan, J9206
Iris Preventix pressure relief/reduction
    mattress, E0184
Iris therapeutic overlays, E0199
IRM ankle-foot orthosis, L1950
Irodex, J1750
Iron dextran, J1750
Irrigation
    solution, A4319
Irrigation/evacuation system, bowel
    control unit, E0350
    disposable supplies for, E0352
Irrigation supplies, A4320, A4322,
        A4323, A4355, A4397–A4400
    Solution, A4319
    Surfit
        irrigation adapter face plate, A4361
        irrigation sleeve, A4397
        night drainage container set, A5102
    Visi-flow irrigator, A4398, A4399
Irvine Inquiry Steerable
    Electrophysiology 6F Catheter,
    C2002-C2003
Isocaine HCl, J0670
Isocal, enteral nutrition, B4150
    HCN, B4152
Isoetharine
    HCl, J7650–J7655
    inhalation solution
        concentrated, J7648
        unit dose, J7649
Isolated limb perfusion, S8048
Isolates, B4150, B4152
IsoMed Infusion Pump Model 8472-20,
        8472-35, 8472-60, C1337
Isoproterenol HCl, inhalation solution
        concentrated, J7658
        unit dose, J7659
Isotein, enteral nutrition, B4153
Isuprel, J7660, J7665
Itraconazole, S0096
IUD, J7300
IV pole, E0776, K0105
IV therapy, S9550, S9555

J-cell battery, replacement for blood glucose monitor, A4254
Jace tribrace, L1832
Jacket
　body (LSO) (spinal), L0500–L0565
　scoliosis, L1300, L1310
Jade II S pacemaker, C1183
Jenamicin, J1580
Jewett, spinal orthosis, L0370
Johnson's orthopedic wrist hand cock-up splint, L3914
Johnson's thumb immobilizer, L3800
Joystick, power add-on, K0460
Jupiter PTA Balloon Dilatation Catheter, C1941

Kabikinase, J2995
Kairos dual chamber pacemaker, C4307
Kaleinate, J0610
Kaltostat, alginate dressing, A6196–A6199
Kanamycin sulfate, J1840, J1850
Kantrex, J1840, J1850
Kartop Patient Lift, toilet or bathroom (see also Lift), E0625
Keflin, J1890
Kefurox, J0697
Kefzol, J0690
Kenaject -40, J3301
Kenalog (-10,-40), J3301
Keratectomy photorefractive, S0810
Kestrone-5, J1435
Keto-Diastix, box of 100 glucose/ketone urine test strips, A4250
Ketorolac thomethamine, J1885
Key-Pred
　-SP, J2640
　-25,-50, J2650
K-Flex, J2360
Kidney
　ESRD supply, A4650–A4927
　system, E1510
　wearable artificial, E1632
Kingsley gloves, above hands, L6890
Kits
　continuous ambulatory peritoneal dialysis (CAPD), A4900
　continuous cycling peritoneal dialysis (CCPD), A4901
　dialysis, A4820, A4910, A4914
　enteral feeding supply (syringe) (pump) (gravity), B4034–B4036

Kits — continued
　fistula cannulation (set), A4730
　intermittent peritoneal dialysis (IPD) supply, A4905
　parenteral nutrition, B4220–B4224
　surgical dressing (tray), A4550
　tracheostomy, A4625
Klebcil, J1840, J1850
Knee
　Adjustabrace™ 3, L2999
　disarticulation, prosthesis, L5150-L5160
　immobilizer, L1830
　joint, miniature, L5826
　Knee-O-Prene™ Hinged Knee Sleeve, L1810
　Knee-O-Prene™ Hinged Wraparound Knee Support, L1810
　locks, L2405-L2425
　Masterbrace™ 3, L2999
　Masterhinge Adjustabrace™ 3, L2999
　orthosis (KO), E1810, L1800-L1885
　Performance Wrap™ (KO), L1825
Knee-ankle-foot orthosis (KAFO), L2000–L2039, L2122–L2136
Knee-O-Prene™ Hinged Knee Sleeve, L1810
Knee-O-Prene™ Hinged Wraparound Knee Support, L1810
Knight apron-front, spinal orthosis, L0330, L0520
Knight-Taylor apron-front, spinal orthosis, L0330
KnitRite
　prosthetic
　　sheath, L8400–L8415
　　sock, L8420–L8435
　stump sock, L8470–L8485
KoalaKair mattress overlay, with pump, E0180
Kodel clavicle splint, L3660
Kogenate, J7192
Konakion, J3430
Konyne-HT, J7194
Kutapressin, J1910
K-Y Lubricating Jelly, A4402, K0281
Kyphosis pad, L1020, L1025
Kytril, J1626

Laboratory tests
　chemistry, P2028–P2038
　microbiology, P7001

Index

Lodging, recipient, escort
  nonemergency transport, A0180,
  A0200
Lonalac powder, enteral nutrition,
  B4150
Lorazepam, J2060
Lovenox, J1650
Low Profile therapeutic dry flotation
  cushion, E0964
Lower limb, prosthesis, addition, L5968
LSO, L0500–L0565
Lubricant, A4402, K0281
Lufyllin, J1180
Luge PTCA guidewire, C3551
Lumbar
  criss-cross (LSO), L0500
  EZ Fit LSO, L0500
  flexion, L0540
  pad, L1030, L1040
  -sacral orthosis (LSO), L0500-L0565
Luminal sodium, J2560
Lupron, J9218
  depot, J1950
Lymphedema therapy, S8950
Lymphocyte immune globulin, J7504

Macausland apron-front, spinal orthosis,
  L0530
Madamist II medication
  compressor/nebulizer, E0570
Magnacal, enteral nutrition, B4152
Magnesium sulphate, J3475
Magnetic source imaging, S8035
Magnuson apron-front, spinal orthosis,
  L0340
Mailman PTCA guidewire, C3551
Maintenance contract, ESRD, A4890
Malibu cervical turtleneck safety collar,
  L0150
Mammotome
  HH Hand-Held Probe with Smartvac
    Vacuum System, C1176
  Probe with Vacuum Cannister, C1177,
    C1179
Mammotome Probe with vacuum
  cannister, C1177, C1179
Mannitol, J2150
Mapping, topographic brain, S8040
Marmine, J1240
Mask
  cushion, K0184
  oxygen, A4620, A4621

Mastectomy
  bra, L8000
  form, L8020
  prosthesis, L8015, L8030, L8035,
    L8600
  sleeve, L8010
Masterbrace™ 3, L2999
Masterfoot™ Walking Cast Sole, L3649
Masterhinge Adjustabrace™ 3, L2999
Masterhinge™ Elbow Brace 3, L3999
Masterhinge™ Hip Hinge 3, L2999
Masterhinge™ Shoulder Brace 3, L3999
Maternity support, L0920, L0930
Mattress
  air pressure, E0176, E0186, E0197
  alternating pressure, E0277
    pad, Bio Flote, E0181
    pad, KoalaKair, E0181
  AquaPedic Sectional, E0196
  decubitus care, E0196
  dry pressure, E0184
  flotation, E0184
  gel pressure, E0196
  hospital bed, E0271, E0272
    non-powered, pressure reducing,
      E0373
  Iris Preventix pressure relief/reduction,
    E0184
  Overlay, E0371-E0372
  TenderFlor II, E0187
  TenderGel II, E0196
  water pressure, E0177, E0187, E0198
    powered, pressure reducing, E0277
Maxillofacial dental procedures,
  D5911–D5999
Maxxum, NC catheter, C1981
MCP, multi-axial rotation unit, L5986
MCT Oil, enteral nutrition, B4155
Measuring cylinder, dialysis, A4921
Mechlorethamine HCl, J9230
Medical and surgical supplies,
  A4206–A6404
Medical conference, S0220-S0221
Medical food, S9435
Medi-Jector injection device, A4210
MediSense 2 Pen blood glucose
  monitor, E0607
Medralone 40, J1030
  80, J1040
Medrol, J7509
Medroxyprogesterone acetate, J1050,
  J1055

Monitor — *continued*
blood glucose, E0607, E0609
Accu-Check, E0607
One Touch II, E0609
Re Flotron Plus Analyzer, E0609
Tracer II, E0607
blood pressure, A4670
pacemaker, E0610, E0615
ventilator, E0450
Monitoring and recording, EKG,
G0004–G0007
Monoclonal antibodies, J7505
Monoject disposable insulin syringes, up
to 1cc, per syringe, A4206
Monojector lancet device, A4258
Mononine, Q0160
Morcellator, C1073
Morphine sulfate, J2270, J2271
sterile, preservative-free, J2275
Mouthpiece (for respiratory equipment),
A4617
M-Prednisol-40, J1030
-80, J1040
MRI contrast material, A4643
Mucoprotein, blood, P2038
Multilink Tetra coronary stent system,
C5045
Multiple post collar, cervical,
L0180–L0200
Muse, J0275
Mutamycin, J9280
Mycophenolate mofetil, J7517
Myochrysine, J1600
Myolin, J2360

Nafcillin sodium, S0032
Nail trim, G0127
Nalbuphine HCl, J2300
Naloxone HCl, J2310
Nandrobolic, J0340
L.A., J2321
Nandrolone
decanoate, J2320–J2322
phenpropionate, J0340
Narcan, J2310
Narrowing device, wheelchair, E0969
Nasahist B, J0945
Nasal
application device (for CPAP device),
K0183
pillows/seals (for nasal application
device), K0184
vaccine inhalation, J3530

Nasogastric tubing, B4081, B4082
National Emphysema Treatment Trial
(NETT) codes, G0110–G0116
Navane, J2330
Navelbine, J9390
Navi-Star diagnostic/ablation catheter,
C2016-C2017
NC Big Ranger catheter, C1981
ND Stat, J0945
Nebcin, J3260
Nebulizer, E0570–E0585
aerosol compressor, K0501
aerosol mask, A7015
aerosols, E0580
Airlife Brand Misty-Neb, E0580
Power-Mist, E0580
Up-Draft Neb-U-Mist, E0580
Up-Mist hand-held nebulizer, E0580
compressor, with, E0570
Madamist II medication
compressor/nebulizer, E0570
Pulmo-Aide compressor/nebulizer,
E0570
Schuco Mist nebulizer system,
E0570
corrugated tubing
disposable, A7010, A7018
non-disposable, A7011
distilled water, A7018
drug dispensing fee, E0590
filter
disposable, A7013
non-disposable, A7014
heater, E1372
large volume
disposable, prefilled, A7008
disposable, unfilled, A7007
not used with oxygen
durable glass, A7017
pneumatic, administration set, A7003,
A7005, A7006
pneumatic, nonfiltered, A7004
saline solution, A7019
small volume, A7004
sterile water/saline, A7020
ultrasonic, dome and mouthpiece,
A7016
ultrasonic, reservoir bottle
non-disposable, A7009
water, A7018-A7020

Index

NuHope — *continued*
   regular adhering tape strips
     (100/pkg), A4454
   regular pink adhering tape strips
     (100/pkg), A4454
   round post-op drainables, A5064
   round post-op urinary pouches,
     A5074
   support belt, L0940
   thinning solvent, A4454
Nulicaine, J2000
Numorphan H.P., J2410
Nursing care, in home
   licensed practical nurse, S9124
   registered nurse, S9123
Nursing services, S9200-S9225
Nutri-Source, enteral nutrition, B4155
Nutrition
   counseling, dental, D1310, D1320
   enteral infusion pump, B9000, B9002
   enteral formulae, B4150–B4156
   guidance, NETT pulmonary rehab
     initial, G0112
     subsequent, G0113
   parenteral infusion pump, B9004,
     B9006
   parenteral solution, B4164–B5200
Nutritional counseling, dietition visit,
   S9470
NYU, hand prosthesis, child, L6872

Oasis Thrombectomy catheter, C1051
Obturator prosthesis
   definitive, D5932
   interim, D5936
   surgical, D5931
Occipital/mandibular support, cervical,
   L0160
Occupational therapist
   home health setting, G0152
Occupational therapy, G0129, S9129
Ocular prosthetic implant, L8610
Oculinum, J0585
Odansetron HCl, J2405, Q0179
Office service, M0064
Offobock cosmetic gloves, L6895
O-Flex, J2360
Ofloxacin, S0034
Ohio Willow
   prosthetic sheath
     above knee, L8410
     below knee, L8400
     upper limb, L8415

Ohio Willow — *continued*
   prosthetic sock, L8420–L8435
   stump sock, L8470–L8485
Omnipen-N, J0290
Oncaspar, J9266
Oncoscint, A4642
Oncovin, J9370
One arm drive attachment, K0101
One-Button foldaway walker, E0143
One Touch
   Basic blood glucose meter, E0607
   Basic test strips, box of 50, A4253
   Profile blood glucose meter, E0607
On-Q Pain management system, C1368
On-Q Soaker pain management system,
   C1368
Ontak IV, C1084
O & P Express
   above knee, L5300, L5210
   ankle-foot orthosis with bilateral
     uprights, L1990
   anterior floor reaction orthosis, L1945
   below knee, L5105
   elbow disarticulation, L6200
   hip disarticulation, L5250
     endoskeletal, L5330
   hip-knee-ankle-foot orthosis, L2080
   interscapular thoracic, L6370
   knee-ankle-foot orthosis, L2000,
     L2010, L2020, L2036
   knee disarticulation, L5150, L5160
   Legg Perthes orthosis, Patten, L1755
   Legg Perthes orthosis, Scottish Rite,
     L1730
   partial foot, L5000, L5020
   plastic foot drop brace, L1960
   supply/accessory/service, L9900
Opium alkaloids, hydrochlorides of,
   J2480
Oppenheimer, wrist-hand-finger
   orthosis, L3924
Oprelvekin, J2355
Opti-Plast Centurion 5.5F PTA catheter,
   shaft length 50cm to 120cm,
   C1933
Opti-Plast XL 5.5F PTA catheter, shaft
   length 75 cm to 120cm, C1933
Oral and maxillofacial surgery,
   D7110–D7999
Oral examination, D0120–D0160
Oral orthotic treatment for sleep apnea,
   S8260
Oraminic II, J0945

Oratec SpineCath intradiscal catheter, C2607
Oratec SpineCath XL intradiscal catheter, C2606
Orbiter ST Steerable electrode catheter, C2000
Ormazine, J3230
Oropharyngeal suction catheter, A4628
Orphenadrine, J2360
Orphenate, J2360
Orthodontics, D8010–D8999
Ortho-Ease forearm crutches, E0111
Orthoflex™ Elastic Plaster Bandages, A4580
Orthoguard hip orthosis, L1685
Orthomedics
  ankle-foot orthosis, L1900
  pediatric hip abduction splint, L1640
  plastic foot drop brace, L1960
  single axis shoe insert, L2180
  ultralight airplane arm abduction splint, L3960
  upper extremity fracture orthosis
    combination, L3986
    humeral, L3980
    radius/ulnar, L3982
Orthomerica
  below knee test socket, L5620
  pediatric hip abduction splint, L1640
  plastic foot drop brace, L1960
  single axis shoe insert, L2180
  upper extremity fracture orthosis
    humeral, L3980
    radius/ulnar, L3982
  wrist extension cock-up, L3914
Orthopedic devices, E0910-E0948
  cervical
    Diskard head halters, E0942
    Turtle Neck safety collars, E0942
Orthopedic shoes
  arch support, L3040–L3100
  footwear, L3201–L3265
  insert, L3000–L3030
  lift, L3300–L3334
  miscellaneous additions, L3500–L3595
  positioning device, L3140–L3170
  transfer, L3600–L3649
  wedge, L3340–L3420
Orthoplast™ Splints (and Orthoplast™ II Splints), A4590
Orthotic additions
  carbon graphite lamination, L2755
  fracture, L2180–L2192, L3995

Orthotic additions — continued
  halo, L0860
  lower extremity, L2200–L2999
  ratchet lock, L2430
  scoliosis, L1010–L1120, L1210–L1290
  shoe, L3300–L3595, L3649
  spinal, L0970–L0999
  upper extremity joint, L3956
  upper limb, L3810–L3890, L3970–L3974, L3995
Orthotic devices
  ankle-foot (see also Orthopedic shoes), E1815, E1830, L1900–L1990, L2102–L2116, L3160
  anterior-posterior, L0320, L0330, L0530
  anterior-posterior-lateral, L0520, L0550–L0565, L0700, L0710
  anterior-posterior-lateral-rotary, L0340–L0440
  cervical, L0100–L0200
  cervical-thoracic-lumbar-sacral, L0700, L0710
  elbow, E1800, L3700–L3740
  fracture, L2102–L2136, L3980–L3986
  halo, L0810–L0830
  hand, E1805, E1825, L3800–L3805, L3900–L3954
  hip, L1600–L1686
  hip-knee-ankle-foot, L2040–L2090
  interface material, E1820
  knee, E1810, L1800–L1885
  knee-ankle-foot, L2000–L2038, L2122–L2136
  Legg Perthes, L1700–L1755
  lumbar flexion, L0540
  lumbar-sacral, L0500–L0565
  lumbar-sacral, hip, femur, L1690
  multiple post collar, L0180–L0200
  not otherwise specified, L0999, L1499, L2999, L3999, L5999, L7499, L8039, L8239
  pneumatic splint, L4350–L4380
  repair or replacement, L4000–L4210
  replace soft interface material, L4392–L4394
  sacroilliac, L0600–L0620
  scoliosis, L1000, L1200, L1300–L1499
  shoe, see Orthopedic shoes
  shoulder, L3650–L3675
  shoulder-elbow-wrist-hand, L3960–L3969

Orthotic devices — *continued*
  spinal, cervical, L0100–L0200
  spinal, DME, K0112–K0116
  thoracic, L0210
  thoracic-hip-knee-ankle, L1500–L1520
  thoracic-lumbar-sacral, L0300–L0440
  toe, E1830
  torso supports, L0900–L0690
  transfer (shoe orthosis), L3600–L3640
  wrist-hand-finger, E1805, E1825,
    L3800–L3805, L3900–L3954
Or-Tyl, J0500
Osgood apron-front, sacroiliac orthosis,
  L0620
Osmolite, enteral nutrition, B4150
  HN, B4150
Ossicula prosthetic implant, L8613
Osteogenic stimulator, E0747–E0749,
  E0760
Osteotomy, segmented/subapical,
  D7944
Ostomy
  accessories, A5093
  adhesive remover wipes, A4365
  appliance belt, A4367
  filter, A4368
  irrigation supply, A4398, A4399
  supplies, A4361–A4421,
    A5051–A5093
    pediatric one-piece system, A5061,
      A5062
    pediatric two-piece drainable
      pouch, A5063
    pediatric two-piece system with
      cut-to-fit synthetic skin barrier,
      A5123
Otto Bock prosthesis
  battery, six volt, L7360
  battery charger, six volt, L7362
  electronic greifer, L7020, L7035
  electronic hand, L7010, L7025
  hook adapter, L6628
  lamination collar, L6629
  pincher tool, L6810
  wrist, L6629, L7260
Overlay, mattress, E0371–E0373
Over-the-Wire balloon dilatation
  catheter, C1810
Owens & Minor
  cervical collar, L0140
  cervical helmet, L0120
Oxacillin sodium, J2700
Oximeter, S8105, S8405

Oxi-Uni-Pak, E0430
Oxygen
  ambulance, A0422
  chamber, hyperbaric, topical, A4575
  concentrator, E1390
  hyperbaric treatment, G0167
  mask, A4620, A4621
  medication supplies, A4611–A4627
  rack/stand, E1355
  regulator, E1353
  respiratory equipment/supplies,
    A4611–A4627, E0424–E0480
    Argyle Sentinel seal chest drainage
      unit, E0460
    Oxi-Uni-Pak, E0430
  supplies and equipment,
    E0425–E0444, E0455,
    E1353–E1406
  tent, E0455
  tubing, A4616
  water vapor enriching system, E1405,
    E1406
Oxymorphone HCl, J2410
Oxytetracycline HCl, J2460
Oxytocin, J2590

Pacemaker
  dual chamber, C4300-C4317
  single chamber, C1180-C1184,
    C4005
Pacemaker, dual chamber, rate-
  responsive, C1135-C1136
Pacemaker monitor, E0610, E0615
Pacemaker, single chamber, C4000-
  C4005
Pacemaker, single chamber, Kairos single
  chamber pacemaker, C4003
Pacer manual wheelchair, K0003
Paclitaxel, J9265
Pad
  abdominal, L1270
  adhesive, A6203–A6205,
    A6212–A6214, A6219–A6221,
    A6237–A6239, A6245–A6247,
    A6254–A6256
  air pressure, E0178, E0179
  alginate, A6192–A6199
  alternating pressure, E0180, E0181
  arm, K0019
  asis, L1250

Pad — *continued*
  calf, K0049
  condylar, L2810
  crutch, A4635
  gel pressure, E0178, E0185, E0196
  gluteal L2650
  heating, E0210, E0215, E0217,
    E0238, E0249
  heel, L3480, L3485
  knee, L1858
  kyphosis, L1020, L1025
  lumbar, L1030, L1040, L1240
  nonadhesive (dressing),
    A6209–A6211, A6216–A6218,
    A6222–A6224, A6228–A6230,
    A6234–A6236, A6242–A6244
  orthotic device interface, E1820
  rib gusset, L1280
  sheepskin, E0188, E0189
  shoe, L3430–L3485
  stabilizer, L3170
  sternal, L1050
  thoracic, L1060, L1260
  torso support, L0960
  triceps, L6100
  trocanteric, L1290
  truss, L8320, L8330
  water circulating, cold, with pump,
    E0218
  water circulating, heat, with pump,
    E0217
  water circulating, heat, unit, E0249
  water pressure, E0177, E0198
  wheelchair, low pressure and
    positioning, E0192
Padden Shoulder Immobilizer, L3670
Pail, for use with commode chair, E0167
Pain management, S9533
Pain therapy, S5018
PainBuster Pain Management System,
  C1368
Palate Somnoplasty coagulating
  electrode, C1321
Palicizumab RSV IgM, C9003
Palmer, wrist-hand-finger orthosis,
  L3936
Pamidronate disodium, J2430
Pan, for use with commode chair, E0167
Panglobulin, J1561
Pantopon, J2480
Papanicolaou (Pap) screening smear,
  P3000, P3001, Q0091
Papaverine HCl, J2440

Paraffin, A4265
  bath unit, E0235
Paragard T 380 A, IUD, J7300
Paramagnetic contrast material,
  (Gadolinium), A4647
Paranasal sinus ultrasound, S9024
Paraplatin, J9045
Parapodium, mobility frame, L1500
Parenteral nutrition
  administration kit, B4224
  pump, B9004, B9006
  solution, B4164–B5200
  supplies, not otherwise classified,
    B9999
  supply kit, B4220, B4222
Parking fee, nonemergency transport,
  A0170
Paste, conductive, A4558
Pathology and laboratory tests,
  miscellaneous, P9010–P9615
Patriot, PTCA guidewire, C3551
Patten Bottom, Legg Perthes orthosis,
  L1755
Pavlik harness, hip orthosis, L1650
Peak expiratory flow meter, S8110
Peak flow meter, portable, S8096
PEFR, peak expiratory flow rate meter,
  A4614
Pegademase bovine, Q2012
Pegaspargase, J9266
Peg-L-asparaginase, J9266
Pediatric hip abduction splint
  Orthomedics, L1640
  Orthomerica, L1640
Pelvic and breast exam, G0101
Pelvic belt/harness/boot, E0944
Pelvicol Acellular collagen Matrix,
  C6012-C6016
Penicillin G
  benzathine and penicillin G procaine,
    J0530–J0580
  potassium, J2540
  procaine, aqueous, J2510
Penlet lancet device, A4258
Penlet II lancet device, A4258
Pentagastrin, J2512
Pentamidine isethionate, J2545, S0080
Pentastarch, Q2013
Pentazocine HCl, J3070
Pentobarbital sodium, J2515
Pentostatin, J9268
Peptavlon, J2512
Percussor, E0480

Percutaneous access system, A4301
Perfluoron, C8890-C8891
Performance Wrap™ (KO), L1825
Periapical service, D3410–D3470
Periodontal procedures, D4210–D4999
Peripherally inserted central venous
    catheter (PICC) insertion, S9527
Perlstein, ankle-foot orthosis, L1920
Permapen, J0560–J0580
Peroneal strap, L0980
Peroxide, A4244
Perphenazine, J3310, Q0175–Q0176
Persantine, J1245
Personal comfort item, A9190
Pessary, A4561-A4562
PET
    lung, imaging, G0125, G0126
    myocardial perfusion imaging,
        G0030–G0047
    whole body
        colorectal metastatic cancer, G0163
        lymphoma, G0164
        melanoma, G0165
        melanoma metastatic cancer,
            G0165
Pfizerpen, J2540
    A.S., J2510
PGE₁, J0270
Pharmaplast disposable insulin syringes,
    per syringe, A4206
Phelps, ankle-foot orthosis, L1920
Phenazine (25, 50), J2550
Phenergan, J2550
Phenobarbital sodium, J2560
Phentolamine mesylate, J2760
Phenylephrine HCl, J2370
Phenytoin sodium, J1165
Philadelphia™ tracheotomy cervical
    collar, L0172
Philly™ One-piece™ Extrication collar,
    L0150
Philos
    dual chamber pacemaker, C4311
    single chamber pacemaker, C4005
PHisoHex solution, A4246
Photofrin, J9600
Photon DR V-230HV3 dual chamber
    defibrillator, C1364
Phototherapy light, E0202
Physical therapy/therapist
    evaluation/treatment, Q0086
    home health setting, G0151

Physician services
    peak expiratory flow rate, S8110
Phytonadione, J3430
Pillo pump, E0182
Pillow
    abduction, E1399
    cervical, E0943
Pin retention, per tooth, D2951
Pinworm examination, Q0113
Piperacillin sodium, S0081
Pitocin, J2590
Plasma
    multiple donor, pooled, frozen, P9023
    protein fraction, P9043
    single donor, fresh frozen, P9017
Plastazote, L3002, L3252, L3253, L3265,
    L5654–L5658
Plaster
    bandages
        Orthoflex™ Elastic Plaster
            Bandages, A4580
        Specialist™ Plaster Bandages,
            A4580
    Genmould™ Creamy Plaster, A4580
    Specialist™ J-Splint™ Plaster Roll
        Immobilizer, A4580
    Specialist™ Plaster Roll Immobilizer,
        A4580
    Specialist™ Plaster Splints, A4580
Platelet
    concentrate, each unit, P9019
    leukoreduced concentrate, C1011-
        C1017
    rich plasma, each unit, P9020
Platelets, P9032-P9040
Platform, for home blood glucose
    monitor, A4255
Platform attachment
    forearm crutch, E0153
    walker, E0154
Platinol, J9060, J9062
Plicamycin, J9270
Plumbing, for home ESRD equipment,
    A4870
Pneumatic
    appliance, E0655–E0673,
        L4350–L4380
    compressor, E0650–E0652
    splint, L4350–L4380
    tire, wheelchair, E0953
Pneumatic nebulizer
    administration set
        small volume
            filtered, A7006

Pneumatic nebulizer — *continued*
administration set — *continued*
small volume — *continued*
non-filtered, A7003
non-disposable, A7005
small volume, disposable, A7004
Podiatric service, noncovered, A9160
Polaris T ablation catheter, C2018
Polocaine, J0670
Polycillin-N, J0290
Polycose, enteral nutrition,
liquid, B4155
powder, B4155
Polygam SD, J1562
Polyrox pacemaker lead, C4600
Pontics, D5281, D6210–D6252
Porfimer, J9600
Pork insulin, J1820
Portable
equipment transfer, R0070–R0076
hemodialyzer system, E1635
x-ray equipment, Q0092
Portagen Powder, enteral nutrition,
B4150
Posey restraints, E0700
Post-coital examination, Q0115
Post-voiding residual, ultrasound, G0050
Postural drainage board, E0606
Potassium
chloride, J3480
hydroxide (KOH) preparation, Q0112
Pouch
Active Life convex one-piece
urostomy, A4421
closed, A5052
drainable, A5061
fecal collection, A4330
Little Ones Surfit mini, A5054
ostomy, A4375–A4378,
A5051–A5054, A5061–A5065
pediatric, drainable, A5061
post-op urinary, A5074
Pouchkins pediatric ostomy system,
A5061, A5062, A5073
Sur-Fit, drainable, A5063
urinary, A4379–A4383, A5071–A5075
urosotomy, A5073
Power mist nebulizer, E0580
Pralidoxime chloride, J2730
Precision, enteral nutrition
HN, B4153
Isotonic, B4153

Precision, enteral nutrition — *continued*
LR, B4156
Predalone-50, J2650
TBA, J1690
Predcor (-25, -50), J2650
Predicort-50, J2650
Prednisol TBA, J1690
Prednisolone
acetate, J2650
oral, J7506, J7510
sodium phosphate, J2640
tebutate, J1690
Prednisone, J7506
Predoject-50, J2650
Prefabricated crown, D2930–D2933
Preface braided guiding sheath (anterior
curve, multipurpose curve,
posterior curve), C6500
Pregnyl, J0725
Premarin IV, J1410
Premium knee sleeve, L1830
Preparation kit, dialysis, A4914
Preparatory prosthesis, L5510–L5595
Prescription drug, J3490, J7140, J8499
chemotherapy, J7150, J8999, J9999
nonchemotherapy, J8499
Pressure
alarm, dialysis, E1540
pad, A4640, E0176–E0199
PressureGuard II, E0186
PressureKair mattress overlay, E0197
Prestige blood glucose monitor, E0607
Pre-Vent heel and elbow protector,
E0191
Preventive dental procedures,
D1000–D1999
Primacor, J2260
Primaxin, J0743
Priscoline HCl, J2670
Probe
Microvasive Swiss F/G Lithoclast
Flexible, C6600
Procainamide HCl, J2690
Processed fascia lata, C1853-C1857
Prochlorperazine, J0780, Q0164–Q0165
Procuren, S9055
Pro-Depo, J1739, J1741
Profasi HP, J0725
Profilnine Heat-Treated, J7194
Progestaject, J2675
Progesterone, J2675

Index

Prograf, J7507, J7508
Prolastin, J0256
Proleukin, J9015
Prolixin decanoate, J2680
Prolotherapy, M0076
Promazine HCl, J2950
Promethazine HCl, J2550,
    Q0169–Q0170
Promethazine and meperdine, J2180
Promix, enteral nutrition, B4155
Pronestyl, J2690
Propac, enteral nutrition, B4155
Propiomazine, J1930
Proplex (-T and SX-T), J7194
Propranolol HCl, J1800
Prorex (-25, -50), J2550
Prostaglandin E$_1$, J0270
Prostaphlin, J2700
Prosthesis
    adhesive, used for facial
        liquid, K0450
        remover, K0451
    auricular, D5914, L8045
    breast, C3001, C3401, L8000–L8035,
        L8600
    dental, fixed, D6210–D6999
    dental, removable, D5110–D5899
    eye, L8610, V2623–V2629
    fitting, L5400–L5460, L6380–L6388
    hand, L6000–L6020
    hemifacial, L8044
    implants, L8600–L8699
    larynx, L8500
    lower extremity, L5700–L5999, L8642
    midfacial, L8041
    miscellaneous service, L8499
    nasal septal, L8047
    obturator, D5931–D5933, D5936
    ocular, V2623–V2629
    orbital, L8042
    partial facial, L8046
    penile, C1007, C3500
    repair, K0449, L7520
    repair or modification, maxillofacial,
        L8048
    socks (shrinker, sheath, stump sock),
        L8400–L8480
    tracheostomy speaking, L8501
    upper extremity, L6000–L6915

Prosthesis — *continued*
    upper facial, L8043
    vacuum erection system, L7900
Prosthetic additions
    lower extremity, L5610–L5999
    upper extremity, L6600–L7274
Prosthetic shrinker, L8440-L8465
Prosthodontic procedures
    fixed, D6210–D6999
    removable, D5110–D5899
Prostigmin, J2710
Prostin VR Pediatric, J0270
Protamine sulfate, J2720
Protectant, skin, A6250
Protector, heel or elbow, E0191
Protirelin, J2725
Protopam chloride, J2730
Protropin, S5022
Prozine-50, J2950
PT Graphix intermediate PTCA
    guidewire, C3551
PTCA
    catheter, C1101
    guidewire, C1100, C3551
Pulmo-Aide compressor/nebulizer,
    E0570
Pulp capping, D3110, D3120
Pulpotomy, D3220
    vitality test, D0460
Pulsar SSI pacemaker, C1182
Pump
    alternating pressure pad, E0182
    ambulatory infusion, E0781
    ambulatory insulin, E0874
    Bio Flote alternating pressure pad,
        E0182
    blood, dialysis, E1620
    Broncho-Cath endobronchial tubes,
        with CPAP, E0601
    enteral infusion, B9000, B9002
    Gomco lightweight mobile aspirator,
        E0600
    Gomco portable aspirator, E0600
    heparin infusion, E1520
    implantable infusion, E0782, E0783
    implantable infusion, refill kit, A4220
    infusion, supplies, A4230–A4232
    insulin, external, E0784
    parenteral infusion, B9004, B9006
    Pillo alternating pressure pad, E0182
    suction, CPAP, E0601

Pump — *continued*
   suction, portable, E0600
   TenderCloud alternating pressure pad,
      E0182
   water circulating pad, E0217, E0218,
      E0236
Purification system, A4880, E1610,
   E1615
Purified pork insulin, J1820

Quad cane, E0105
Quadri-Poise canes, E0105
Quantum Ranger, catheter, C1981
Quelicin, J0330
Quick Check blood glucose test strips,
   box of 50, A4253
Quick release restraints, E0700
Quikfit crutch, E0114
Quik-Fold Walkers, E0141, E0143
Quinoprestin, C1024, J2770

Rack/stand, oxygen, E1355
Racrolimus, C9006
Radiation therapy, intraoperative, S8049
Radioelements for brachytherapy,
   Q3001
Radiograph, dental, D0210–D0340
Radioimmunoscintigraphy, S8080
Radiology service, R0070–R0076
Radiopharmaceutical
   diagnostic imaging agent, A4641,
      A4642, A9500–A9505
   Technetium Tc 99m Apcitide, A9504
   therapeutic, A9600
Radius 20mm self expanding stent with
   over the wire delivery system,
   C5046
Rail
   bathtub, E0241, E0242, E0246
   bed, E0305, E0310
   toilet, E0243
RAMP guiding introducer, C1004
Rancho hip action, hip orthosis, L1680
Ranger catheter, C1981
Rapid Exchange single-use biliary stent
   system, C5010
Raptor PTCA dilatation catheter, C1939
Rascal, power wheelchair, K0010
Re Flotron Plus analyzer, E0609
Ready-For-Use wooden crutches, E0113
Recement
   crown, D2920
   inlay, D2910

Reciprocating peritoneal dialysis system,
   E1630
Recombinant
   ankle splints, L4392–L4398
   DNA insulin, J1820
Recombinate, J7192
Reconstruction patch, C6034-C6041
Red blood cells, P9038-P9040
Red blood cells, each unit, P9021,
   P9022
Red Dot
   crutches, E0114
   folding walkers, E0135, E0143
Redisol, J3420
Regitine, J2760
Reglan, J2765
Regular insulin, J1820
Regulator, oxygen, E1353
Relefact TRH, J2725
Remicade, J1745
Renacidin, Q2004
RenAmin, parenteral nutrition, B5000
Renu, enteral nutrition, B4150
ReoPro, TRH, J0130
Repair
   contract, ERSD, A4890
   dental, D2980, D3351–D3353,
      D5510–D5630, D6090, D6980,
      D7852, D7955
   durable medical equipment, E1340
   hearing aid, V5014, V5336
   home dialysis equipment, A4890
   orthotic, L4000–L4130
   prosthetic, L7500, L7510, L7520
   skilled technical, E1350
Replacement
   battery, A4254, A4630, A4631
   components, ESRD machine, E1640
   handgrip for cane, crutch, walker
      A4636
   ostomy filters, A4421
   pad (alternating pressure), A4640
   tanks, dialysis, A4880
   tip for cane, crutch, walker, A4637
   underarm pad for crutch, A4635
Repliform Tissue regeneration matrix,
   C1850
Rep-Pred
   40, J1030
   80, J1040
ResCap headgear, K0185
Reservoir
   metered dose inhaler, A4627

Sargramostim (GM-CSF), J2820
Satumomab pendetide, A4642
Scale, dialysis, A4910
Schuco
    mist nebulizer system, E0570
    vac aspirator, E0600
SciMed 6F Wiseguide Guide Catheter,
    C2608
SciMed Remedy coronary balloon
    dilatation infusion catheter
    (20mm), C1932
Scintimammography, S8080
Scissors, dialysis, A4910
Scoliosis, L1000, L1200, L1300–L1499
    additions, L1010–L1120,
        L1210–L1290
Scott ankle splint, canvas, L1904
Scott-Craig, stirrup orthosis, L2260
Scottish-Rite, Legg Perthes orthosis,
    L1730
Screening
    newborn metabolic, S3620
Screening examination
    cervical or vaginal, G0101
    colorectal cancer, G0104-G0017,
        G0120-G0122
    digital rectal, annual, S0605
    gynecological
        established patient, S0612
        new patient, S0610
    ophthalmological, including refraction
        established patient, S0621
        new patient, S0620
    proctoscopy, S0601
    prostate
        digital, rectal, G0102
    prostate specific antigen test (PSA),
        G0103
Sealant
    skin, A6250
    tooth, D1351
Seat
    attachment, walker, E0156
    insert, wheelchair, E0992
    lift (patient), E0621, E0627–E0629
    upholstery, wheelchair, E0975
Seattle Carbon Copy II, foot prosthesis,
    L5976
Secobarbital sodium, J2860
Seconal, J2860
Secure-All
    restraints, E0700
    universal pelvic traction belt, E0890

Selestoject, J0704
Semen analysis, G0027
Semilente insulin, J1820
Sensitivity study, P7001
SEPT, C1004
Sermorelin acetate, Q2014
Serum clotting time tube, A4771
SEWHO, L3960–L3974
Sexa, G0130
Sheath
    guiding, C6500
Sheath, tips, C6501
Sheepskin pad, E0188, E0189
Shoes
    arch support, L3040–L3100
    for diabetics, A5500–A5508
    insert, L3000–L3030
    lift, L3300–L3334
    miscellaneous additions, L3500–L3595
    orthopedic (see Orthopedic shoes),
        L3201–L3265
    positioning device, L3140–L3170
    post-operative
        Specialist™ Health/Post Operative
            Shoe, A9270
        Specialist™ Trainer, L3218
            (women), L3223 (men)
    transfer, L3600–L3649
    wedge, L3340–L3485
Shoulder
    abduction positioner, L3999
    braces, L3999
        Masterhinge™ Shoulder Brace 3,
            L3999
    disarticulation, prosthetic, L6300-
        L6320, L6550
    orthosis (SO), L3650–L3675
        elastic shoulder immobilizer, L3670
        Padden Shoulder Immobilizer,
            L3670
        Sling and Swathe, L3670
        Velpeau Sling Immobilizer, L3670
    spinal, cervical, L0100-L0200
Shoulder-elbow-wrist-hand orthosis
    (SEWHO), L3960–L3969
Shunt accessory for dialysis, A4740
    aqueous, L8612
Sierra wrist flexion unit, L6805
Sigma 200 S pacemaker, C1183-C1184
Sigmoidoscopy, cancer screening,
    G0104, G0106

Sildenafil citrate, S0090
Silicate dental restorations, D2210
Single bar "AK," ankle-foot orthosis,
    L2000, L2010
Single bar "BK," ankle-foot orthosis,
    L1980
Single use device for treatment of
    female stress urinary incontinence,
    C1370
Sinusol-B, J0945
Sirolimus, C9106, J7520
Sitz bath, E0160–E0162
Skilled nurse
    home health setting, G0154
Skilled nursing, G0128
Skin
    barrier, ostomy, A4362,
        A4369–A4374, A4385–A4386
    bond or cement, ostomy, A4364
    gel protective dressing wipes, A5119
    grafts, cultured, G0170, G0171
    sealant, protectant, moisturizer,
        A6250
    test, collagen, G0025
Sling, A4565
    axilla, L1010
    Legg Perthes, L1750
    lumbar, L1090
    patient lift, E0621, E0630, E0635
    pelvic, L2580
    Sam Brown, L1750
    SEWHO, L3969
    trapezius, L1070
Sling and Swathe, orthosis (SO), L3670
Sling fixation system
    stress urinary incontinence, C1028
    female, C6050
    male, C6080
Smart Cordis Nitinol stent and delivery
    system, C1372
Smoking cessation program, S9075
SO, vest type abduction retrainer, L3675
Social worker
    home health setting, G0155
    nonemergency transport, A0160
    visit in home, S9127
Sock
    body sock, L0984
    prosthetic sock, L8420–L8435, L8480,
        L8485
    stump sock, L8470–L8485

Sodium
    chloride injection, J2912
    chromate Cr51, C9000, C9102
    ferric gluconate complex, J2915
    ferric gluconate in sucrose, S0098
    hyaluronate, J7315
    iodide 1-123, C1087
    iothalamate I-125, C9103
    succinate, J1720
Sof-Rol™ Cast Padding, (not separately
    reimbursable from the casting
    procedure or casting supplies
    codes)
Soft Tip Sheaths, C6501
Soft Touch lancets, box of 100, A4259
Softclix lancet device, A4258
Softop helmet, L0110
Soft Touch II lancet device, A4258
Solganal, J2910
Solo, power attachment (for
    wheelchair), E1065
Solo™ Cast Sole, L3540
Solu-Cortef, J1720
Solu-Medrol, J2920, J2930
Solurex, J1100
Solurex LA, J1095, J1100
Solution
    calibrator, A4256
    dialysate, A4700, A4705, A4760
    enteral formulae, B4150–B4156
    irrigation, A4323
    parenteral nutrition, B4164–B5200
Somatrem, Q2015, S0010
Somatropin, Q2016, S0011
S.O.M.I. brace, L0190, L0200
Somi multiple-post collar, cervical
    orthosis, L0190
Sorbent cartridge, ESRD, E1636
Sorbsan, alginate dressing,
    A6196–A6198
Sparine, J2950
Spasmoject, J0500
Specialist™ Ankle Foot Orthosis, L1930
Specialist™ Cast Padding, (not
    separately reimbursable from the
    casting procedure or casting
    supplies codes)
Specialist™ Closed-Back Cast Boot,
    L3260
Specialist™ 100 Cotton Cast Padding,
    (not separately reimbursable from
    the casting procedure or casting
    supplies codes)

Specialist™ Gaitkeeper™ Boot, L3260
Specialist™ Health/Post Operative Shoe,
    A9270
Specialist™ Heel Cups, L3485
Specialist™ Insoles, L3510
Specialist™ J-Splint™ Plaster Roll
    Immobilizer, A4580
Specialist™ Open-Back Cast Boot, L3260
Specialist™ Orthopaedic Stockinet, (not
    separately reimbursable from the
    casting procedure or casting
    supplies codes)
Specialist™ Plaster Bandages, A4580
Specialist™ Plaster Roll Immobilizer,
    A4580
Specialist™ Plaster Splints, A4580
Specialist™ Pre-Formed Humeral
    Fracture Brace, L3980
Specialist™ Pre-Formed Ulnar Fracture
    Brace, L3982
Specialist™ Thumb Orthosis, L3800
Specialist™ Tibial Pre-formed Fracture
    Brace, L2116
Specialist™ Toe Insert for Specialist™
    Closed-Back Cast Boot and
    Specialist™ Health/Post Operative
    Shoe, A9270
Specialist™ Trainer, shoe, post-operative
    men, L3223
    women, L3218
Specialist™ Wrist/Hand Orthosis, L3999
Specialist™ Wrist-Hand-Thumb-orthosis,
    L3999
Specialty absorptive dressing,
    A6251–A6256
Spectinomycin HCl, J3320
Spectranetics
    Concentric laser catheter, C2602-
        C2604
    Extreme laser catheter, C2605
Speech and language pathologist
    home health setting, G0153
Speech assessment, V5362–V5364
Speech communication device, E1900
Speech generating device
    accessory, K0546-K0547
    digitized, K0541-K0542
    software, K0545
    synthesized, K0543-K0544
Speech therapy, S9128
Spenco shoe insert, foot orthosis, L3001

Spinal orthosis,
    anterior-posterior, L0320, L0330,
        L0530
    anterior-posterior-lateral, L0520,
        L0550–L0565
    anterior-posterior-lateral-rotary,
        L0340–L0440
    Boston type, L1200
    cervical, L0100–L0200
    cervical-thoracic-lumbar-sacral
        orthosis (CTLSO), L0700, L0710,
        L1000
    DME, K0112–K0116
    halo, L0810–L0830
    lumbar flexion, L0540
    lumbar-sacral (LSO), L0500–L0565
    Milwaukee, L1000
    multiple post collar, L0180–L0200
    sacroilliac, L0600–L0620
    scoliosis, L1000, L1200, L1300–L1499
    torso supports, L0900–L0999
Splint, A4570, L3100, L4350-L4380
    ankle, L4392-L4398
    dynamic, E1800, E1805, E1810,
        E1815
    footdrop, L4398
    Orthoplast™ Splints (and
        Orthoplast™ II Splints), A4590
    Specialist™ Plaster Splints, A4580
    Thumb-O-Prene™ Splint, L3999
    toad finger, A4570
    Wrist-O-Prene™ Splint, L3800
Spoke protectors, each, K0065
Sports supports hinged knee support,
    L1832
STAAR elastic ultraviolet-absorbing
    silicone posterior chamber
    intraocular lens, toric, C3851
Staphcillin, J2970
Star Lumen tubing, A4616
Steeper, hand prosthesis, L6868, L6873
Steindler apron-front, spinal orthosis,
    L0340
Sten, foot prosthesis, L5972
Stent
    biliary, C1042, C1371, C5002-C5018
    colon, C5130
    colorectal, C5131-C5133
    coronary, C1375, C5030-C5032,
        C5038, C5041-C5046
    enteral, C1319
    iliac, C1320
    peripheral, C5039-C5040

Stent — *continued*
  self-expandable for creation of
    intrahepatic shunts, C1040,
    C5283
  tracheobronchial, C1039, C5281–
    C5282, C5284
  ureteral, C5280
Step 'N Rest folding walker, E0145
Sterile cefuroxime sodium, J0697
Stilphostrol, J9165
Stimulators
  neuromuscular, E0744, E0745
  osteogenesis, electrical, E0747–E0749
  salivary reflex, E0755
  ultrasound, E0760
Stocking
  Delta-Net™ Orthopaedic Stockinet,
    (not separately reimbursable
    from the casting procedure or
    casting supplies codes)
  gradient compression, L8100–L8239
  Specialist™ Orthopaedic Stockinet,
    (not separately reimbursable
    from the casting procedure or
    casting supplies codes)
Stoma
  cap, A5055
  catheter, A5082
  cone, A4399
  plug, A5081
Stomach tube, B4083
Stomahesive
  skin barrier, A4362, A5122
  sterile wafer, A4362
  strips, A4362
Storm Arrow power wheelchair, K0014
Storm Torque power wheelchair, K0011
Straight-In Fixation system with electric
    inserter male, C6080
Stratasis urethral sling, 20/40 cm,
    C6051, C6052
Streptase, J2995
Streptokinase, J2995
Streptomycin sulfate, J3000
Streptozocin, J9320
Strip(s)
  blood, A4253
  glucose test, A4253, A4772
  Nu-Hope
    adhesive, 1 oz bottle with
      applicator, A4364

Strip(s)
  Nu-Hope — *continued*
    adhesive, 3 oz bottle with
      applicator, A4364
    extra long adhering tape strips
      (100/pkg), A4454
    extra long pink adhering tape strips
      (100/pkg), A4454
    extra wide adhering tape strips
      (100/pkg), A4454
    extra wide pink adhering tape strips
      (100/pkg) , A4454
    regular adhering tape strips
      (100/pkg), A4454
    regular pink adhering tape strips
      (100/pkg), A4454
  urine reagent, A4250
Strontium-89 chloride, A9600
Study, gastrointestinal fat absorption,
    S3708
Stump sock, L8470–L8485
Stylet, A4212
Sublimaze, J3010
Succinylcholine chloride, J0330
Sucostrin, J0330
Suction pump
  portable, E0600
Sulfamethoxazole and trimethoprim,
    S0039
Sullivan
  V, E0601
  V Elite, E0601
  VPlus, E0601
Sumacal, enteral nutrition, B4155
Sumatriptan succinate, J3030
Sunbeam moist/dry heat pad, E0215
Supply/accessory/service, A9900
Support
  arch, L3040–L3090
  cervical, L0100–L0200
  elastic, L8100–L8239
  maternity, L0920, L0930
  spinal, L0900–L0960
  vaginal, A4560
Supreme bG Meter, E0607
SureStep blood glucose monitor, E0607
Sur-Fit
  closed-end pouch, A5054
  disposable convex inserts, A5093
  drainable pouch, A5063
  flange cap, A5055

Terramycin IM, J2460
Terry Treads slipper, E0690
Terumo disposable insulin syringes, up to 1cc, per syringe, A4206
Testadiate-Depo, J1080
Testaqua, J3140
Testa-C, J1080
Test-Estra-C, J1060
Test-Estro Cypionates, J1060
Test lead kit
  sacral nerve stimulation, S8300
Testex, J3150
Testoject
  -50, J3140
  -LA, J1070, J1080
Testone LA 100, J3120
  LA 200, J3130
Testosterone
  aqueous, J3140
  cypionate and estradiol cypionate, J1060
  enanthate and estradiol valerate, J0900, J3120, J3130
  propionate, J3150
  suspension, J3140
Testradiate, J0900
Testradiol 90/4, J0900
Testrin PA, J3120, J3130
Tetanus immune globulin, human, J1670
Tetracycline, J0120
Thalamus stimulation, S8001
Thallous chloride TL 201, A9505
Theelin aqueous, J1435
Theophylline, J2810
TheraCys, J9031
Therapeutic agent, A4321
Therapy
  activity, Q0082
  lymphedema, S8950
  physical, evaluation/treatment, Q0086
Thermalator T-12-M, E0239
Thermometer, dialysis, A4910
Thiethylperazine maleate, J3280, Q0174
Thinning solvent, NuHope, 2 oz bottle, A4455
Thiotepa, J9340
Thiothixene, J2330
Thomas
  heel wedge, foot orthosis, L3465, L3470
  suspension, wrist-hand-finger orthosis, L3926

Thoracic-hip-knee-ankle (THKO), L1500–L1520
  Big Hug, L1510
  Chameleon, L1510
  Easy Stand, L1500
  Little Hug, L1510
  Tristander, L1510
Thoracic-lumbar-sacral orthosis (TLSO)
  scoliosis, L1200–L1290
  spinal, L0300–L0440
Thoracic orthosis, L0210
Thorazine, J3230
Thumb
  immobilizer, Johnson's, L3800
  Specialist™ Thumb Orthosis, L3800
Thymoglobulin, J7504
Thumb-O-Prene™ Splint, L3999
Thymol turbidity, blood, P2033
Thypinone, J2725
Thyrotropin (TSH) injection, up to 10 I.U., J3240
Thytropar, J3240
Tibia
  Specialist™ Tibial Pre-formed Fracture Brace, L2116
  Toad finger splint, A4570
Ticarcillin disodium and clavulanate potassium, S0040
Tice BCG, J9031
Ticon, J3250
Tigan, J3250
Tiject-20, J3250
Tiller control, power add-on, K0461
Tip (cane, crutch, walker) replacement, A4637
Tire, wheelchair, E0996, E0999, E1000
Tissue-based surgical dressings, Q0183–Q0185
Tissue marker, C1057
TLSO, L0300–L0440, L1200–L1290
Tobramycin
  inhalation solution, J7682
  sulfate, J3260
  unit dose, J7682
Toe
  Specialist™ Toe Insert for Specialist™ Closed-Back Cast Boot and Specialist™ Health/Post Operative Shoe, A9270
Tofranil, J3270

Index

Travasorb, enteral nutrition — *continued*
STD, B4156
Traveler manual wheelchair, K0001
Tray
insertion, A4310–A4316, A4354
irrigation, A4320
surgical (see also kits), A4550
wheelchair, E0950
Treatment program
partial hospitalization, G0172
Triam-A, J3301
Triamcinolone
acetonide, J3301
diacetate, J3302
hexacetonide, J3303
inhalation solution
concentrated, J7683
unit dose, J7684
Triethylperazine maleate, J3280
Trifocal, glass or plastic, V2300–V2399
Trifupromazine HCl, J3400
Trigeminal division block anesthesia,
D9212
Tri-Kort, J3301
Trilafon, J3310
Trilog, J3301
Trilone, J3302
Trim nails, G0127
Trimethaphan, J0400
Trimethobenzamide HCl, J3250, Q0173
Trimetrexate glucoronate, J3305
Trismus appliance, D5937
Trobicin, J3320
Trooper PTCA guidewire, C3551
Trovan, J0200
Truform prosthetic shrinker, L8440-
L8465
Truss, L8300–L8330
Tube/Tubing
anchoring device, A5200
blood, A4750, A4755
CPAP device, K0187
gastrostomy, B4084, B4085
irrigation, A4355
larynectomy, A4622
nasogastric, B4081, B4082
oxygen, A4616
serum clotting time, A4771
stomach, B4083
suction pump, each, A7002
tire, K0064, K0068, K0078, K0091,
K0093, K0095, K0097

Tube/Tubing — *continued*
tracheostomy, A4622
urinary drainage, K0280
Turbinate Somnoplasty coagulating
electrode, C1322
Turtle Neck safety collars, E0942

Ultra Blood Glucose
monitor, E0607
test strips, box of 50, A4253
Ultra ICE catheter, C1035
UltraCare vest-style body holder, E0700
UltraCross coronary imaging catheter,
C1038
Ultrafast computed tomography, S8092
Ultrafine disposable insulin syringes, per
syringe, A4206
Ultraflex Diamond biliary stent system,
C1042
UltraFlex Tracheobronchial
endoprosthesis, C5284
Ultralente insulin, J1820
Ultrasound
bladder capacity test, G0050
paranasal sinus, S9024
Ultraverse 3.5F Balloon dilatation
catheter, C1934
Ultraviolet cabinet, E0690
Ultrazine-10, J0780
Unasyn, J0295
Unclassified drug, J3490
Undercasting (not separately
reimbursable from the casting
procedure or casting supplies
codes)
Underpads, disposable, A4554
Unilet lancet device, A4258
Unipuncture control system, dialysis,
E1580
Unistik lancet device, A4258
Universal
remover for adhesives, A4455
socket insert
above knee, L5694
below knee, L5690
telescoping versarail bed rail, E0310
Up-Draft Neb-U-Mist, E0580
Upper extremity addition, locking
elbow, L6693
Upper extremity fracture orthosis,
L3980–L3999
Upper limb prosthesis, L6000–L7499
Urea, J3350

Ureaphil, J3350
Urecholine, J0520
Ureterostomy supplies, A4454–A4590
Urethral sling, C6051-C6052
Urethral suppository, Alprostadil, J0275
Urgent care, S9088
Urinal, E0325, E0326
Urinary
    catheter, A4338–A4346,
        A4351–A4353, K0410, K0411
    catheter irrigation, A4321
    collection and retention (supplies),
        A4310–A4359, K0407, K0408,
        K0410, K0411
    leg bag, A5105, A5112
    tract implant, collagen, L8603
Urine
    collector, A4335
    sensitivity study, P7001
    tests, A4250
Urofollitropin, Q2018
Urokinase, J3364, J3365
Urolume, C1008
Uromax Ultra high pressure balloon
    dilatation catheter with Hydroplus
    coating, C1936
Urostomy pouch, A5073
USMC
    hinged Swedish knee cage, L1850
    universal knee immobilizer, L1830
U-V lens, V2755

Vabra aspirator, A4480
Vaccination, administration
    hepatitis B, G0010
    influenza virus, G0008
    pneumococcal, G0009
Vacuum erection system, L7900
Valergen (10, 20, 40), J0970, J1380,
    J1390
Valertest No. 1, 2, J0900
Valium, J3360
Valrubicin, J9357
Valstar, J9357
Vancocin, J3370
Vancoled, J3370
Vancomycin HCl, J3370
Vaporizer, E0605
VAPR electrode, VAPR T thermal
    electrode, C1323

Vascular
    catheter (appliances and supplies),
        A4300–A4306
    closure device, C1145
    graft material, synthetic, L8670
        closing device, C5600
VasoSeal ES device, C5600
Vasoxyl, J3390
Vaxcel chronic dialysis catheter, C1037
Velban, J9360
Velosulin, J1820
Velpeau Sling Immobilizer, L3670
Velsar, J9360
Venipuncture, routine specimen
    collection, G0001
Venous
    access port/reservoir, C1036
    pressure clamp, dialysis, A4918
Ventak defibrillator, C1076-C1078
Ventilator
    battery, A4611–A4613
    moisture exchanger, disposable,
        A4483
    negative pressure, E0460
    volume, stationary or portable, E0450
VePesid, J8560, J9181, J9182
Veripath peripheral guiding, C2151
Versa-Pole IV pole, E0776
Versed, J2250
Vertebral axial decompression, S9090
Vesprin, J3400
Vest, safety, wheelchair, E0980
    chest compression, S8200
        system generator and hoses, S8205
V-Gan (25, 50), J2550
Vigor
    DR pacemaker, C1315
    SR pacemaker, C1180
Vinblastine sulfate, J9360
Vincasar PFS, J9370
Vincristine sulfate, J9370–J9380
Vinorelbine tartrate, J9390
Visi wheelchair tray, E0950
Visi-flow
    irrigation, A4367, A4397, A4398,
        A4399, A4402, A4421, A5123
    stoma cone, A4399
Vision Record wheelchair, K0005
Vision service, V2020–V2799
Vision Tek protective eyewear, E0690
Vistaject, J3410
Vistaril, J3410

Vistide, J0740
Vitajet, A4210
Vital HN, enteral nutrition, B4153
Vitamin B$_{12}$ cyanocobalamin, J3420
Vitamin B$_{17}$, J3570
Vitamin K, J3430
Vitaneed, enteral nutrition, B4151
Vitrasert, J7310
Viva/Long Viva, catheter, C1981
Vivonex, enteral nutrition
    HN, B4153
    STD, B4156
    T.E.N., B4153
Voice Touch blood glucose monitor,
    E0609
Von Rosen, hip orthosis, L1630
Von Willebrand factor complex, Q2022
Vortex power wheelchair, K0014

Wafer, Little Ones Surfit flexible, A5123
Walker, E0130–E0147, K0458, K0459
    accessories, A4636, A4637
    attachments, E0153–E0159
    enclosed with wheels, E0144
    folding
        Auto-Glide, E0143
        Easy Care, E0143, E0146
        framed with wheels, E0144
        One-Button, E0143
        Quik-Fold, E0141, E0143
        Red Dot, E0135, E0143
        Step 'N Rest, E0145
        Sure-Gait, E0141, E0143
Wallgraft Tracheobronchial
    endoprosthesis with Unistep
    delivery system, C5281-C5282
Wallstent
    biliary endoprosthesis, C1042, C5016-
        C5018
    iliac endoprosthesis, C1320
    interal endoprosthesis, C1319, C5134
    tracheobronchial endoprosthesis,
        C1039
    transjugular intrahepatic
        portosystemic shunt (TIPS),
        C1040, C5283
Wallstent Enteral Wallstent
    endoprosthesis and Unistep delivery
    system (60mm in length), C1319

Water
    ambulance, A0050
    distilled (for nebulizer), A7018
    for nebulizer, A7018-A7020
    pressure pad/mattress, E0177, E0187,
        E0198
    purification system (ESRD), E1610,
        E1615
    softening system (ESRD), E1625
    sterile, A7019-A7020
    tanks (dialysis), A4880
    treated, A4714
Wedges, shoe, L3340–L3420
Wehamine, J1240
Wehdryl, J1200
Wellcovorin, J0640
Wet mount, Q0111
Wheel attachment, rigid pickup walker,
    E0155
Wheelchair, E0950–E1298,
    K0001–K0108
    accessories, E0192, E0950–E1001,
        E1065–E1069
    cushions, E0963-E0965
        High Profile, 4-inch, E0965
        Low Profile, 2-inch, E0963
        tray, E0950
        Visi, E0950
    amputee, E1170–E1200
    back, fully reclining, manual, K0028
    battery, A4631
    bearings, any type, K0452
    component or accessory, NOS, K0108
    heavy-duty
        Tracer, E1280, E1285, E1290,
            E1295
    lightweight, E1240-E1270
        Ez Lite, E1250
        Tracer, E1240, E1250, E1260,
            E1270
    motorized, E1210–E1213
    narrowing device, E0969
    power add-on, K0460–K0461
    specially sized, E1220–E1230
    tire, E0996, E0999, E1000
    transfer board or device, E0972
    tray, K0107
    van, nonemergency, A0130
    youth, E1091
WHFO, with inflatable air chamber,
    L3807
Whirlpool equipment, E1300–E1310
WHO, wrist extension, L3914

Wig, S8095
Wilcox apron-front, spinal orthosis, L0520
Williams, spinal orthosis, L0540
Wilson-Cook colonic Z-stent, C5130
Win RhoSD, J2792
Wipes, A4245, A4247
  Allkare protective barrier, A5119
WIZZ-ard manual wheelchair, K0006
WorkHorse PTA balloon catheter, C1935
Wound cleanser, A6260
Wound cover
  alginate dressing, A6196–A6198
  collagen dressing, A6021–A6024
  foam dressing, A6209–A6214
  hydrocolloid dressing, A6234–A6239
  hydrogel dressing, A6242–A6248
  specialty absorptive dressing, A6251–A6256
Wound filler
  alginate, A6199
  foam, A6215
  hydrocolloid, A6240–A6241
  hydrogel, A6248–A6249
  not elsewhere classified, A6261–A6262
Wound healing
  other growth factor preparation, S9055
  Procuren, S9055
Wound pouch, A6154
Wrist
  brace, cock-up, L3908
  disarticulation prosthesis, L6050, L6055
  hand/finger orthosis (WHFO), E1805, E1825, L3800-L3954
  Specialist™ Pre-Formed Ulnar Fracture Brace, L3982
  Specialist™ Wrist/Hand Orthosis, L3999
  Specialist™ Wrist-Hand-Thumb-orthosis, L3999
  Splint, lace-up, L3800
  Wrist-O-Prene™ Splint, L3800
WWMT Brachytherapy needle, MD Tech P.S.S. prostate seeding set (needle), C1702
Wyamine sulfate, J3450
Wycillin, J2510
Wydase, J3470

Xcaliber power wheelchair, K0014
Xenon regional cerebral blood-flow studies, S9023
Xenon Xe 133, Q3004
Xylocaine HCl, J2000
X-ray equipment, portable, Q0092, R0070, R0075

Zantac, J2780
Zemplar, J2500
Zenapax, J7513
Zetran, J3360
Zidovudine, J3485
Zinacef, J0697
Zinecard, J1190
Zithromax I.V., J0456
Zofran, J2405
Zoladex, J9202
Zolicef, J0690
Zosyn, J2543

Index